Pick Up and Oocyte Management

Antonio Malvasi · Domenico Baldini

Editors

Pick Up and Oocyte Management

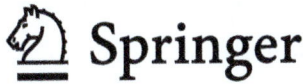 Springer

Editors
Antonio Malvasi
Department of Obstetrics and Gynecology
Santa Maria Hospital
GVM Care and Research
Bari
Italy

Domenico Baldini
Center of Medically Assisted Procreation
MOMO' fertiLIFE Srl
Bisceglie
Italy

Laboratory of Human Physiology
Phystech BioMed School
Faculty of Biological and Medical Physics
Moscow Institute of Physics and Technology
(State University)
Dolgoprudny
Moscow Region
Russia

Santa Maria della Misericordia University Hospital
Perugia
Italy

ISBN 978-3-030-28743-6   ISBN 978-3-030-28741-2   (eBook)
https://doi.org/10.1007/978-3-030-28741-2

This Springer imprint is published by the registered company Springer Nature Switzerland AG
The registered company address is: Gewerbestrasse 11, 6330 Cham, Switzerland

I dedicated this book to my beloved mother and father for their sacrifices and love towards me.
I also devote my work to my brother who has always been close to me, even in difficult moments. To my hometown which give me its Roman-Greek ancient culture.

Antonio Malvasi

To my family, to my wife Derna, to my son Giorgio and to my son Marco who looks at me from up there;
To my parents and to those who have contributed to my professional growth.

Domenico Baldini

Acknowledgments

The authors sincerely thank Antoni Dell'Aquila for the realization of some wonderful images for this book. These pictures are the result of the long collaboration between Prof. Antonio Malvasi and Antonio Dell'Acquila into the medical graphics academy, founded by them.

Contents

A Short History of Oocyte Pick-up

1

Ettore Cittadini and Giorgio Maria Baldini

Contents

Before talking about the history of ovarian pick-up, it is important to have a look at the history of the medicine, especially to take into account the part concerning female reproductive system anatomy. The anatomical and physiological description of the ovary, the most important reproductive organ, takes place in a recent historical period with respect to other human organs. Before the fourteenth century, the ovary was considered as a female testis and the uterus as an empty penis.

In 1543, Andreas Vesalius (Fig. 1.1) published De Humani Corporis Fabrica; with its extensive account of the anatomy of the generative organs, he carefully and systematically introduced the structure of the human body in a way that was truthful to the findings of human dissection that had never been accomplished before [1, 2].

E. Cittadini (✉)
Faculty of Medicine, Department of Obstetrics and Gynecology, University of Palermo, Palermo, Italy
e-mail: info@ettorecittadini.it

G. M. Baldini
Center of Medically Assisted Procreation, MOMO' fertiLIFE, Bisceglie, Italy

He noted the disposition of the Fallopian tubes but failed to clarify their specific function [3].

Instead, he considered their relationship with the ovaries was analogous to that of the male ducts with the testes, so he illustrated the ducts as coiled round the "female testes."

In 1721, an Italian scientist, Antonio Vallisneri (1661–1730), with this expressive description: "Young peasant woman, married, moderately plump, infertile, with ovaries larger than normal, like doves' eggs, lumpy, shiny and whitish," (Fig. 1.2) described for the first time the clinical and pathological features of the "polycystic" or "micropolycystic" ovary [4].

He was a student of Marcello Malpighi (1628–1694), one of the first ovary researcher. Malpighi had made his first known drawing of a monkey ovary in 1666 and had noted the Graafian follicles.

He had reasoned that the actual egg is within the ovary. In contrast to the Graaf's theories that the follicle was the egg, Malpighi proposed in 1681 that the egg was derived from the luteal tissue present in a mature mammalian ovary [5, 6] (Fig. 1.3).

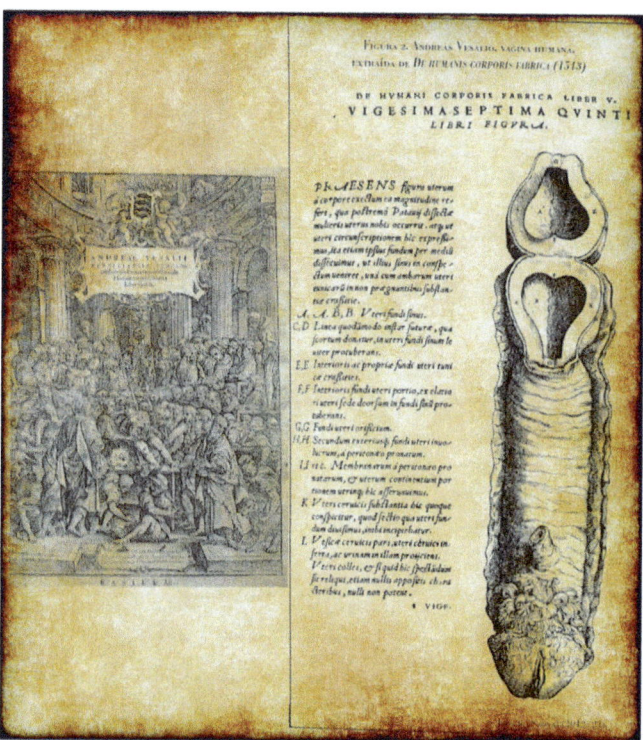

Fig. 1.1 In 1543, Andreas Vesalius published De Humani Corporis

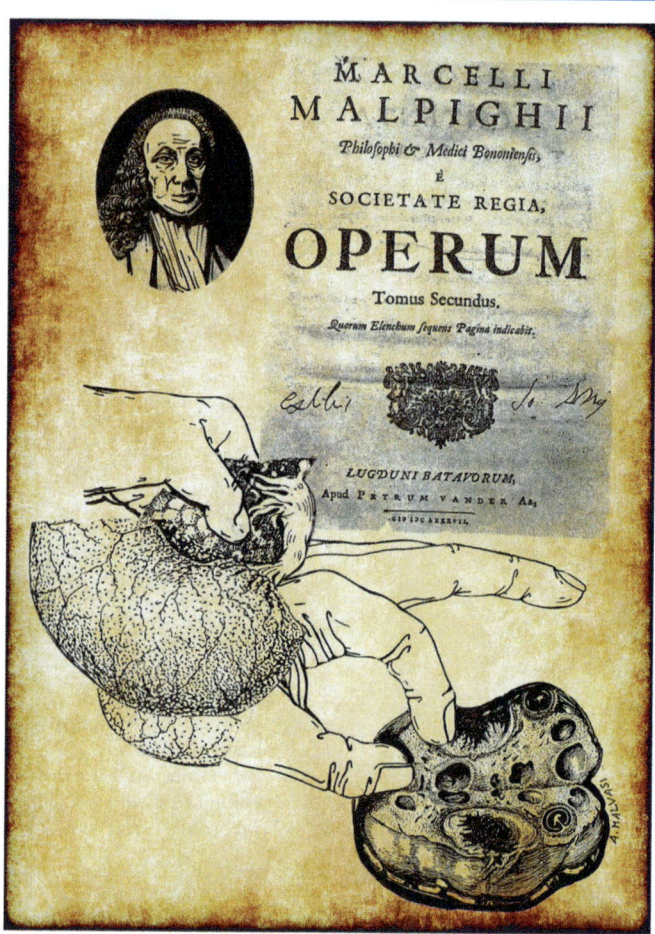

Fig. 1.3 Marcello Malpighi (1628–1694), italian medical. He performed studies on ovary pathology

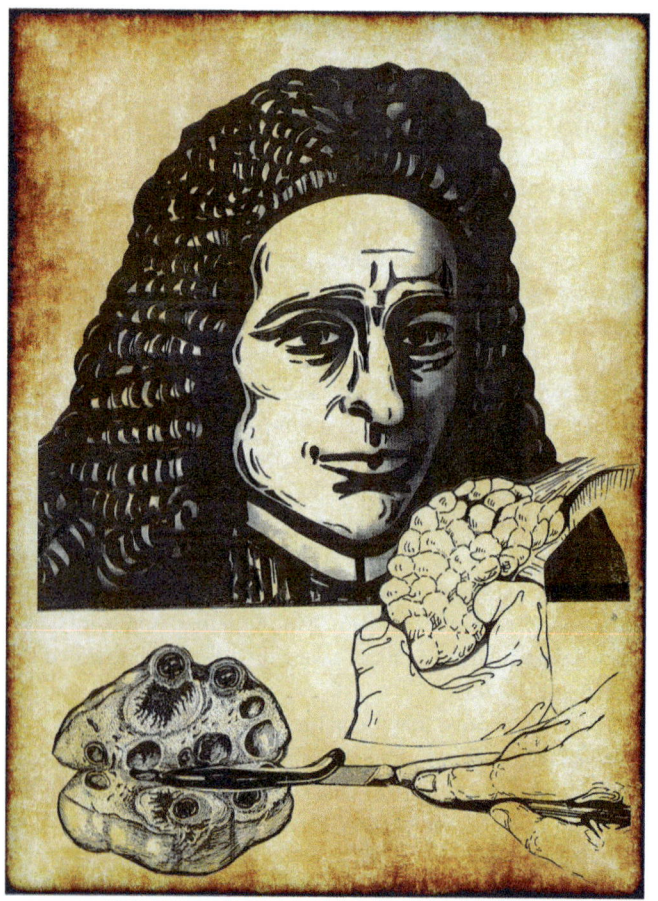

Fig. 1.2 Antonio Vallisneri (1661–1730), an Italian medical scientist, studied and described in 1721 the ovary with PCOS

Gabriele Fallopio (1523–1562) (Fig. 1.4), one of the greatest anatomists of the sixteenth century, had noticed the follicles previously but he didn't recognize its reproductive significance [7]. Moreover, he was able to prove that the Fallopian tube is a unique organ that connects the uterine horn to the ovary [8] (Fig. 1.5).

It is noticeable to underline that the only approach in vivo to understand the female reproductive system was the manual abdominal examination [9, 10]. In fact, the most fundamental diagnostic instrument in the past was the hand.

Trotula de' Ruggiero of the famous school of Salerno was the first female physician in the history of medicine and the first female professor of medicine [11]. She was one of the first physicians to describe a number of obstetrical and gynaecological conditions and also wrote on male infertility.

De passionibus mulierum was probably her most famous work, and she was included in the "famous quartet of Salerno" in the eleventh century by several medical historians [12] (Fig. 1.6). Trotula's chapter on the causes of infertility is noteworthy as she recognizes both female and male infertility.

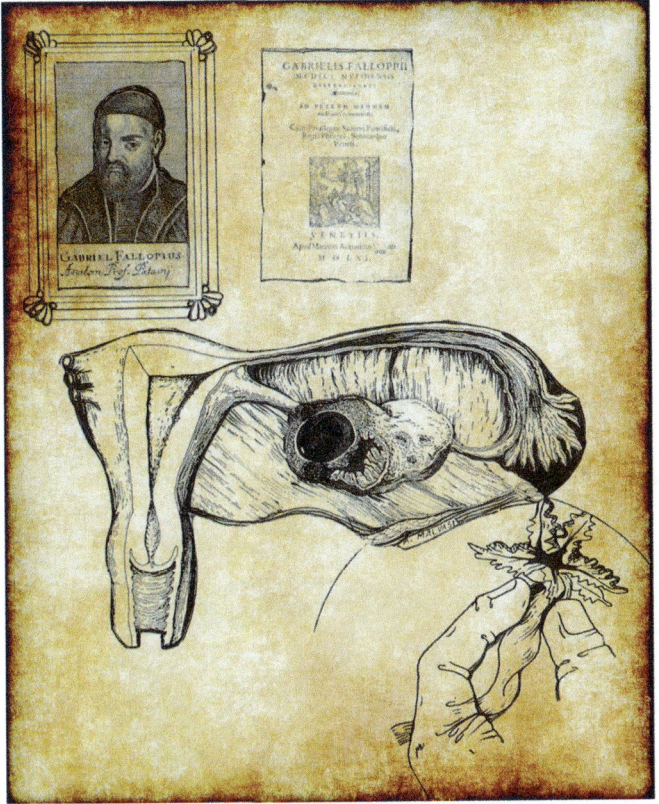

Fig. 1.4 Gabriele Fallopio (1523–1562), one of the greatest anatomists of the sixteenth century, had noticed the follicles previously but he didn't recognize its reproductive significance

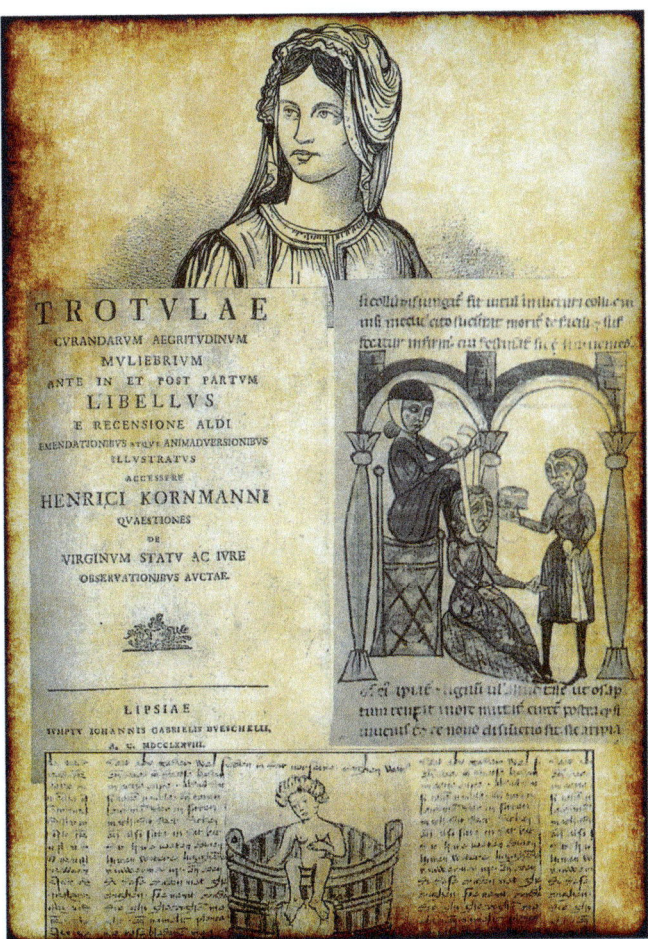

Fig. 1.6 Trotula de' Ruggiero of the famous school of Salerno was the first female physician in the history of medicine and the first female professor of medicine

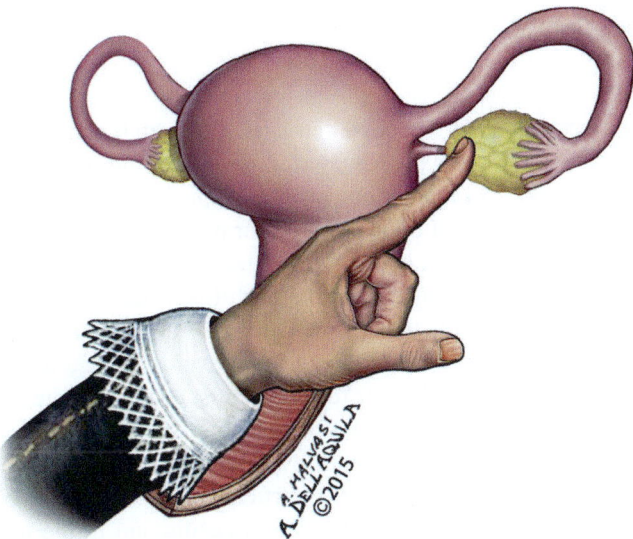

Fig. 1.5 During seventeenth and eighteenth centuries the only diagnostic instrument of the ovary: the hand

Trotula writes that some women "have a womb so soft and slippery that the seed having been received cannot be retained in it. Sometimes this happens through a defect of the male who has seed so thin that when it is poured into the vagina it slips out because of its own liquidness." [13].

For many years, the gynaecological examination was the only way to evaluate ovarian conditions (Fig. 1.7).

Only with the discovery of ultrasound the evaluation of the anatomy of the ovaries and their function has taken a considerable step forward (Fig. 1.8).

Oocyte pick-up may be defined as the process of the aspiration of follicular fluid, and the oocytes contained therein, directly from the ovaries of a woman, before them being released spontaneously from the ovarian follicles.

Aside from the occasional warnings from Palmer and Klein [14] regarding the retrieval of human oocytes using laparoscopy for the cytological evaluation of their quality—it is only with advances in the technologies of assisted reproduction, that the need has been recognized for timed retrieval of initially mature oocytes (1969) via laparoscopy (and usually after the induction of multiple follicular growth). Although this possibility became popular with the famed collaboration between Patrick Steptoe and Robert Edwards in 1969, it is also important for us to remember that, in 1964, 5 years earlier, Steptoe had already presented recordings made with ANSCO film with pictures of laparoscopic

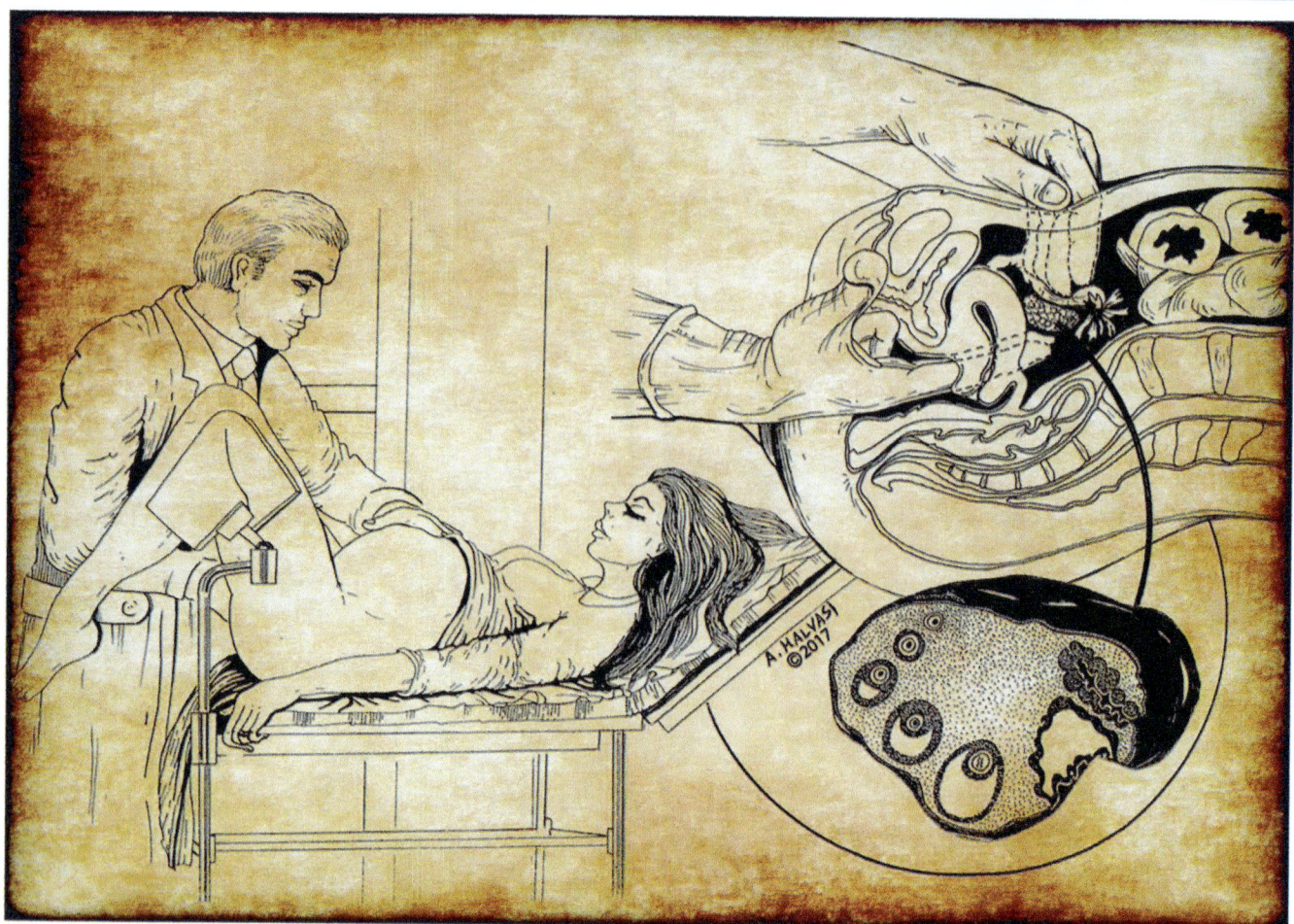

Fig. 1.7 Bimanual palpation at the beginning of nineteenth century for normal and pathological ovaries

retrieval of human oocytes [15], at the "First World Congress on Gynecological Coelioscopy" (Palermo, November 1964).

In 1971 the pioneering work of Steptoe and Edwards brought to the first embryonic transfer after laparoscopic pick-up with different types of ovarian stimulation. After 32 failures, the first pregnancy achieved in 1975 turned out to be ectopic [16, 17]. The first successful outcome of IVF was achieved on 27th July 1978 with the birth of Louise Brown in Manchester from a laparoscopic retrieval on the spontaneous cycle of a single ovarian follicle. In the years after that, following on from the excellent results achieved by Steptoe, oocyte pick-up was carried out using the laparoscopic technique, with hospitalization and general anaesthesia.

It is worth noting that, despite the introduction of abdominal transducers and vaginal scanners in the mid-1980s, which allowed for the echographic pick-up of oocytes, Patrick Steptoe was a proponent of laparoscopic retrieval until his death in 1988 and he staunchly defended its main advantages. These can be summarized as follows: (1) the possibility of carrying out a complete pelvic diagnostic exploration contemporaneous to oocyte retrieval; (2) A high percentage of oocyte retrieval; (3) the possibility of carrying out procedures on the fallopian tubes, such as salpingolysis and tubular disagglutination immediately after pick-up.

The laparoscopic technique utilized for oocyte pick-up does not differ greatly from the traditional method—aside from certain details that can be listed as: (1) no instruments are inserted into the uterine so as to avoid damage to the endometrium, which after few days must accommodate the developing embryo; (2) the patient may be positioned on the operating table with the lower limbs lying flat, as in most normal procedures; (3) particular attention must be placed when introducing the Veress needle and to the trocars for access since we are dealing with patients undergoing multiple operations; (4) the gas in pneumoperitoneum which is safe for the oocytes, such as a mix of 90% nitrogen, 5% oxygen, and 5% carbon dioxide, is used in oocyte culturing; (5) a choice of aspiration needles which takes into consideration the size of the cumulus oophorus, the adhesive nature of this structure, as well as the need to utilize the minimum space for the liquids and the maximum

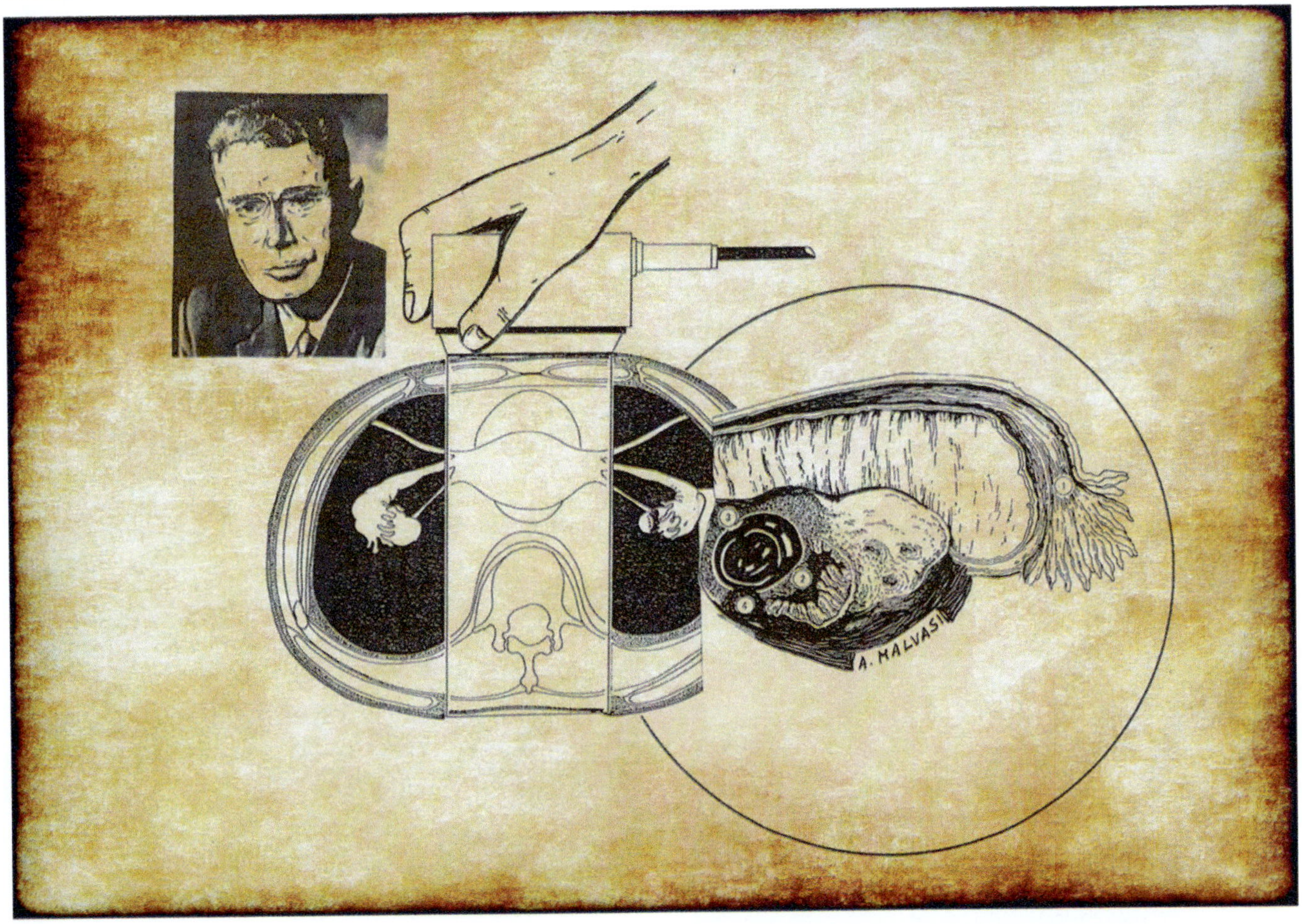

Fig. 1.8 Ian Donald pioneer of ultrasound; The ultrasound represented the greatest change in the diagnosis and treatment of the genital apparatus

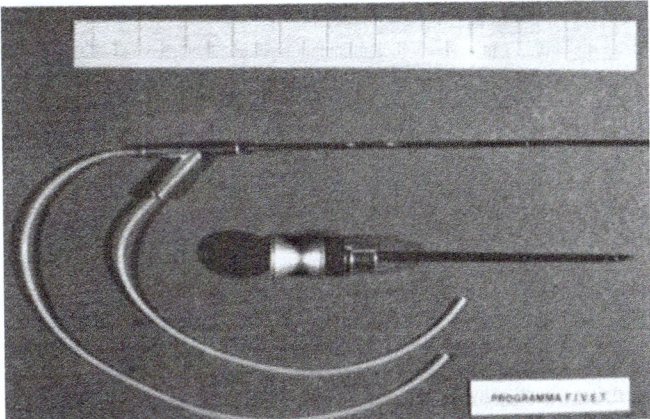

Fig. 1.9 The double-cannula needle used by Steptoe and its trocar

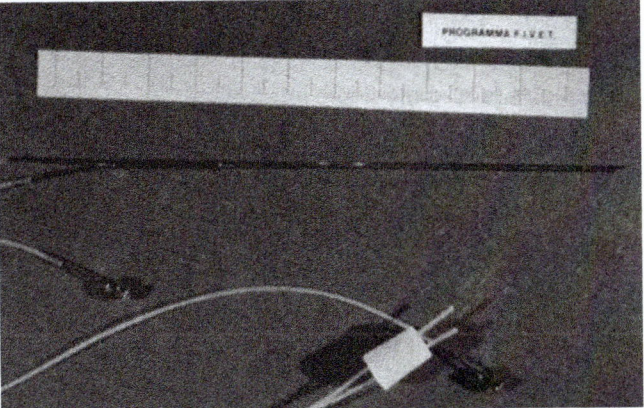

Fig. 1.10 The double-cannula needle

flow rate inside the system [18]. This flow must be continuous to minimize the liquid turbulence, so as to avoid oocyte adhesion and the damage caused during its transposition. Steptoe used a double-cannula needle (Figs. 1.9 and 1.10) and soon after nearly all groups active in Italy were using Craft double-cannula or the Renou single-cannula needles (Fig. 1.11), or different models (Figs. 1.12 and 1.13).

Follicle aspiration must be done using general aspiration systems but with intermediate reducers attached to them, or using a suitable aspirator with micro-regulation, such as that

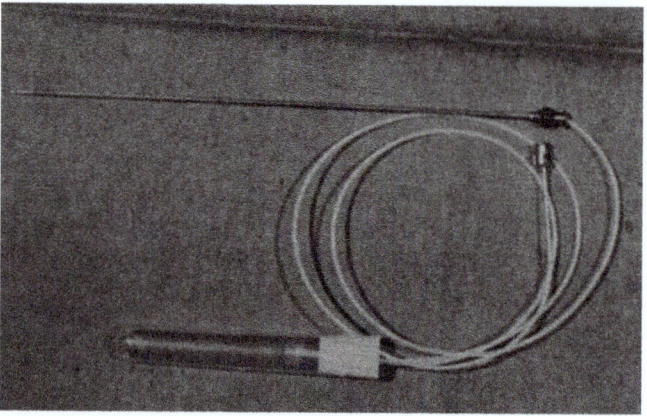

Fig. 1.11 The mono-cannula needle of Renou with its Teflon covering, the silicon stopper, and the recovery tube

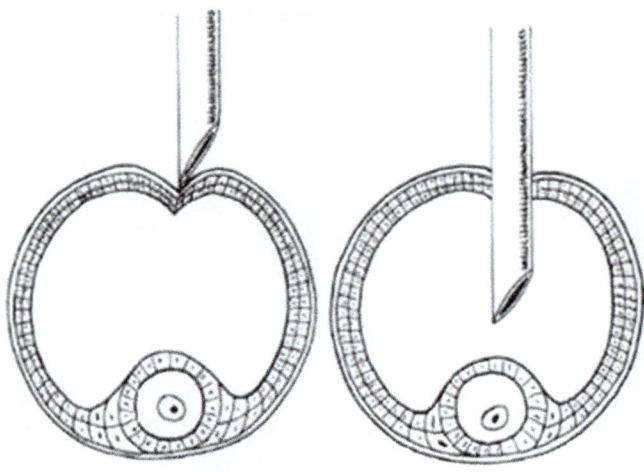

Fig. 1.13 The follicle distortion under the needle's pressure and the needle inside the follicle

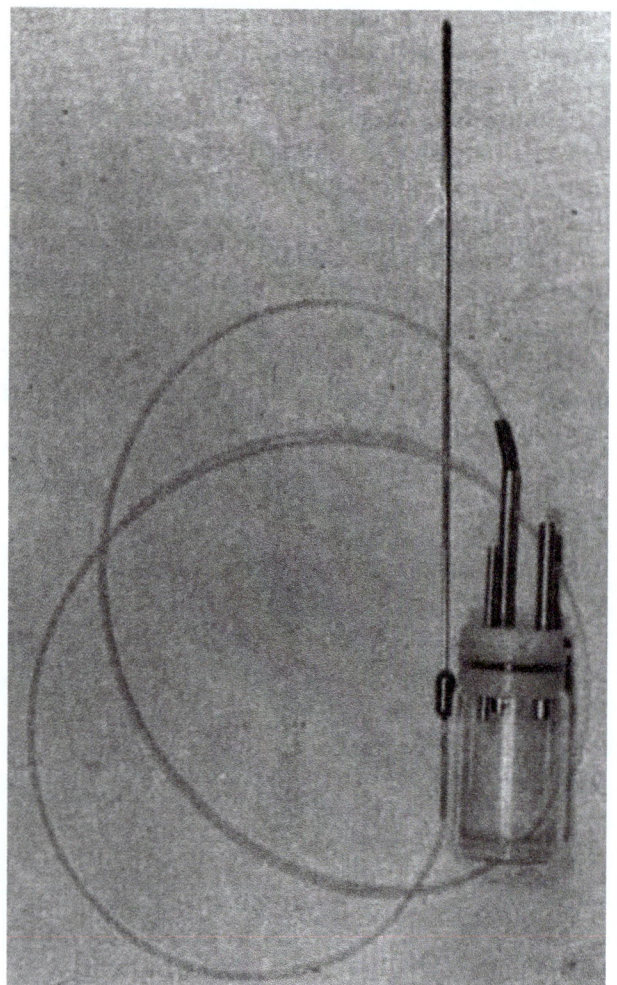

Fig. 1.12 The needle utilized by our group

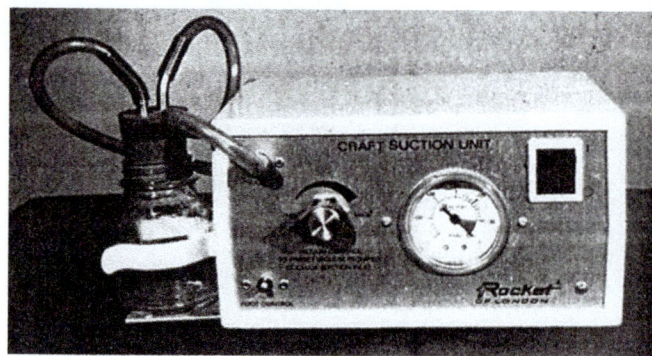

Fig. 1.14 Schematic view of the aspiration system

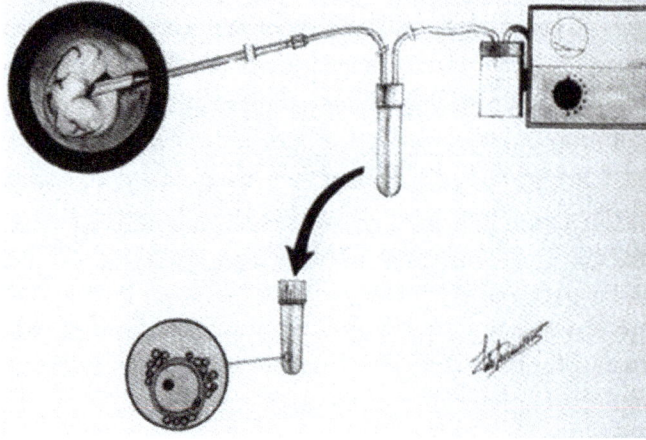

Fig. 1.15 The Craft aspirator for oocyte pick-up

of Craft. Optimal pressure for the aspiration is between 60 and 100 mmHg (Figs. 1.14 and 1.15).

The procedure begins by puncturing the largest follicle in one of the two ovaries and penetrating them by about 5 mm (Fig. 1.16) [19].

The majority of the literature suggests an apical puncture of the follicle, whereas others (Cittadini) prefer to make the puncture towards the base since apical puncture takes place at the most eroded point, can, on occasion, mean a hole larger than the needle and the consequent leak of follicular fluid and the possible loss of the oocyte [20–22]. Furthermore, the

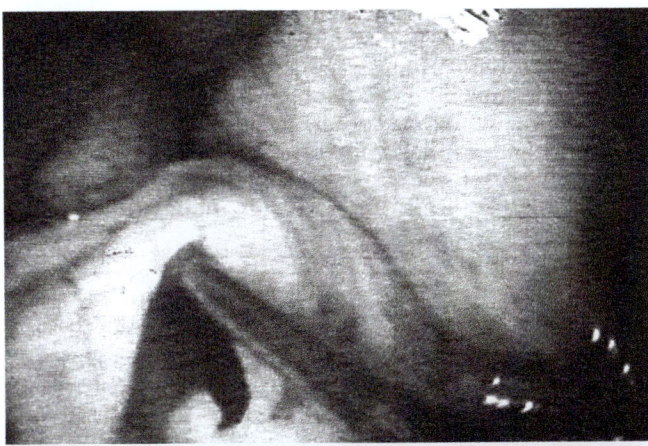

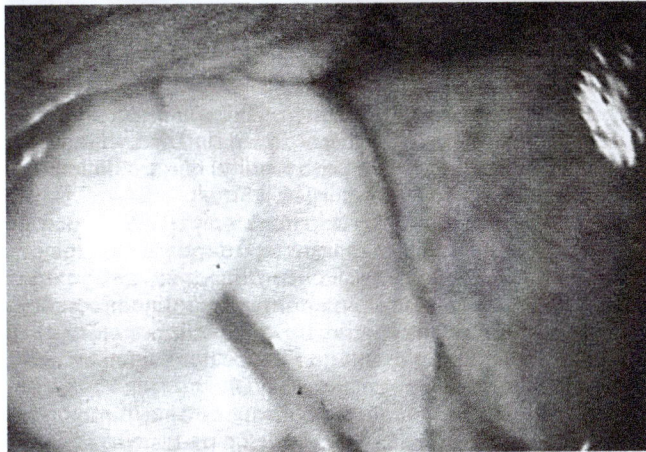

Fig. 1.16 Follicle puncture and aspiration

technique involves a greater risk of leaving the oocyte behind in the follicle and then have to retrieve it via washing or flushing. The aspirator, controlled via a pedal, must be switched off prior to the penetration of the oocyte by the needle so that the increase of the intra-follicular pressure is rapidly decreased which is determined at the moment of entry and can cause the breakage of the follicle. As the aspiration takes places, the tension of the follicle gradually reduces thus it is opportune to create a hollow with the needle, in which the residual follicular liquid and eventual oocyte can be collected. Once the follicular liquid has been completely aspirated it is standard practice to clean the needle by aspirating in the middle of the collection, with the aim of preventing the formation of internal coagulations whilst removing the oocyte which may have remained attached to the walls. Employing this technique, Cittadini has a retrieval percentage of 90–95% without the need for flushing, whilst the Australian groups obtain this percentage only after the fourth or fifth flushing. Many authors prefer an oblique vision telescope (30°) for an easier vision of the ovarian walls (Figs. 1.17 and 1.18).

The aspiration is interrupted when a small opaque mass is visible as it could contain the oocyte and cumulus oophorus. The needle is kept on site until the laboratory provides a response.

Normally, only follicles with a diameter superior to 15 mm are punctured for two main reasons: firstly because follicles with a diameter inferior to 15 mm generally do not contain mature oocytes and secondly due to the fact that the aspiration of all the follicles present in the gonads has a direct effect on the quality of the corpus luteum. Therefore, it is easy to establish an insufficiency in the second phase of the cycle which could have serious repercussions in the initial stages of an eventual pregnancy. It has been noted that pregnancies generally develop from oocytes aspirated with at least 3–8 mL of follicular fluid.

If, at the moment of laparoscopy, a burst follicle has already been detected, then it is possible to aspirate the Douglas space first and then the follicle bed in an attempt to pick up the oocyte. The occasional discovery of a burst follicle in the presence of numerous mature follicles can act as an indicator of oocyte maturity (viscous follicular fluid, more layers of radiate crown, etc.).

Furthermore, if a series of patients never display a burst follicle, it can be presumed that the timing of the laparoscopy, adopted by the group, is too early.

Sometimes during the aspiration of the oocyte, there can be certain difficulties which are usually overcome, unless the ovaries are completely inaccessible. It should be noted, however, that conceptions and pregnancies have been obtained with oocytes aspirated by Douglas, often among adhesions and blood clots. When there are delays in the collection of the oocyte, more than 50 min after the administration of anaesthetic they are accompanied by normal pregnancies. This confirms that neither the prolonged use of general anaesthetic nor the presence of intraperitoneal carbon dioxide are seriously damaging for the oocyte.

With the advances of **gynaecological echography imaging** in the 1980s, many reports were published describing the actual effectiveness of ultrasonically guided oocyte pick-up.

Laparoscopic pick-up, therefore, seemed complicated and produced a rate of success less than 50% per follicle, both for the pick-up of mature oocytes and for the rates of fertilization. In addition, the efficacy of the technique may be obstructed by multiple adhesions or tubal pathologies which block the access to the ovary for the laparoscopic instruments [21, 22].

Transvesical techniques: in 1982, Lenz S., Lauritsen J.G. [23] showed that ultrasounds could be used not only for diagnostic purposes, but also for operative ones. Danish gynaecologists were the first to experiment the efficiency of a new ultrasonically guided percutaneous aspiration method in reaching ovarian follicles and carrying out oocyte pick-up (Fig. 1.19).

In the original work of Lenz, the echographic pick-up was carried out using a handmade guide positioned on a linear transductor, a line showing the angle of the needle in relation to the scansion surface of the transductor was displayed on the monitor via a goniometer. Currently, the increasingly

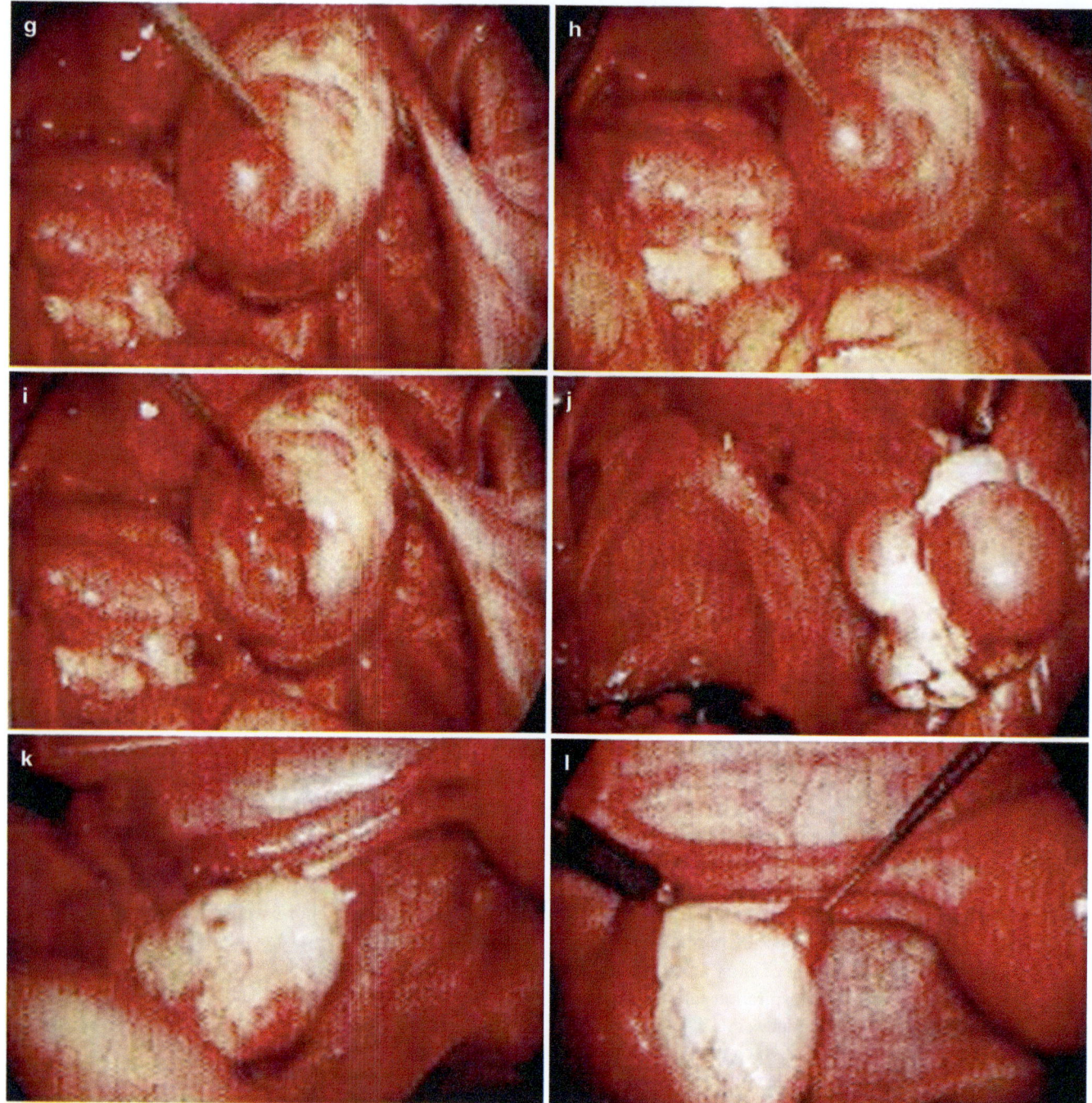

Fig. 1.17 The steps of laparoscopic oocyte retrieval according to Mettler et al. 1982

IN VITRO FERTILIZATION OF HUMAN OVA

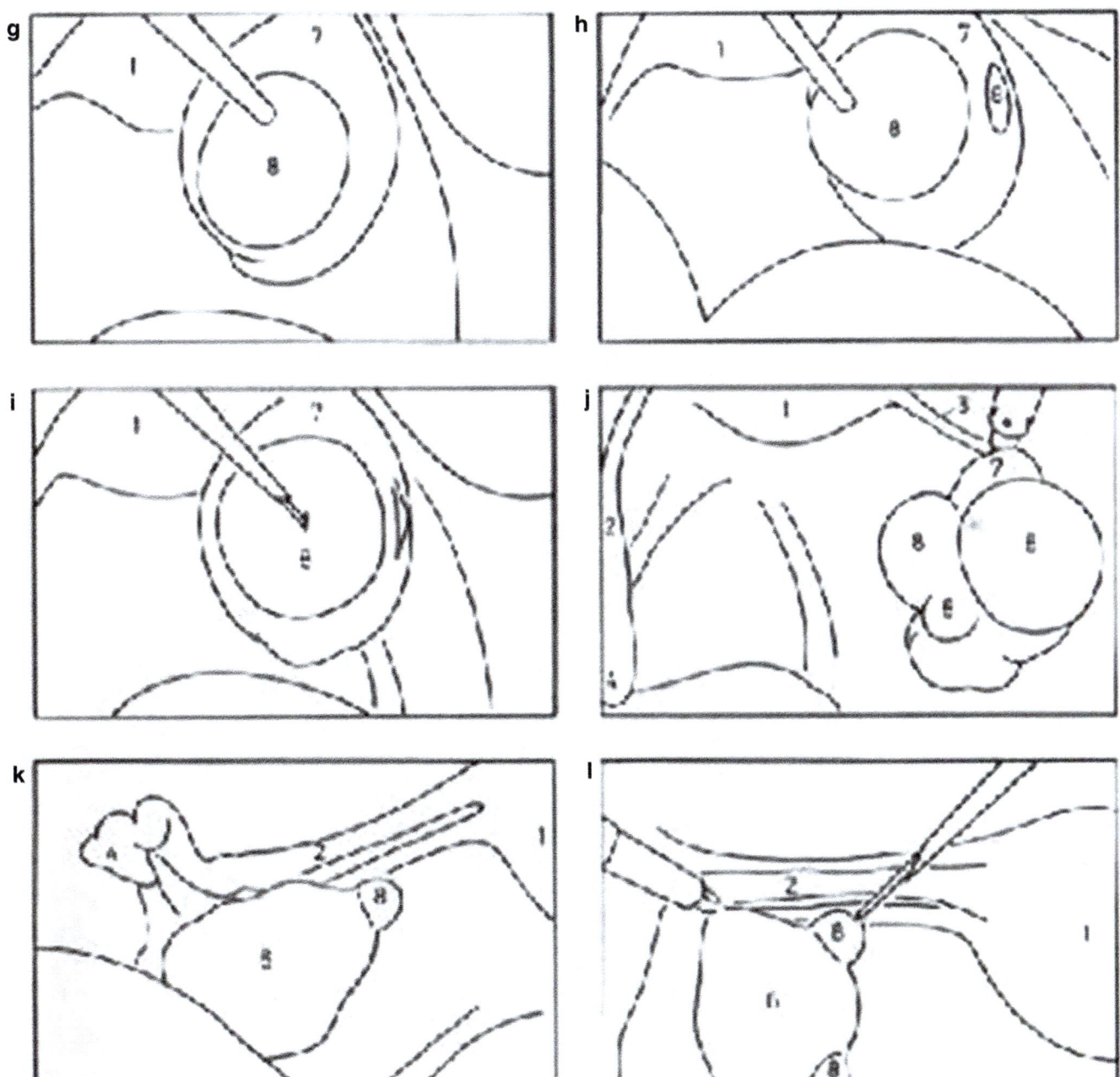

Fig. 1.17 (continued)

Fig. 1.18 Advantages of an oblique vision telescope (30°) of the ovary

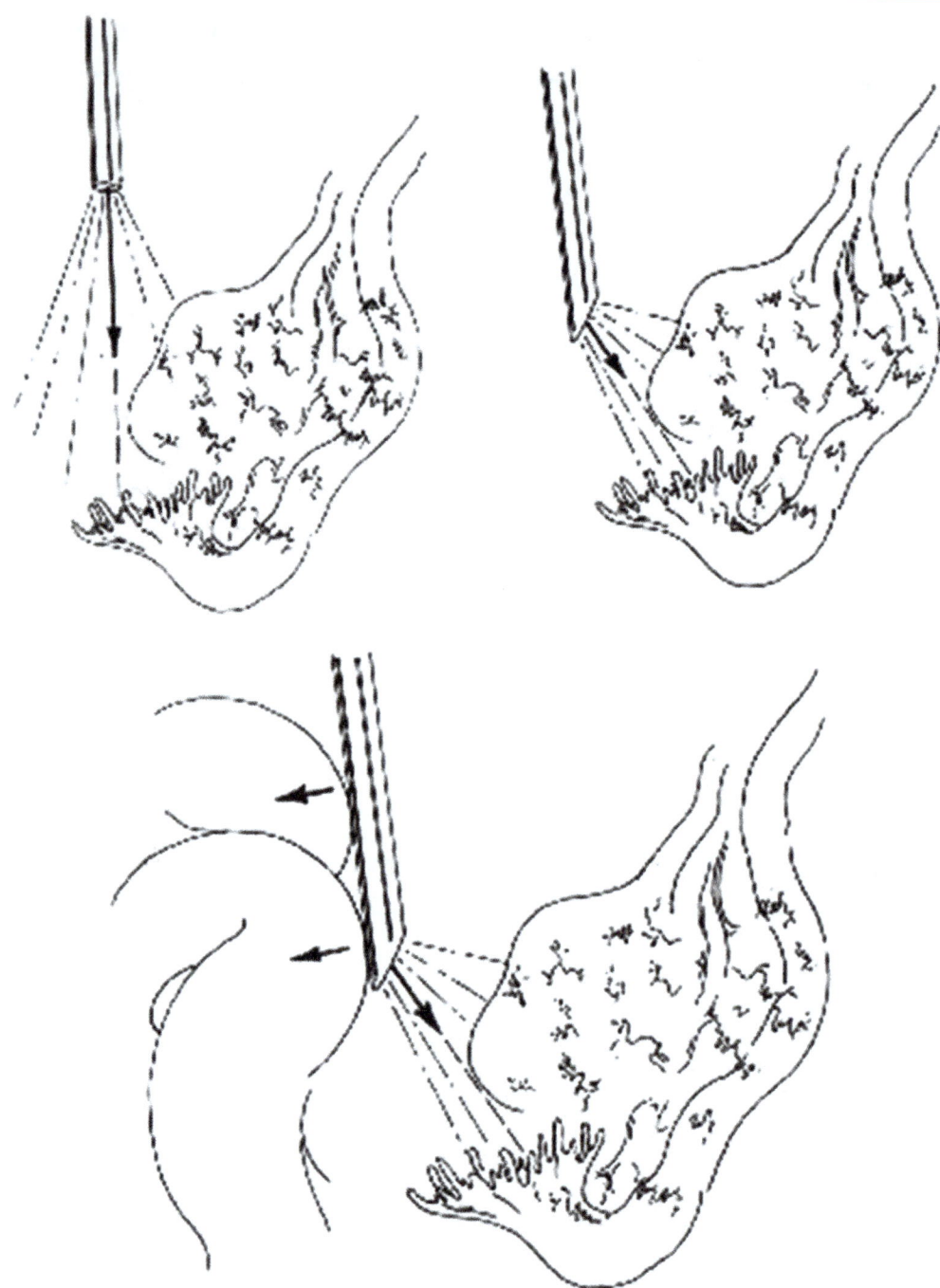

widespread and repeated use of echography in needle biopsies, also for deeper organs, was due to the production of easy-assembly guides for various types of transducers. Moreover, due to their lack of problems and ease of use, for field-relevant transducers, there is the possibility of seeing different lines of biopsy onscreen simultaneously, and different angles via a luminous tracing line, equipped with a marker which allows for the immediate measurement of the depth of the organ to be reached.

In some cases, this same result can be obtained using a manual handle via the vaginal canal, or combined abdominal-vaginal, with the aim of bringing and keeping the ovary in the required position. Obviously, in cases one may try to puncture the ovary via the vaginal canal through the posterior fornix, but always using ultrasonography.

This method is also used in cases in which one wishes to aspirate from the Douglas pouch any oocytes fallen there after ovulation.

During this procedure, the needle, attached to an abdominal transducer, was inserted percutaneously into the antral follicle, going through the abdominal wall and the urinary bladder.

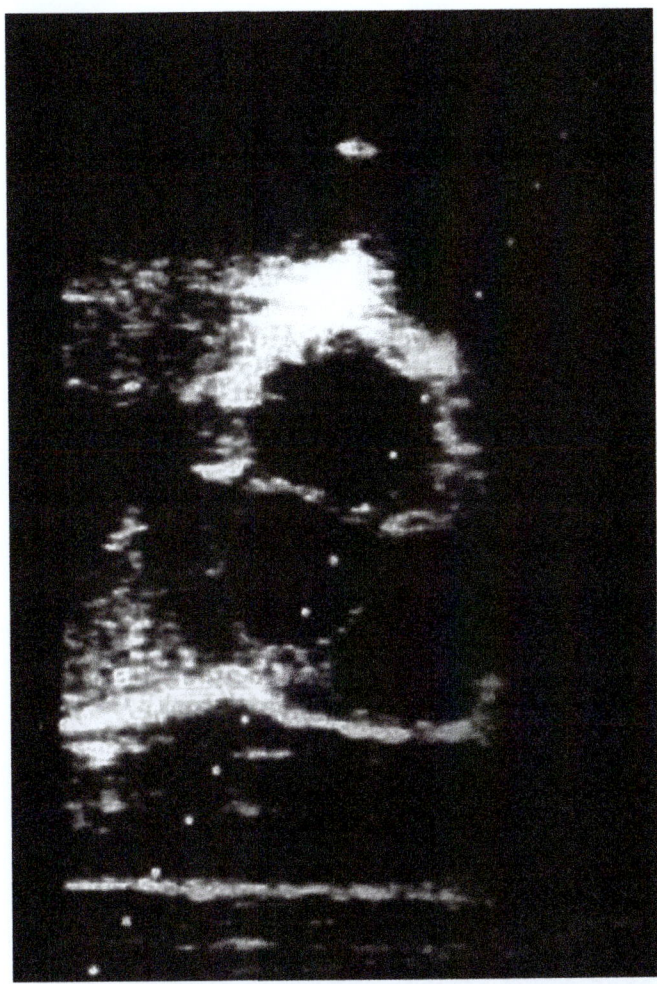

Fig. 1.19 View of the follicles under the bright track of the echographic screen

The needle used is different to that used in laparoscopic retrieval. It has a length of 22.5 cm with an external diameter of 1.5 mm. It is entirely coated in Teflon which reduces its LUMEN to 1.3 mm. At the distal extremity, there are some incisions which increase its echo-reflectivity on the echographic screen. The needle has an angulation of 60° with respect to the screened surface.

The patient is placed in the gynaecological position on the surgical table, which allows for the emptying of any residual urine. Next, one proceeds with filling the bladder with 300–400 mL of NaCL sterile solution at 9%, to which some prefer to add 5 mL of methylene blue. By these means, it is possible to get a better view (when the bladder is full it becomes an effective acoustic window) of the pelvic organs, particularly the ovaries. At the same time, the presence of a dye (methylene blue) in the bladder, allows for the certainty, once the needle has been introduced, that follicular, rather than vesicular fluid, is being aspirated. Furthermore, this technique guarantees the sterility of the culture, unlike the Danish method, which exploits the same urine of the

patient and not the NaCL solution. As soon as the follicle has been located using echography, one attempts to position it under the luminous line of the monitor. The needle is inserted, therefore, under guide and it is introduced into the abdominal cavity via the trans-vesical route, until the surface of the ovarian follicle is reached. When, through observation of the echography display, it is noted that the tip of the needle (which is echo-reflective) begins to warp the edges of the follicular wall—only then can the process of aspiration begin (the aspiration pressure must be maintained at around 90–100 mmHg) and the internal is penetrated.

The follicle's collapse is seen on the echography display and the follicle liquid is seen in the collecting tube almost simultaneously. Usually, it is possible to do one or two flushings without moving the needle from its position. In cases where the ovaries are positioned behind the uterus, it is possible to reach the follicles by completely crossing the uterus with the needle or, utilizing forceps positioned on the cervix and applying traction to the bladder—until the ovary is in the desired position (Fig. 1.20).

In the study, 30 infertile women underwent the procedure—18 under local anaesthetic, 13 under general anaesthetic—with a retrieval success rate of 52%. The presence of adhesions did not impede the procedure although the risk of bleeding and of the lower urinary tract was high.

The harvest of oocytes collected was comparable to that of the laparoscopic approach, but with a lower rate of complications and with easier access to the ovaries. The procedure could not be conducted with short-lasting general anaesthetic or local in an outpatient capacity.

The reduction in risk and cost of oocyte retrieval using echography convinced the scientific community to abandon the laparoscopic technique and to develop further the former [22, 23].

One year later, another group from northern Europe, led by the gynaecologists L. Hamberger and M. Wikland in

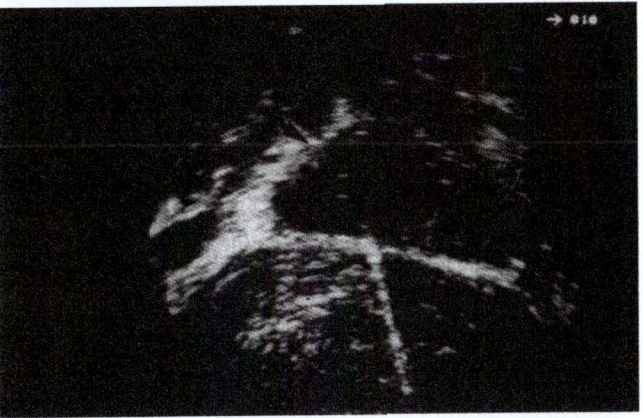

Fig. 1.20 The needle across the entire endometrial width to reach the ovary

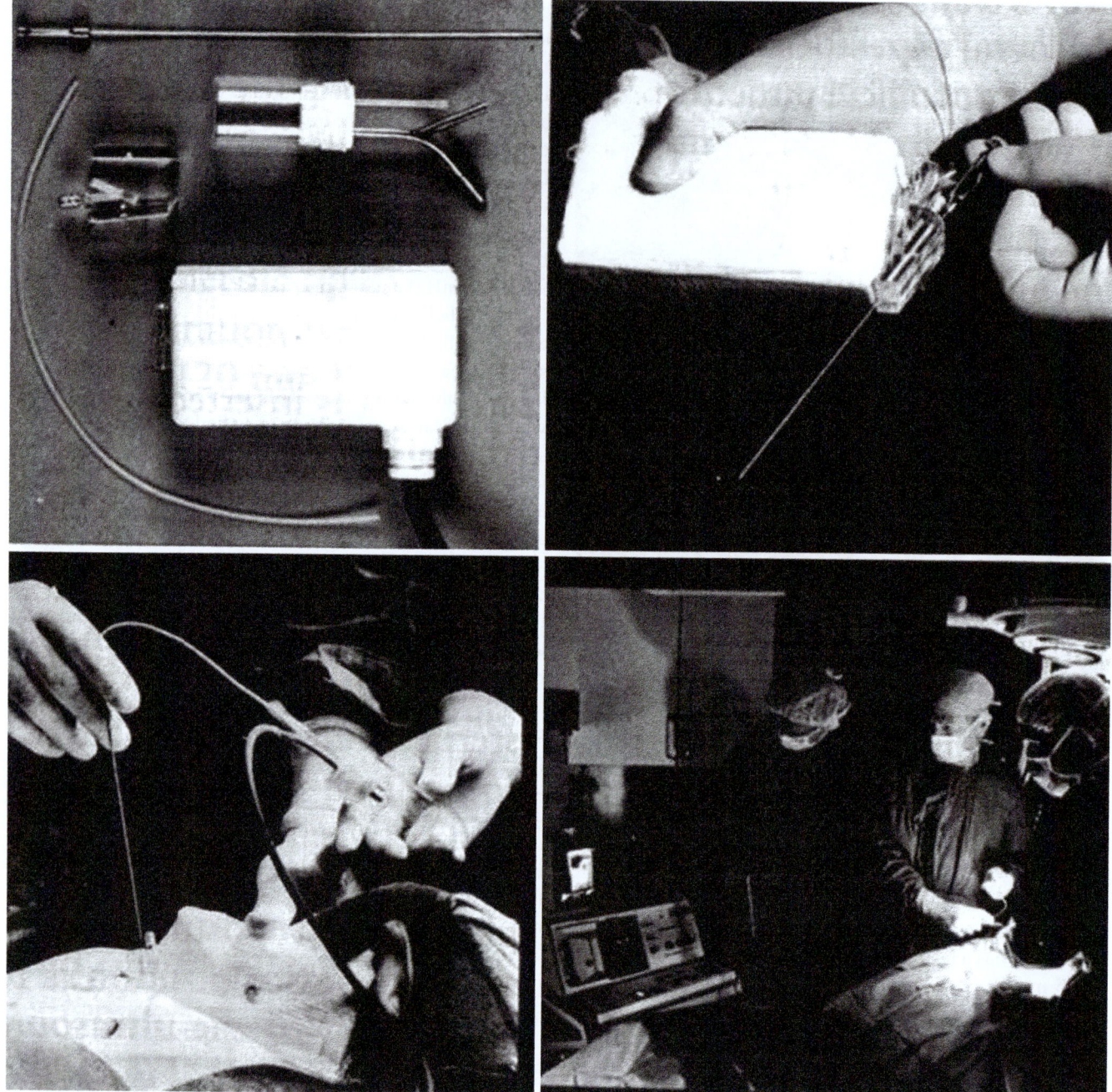

Fig. 1.21 Follicular puncture procedure utilizing a real-time linear-array equipment

Gothenburg, Sweden, described for the first time, the possibility of using an echographic vaginal probe in oocyte retrieval (Figs. 1.21, 1.22, and 1.23).

A needle was guided along the echographic vaginal probe to carry out a precise hole in the follicle and recover the follicular fluid [24, 25].

The puncturing direction was indicated by a line on the screen of the monitor of the ultrasound equipment. The exact angle and direction of this line were calibrated by holding the transducer with the needle guide and the needle in position on the surface of a bath containing a solution of 20% ethanol at 37 °C.

The sector scanner can also be equipped with a computerized pre-calibration of the puncturing line allowing the use of various needle directions (Sonotron Ltd., Malmoe, Sweden). A detailed description of the ultrasound-guided puncture of ovarian follicles using the linear-array equipment was recently published by our group [19].

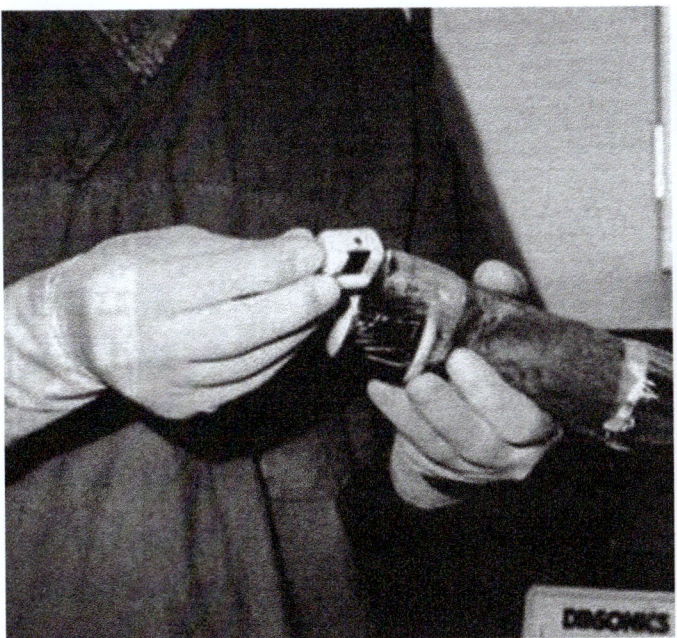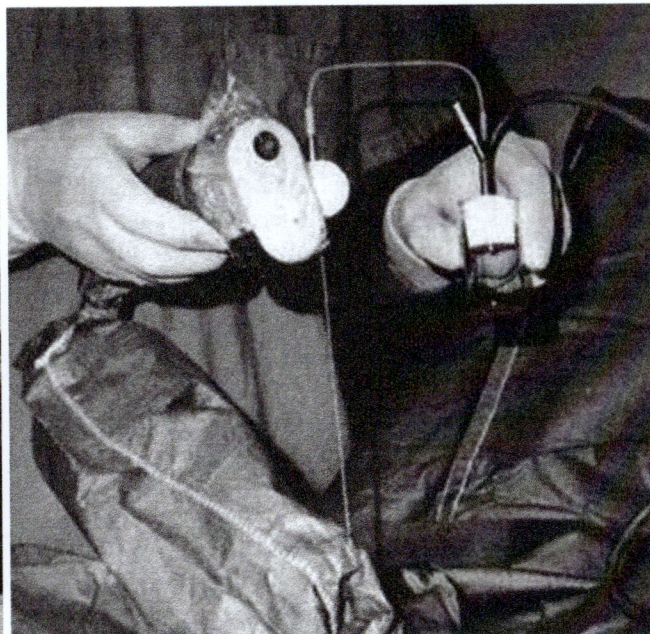

Fig. 1.22 Steering device for puncturing needle into a sector scanner transducer

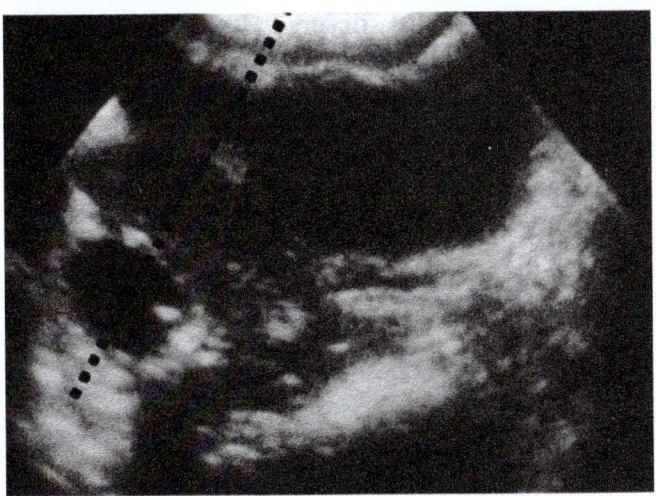

Fig. 1.23 Puncturing line crossing a preovulatory follicle

1.1 Puncturing Needles

Siliconized (Sigma coat) stainless steel needles varying in inner diameter between 1.0 and 1.8 mm have been tested. The optimal inner diameter with regard to oocyte recovery rate was found to be 1.2–1.4 mm. In order to amplify the echo and the visualization of the needle tip, shallow circumferential grooves were drilled close to the needle tip (Figs. 1.20 and 1.21). The needles utilized were manufactured by Allmekano Ltd., Goteborg, Sweden.

The punctures were performed either under light general or local anaesthesia, depending on the patient's preferences and/ or upon the number of follicles to be punctured. If, on examination immediately prior to the puncture, more than two preovulatory follicles were found in an optimal position for a transvesical puncture, general anaesthesia was often preferred. Without general anaesthesia, total pain relief cannot be guaranteed when the route chosen for follicle puncture necessitates passing the needle through the posterior wall of the bladder and the peritoneum. In cases where the position of the ovaries behind the uterus made transvaginal puncture more preferable, local anaesthesia was generally quite sufficient.

1.2 Puncturing Procedure

Prior to puncture, a rubber urinary catheter was inserted and the patient was placed in a gynaecological or horizontal position. The bladder was completely emptied and refilled with sterile solution to a total volume varying between 200 and 500 mL. Caution must be taken to fill the bladder slowly in order to avoid translocation of the ovaries to a position close to the abdominal wall since this ovarian position is unfavourable when using low-energy transducers with poor resolution in the near field.

The transducer was covered by a sterile, thin-walled plastic bag. In order to optimize the sound transmission, a thin layer of aquasonic gel (Lederle Ltd., New Jersey, USA) was placed between the transducer surface and the plastic bag.

The steering device for the needle was then attached to the transducer which, in turn, was placed in a position for optimal visualization of the follicle to be punctured. When this position is reached, the puncturing line (on the screen of the monitor of the ultrasound unit) should pass through the maximal diameter of the follicle.

This method appeared simple and effective in that a better view of the follicles, even of the smaller ones, was associated with a better rate of collection compared with the abdominal approach. Furthermore, the technique was less traumatic and could be done using only light local anaesthetic and the patient could usually leave the hospital an hour or two later.

Later studies showed a greater preference for it, both on the part of doctors and specialists, compared to the transvaginal approach, because of the better view of the pelvic organs, of the monitoring of follicles and therefore, of the oocyte aspiration. The first vaginal transducer was designed and developed by the Danish company Bruel and Kjaer in collaboration with Wikland's group (Fig. 1.24).

Soon, guides were made for specific types of needles— puncture needles and other accessories for this new technique by a Swiss biotech company, SweMed Lab, created in Gothenburg to this end. Once an initial fear relating to the danger of oocyte alteration and ultrasound was overcome, the transvaginal technique, thanks to its simplicity and efficacy, became widespread and now, having been carried out for more than 30 years, has become the default choice for the retrieval of oocytes for in vitro fertilization (Figs. 1.25 and 1.26).

The needle, connected to the collection and suction unit, was then advanced until its tip reached the level of the follicular wall. Prior to puncture, an ideal position for the needle tip can

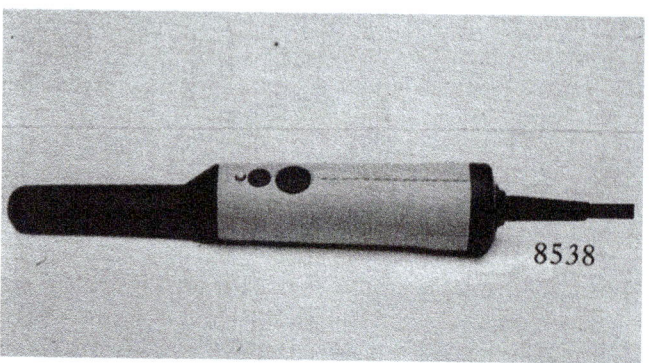

Fig. 1.24 The Bröel and kjaer probe

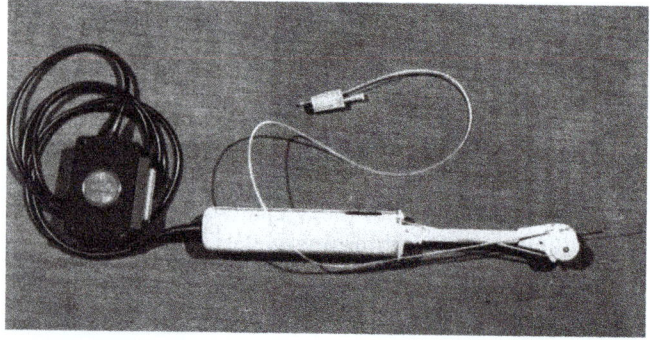

Fig. 1.25 The Kretz probe

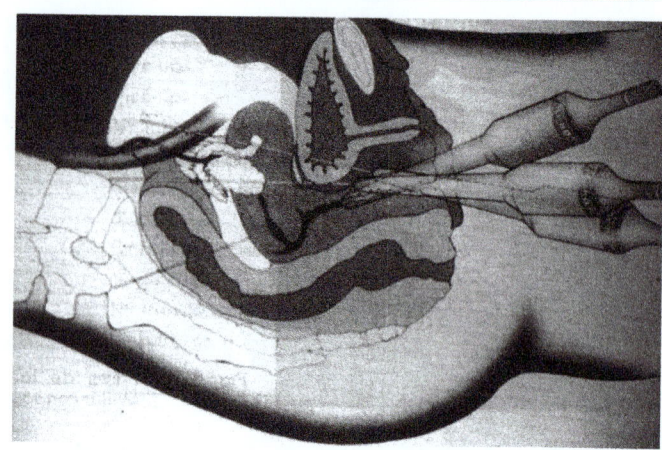

Fig. 1.26 The section shows the relationship between the vaginal probe and the observed organ

be guaranteed only by visualization of an inward bulging movement of the follicle wall in response to slight mechanical pressure from the needle tip. The puncture was then performed by a rapid, firm, and sharp insertion of the needle for 5–10 mm. The echo of the needle tip can usually be visualized clearly in the antrum of the follicle. Aspiration was then performed rapidly by applying a negative pressure of 100–120 mmHg. Small amounts of sterile saline may have filled part of the needle during its passage through the bladder since no stilette is utilized.

The needle was maintained in this position within the follicle until an oocyte was recovered. It may happen that repeated irrigation of the follicle is necessary. Double-cannula needles have not been found optimal for ultrasound aspiration.

For puncturing more than one follicle in the same ovary, the needle is withdrawn to the bladder and the transducer is focused on the next follicle. If an optimal position for the needle cannot be attained, the needle is totally withdrawn and reinserted.

Transuretral technique: the use of echography in transabdominal and transvesical oocyte retrieval led the way for the development of other techniques, such as transuretral. This technique was carried out with the needle inserted via the urethra and guided by echography by a probe sent into the woman's abdomen (Figs. 1.27 and 1.28).

Utrasonically guided transuretral puncture: the two methods of oocyte retrieval described above resulted in some problems, especially related to the dislocation of the ovaries. In 1985, in an attempt to solve some of these problems, Parson [26] proposed a transuterine technique of oocyte retrieval.

The patient was placed in the lithotomy position with the bladder filled with Hartmann's solution.

Earlier, a metal catheter was used to protect the urethra during the passage of the needle, currently however, it is preferred to use a Foley catheter and "hide" the tip of the needle in one of the holes situated at the end of the same catheter, thus inserting the catheter and the needle simultaneously. Over the years, various groups have further outlined an echography-guided transvaginal technique in oocyte retrieval.

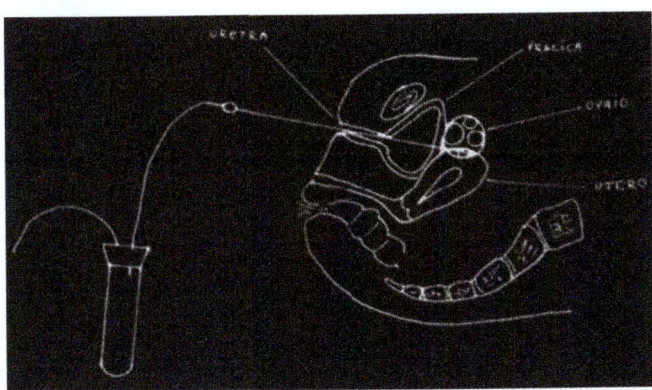

Fig. 1.27 Follicular aspiration by transuretral puncture according to Parson

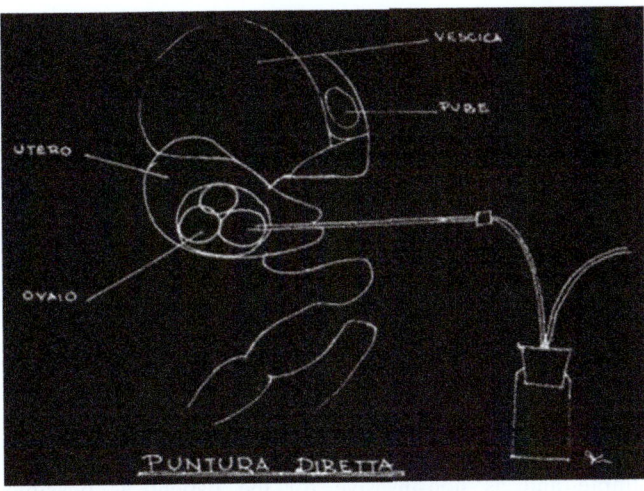

Fig. 1.29 Schematic view of follicular aspiration by transvaginal approach and under abdominal probe control. Dellenbach 1985

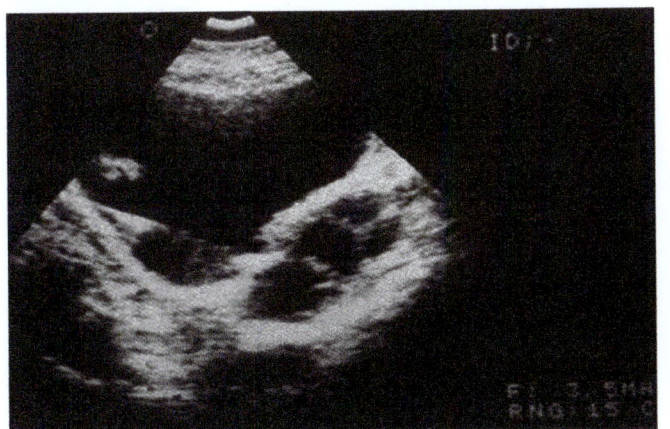

Fig. 1.28 Oocyte aspiration by transuretral puncture: on the left side the needle point and above the Foley balloon; on the right the follicles

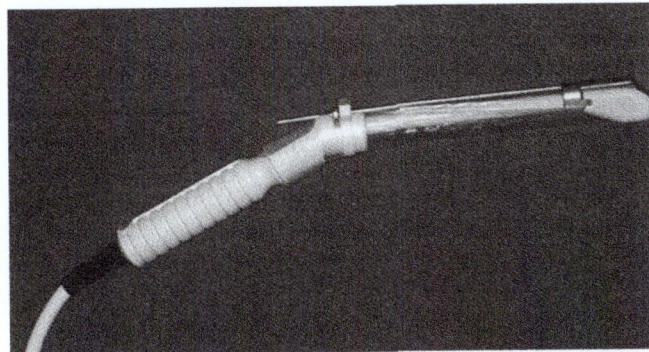

Fig. 1.30 The vaginal probe is overflowed from the needle's guide for oocyte pick-up (Feichtinger 1986)

In 1985, Dellenbach and Coll published a study of 100 patients, comparing the transvaginal approach with the other techniques put forward up until then [27]. With the new technique, the ultrasonic probe was positioned on the patient's abdomen and the needle was introduced via the posterior fornix in the ovary's cul-de-sac (Fig. 1.29).

The technique, put forward as non-painful and easy to learn and carry out, could be effectuated also on outpatients, avoiding the risk, cost, and general anaesthetic that laparoscopy entailed, or the discomfort of trans-abdominal transvesical access. The number and the quality of oocytes was comparable to the previous approaches, the only complications were traceable to the involuntary puncture of a venous structure, but it was without repetition.

The technique had great advantages compared to the previous methods, despite the fact that the distance between the ultrasonic guide and the ovaries remained high. The changing-point came with the introduction of vaginal probes which allowed for a more immediate approach, thanks to their use of high-frequency waves and better special resolution [24, 25, 28].

Puncture with vaginal probe: the development of small-sized (causing little discomfort) vaginal probes has allowed

for the use of the probe in the FIVET for oocyte retrieval from the vaginal fornices (Fig. 1.30) [29].

The possibility of having a clearer image of the pelvic structures by using higher frequency transducers (7–7.5 mHz) placed at a closer distance to the organ to be examined has opened up new developments in the field of ultrasonic diagnosis. The advantages of this new approach are many: firstly, it means we can see and aspirate follicle with a diameter of less than a centimetre, without creating problems for the patient, giving furthermore a greater guarantee to the operator of accurately locating the pelvic vessels.

With this technique, the endovaginal transducer is covered with a sterile plastic (or latex) coating and the guide is connected to this by biopsy. After introducing the needle into the guide, one proceeds to the puncture of the follicles. The patient is premedicated with benzodiapezine and with painkillers and is placed in the lithography position. The vagina is well disinfected with antibacterial agents, for example, povidone at 1%, florhexidine acetate or Betadine and washed with culture medium.

Next, one proceeds with the paracervical anaesthesia with lidocaine at 1%. Many patients accept the injection without any local anaesthetic: Although it is rather rare for patients to request general anaesthetic, they must be prepared for this in these cases. Before introducing the transducer into the vagina, one puts some millilitres of culture medium into the vaginal fornices to obtain the maximum amount of contact between the vaginal wall and the transducer. The vaginal probe is introduced and oriented towards the ovary. After the follicle has been positioned inside the luminous tracing on the display, the needle is rapidly inserted towards the vaginal wall and the ovarian tissue. As soon as the tip of needle is observed to have penetrated the follicle (Fig. 1.31), aspiration can begin. Subsequently, the adjacent follicle is punctured using swift movements of the probe without extracting the needle. Using this technique, the collection procedure is simple and as non-invasive for the patient as possible (Fig. 1.32). In cases with the ovary behind a uterus which is difficult to move, it is sometimes necessary to traverse the entire thickness of the myometrium in order to reach the fol-

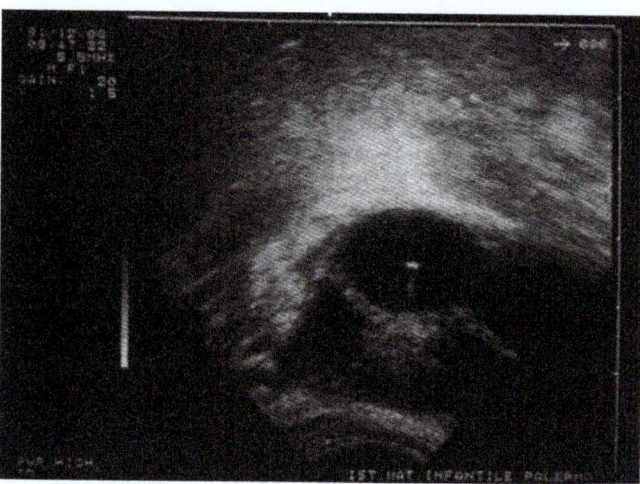

Fig. 1.31 The point of the needle is in central part of the follicle

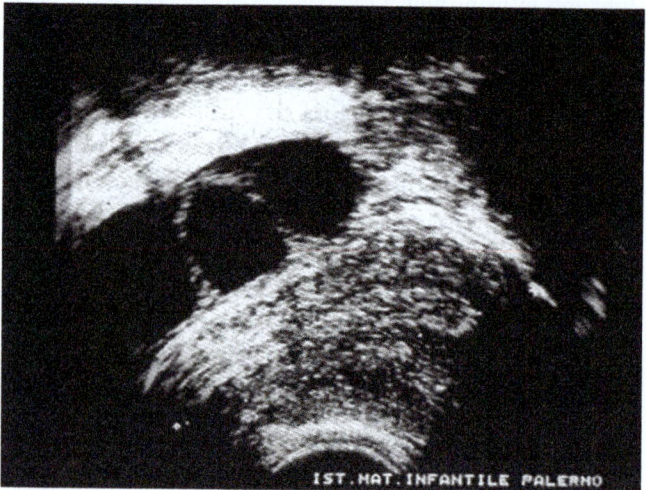

Fig. 1.32 The follicles are put in row for an easier aspiration

licles. The percentage of oocytes collected per patient is high, thanks to the possibility of reaching the small-sized follicles.

The average rate of oocyte recovery using ultrasound-guided sampling appears to be in congruence with laparoscopic retrieval in the majority of cases reported [25, 30].

1.3 The Present Transvaginal Technique

In the last years, just a few and small alterations in the initially proposed techniques have been realized [29, 31], i.e., the antibiotic profilaxis [32] and the elimination of vaginal disinfectants that could have a negative action on harvested oocytes. The choice of anaesthesia is in favour of a simple sedation [33, 34], more than a local, spinal [35], epidural, or a general one, avoiding drugs that could be toxic for oocytes. The choice of the needle to apply on the probe should be carefully considered: not so thin to be able to damage the oocytes and not too thick to increase the pain. The negative pressure depends upon the follicular size, from 90 to 120 mmHg for the largest ones and from 40 to 60 for the smallest ones (Figs. 1.23 and 1.24).

1.4 Flushing

Since the beginning of the transition from the laparoscopic to the transvaginal oocytes recovery, the correlation between harvested oocytes and obtained embryos appeared clear [36–38]. With the aim of increasing these numbers, the follicular flushing following the direct aspiration has been proposed [39–41]. Various double channel needles, ad hoc designed, were proposed, allowing at the same time the follicular aspiration in a channel, the follicular washing in a second one, and a final re-aspiration of washing liquid without extracting the needle from the follicle [42] (Figs. 1.9, 1.10, and 1.11).

The potential benefits of follicular flushing consist in the possibility of overpassing the oocyte retention inside the follicle or in the harvesting and recovery system [43].

Updated reviews based on randomized clinical studies of normospermic patients have concluded that the follicular flushing shouldn't be routinely utilized as no benefit in terms of harvested oocytes, clinical pregnancy rates, and live births has been proved [44]. Anymore, the procedure time is increased with, as a consequence, a longer anaesthesia duration. It should be noted that in the past time the choice of flushing has been supported by prospective non-randomized studies in which an increased number of harvested oocytes using the double channel needles was observed in comparison with the direct aspiration with single channel needles [45, 46].

Today the flushing is rarely used, except in the oocyte pick-up of "poor responders," in which the final purpose should be the recovery of the maximum number of oocytes. Anyway, a recent study of follicular flushing in a group of poor responders conducted in New York and published [47] in Human Reproduction brought to the conclusion that the follicular flushing in these patients doesn't increase the number of harvested oocytes and that the number of embryos obtained, the implantation, and the pregnancy rates were decreased. The authors affirm that in the same group of poor responders, when a single channel needle has been used, the implantation rates have been of 34%, the clinical pregnancy rates of 36–45% and conclude that the outcome of IVF could be reduced by the systematic use of flushing. On the basis of these conflicting results, the practice of follicular flushing should be adopted with precaution also in poor responders, awaiting the results of more detailed and controlled studies.

1.5   Oocyte Pick-up Complications

Although complications are rare, several complications of transvaginal oocyte collection have been reported. The commonest operative complications are: haemorrhage; trauma to pelvic structures; pelvic infections, tubo-ovarian, or pelvic abscess [48].

1.5.1   Haemorrhage

It can result in vaginal bleeding at and after oocyte collection (open bleeding) or in intra-abdominal bleeding (covert bleeding). The most common external haemorrhage are the colporrhagias and the hemorrhage of the cervix, with an incidence of 1.4%. The incidence of internal haemorrhages varies from 0 to 1.3%. The covert bleeding generally stops spontaneously in a short time; sometimes, a haemo-transfusion is required and in other cases a diagnostic-operative laparoscopy is required. Very rarely they are due to accidental lesions of iliac vessels or other pelvic vessels that represent dramatic surgical emergencies.

1.5.2   Pelvic Infections

These may be caused by transport of germs from vaginal flora into the pelvic-abdominal cavity through the needle utilized for the pick-up. Their incidence is between 0.2 and 0.5% and most of them require hospitalization and antibiotic treatment.

1.5.3   Traumatic Lesions of Internal Organs

Intestinal perforations, vesical and ureteral lesions are extremely rare and often extremely dramatic (Fig. 1.33).

Fig. 1.33 Traumatic lesion of internal organs: bowel

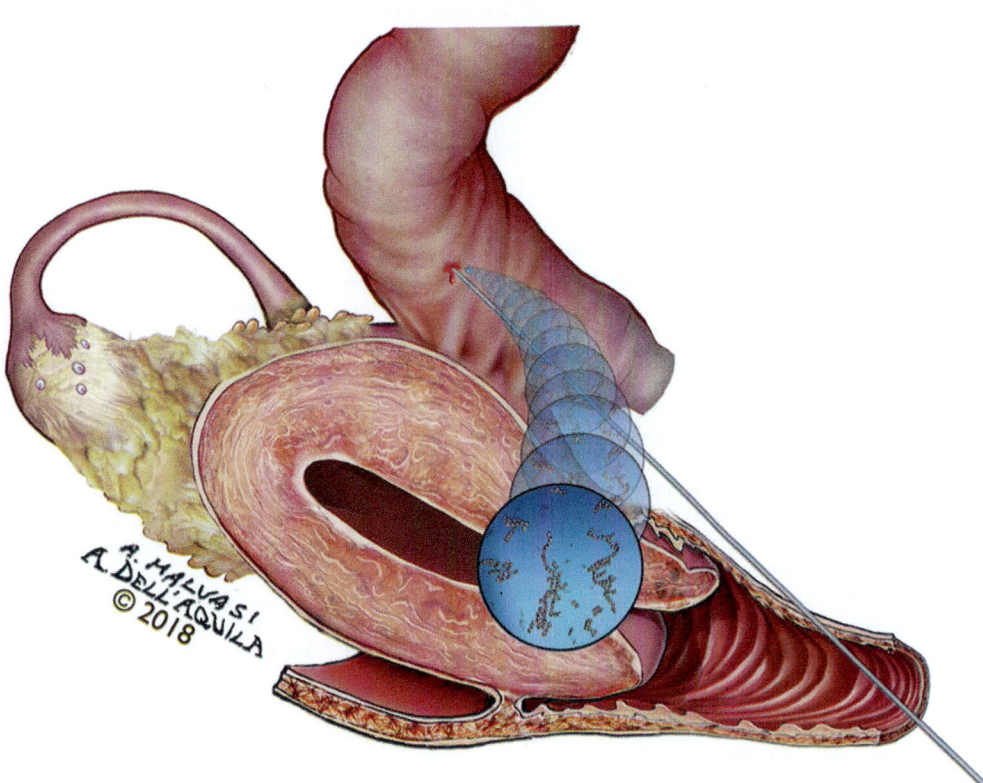

Rarely reported complications include: ovarian torsion, rupture of ovarian endometriomas, appendicitis, ureteral obstructions, and vertebral osteomyelitis.

1.5.4 Technical Aspects and Practical Suggestions

The fundamental rules are:

- To avoid the puncture of ovarian hilum
- To avoid complications at the maximum of possibilities the multiple punctures of the ovary
- To go with the needle's point as close as possible to the follicle to reduce at the minimum the excursions of the needle inside the ovary
- To maintain a visual continuous control of the lateral iliac vessels

References

1. Joutsivuo T. Vesalius and De humani corporis fabrica: Galen's errors and the change of anatomy in the sixteenth century. Hippokrates (Helsinki). 1997;98–112.
2. Toledo-Pereyra LH. De Humani Corporis Fabrica surgical revolution. J Invest Surg. 2008;21(5):232–6.
3. Herrlinger R, Feiner E. Why did Vesalius not discover the fallopian tubes? Med Hist. 1964;8:335–41.
4. Speca S, Napolitano C, Tagliaferri G. The pathogenetic enigma of polycystic ovary syndrome. J Ultrasound. 2007;10(4):153–60.
5. Gilson H. De Formatione Ovi et Pulli (1621), by Girolamo Fabrici. Embryo Project Encyclopedia 2008-09-30.
6. Hunter RHF. Physiology of the Graafian follicle and ovulation. Cambridge University; 2003.
7. Phadnis SV, Irvine LM. Fallopius: the great anatomist, surgeon and botanist. J Obstet Gynaecol. 2013;33(2):107–8.
8. Kothary PC, Kothary SP. Gabriele Fallopio. Int Surg. 1975;60:80–1.
9. Stolberg M. Empiricism in sixteenth-century medical practice: the notebooks of Georg Handsch. Early Sci Med. 2013;18:48.
10. Walker HK, Hall WD, Hurst JW. Clinical methods: the history, physical, and laboratory examinations. 3rd ed. Boston: Butterworths; 1990.
11. Bifulco M, Ciaglia E, Marasco M, Gangemi G. A focus on Trotula dé Ruggiero: a pioneer in women's and children's health in history of medicine. J Matern Fetal Neonatal Med. 2014;27(2):204–5.
12. Hurd-Mead KC. A history of women in medicine. Boston: Milford House; 1973. p. 126.
13. Mason-Hohl E, trans. The diseases of women by Trotula of Salerno. Hollywood: The Ward Ritchie Press; 1940. p. 16.
14. Klein PR. Palmer. La sterilité coniugale, Masson, Paris; 1960.
15. Steptoe PC. Laparoscopy. Ginecological coelioscopy. In: Proc. First World Congress on Gynecological Coelioscopy, Palermo; 1962.
16. Steptoe PC. Laparoscopy in gynecology. Edinburgh: Ed Livingstone; 1967.
17. Steptoe PC, Edwards RG, Purdy M. Clinical aspects of pregnancies established with cleaving embryos grown in vitro. Br J Obstet Gynecol. 1980;7:757–60.
18. Wood C, Leeton J, Talbot JM, Trounson A. Technique for collecting mature human oocytes for in vitro fertilization. Br J Obstet Gynecol. 1981;88:756–60.
19. Mettler L, Seki M, Baukloh, Semm K. Recovery and in vitro fertilization of human ova. In: In vitro fertilization and embryo transfer, by Hafez and Semm. 1982. p. 189–211.
20. Cittadini E, Flamigni C. Evolution de les technicas FIVET y GIFT. Ed: Fondazione per gli Studi sulla riproduzione umana, Palermo; 1989.
21. Cittadini E, Flamigni C, Forleo R, Sbiroli C. Infertilità femminile: Attuali orientamenti tecnici. Palermo: COFESE Ediz; 1986.
22. Cittadini E, Quartararo P. Fecondazione in vitro oggi. Palermo: COFESE Ed; 2000.
23. Lenz S, Lauritsen JG. Ultrasonically guided percutaneous aspiration of human follicles under local anesthesia: a new method for collecting oocytes for in vitro fertilization. Palermo: Cofese Ed; 1982.
24. Gembruch U, Diedrich K, Welker B, Wahode J, van der Ven H, Al-Hasani S, Krebs D. Transvaginal sonographically guided oocyte retrieval for in-vitro fertilization. Hum Reprod. 1988;3:59–63.
25. Dellenbach P, Nisand I, Moreau L, Feger B, Plumere C, Gerlinger P. Transvaginal sonographically controlled ovarian follicle puncture for egg retrieval. Lancet. 1984;1:1467.
26. Parsons J, Riddle A, Booker M, Goswamy R, Wilson L, Akkermans J, Whitehead M, Campbell S. Oocyte retrieval for in-vitro fertilization by ultrasonically guided needle aspiration via the urethra. Lancet. 1985;1(8437):1076–7.
27. Hamberger L, Wikland M. Clinical experience with ultrasound-guided follicle aspiration. In: Recent progress in human in vitro fertilization. Cofese, Ed; 1984.
28. Wikland M, Enk L, Hamberger L. Transvesical approaches for the aspiration of follicles by use of ultrasound. Ann N Y Acad Sci. 1985;442:182–94.
29. Feichtinger W. Current technology of oocyte retrieval. Curr Opin Gynecol. 1992;4:697–701.
30. Wiseman DA, Short WB, Pattinson HA, Taylor PJ, Nicholson SF, Elliot PD, Fleetham JA, Mortimer ST. Oocyte retrieval in an in vitro fertilization-embryo transfer program: comparison of four methods. Radiology. 1898;173:99–102.
31. Cittadini E, Gattuccio F, La Sala GB, Palermo R. La Sterilità Umana, Cofese Edizioni, Palermo; 1990.
32. Meldrum DR. Antibiotics for vaginal oocyte aspiration. J In Vitro Fert Embryo Transf. 1989;6(1):1–2.
33. Soussis I, Boyd O, Paraschost T, Duffy S, Bower S, Troughton P, Lowe J, Grounds R. Follicular fluid levels of midazolam, fentanyl, and alfentanil during transvaginal oocyte retrieval. Fertil Steril. 1995;64(5):1003–7.
34. Kwan I, Bunn F. Effects of prehospital spinal immobilization: a systematic review of randomized trials on healthy subjects. Prehops Disaster Med. 2005;20(1):47–53. Review.
35. Trout SW, Vallerand AH, Kemmann E. Conscious sedation for in vitro fertilization. Fertil Steril. 1998;69(5):799–808. Review.
36. Awonuga A, Waterstone J, Oyesanya O, Curson R, Nargund G, Parsons J. A prospective randomized study comparing needles of different diameters for transvaginal ultrasound-directed follicle aspiration. Fertil Steril. 1996;65(1):109–13.
37. Scott RT, Hofmann GE, Musher SJ, Acosta AA, Kreiner DK, Rosewaks Z. A prospective randomized comparison of single- and double-lumen needles for transvaginal follicular aspiration. J In Vitro Fert Embryo Transf. 1989;6:98–100.
38. Kingsland CR, Taylor CT, Aziz N, Bickerton N. Is follicular flushing necessary for oocyte retrieval? A randomized trial. Hum Reprod. 1991;6:382–3.
39. Tan SL, Waterstone J, Wren M, Paeson J. A prospective randomized study comparing aspiration only with aspiration and flushing

for transvaginal ultrasound-directed oocyte recovery. Fertil Steril. 1992;58:356–60.

40. Wongtra-Ngan S, Vutyavanich T, Brown J. Follicular flushing during oocyte retrieval in assisted reproductive techniques. Cochrane Database Syst Rev. 2010;CD 004634.

41. Haydardedeoglu B, Cok T, Kilicdag EB, Parlakgumus AH, Simsek E, Bagis T. In vitro fertilization-intracytoplasmic sperm injection outcomes in single- versus double-lumen oocyte retrieval needles in normally responding patients: a randomized trial. Fertil Steril. 2011;95:812–4.

42. Levy G, Hill MJ, Ramirez CI, Correa L, Ryan ME, Decherney AH, Levens ED, Whitcomb BW. The use of follicle flushing during oocyte retrieval in assisted reproductive technologies: a systematic review and meta-analysis. Hum Reprod. 2012;27:2373–9.

43. El Hussein E, Balen AH, Tan SL. A prospective study comparing the outcome of oocyte retrieved in the aspirate with those retrieved in the flush during transvaginal ultrasound directed oocyte recovery for in-vitro fertilization. Br J Obstet Gynaecol. 1992;99:841–4.

44. Waterstone JJ, Parsons JH. A prospective study to investigate the value of flushing follicles during transvaginal ultrasound-directed follicle aspiration. Fertil Steril. 1992;57:221–3.

45. Babtharia S, Haloob AR. Is there a benefit from routine follicular flushing for oocyte retrieval? J Obstet Gynaecol. 2005;25: 374–6.

46. Levens ED, Whitcomb BW, Payson MD, Larsen FW. Ovarian follicular flushing among low-responding patients undergoing assisted reproductive technology. Fertil Steril. 2009;91:1381–4.

47. Mok-Lin E, Brauer AA, Schattman G, Zaninovic N, Rosenwaks Z, Spandorfer S. Follicular flushing and in vitro fertilization outcomes in the poorest responders: a randomized controlled trial. Hum Reprod. 2013;28(11):2990–5.

48. Ludwig AK, Glawatz M, Griesinger G, Diedrichk K, Ludwig M. Perioperative and post-operative complications of transvaginal ultrasound-guided oocyte retrieval: prospective study of >1000 oocyte retrievals. Hum Reprod. 2006;21:3235–40.

Anatomy and Physiology of Ovarian Follicle

Marija Dundović, Lada Zibar, and Mariaelena Malvasi

Contents

Female reproductive system is a place of origin of a new human life. It produces female gametes, gives a supportive environment for fertilization and embryo development, ultimately it nurtures a growing fetus for 40 weeks of gestation. Women are born with two ovaries placed on either sides of the uterus in the abdomen. They have a complex role on regulating menstrual cycle, producing hormones and monthly giving a single mature oocyte that is ready for fertilization, subsequently giving a couple a chance for pregnancy. It is the intention of this chapter to describe a structure of a single follicle that is a place of human oocyte origin, its development through various stages of woman's life and menstrual cycle. Also, we will explain the effect of hormones on ovarian tissue and follicle development and how they affect oocyte maturation, what happens to the follicle after the rupture, and what is the significance of various growth factors and chemical signals in physiology of the follicle.

Gametogenesis, oogenesis in this particular case, represents developmental stages of oocytes.

Oogenesis starts before birth when primordial germ cells migrate do gonadal ridge and start their differentiation to oogonia. Oogonia divide by mitosis and reach a number of 7,000,000 by the fifth month of gestation and at the same time some of them differentiate into primary oocytes. By the seventh month of gestation, most of them become atretic and primary oocytes that do survive and enter in prophase of the first meiotic division and become dormant in that form all the way to puberty [1]. Primary oocyte together with its layer of follicular cells makes a primordial follicle. Also, it is well known that a female newborn carries approximately 1–2 million of primary oocytes and that number decreases to 400,000 at puberty and about 400 hundred reach maturation and ovulate. It is interesting to see what happens to all the oocytes that become atretic. Vaskivuo et al. [2] published a paper in 2001 that explained the survival of human ovarian follicles from fetal to adult life and the mechanism of apoptosis in human ovaries. Their results show that a large amount of oocytes degenerate during fetal life through apoptosis, and it is already evident in the 13th week of gestation. Their findings also showed that the rate of apoptosis in the adult ovary increased with growing follicular size and only slightly affected early growing follicles. It is a mechanism for eliminating recruited follicles that do not reach dominant follicle stage. It is also important to notice that during fetal stage

M. Dundović (✉)
Department of Human Reproduction and Assisted Reproductive Techniques, Clinical Hospital Center Osijek, Osijek, Croatia

L. Zibar
Clinical Hospital Merkur, Zagreb, Croatia

M. Malvasi
Department of Anatomical Medical and Histological Science of the Locomotor System, Sapienza University, Rome, Italy

© Springer Nature Switzerland AG 2020
A. Malvasi, D. Baldini (eds.), *Pick Up and Oocyte Management*, https://doi.org/10.1007/978-3-030-28741-2_2

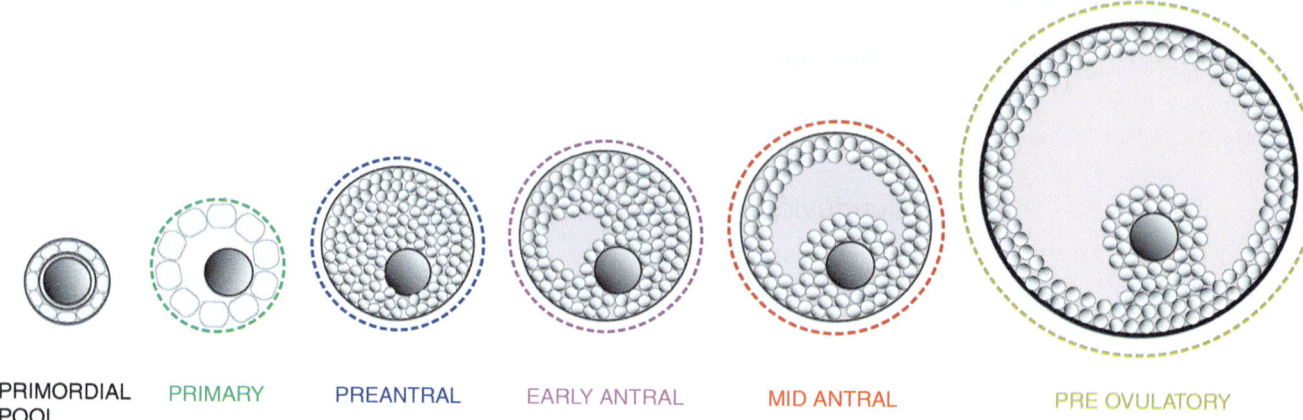

PRIMORDIAL POOL   PRIMARY   PREANTRAL   EARLY ANTRAL   MID ANTRAL   PRE OVULATORY

Fig. 2.1 Stages of development of human ovarian follicles

apoptosis is a mechanism for eliminating oocytes, but in adult life apoptosis is located in granulosa cells and they play a major role in follicular demise.

Ovaries are specific by their structure since at a monthly basis they go through extreme changes and reorganization. Follicles that contain oocytes go through various stages of development that include primordial, primary, secondary, preantral and antral follicles that ultimately give rise to a large follicle called Graafian follicle (Fig. 2.1). This process is controlled by various hormones and growth factors [3].

Environment in which oocyte matures has been proven to influence the quality of the oocyte and subsequently entire embryo and its implantation potential. This is especially interesting to observe from assisted reproductive techniques perspective where a mature oocyte with excellent metabolic activity plays a crucial role in embryo development and its morphology (Fig. 2.2).

Dumesic et al. (2015) [4] have investigated a relationship between follicular fluid and cumulus cells and oocyte health. They found that signaling between oocytes and somatic cells changed intrafollicular environment that controlled follicle growth and which antral follicle was to be selected to ovulate a healthy oocyte. Cellular metabolism is key to a normal meiotic resumption. Maternal ageing or metabolic disease perturb cellular mechanisms within the oocyte, alter macromolecules, and induce mitochondrial mutations which hurts the oocyte.

It is clear that the environment that brings an oocyte to its maturity plays a crucial role and not just in maturity but also in oocye shape and quality (Figs. 2.3 and 2.4). Therefore, there will be a great emphasis on folliculogenesis and how the actual follicles change and what structural changes give rise to a mature oocyte.

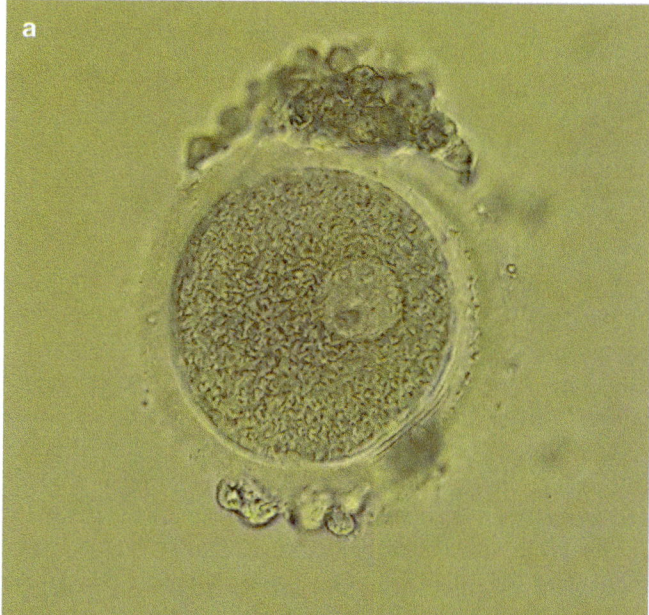

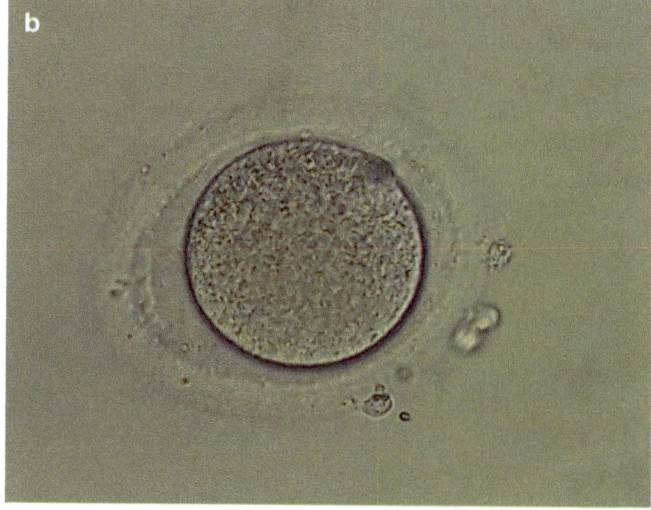

Fig. 2.2 Oocyte maturity: (**a**) germinal vesicle, (**b**) MI—immature oocyte, (**c**) MII—mature oocyte (author: MarijaDundović)

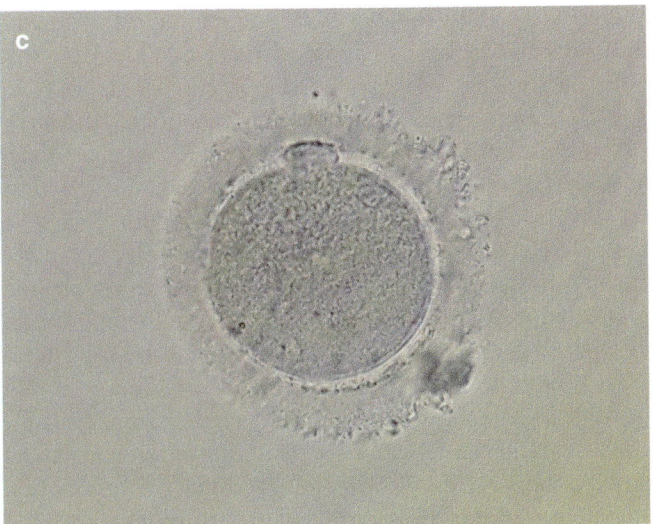

Fig. 2.2 (continued)

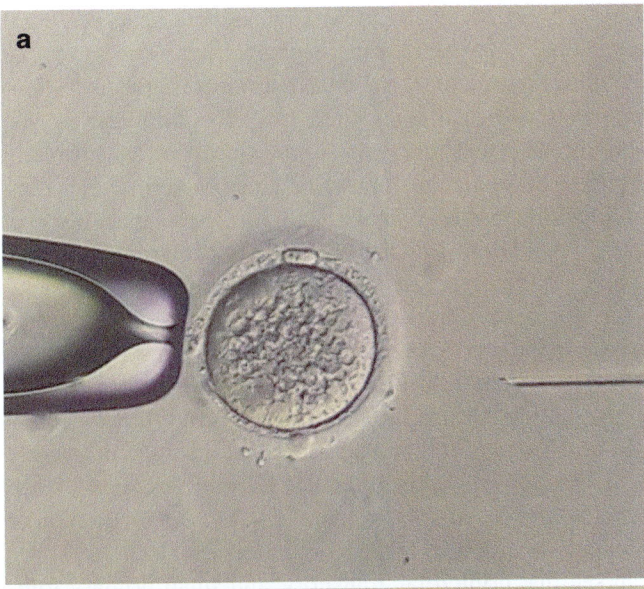

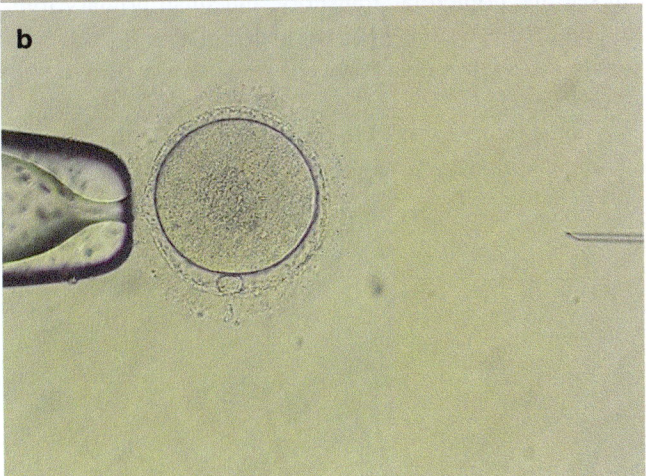

Fig. 2.4 Irregularities in oocyte structure, mainly cytoplasm, seen when performing ICSI (intracytoplasmic injection of sperm) (**a** and **b**) (author: Marija Dundović)

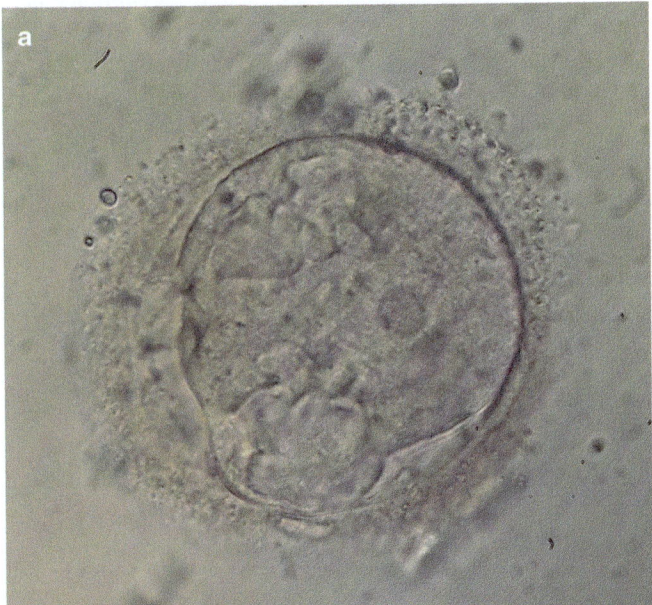

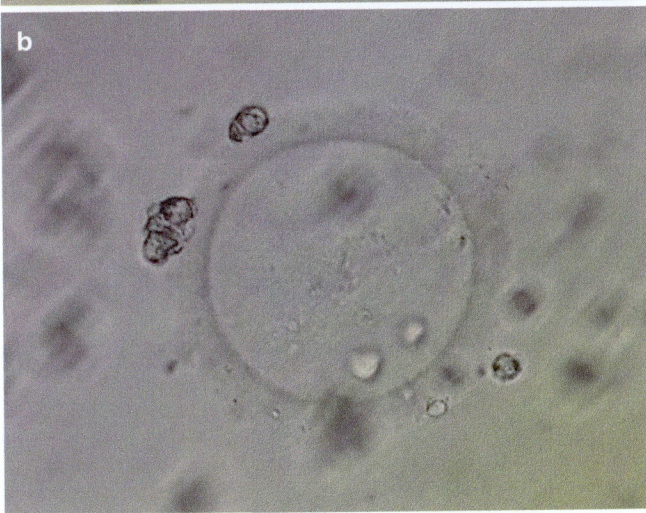

Fig. 2.3 (**a**) Very irregular shaped germinal vesicle, (**b**) zona free—no oocyte retrieved within zona pellucida (author: MarijaDundović)

2.1   Follicle Growth

Changes in structure and size of a follicle that lead to a mature oocyte happen in a process of folliculogenesis. It is a process that takes approximately 1 year in women, and it includes growth of a recruited primordial follicle that develops into a specialized Graafian follicle which will either ovulate to give a mature oocyte or die by atresia.

Mechanisms that regulate folliculogenesis are under control of changing concentrations of hormones and growth factors, at endocrine level they are regulated by the central nervous system, anterior pituitary, and ovary cascade system [5]. It is important to mention the synergy of these two control systems where growth factors can enhance or reduce the action of certain hormones locally—autocrine or paracrine system of control. Interestingly, very similar mechanisms control early embryogenesis and blastocyst implantation.

Atwood and Meethal (2016) [6] examine spatiotemporal regulation of mentioned signals and confirm that hypothalamic-pituitary-gonadal hormones regulate folliculogenesis, follicular quiescence, ovulation, follicular atresia, and corpus luteal functions. After conception and in early embryo development, autocrine and paracrine signaling becomes increasingly important, and these signals are crucial for synthesis of human chorionic gonadotropin which is a proof of embryo existing in female reproductive system. This hormone ultimately has an effect, upon blastocyst arrival in the uterus, on tissue remodeling and supports controlled invasion of the blastocyst in the endometrium.

Regarding the structural changes, human folliculogenesis can be divided into four main steps that include initiation of follicular growth, early follicular growth, selection of one follicle from a pool of selectable follicles, and maturation of preovulatory follicle. In the work of Gougeon (2010) [7], we can see that primordial, transitory, and small primary follicles constitute ovarian reserve, and initiation of follicular growth starts when oocyte nucleus reaches a critical diameter of 19 μm.

After entering the growth phase, granulosa cells proliferate and the oocyte grows at the quickest rate so follicles become secondary follicles with multiple layers of granulosa cells and are around 2 mm in diameter. Selectable follicles measure from 2 to 5 mm and their number ranges from 3 to 11 in an ovary of women 24–33 years of age. Research has shown that the selected follicle is the one that is the healthiest, grows faster than the other ones, and is the most sensitive to FSH (follicle-stimulating hormone). From the time of selection to ovulation, the selected follicle rapidly changes in size from approximately 6 mm up to 18 mm and more, and it is important to point out that in the mid-follicular phase the preovulatory follicle becomes highly vascularized through theca. Theca cells have a very important role in folliculogenesis (Fig. 2.5)—they synthesize androgens, connect granulosa cells and oocyte during development, and provide support for a growing follicle. They are, to simplify, an outer layer of the follicle and have their origin in stromal tissue surrounding the primordial follicle. They are specialized cells that are recruited to surround an activated follicle and provide structural support and acquire a capillary network [8].

Regarding the recruitment of follicles into later stages of development, literature shows the two types: initial and cyclic recruitment. Initial recruitment involves primordial

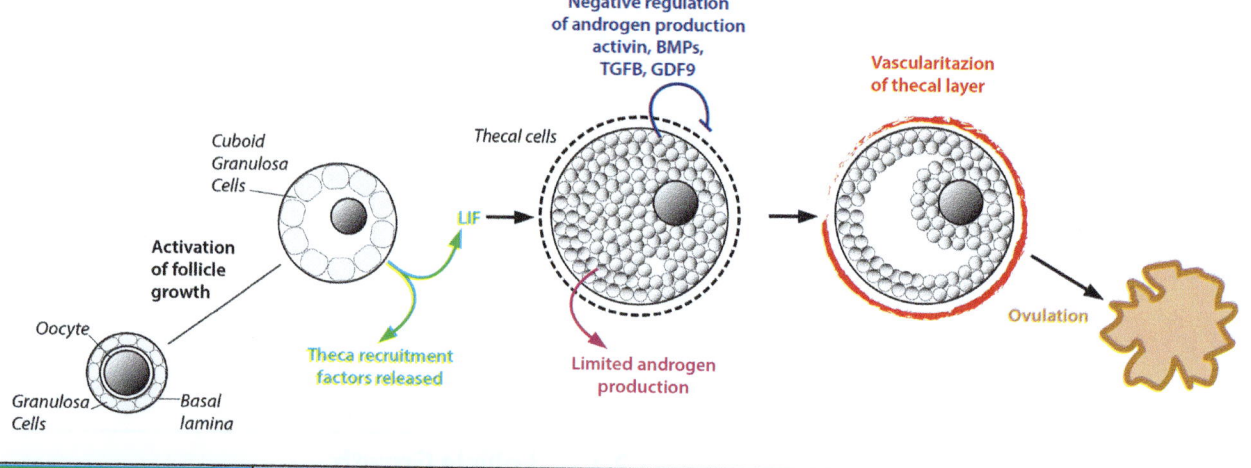

PRIMORDIAL	PRIMARY	PREANTRAL	ANTRAL	CORPUS LUTEUM
No theca	Cuboidal CGs	Thecal cells recruited and begin to differenziate; produce LH receptors, steroidogenics enzymes and small amount of androgens	Theca cells mature and become steroidogenic under control of LH	Theca cells luteinize
Flattened GCs	Signal from follicle to stroma to recruit thacal cells			Transient endocrine gland
Precursor thecal cells in surrounding stroma No Lh expression No ability to produce steroids			Increasing amounts of androgen produced, converted to estradiol in CGs	Change function to produce progesterone
		CGs secrets activin, BMPs, GDF9, inhibin, TGFB to control androgen production		

Fig. 2.5 Development of theca cells

LIFE HISTORY OF OVARIAN FOLLICLES

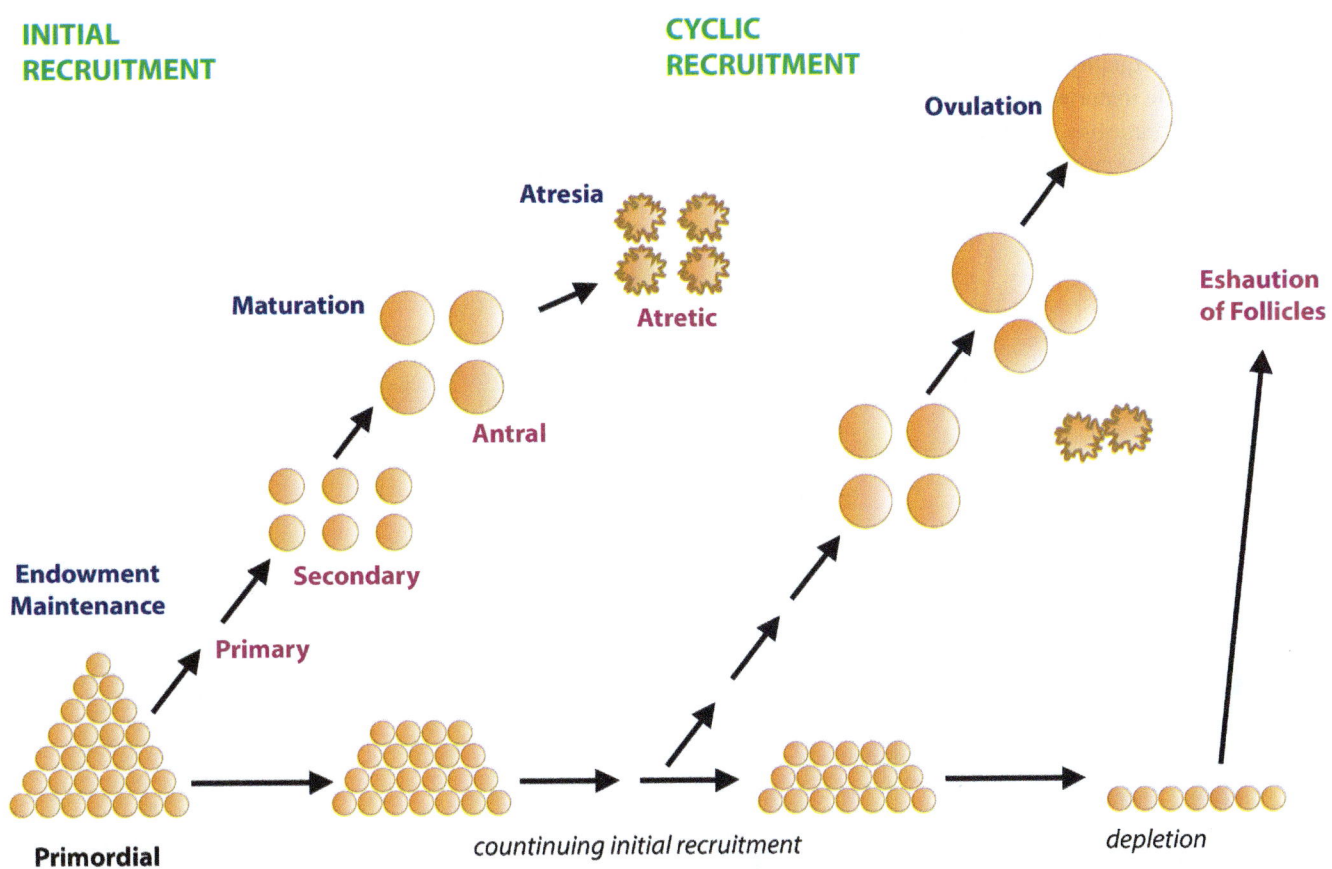

Fig. 2.6 History of ovarian follicles

follicles that aren't under influence of hormones, they remain dormant and this happens continuously throughout life after follicle formation and oocytes have just started to grow. Cyclic recruitment involves antral follicles in growth phase that are under FSH influence, start their recruitment after onset of puberty with grown oocytes, and can undergo apoptosis as a mechanism of cellular death if not selected to reach maturity and ovulate (Fig. 2.6 and Table 2.1) [9].

In addition, Chang et al. (1998) [10] have studied neutrophil—interleukin-8 system in human folliculogenesis and have come to a conclusion that neutrophils and endogenous interleukin-8 are expressed in the theca vasculature during folliculogenesis in normal ovulatory women, being particularly abundant in cohort follicles undergoing atresia. This led them to propose that there could be a system involving these factors that could function as a mechanism for follicle atresia. Many other studies have shown that granulosa cells that surround the oocyte are essential in determining the survival of follicles. Matsuda et al. (2012) [11] described the regulation of follicular growth and atresia by granulosa cells, and the key factor was the appearance of apoptotic granulosa

Table 2.1 Differences between initial and cyclic recruitment of ovarian follicles

Stages	Initial recruitment (initiation of growth)	Cyclic recruitment (escape from atresia)
	Primordial	Antral (human: 2–5 mm in diameter: rodents: 0.2–0.4 mm in diameter)
Hormones involved	Not determined	FSH
Default pathway	Remain dormant	Apoptosis
Timing	Continuous throughout life, begins after follicle formation	Cyclic (human: 28 days, rodents: 4–5 days), starts after puberty onset
Oocyte status	Starting to grow, not capable of undergoing germinal vesicle breakdown	Completed growth, competent to undergo germinal vesicle breakdown

cells in atretic follicles which led to completely apoptotic granulosa in progressed atretic follicles with a disruptive granulosa layer. The deprivation of key survival-promoting factors or stimulation by death ligands caused apoptosis.

Cumulus cells that directly surround the oocyte originate from granulosa cells and have a great role in oocyte maturation and growth (Fig. 2.7).

Transcriptome analysis (mRNA expression) in cumulus cell can indicate quality of the environment the oocyte was exposed to while maturing and give rise to some biomarkers that can be an indicator of oocyte and later embryo fitness resulting in healthy pregnancies [12].

We can say that in terms of structural changes, follicular antrum or cavity certainly has very expansive growth and makes the majority of volume of preovulatory Graafian follicle (Figs. 2.8, 2.9, and 2.10). Rodgers and Irvine-Rodgers (2010) [13] have described the process of follicular antrum and fluid formation in a way that granulosa cells produce hyaluronan and proteoglycan versican generates osmotic gradient that draws fluid from thecal vasculature (Fig. 2.11).

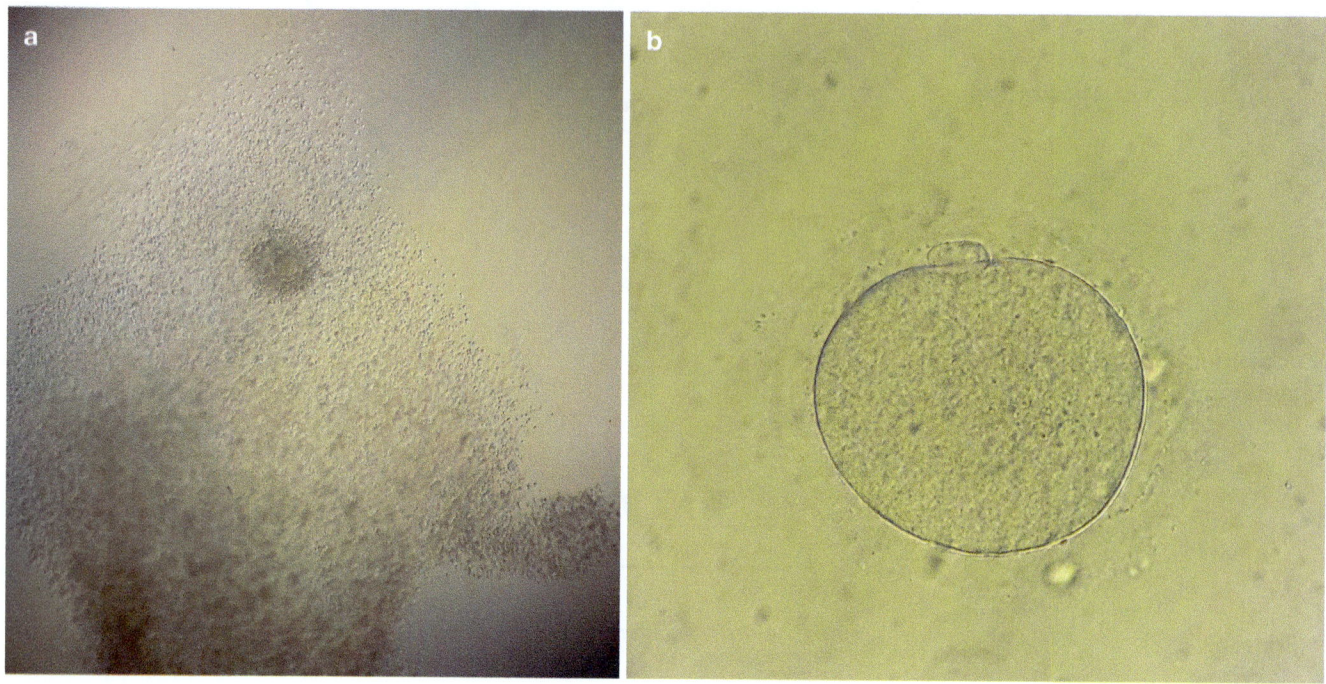

Fig. 2.7 (**a**) Cumulus oocyte complex (COC)—the oocyte is visible and surrounded with cumulus cells, (**b**) oocyte derived from COC in **a**

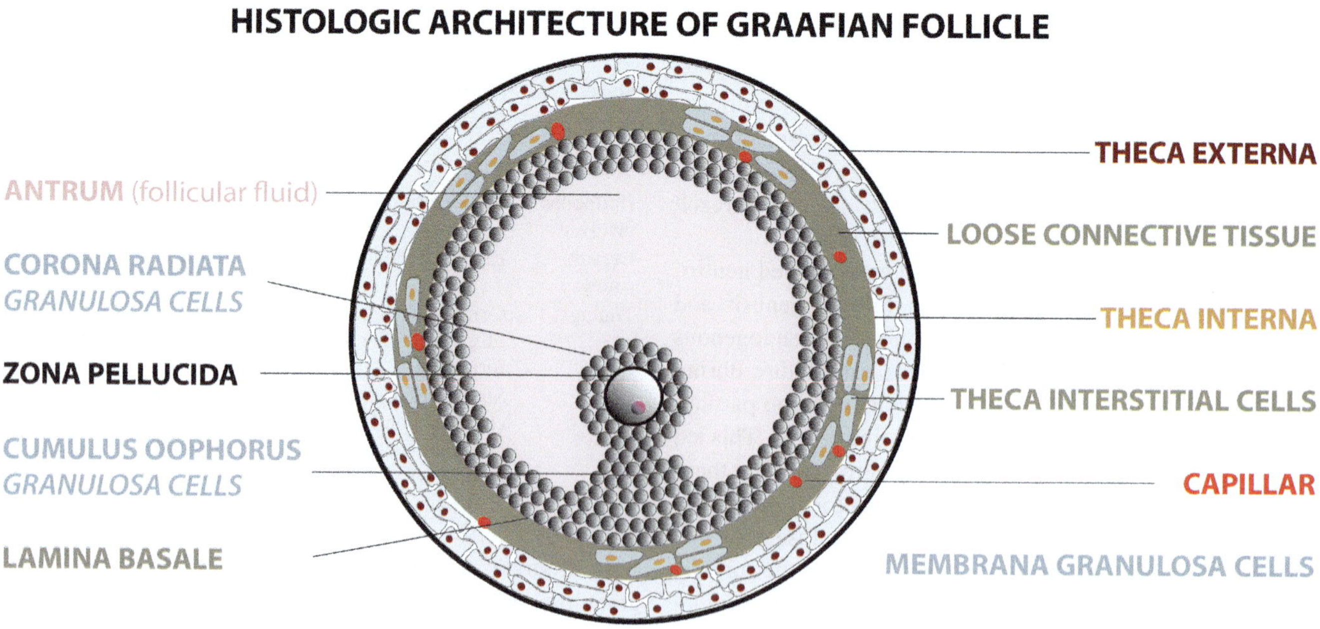

HISTOLOGIC ARCHITECTURE OF GRAAFIAN FOLLICLE

ANTRUM (follicular fluid)

CORONA RADIATA
GRANULOSA CELLS

ZONA PELLUCIDA

CUMULUS OOPHORUS
GRANULOSA CELLS

LAMINA BASALE

THECA EXTERNA

LOOSE CONNECTIVE TISSUE

THECA INTERNA

THECA INTERSTITIAL CELLS

CAPILLAR

MEMBRANA GRANULOSA CELLS

Fig. 2.8 Structure of Graafian follicle

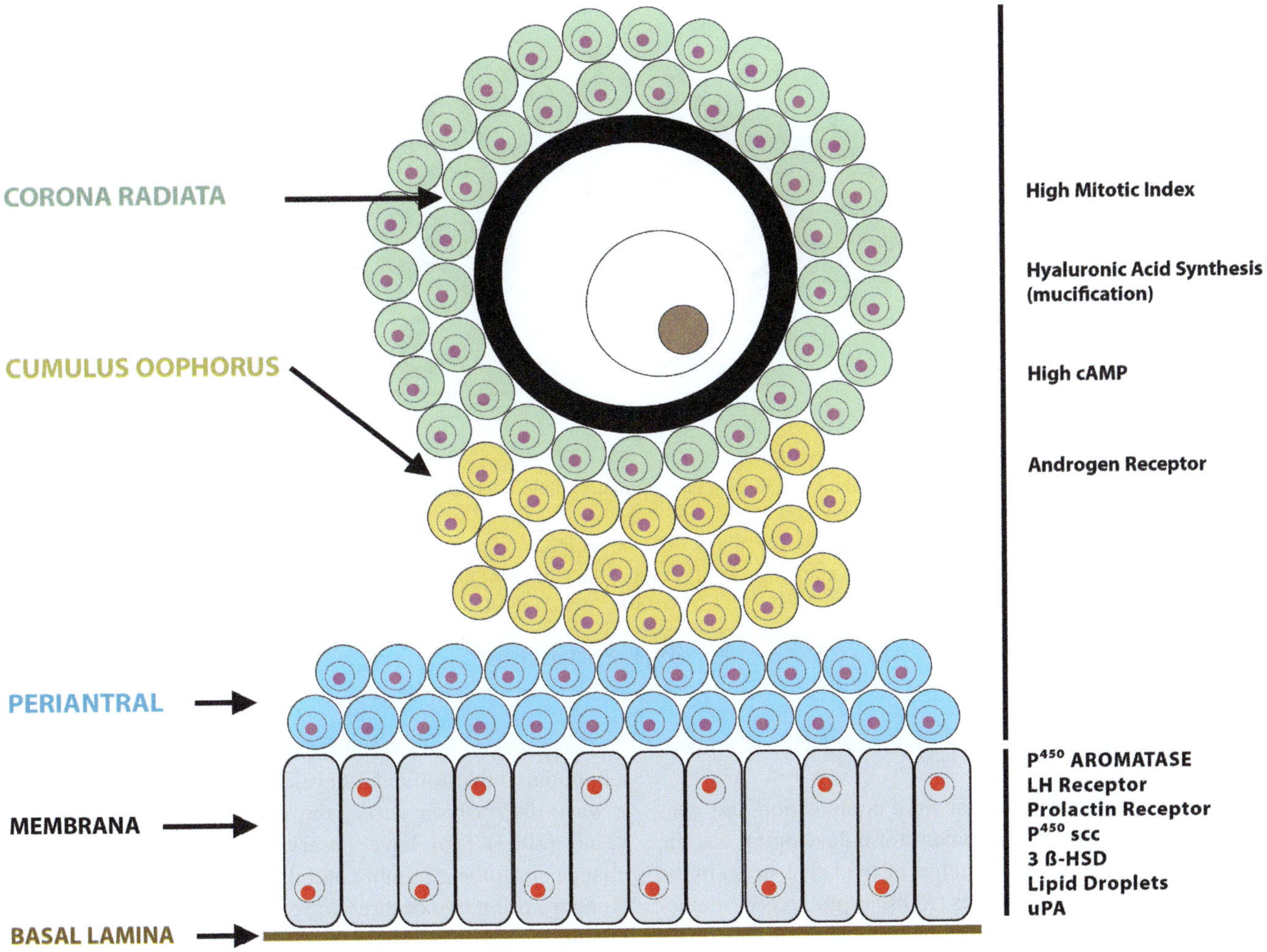

CORONA RADIATA

CUMULUS OOPHORUS

PERIANTRAL

MEMBRANA

BASAL LAMINA

High Mitotic Index

Hyaluronic Acid Synthesis
(mucification)

High cAMP

Androgen Receptor

P^{450} **AROMATASE**
LH Receptor
Prolactin Receptor
P^{450} **scc**
3 ß-HSD
Lipid Droplets
uPA

Fig. 2.9 Structure of cells that surround an oocyte in a Graafian follicle

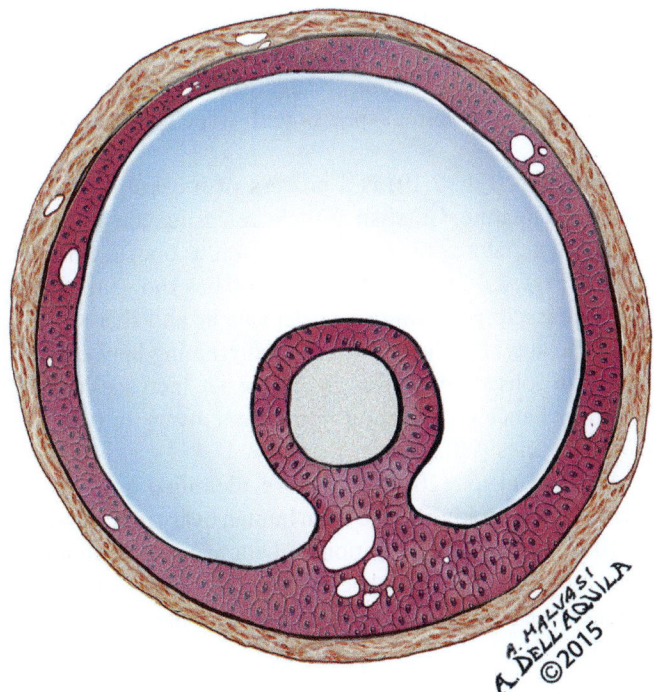

Fig. 2.10 Follicle with oocyte

Aquaporins from granulosa cell could be involved in water transport into the follicle. Follicular fluid is of complex composition that has a significant relevance for developing oocytes. Ambekar et al. (2013) [14] have carried series of tests in order to characterize proteome of human follicular fluid. They report identification of 480 proteins, 320 of which have never been described before in the follicular fluid. The identified proteins include growth factors, hormones, signaling receptors, enzymes, antibodies, and complement. This will help in understanding the process of follicular maturation and in case of IVF patients, some proteins can be used as biomarkers for oocyte quality and eventually IVF success.

Jozwik et al. (2006) [15] aimed to determine amino acids, ammonia, and urea concentrations in human ovarian follicular fluid and compare it to concentrations found in plasma. They found threefold increase of glutamate concentration (Table 2.2) in follicular fluid, higher concentrations of ammonia in follicular fluid, and no significant difference in urea concentration. These findings may reflect utilization of amino acids and transport characteristics of the

Fig. 2.11 Ovarian follicle recruitment

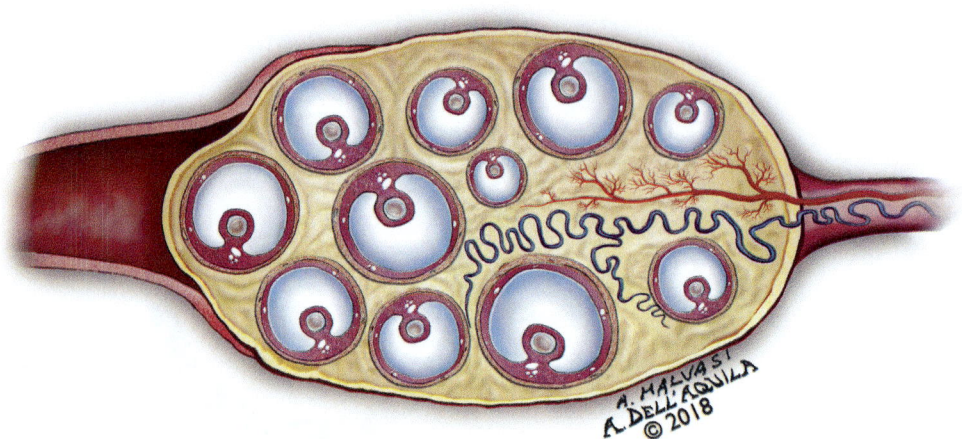

Table 2.2 Comparison of concentrations of ammonia and urea in preovulatory fluid to concentrations of ammonia in whole blood and urea in plasma

Substance	Concentration in blood or plasma	Concentration in follicular fluid	P-value	Difference between blood or plasma and follicular fluid	Blood or plasma-to-follicular fluid ratio
Ammonia (µM)	22.11 ± 1.96 (whole blood)	38.87 ± 2.23	<0.001	−16.77 ± 2.42	0.58 ± 0.05
Urea (mM)	3.37 ± 0.18 (plasma)	3.36 ± 0.22	0.911	0.015 ± 0.063	1.01 ± 0.02

follicular cells which can be an important factor in embryo development.

When speaking of follicular fluid composition and general follicle as a microenvironment for a developing oocyte, it is important to note the existence of oxidative stress in the form of reactive oxygen species (ROS) as products of metabolism within the follicle. Melatonin, generally known as a pineal gland secrete that regulates circadian rhythm and reproduction, is found to be an excellent free radical scavenger in the ovarian follicle. Tamura et al. (2013) [16] summarized new findings related to beneficial effects of melatonin which enters the follicular fluid via blood. It acts as a potent antioxidant (Fig. 2.12) and contributes to oocyte maturation and embryo development.

This chapter also demonstrated usage of melatonin as an infertility treatment since research has shown that it elevates fertilization and pregnancy rates.

With the usage of scanning and transmission electron microscope (SEM and TEM) Makabe, Naguro, and Stallone (2006) [17] were able to demonstrate the fine relationship existing between oocyte and follicular cells during various stages of follicular development (Figs. 2.13, 2.14, 2.15, 2.16, and 2.17).

Oocytes maintain a close relationship throughout the entire follicular development, oocytes form a specialized membrane system that provides a cytoplasmic scaffold inside the zona pellucida and eases the metabolic exchange between oocytes and follicular cells and, lastly, such a structure can be called a syncytium because of the existing complex that finely modulates the oocyte growth (Fig. 2.18).

Dynamics of human follicular growth are explained with a hypothesis that follicular development in women occurs in a wave-like fashion during the menstrual cycle. Baerwald et al. (2003) [18] have observed non-random wave-like changes in follicle number and diameter and confirmed that women exhibit two or three waves of folliculogenesis during an interovulatory interval.

This is opposed to a previously held notion that a single cohort of antral follicles grows only during follicular phase of menstrual cycle. A review paper from Baerwald et al. (2012) [19] concludes increasing evidence that multiple waves of antral follicles develop during the human menstrual cycle and were able to compare the results with those documented in several animal species with some species-specific difference.

Ovulation (Fig. 2.19) is a process of breaking the outer layer of a mature Graafian follicle releasing the follicular fluid with a mature oocyte within a cumulus oocyte complex (COC) (Figs. 2.10 and 2.19). A research has shown that ovulation characteristics were age dependent and that women under the age of 29 have ovulations alternating between two ovaries in consecutive cycles and as the age increases there is a higher chance of ovulation in the same ovary in two consecutive cycles [20].

Al-Alem et al. (2015) [21] have identified a leukocyte attractant, chemokine ligand 20 in human ovary that increases by 40-fold after administration of beta hCG and stimulates leukocyte migration. Leukocyte presence aids to the final ovulatory events and positively contributes to female fertility.

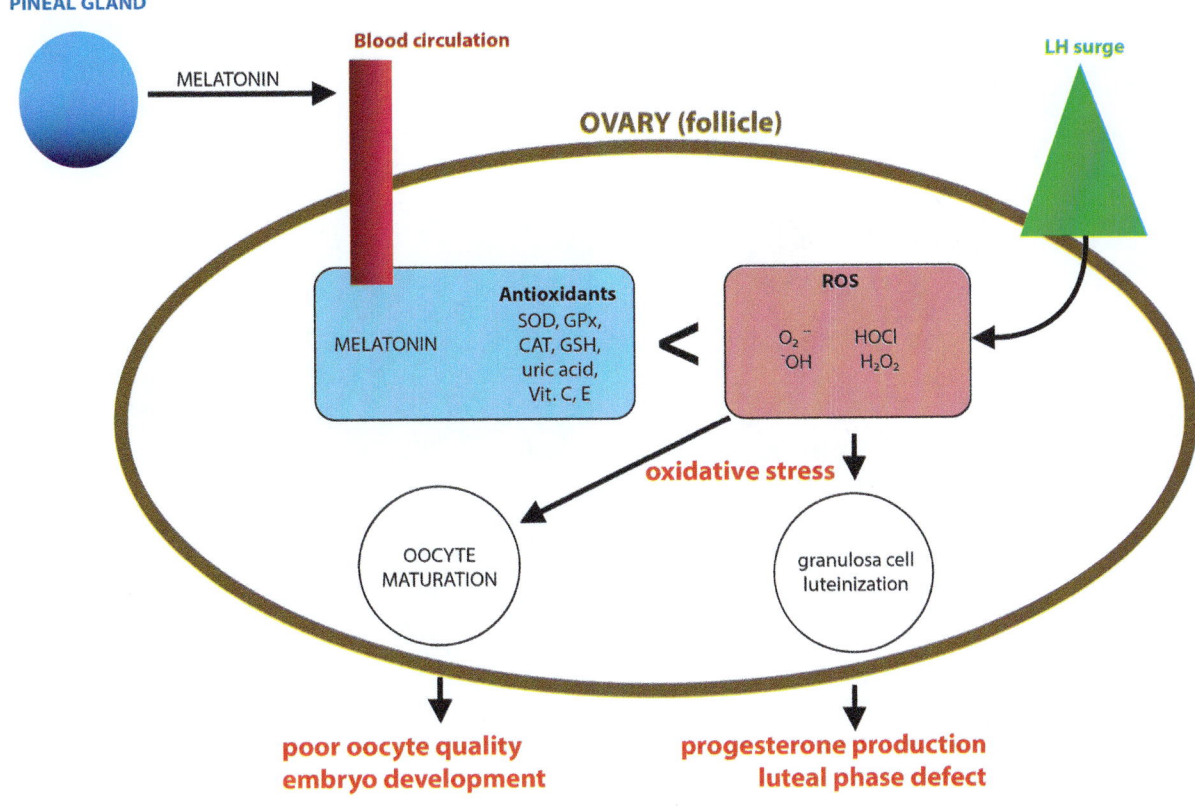

Fig. 2.12 Roles of melatonin

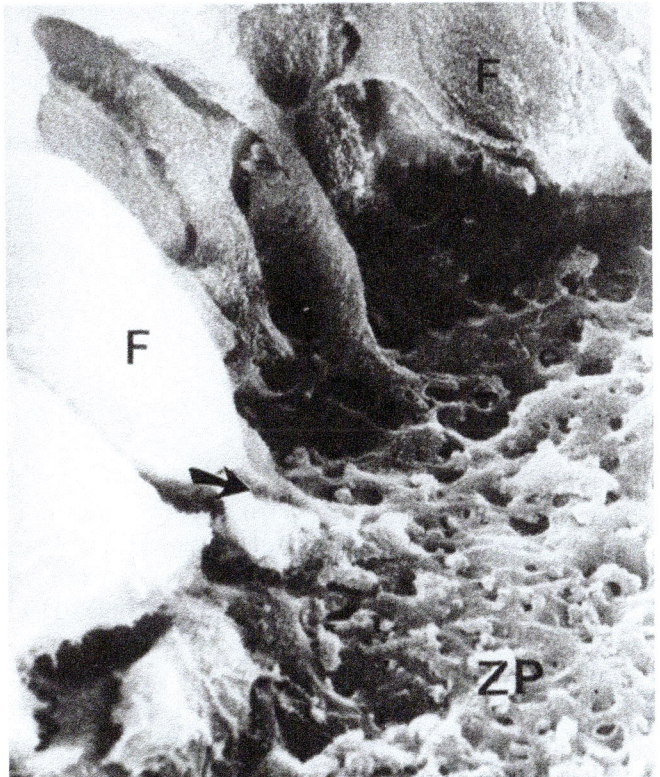

Fig. 2.13 Scanning electron micrograph of mouse ovary (5800 × 1.9). *F* Follicular cells of the radiata corona, the arrows indicate the cytoplasmic prolongations of follicular cells in relationship with the zona pellucida

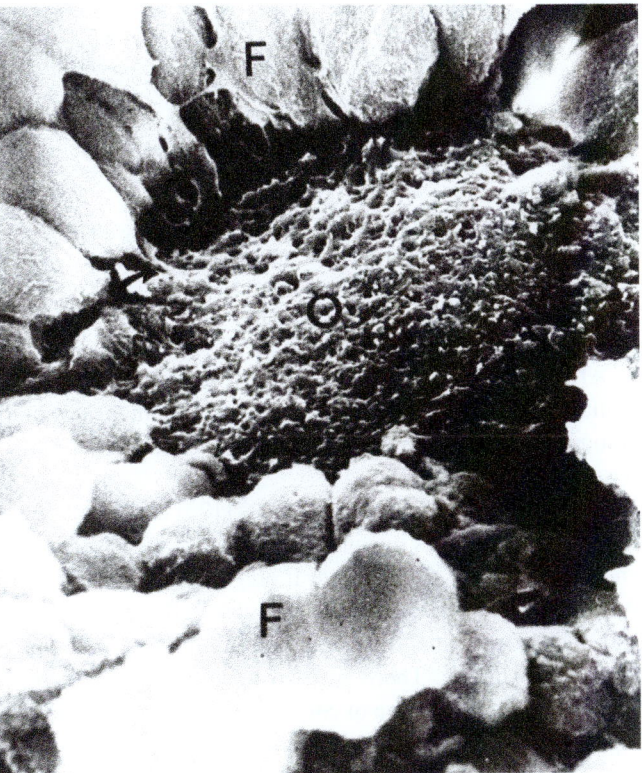

Fig. 2.14 Scanning electron micrograph of mouse ovary (2050 × 1.9). *O* oocyte, *F* follicular cells of the radiata crown. The arrows indicate cytoplasmic prolongations of follicular cells in relation to the zona pellucida

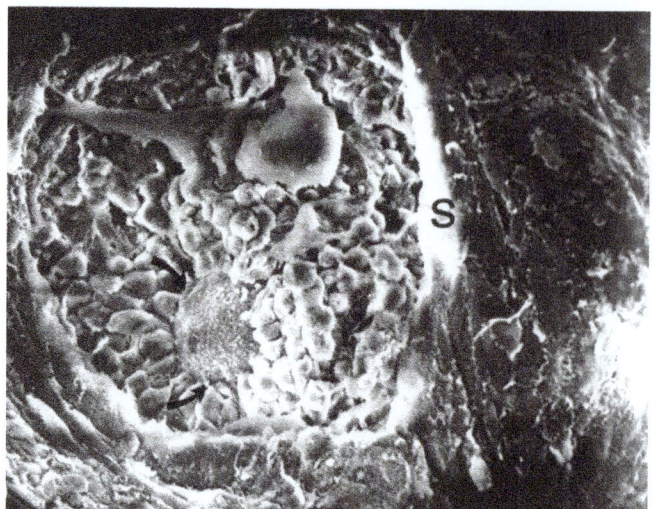

Fig. 2.15 Scanning electron micrograph of mouse ovary (830 × 1.9) Growing follicle *S* ovary surface, within the follicle is observed an oocyte surrounded by cumulus oophorus

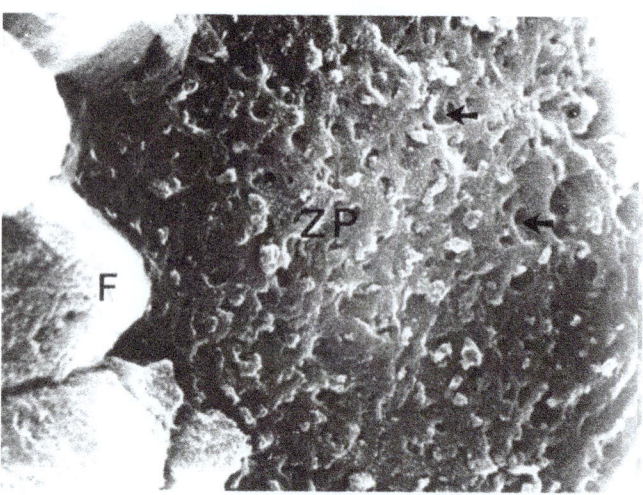

Fig. 2.16 Scanning electron micrograph of mouse ovary (5800 × 1.9). Growing follicle strong enlargement of an oocyte surrounded by follicular cells rounded by cumulus oophorus

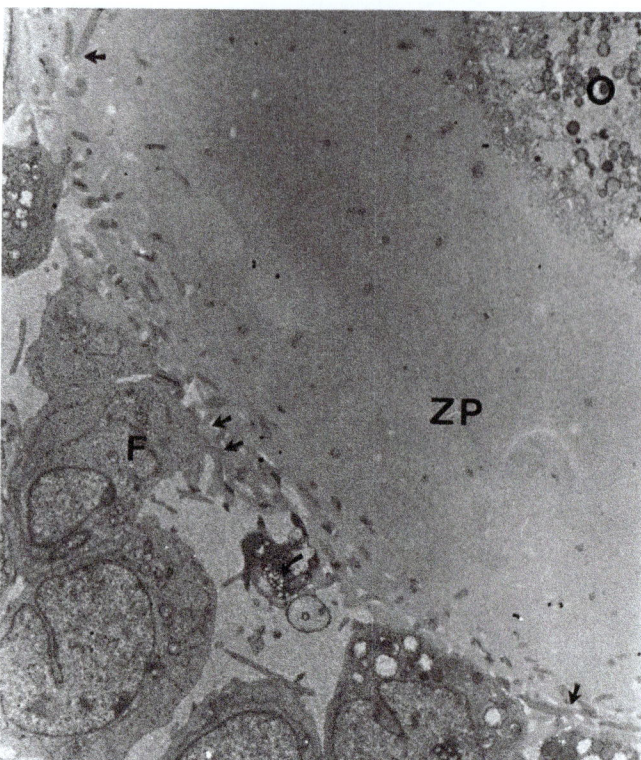

Fig. 2.17 Electronic microphotography with mouse ovary transmission. Cumulus oophorus, *F* follicular cells, *Zp* Pellucida zona, *O* oocyte. The arrows indicate the invagination of follicular cells in relation to the zona pellucida

which is development of capillaries from pre-existing blood vessels in such a way that each cell of corpus luteum is in direct contact with several capillaries giving corpus luteum one of the highest blood rates in the organism.

It is important to preserve the existing pregnancy until placenta is fully developed. In case that pregnancy does not happen, corpus luteum stops with progesterone production and luteal cells die through apoptosis, tissue disintegrates, and changes result in a gland formed of connective tissue called corpus albicans.

2.2 Relevance of Hormones

As previously stated, the ovary is comprised of several cell types (germ and somatic cells) and undergoes dramatic changes in structure during menstrual cycle. Every step of folliculogenesis is controlled by hormones through hypothalamic-pituitary-ovarian axis. Elder and Dale (2011) [24] describe the endocrine control of reproduction that starts in hypothalamus with secretion of gonadotropin-releasing hormone (GnRH) in pulses which stimulates anterior pituitary gland that in turn secretes luteinizing hormone (LH) and follicle-stimulating hor-

After ovulation and exit of a mature oocyte, residual follicular cells form the corpus luteum with a main task of high amounts of progesterone production in order to support a possible pregnancy [22].

In their chapter, Stocco et al. (2007) [23] explained structural origin of corpus luteum, its function in menstrual cycle and fate in case of pregnancy or if pregnancy did not happen. After LH induced ovulation, follicular cells stop dividing and undergo terminal differentiation to luteal cells that produce progesterone. There are two more structural changes that lead to the formation of corpus luteum—tissue remodeling that includes changes in extracellular matrix composition that supports basic cellular processes and vascularization

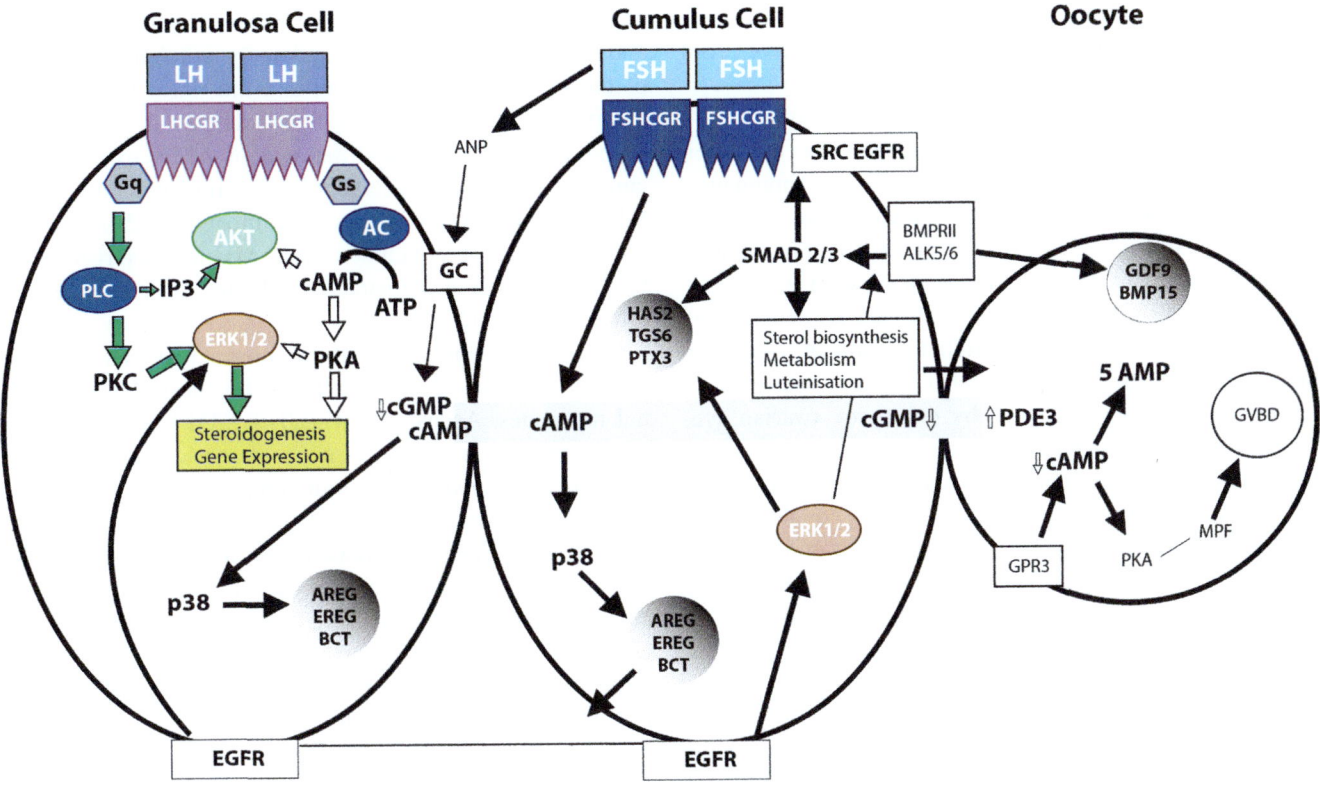

Fig. 2.18 Possible interactions between an oocyte and follicle

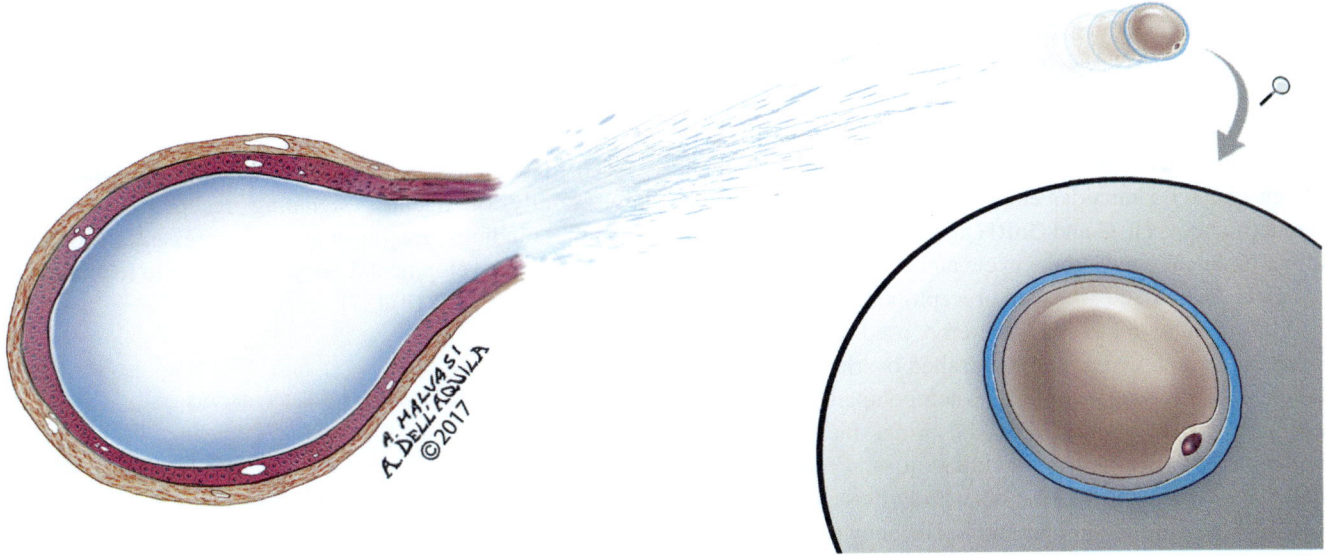

Fig. 2.19 Expulsion of the oocyte from the follicle

mone (FSH). FSH stimulates the growth of follicles, production of granulosa cells, and appearance of LH receptors on granulosa cells. Levels of estrogen produced by granulosa cells rise until threshold is achieved that elicits LH surge which is a trigger for ovulation. It is important to note that low levels of estrogen cause a negative feedback on FSH and LH secretion and high levels of estrogen give

a positive feedback. High levels of progesterone support negative feedback from estrogens and keep FSH and LH levels low. Woodruff and Shea (2011) [25] hypothesized that follicle activation is dependent of physical environment in addition to hormonal pathways. They claimed that the more rigid ovarian cortex the harder the follicle growth and that biochemical environment modulates follicular response to hormones. They found supporting evidence but new tools need to be developed in order to give proof to this theory.

Drummond (2006) [26] reviews the role of steroids in follicular growth. Progesterone regulates granulosa cells, follicle rupture and supports embryo implantation and pregnancy. Androgens appear to promote folliculogenesis in early stages, they enhance FSH-mediated differentiation of granulosa cells and play roles in oocyte maturation and Lebbe et al. (2017) [27] conclude that androgen homeostasis in developing antral and preantral follicle is crucial for growth and oocyte maturation, findings that are very important in treating fertility issues caused by polycystic ovarian syndrome (PCOS). Estrogen promotes follicle growth, facilitating granulosa cells differentiation and induces receptors for FSH and LH. Kolibianakis et al. (2005) [28] concluded that the main role of estrogen in folliculogenesis is enhancement through estrogen receptor b and it appears to regulate cyclic gonadotropin release in occulation process. However, it doesn't seem to have an impact on oocyte quality and developmental potential.

Mechanism for LH surge is very complex and timing is crucial in order to achieve a fully matured and grown oocyte ready for fertilization. Oocytes are dormant in prophase 1 and need to complete first meiotic division in order to be mature for fertilization, they don't have LH receptors so LH surge acts through alternating pathways. Kawamura et al. (2011) [29] have shown a limited number of ligands that are induced by the LH surge to promote germinal vesicle breakdown and resumption of meiosis.

It is interesting to analyze the effect of ovulation triggering in controlled ovarian hyperstimulation protocols. In their review chapter, Humaidan et al. (2012) [30] describe the differences in beta HCG and GnRH agonist triggering and their effect on luteal phase of the cycle and endometrial receptivity. Beta HCG shares the same receptors as LH owing it to similar structure to LH and is therefore used as a trigger ovulation in women undergoing controlled ovarian hyperstimulation. It has a longer half-life when compared to LH and causes multiple corpora lutea and brings the patient to a higher risk of ovarian hyperstimulation syndrome, a potentially dangerous state for a patient with serious consequences. GnRH triggering as an alternative has shown a significant reduction and sometimes complete elimination of OHSS symptoms.

Anti-Müllerian hormone (AMH) is produced by developing oocytes and granulosa cells, it exerts a negative inhibitory effect on primordial follicles transitioning to primary follicles, and it is an indirect marker for ovarian reserve [31]. De Vet et al. (2002) [32] monitored AMH serum levels and concluded that its concentrations declined over time and it correlates with antral follicle count and age and that it is a good marker for ovarian reserve. Weenen et al. (2004) [33]

confirmed the role of AMH in initial and cyclic recruitment and suggest that AMH may regulate the efficiency of the use of the primordial follicle pool and thus have a role in the determination of menopause. Grondahl et al. (2011) [34] found that there was a difference of AMH expressed in cumulus and granulosa cells of large antral and preovulatory follicles and cumulus cells had significantly higher levels of AMH. They have concluded that AMH may exert intrafollicular functions in preovulatory follicles and can be related to follicular health.

There are some external hormones that can have an effect on estrous cycle and folliculogenesis besides sexual hormones. Asensio et al. (2018) [35] have found that allopregnanolone, which is a neurosteroid, effects sexual behavior and anxiety and can have an effect on estrous cycle by interfering with regression of corpus luteum prolonging its existence, decreasing the number of developing follicles. Since ovaries have receptors for cortisol, they are susceptible to its effects. There is evidence for free cortisol accumulation in preovulatory follicle and that cortisol may reduce inflammatory reactions after ovulation and that corpus luteum benefits from it too [36].

2.3 Growth Factors Influencing Ovarian Follicles

Even though folliculogenesis is controlled by hypothalamic-pituitary-ovarian axis, there are new findings that show significant influence of several growth factors and signaling pathways (Table 2.3).

TGF-β (tumor growth factor β) superfamily represent a large family of ligands, signaling receptors, and non-signaling binding proteins that are expressed by ovarian somatic cells developmental oocytes in order to regulate folliculogenesis (Fig. 2.18) [37].

Table 2.3 Follicle development regulatory factors

Regulatory factor	Cellular source	Cellular site of action
Tumor necrosis factor-alpha	Oocyte	Oocyte
Basic fibroblast growth factor	Oocyte	Granulosa, theca, stroma
Kit ligand	Granulosa	Oocyte, theca, stroma
Leukemia inhibitory factor	Granulosa	Oocyte, granulosa
Keratinocyte growth factor	Theca	Granulosa
Bone morphogenic protein-4	Theca/stroma	Granulosa
Bone morphogenic protein-7	Stroma	Granulosa
Insulin	Endocrine	Oocyte
Progesterone	Endocrine	Oocyte
Müllerian inhibitory substance	Antral follicle	Primordial follicle

Richards and Pangas (2010) [38] discuss clinical evidence of various powerful ovarian regulators that include FSH signaling pathways, for example.

In the early stages of folliculogenesis, FSH promotes growth of granulosa cells by activating adenylyl cyclase leading to production of cAMP and activating protein kinase A, but it also activates pathways that do not include cAMP. In the later stages of folliculogenesis, estradiol enhances the FSH actions through suppression of phosphodiesterase 1C, which increases levels on intracellular cAMP induced by FSH. High levels of intracellular cAMP keep the oocyte meiotically arrested by suppressing maturation-promoting factor [39].

FSH also works in synergy with insulin-like growth factor-1 (IGF-1) to stimulate steroidogenesis in granulosa cells [40]. Insulin and IGF have an important role in folliculogenesis and steroidogenesis, they are linked to adiponectin—adipokine that is involved in insulin resistance in patient with polycystic ovarian syndrome and research has shown that it decreases steroidogenesis in theca cells [41]. There are also findings that the reduction of IGF bioavailability results in atresia of follicles not selected in the cohort for dominance [42].

The assembly of primordial follicles early in prenatal development and their transition to primary oocytes is crucial as it sets the number of available oocytes in a woman's adult age.

There are multiple types of growth factors that are involved in transition of primordial follicles to primary ones. Kit ligand stimulates theca cell growth and androgen production; basic fibroblast growth factor acts on ovarian somatic cells to influence primordial follicle development; keratinocyte growth factor is produced in precursor theca cells adjacent to developing granulosa cells and promotes primordial follicle development, and AMH represents the only known negative regulatory factor for primordial follicle development [43]. Besides having a negative effect on primordial follicles, AMH inhibits FSH-dependent cycle recruitment and plays a role throughout gonadotropin-independent follicle growth [44]. Kit ligand plays an important role not only in early stages of follicular development but in oocyte survival and growth, theca cell recruitment and maintenance of meiotic arrest [45]. Primordial follicles need to be dormant in order to give a reserve of oocytes for a normal length of female reproductive life. Intraoocyte signaling molecules that maintain primordial follicle dormancy are PTEN tumor suppressor and Tsc tumor suppressor and they appear to work in synergistic manner [46].

The oocyte secretes several types of growth factors that are key and that if in absence (e.g., growth differentiation factor 9—GDF-9) folliculogenesis is blocked at primary preantral stage [47]. GDF-9 is expressed abundantly in primary follicles and is not expressed in small primary follicles but in

late ones [48]. Pangas et al. (2002) [49] have also found activine, member of TGF-β family, activated in some stages of folliculogenesis. Global analysis of gene expression of oocytes in early folliculogenesis identified the appearance of 6301 unique genes, GDF-9 was expressed in small quantities which is consistent with other findings [50]. GDF-9 with BMP-6 and BMP-15 (bone morphogenic factor 6 and 15) works within antral follicles to prevent premature luteinization while supporting follicular growth [51]. Research has also shown that oocytes communicate with granulosa cells through paracrine-activating factors and share small molecules with the help of gap junctions; these two ways regulate oocyte growth and granulosa cell proliferation [52]. Kidder and Mhawi (2002) [53] described the role of gap junctions in folliculogenesis and stated that gap junctions that connect the oocyte with granulosa cells contain predominantly connexin 43 and that loss of connexin negatively affects development of antral follicles.

In context of ovulation, LH surge stops the FSH-dependent steroidogenesis and promotes differentiation of somatic cells to luteal cells, it induces multiple signaling cascades that lead to oocyte maturation and ovulation that include inositol phosphate signaling, regulates protein kinase 3, regulates cGMP levels in the follicle and activates epidermal growth factor signaling [54]. Epidermal growth factor network downregulates cGMP, and it provides meiotic inducing signals [55]. LH surge also induces EGF-like factors in granulosa cells like amphiregulin, beta-cellulin, and epiregulin through protein kinase A that bind to granulosa and cumulus cells and lead to ovulation. Zamah et al. (2010) [56] examined the relationship of LH and amphiregulin in gonadotropin-stimulated cycles. Their findings support the role of amphiregulin as intrafollicular signal and may have a role in healing ovarian surface tissue after ovulation. It is possible to compare ovulation and inflammation since there is a rupture of ovarian tissue on the site of ovulation, and besides amphiregulin, research has shown that granulosa cells produce granulocyte-colony-stimulating factor that induces leukocyte accumulation in follicular wall and after the LH surge, they produce proteolytic enzymes that are a major factor in the rupture of follicle [57].

After follicular rupture, granulosa cells become luteal cells and express a high amount of vascular endothelial growth factor (VEGF) which is involved in angiogenesis that is happening in the formation of corpus luteum [58].

2.4 Applications in Assisted Reproduction Techniques (ART)

Understanding of follicular growth and factors affecting it plays an incredibly important role in determining the right stimulation protocol for women undergoing ART treatments.

The development of more than one waves of folliculogenesis influenced new ART regiments [59]. Analysis of genes expressed in cumulus cells, especially gene GREM1 could accurately predict maturity and fertilization potential of oocytes collected and embryo quality [60]. Also, research has shown that FSH receptor genotype has a direct association to menstrual cycle dynamics and influences its length [61], a fact that is important to clinicians in ART. Polycystic ovarian syndrome (PCOS) is a common endocrine and metabolic disorder that causes fertility problems and includes multiple symptoms that cause anovulatory cycles, higher levels of androgens and increased body weight. Factors characterizing PCOS can be extraovarian-like FSH deficiency, hypersecretion of LH, hyperandrogenemia, and hyperinsulinemia [62]. Intraovarian factors include multitude of growth factors and cytokines described in the previous section and together with extraovarian factors make a complex problem that often brings a patient to ART procedures in order to conceive a baby.

All the accessible knowledge on ovarian function, folliculogenesis and growth factors applies in oncofertility patients. Women that went through chemotherapy have smaller chances of conceiving and sometimes it is impossible to do hormonal stimulation in attempt to collect oocytes in order to cryopreserve them since some tumors are influenced by hormones. Cryopreservation of ovarian tissue and later transplanting it back to the same patient after successful cancer treatment resulted in 20% cases leading to childbirth [63]. Freezing of ovarian tissue does not appear to have a significant impact on early stages of folliculogenesis [64]. Xiao et al. (2015) [65] have even managed to produce meiotically competent and mature oocytes after in vitro maturation and in vitro follicular growth by applying two-step follicle culture strategy, and this treatment can prevent adverse effects of hormone therapy on cancer patients. Aziz et al. (2017) [66] were also able to successfully culture a single human preantral follicle encapsulating it in a microfluidic chip with the usage of calcium alginate microbeads. Collagen hydrogel proved to be a good substrate for in vitro growth of ovarian follicles [67].

Xenografting human ovarian tissue in mice has been proven as a good technique for research of follicle development in vivo and has produced mature human follicles with mature MII oocytes, and it can be a technique used in restoring fertility but still has a lot of ethical issues [68]. Kim et al. (2002) [69] have also shown that after xenotransplantation of human ovarian tissue on host animal, human ovarian follicle can be matured to ovulation and later form corpus luteum.

Isolation of ovarian stem cells and later intraovarian transplantation has generated functional oocytes in a mouse that were successfully fertilized and gave a hatching blastocyst (Fig. 2.20) [70].

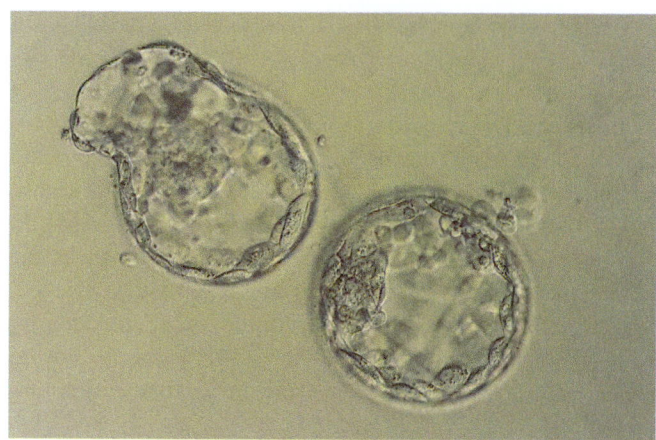

Fig. 2.20 Hatching blastocyst on day 5 of development (on the left) (author: Marija Dundović)

This method may be the right treatment for women of reproductive age that are cancer survivors and plan on having children since this may be an elegant way of restoring ovarian functions without removing parts of reproductive system.

References

1. Sadler TW. Langman's medical embryology. 12th ed. Wolters Kluwer, Lippincott Williams & Wilkins, printed in China; 2011. 384 pp.
2. Vaskivuo TE, Anttonen M, Herva R, Billig H, Dorland M, Velde ER, Stenback F, Heikinheimo M, Tapanainen JS. Survival of human ovarian follicles from fetal to adult life: apoptosis, apoptosis-related proteins, and transcription factor GATA-4. J Clin Endocrinol Metabol. 2001;86(7):3421–9.
3. Coward K, Wells D. Textbook of clinical embryology. Cambridge: Cambridge University Press; 2013. 391 pp.
4. Dumesic DA, Meldrum DR, Katz-Jaffe MG, Krishner RL, Schoolcraft WB. Oocyte environment: follicular fluid and cumulus cells are critical for oocyte health. Fertil Steril. 2015;103(2):303–16.
5. Erickson GF. Glob Libr Women's Med. Follicle growth and development. (ISSN: 1756-2228) 2008. https://doi.org/10.3843/GLOWM.10289.
6. Atwood CS, Meethal SV. The spatiotemporal hormonal orchestration of human folliculogenesis, early embryogenesis and blastocyst implantation. Mol Cell Endocrinol. 2016;430:33–48. https://doi.org/10.1016/j.mce.2016.03.039.
7. Gougeon A. Human ovarian follicular development: from activation of resting follicles to preovulatory maturation. Ann Endocrinol. 2010;71:132–43.
8. Young JM, McNeilly AS. Theca: the forgotten cell of the ovarian follicle. Reproduction. 2010;140:489–504.
9. McGee EA, Hsueh AJW. Initial and cyclic recruitment of ovarian follicles. Endocr Rev. 2000;21(2):200–14.
10. Chang JR, Gougeon A, Erickson GF. Evidence for a neutrophil–interleukin-8 system in human folliculogenesis. Am J Obstet Gynecol. 1998;178(4):650–7.
11. Matsuda F, Inoue N, Manabe N, Ohkura S. Follicular growth and atresia in mammalian ovaries: regulation by survival and death of granulosa cells. J Reprod Dev. 2012;50(1):44–50.

12. Huang Z, Wells D. The human oocyte and cumulus cells relationship: new insights from the cumulus cell transcriptome. Mol Hum Reprod. 2010;16(10):715–25.

13. Rodgers RJ, Irvine-Rodgers HF. Formation of the ovarian follicular antrum and follicular fluid. Biol Reprod. 2010;82:1021–9.

14. Ambekar AS, Nirujogi RS, Srikants SM, Chavan S, Kelkar DS, Hinduja I, Zaveri K, Keshava Prasad TS, Harsha HC, Pandey A, Mukherjee S. Proteomic analysis of human follicular fluid: a new perspective towards understanding folliculogenesis. J Proteome. 2013;87:68–77.

15. Jozwik M, Jozwik M, Teng C, Battaglia C. Amino acid, ammonia and urea concentrations in human pre-ovulatory ovarian follicular fluid. Hum Reprod. 2006;21(11):2776–82.

16. Tamura H, Taksaki A, Taketami T, Tanabe M, Kizuka F, Lee L, Tamura I, Maekawa R, Asada H, Yamagata Y, Sugino N. Melatonin as a free radical scavenger in the ovarian follicle. Endocr J. 2013;60(1):1–13.

17. Makabe S, Naguro T, Stallone T. Oocyte–follicle cell interactions during ovarian follicle development, as seen by high resolution scanning and transmission electron microscopy in humans. Microsc Res Tech. 2006;69:436–49.

18. Baerwald AR, Adams GP, Pierson RA. A new model for ovarian follicular development during the human menstrual cycle. Fertil Steril. 2003;80(1):116–22.

19. Baerwald AR, Adams GP, Pierson RA. Ovarian antral folliculogenesis during the human menstrual cycle: a review. Hum Reprod Update. 2012;18(1):73–91.

20. Fukuda M, Fukuda K, Andersen KY, Byskov AG. Characteristics of human ovulation in natural cycles correlated with age and achievement of pregnancy. Hum Reprod. 2001;16(12):2501–7.

21. Al-Alem L, Puttabyatappa M, Rosewell K, Brannstrom M, Akin J, Boldt J, Muse K, Curry TE. Chemokine ligand 20: a signal for leukocyte recruitment during human ovulation? Endocrinology. 2015;156(9):3358–69.

22. Niswender GD, Juengel JL, Silva PJ, Rollyson MK, McIntush EW. Mechanisms controlling the function and life span of the corpus luteum. Physiol Rev. 2000;80(1):1–29.

23. Stocco C, Telelria C, Gibori G. The molecular control of corpus luteum formation, function and regression. Endocr Rev. 2007;28(1):117–49.

24. Elder K, Dale B. In-vitro fertilization. 3rd ed. Cambridge: Cambridge University Press; 2011. 277 pp.

25. Woodruff TK, Shea LD. A new hypothesis regarding ovarian follicle development: ovarian rigidity as a regulator of selection and health. J Assist Reprod Genet. 2011;28:3–6.

26. Drummond A. The role of steroids in follicular growth. Reprod Biol Endocrinol. 2006;4:16.

27. Lebbe M, Taylor AE, Visser JA, Kirkman-Brown JC, Woodruff TK, Arlt W. The steroid metabolome in the isolated ovarian follicle and its response to androgen exposure and antagonism. Endocrinology. 2017;158(5):1474–85.

28. Kolibianakis EM, Papanikolaou EG, Fatemi HM, Devroey P. Estrogen and folliculogenesis: is one necessary for the other? Curr Opin Obstet Gynecol. 2005;17:249–53.

29. Kawamura K, Cheng Y, Kawamura N, Takae S, Okada A, Kawagoe Y, Mulders S, Terada Y, Hsueh AJW. Pre-ovulatory LH/hCG surge decreases C-type natriuretic peptide secretion by ovarian granulosa cells to promote meiotic resumption of pre-ovulatory oocytes. Hum Reprod. 2011;26(11):3094–101.

30. Humaidan P, Papanikolau EG, Kyrou D, Alsbjerg B, Polyzos NP, Devroey P, Fatemi HM. The luteal phase after GnRH-agonist triggering of ovulation: present and future perspectives. Reprod Biomed Online. 2012;24:134–41.

31. Wallace WHB, Kelsey TW. Human ovarian reserve from conception to menopause. PLoS One. 2010;5(1):e8772.

32. De Vet A, Laven JSE, de Jong FH, Themmen APN, Fauser BCJM. Antimullerian hormone serum levels: a putative marker for ovarian aging. Fertil Steril. 2002;77(2):357–62.

33. Weenen C, Laven JSE, von Bergh ARM, Cranfield M, Groome NP, Visser JA, Kramer P, Fauser BCJM, Themmen APN. Anti-Mullerian hormone expression pattern in the human ovary: potential implications for initial and cyclic follicle recruitment. Mol Hum Reprod. 2004;10(2):77–83.

34. Grondahl ML, Nielsen ME, Dal Canto MB, Fadini R, Rasmussen IA, Westergaard LG, Kristensen SG, Andersen CY. Anti-Mullerian hormone remains highly expressed in human cumulus cells during the final stages of folliculogenesis. Reprod Biomed Online. 2011;22:389–98.

35. Asensio JA, Cacares ARR, Pelegrina LT, Sanhuenza MA, Scotti L, Parborelli F, Laconi MR. Allopregnanolone alters follicular and luteal dynamics during the estrous cycle. Reprod Biol Endocrinol. 2018;16:35.

36. Andersen CY. Possible new mechanism of cortisol action in female reproductive organs: physiological implications of the free hormone hypothesis. J Endocrinol. 2002;173:211–7.

37. Knight PG, Glister C. TGF-b superfamily members and ovarian follicle development. Reproduction. 2006;132:191–206.

38. Richards AJ, Pangas SA. The ovary: basic biology and clinical implications. J Clin Invest. 2010;120(4):963–72.

39. Gilchrist RB. Recent insights into oocyte—follicle cell interactions provide opportunities for the development of new approaches to in vitro maturation. Reprod Fertil Dev. 2011;23:23–31.

40. Giudice LS, Milki AA, Milkowski DA, Danasouri I. Human granulosa contain messenger ribonucleic acids encoding insulin-like growth factor-binding proteins (IGFBPs) and secrete IGFBPs in culture. Fertil Steril. 1991;56(3):475–80.

41. Lagaly DV, Aad PY, Grado-Ahuir AJ, Hulsey LB, Spicer LJ. Role of adiponectin in regulating ovarian theca and granulosa cell function. Mol Cell Endocrinol. 2008;284:38–45.

42. Guidice LC. Insulin like growth factor family in Graafian follicle development and function. J Soc Gynecol Investig. 2001;8(1):26–9.

43. Skinner M. Regulation of primordial follicle assembly and development. Hum Reprod Update. 2005;11(5):461–71.

44. Dewailly D, Robin G, Peigne M, Decanter C, Pigny P, Catteau-Jonard S. Interactions between androgens, FSH, anti-Mullerian hormone and estradiol during folliculogenesis in the human normal and polycystic ovary. Hum Reprod Update. 2016;22(6):709–24.

45. Hutt KJ, McLaughlin EA, Holland MK. Kit ligand and c-Kit have diverse roles during mammalian oogenesis and folliculogenesis. Mol Hum Reprod. 2006;12(2):61–9.

46. Reddy P, Zheng W, Liu K. Mechanisms maintaining the dormancy and survival of mammalian primordial follicles. Trends Endocrinol Metab. 2009;21(2):96–103.

47. Erickson GF, Shimasaki S. The physiology of folliculogenesis: the role of novel growth factors. Fertil Steril. 2001;76(5):943–9.

48. Aaltonen J, Laitinen MP, Vuojolainen K, Jaatinen R, Horelli-Kuitunen N, Seppa L, Louhio H, Tuuri T, Sjober J, Butzow R, Hovatta O, Dale L, Ritvos O. Human growth differentiation factor 9 (GDF-9) and its novel homolog GDF-9B are expressed in oocytes during early folliculogenesis. J Clin Endocrinol Metabol. 1999;84(9):2744–50.

49. Pangas SA, Rademaker AW, Fishman DA, Woodruff TK. Localization of the activin signal transduction components in normal human ovarian follicles: implications for autocrine and paracrine signaling in the ovary. J Clin Endocrinol Metabol. 2002;87(6):2644–57.

50. Markholt S, Grondahl ML, Ernst EH, Yding Andersen C, Ernst E, Lykke-Hartmann K. Global gene analysis of oocytes from early stages in human folliculogenesis shows high expression of novel genes in reproduction. Mol Hum Reprod. 2013;18(2):96–110.

51. Oktem O, Urman B. Understanding follicular growth in vivo. Hum Reprod. 2010;25(12):2944–54.
52. Kidder GM, Vanderhyden BC. Bidirectional communication between oocytes and follicle cells: ensuring oocyte developmental competence. Can J Physiol Pharmacol. 2010;88:399–413.
53. Kidder GM, Mhawi AA. Gap junctions and ovarian folliculogenesis. Reproduction. 2002;123:613–20.
54. Conti M, Hsieh M, Zamah AM, Oh JS. Novel signaling mechanisms in the ovary during oocyte maturation and ovulation. Mol Cell Endocrinol. 2012;356:65–73.
55. Richani D, Gilchrist RB. The epidermal growth factor network: role in oocyte growth, maturation and developmental competence. Hum Reprod Update. 2018;24(1):1–14.
56. Zamah AM, Hsieh M, Chen J, Vigne JL, Rosen MP, Cedars MI, Conti M. Human oocyte maturation is dependent on LH-stimulated accumulation of the epidermal growth factor-like growth factor, amphiregulin. Hum Reprod. 2010;25(10):2569–78.
57. Makinoda S, Waseda T, Tomizawa H, Fujii R. Granulocyte colony-stimulating factor (G-CSF) in the mechanism of human ovulation and its clinical usefulness. Curr Med Chem. 2008;15:604–13.
58. Yamamoto S, Konishi I, Tsuruta Y, Nanbu K, Mandai M, Kuroda H, Matsushita K, Hamis AA, Yura Y, Mori T. Expression of vascular endothelial growth factor (VEGF) during folliculogenesis and corpus luteum formation in the human ovary. Gynecol Endocrinol. 1997;11:371–81.
59. Yang DZ, Yang W, Li Y, He Z. Progress in understanding human ovarian folliculogenesis and its implications in assisted reproduction. J Assist Reprod Genet. 2013;30:213–9.
60. McKenzie LJ, Pangas SA, Carson SA, kovanci E, Cisneros P, Buster JE, Amato P, Matzuk MM. Human cumulus granulosa cell gene expression: a predictor of fertilization and embryo selection in women undergoing IVF. Hum Reprod. 2004;19(12):2869–74.
61. Greb RR, Grieshaber K, Gromoll J, Sonntag B, Nieschlag E, Kiesel L, Simoni M. A common single nucleotide polymorphism in exon 10 of the human follicle stimulating hormone receptor is a major determinant of length and hormonal dynamics of the menstrual cycle. J Clin Endocrinol Metab. 2005;90(8):4866–72.
62. Qiao J, Feng HL. Extra- and intraovarian factors in polycystic ovary syndrome: impact on oocyte maturation and embryo developmental competence. Hum Reprod Update. 2011;17(1):17–33.
63. Smitz J, Dolmans MM, Donnez J, Fortune JE, Hovatta O, Jewgenow K, Picton HM, Plancha C, Shea LD, Stouffer RL, Telfer EE, Woodruff TK, Zelinski MB. Current achievements and future research directions in ovarian tissue culture, in vitro follicle development and transplantation: implications for fertility preservation. Hum Reprod Update. 2010;16(4):395–414.
64. David A, Dolmans M, van Langendonckt A, Donnez J, Amorin CA. Immunohistochemical localization of growth factors after cryopreservation and 3 weeks' xenotransplantation of human ovarian tissue. Fertil Steril. 2011;95(4):1241–6.
65. Xiao S, Zhang J, Romero MM, Smith KN, Shea LD, Woodruff TK. In vitro follicle growth supports human oocyte meiotic maturation. Sci Rep. 2015;5:17323.
66. Aziz AUR, Fu M, Deng J, Geng C, Luo Y, Lin B, Yu X, Liu B. A microfluidic device for culturing an encapsulated ovarian follicle. Micromachines. 2017;8:335.
67. Joo S, Oh S, Sittadjody S, Opara EC, Jasckson JD, Lee SJ, Atala A. The effect of collagen hydrogel on 3D culture of ovarian follicles. Biomed Mater. 2016;11:065009.
68. Dittrich R, Lotz L, Fehm T, Krussel J, von Wolff M, Toth B, van der Ven H, Schuring AN, Wurfel W, Hoffmann I, Beckmann MQ. Xenotransplantation of cryopreserved human ovarian tissue—a systematic review of MII oocyte maturation and discussion of it as a realistic option for restoring fertility after cancer treatment. Fertil Steril. 2015;103(6):1557–65.
69. Kim SS, Soules MR, Battaglia DE. Follicular development, ovulation, and corpus luteum formation in cryopreserved human ovarian tissue after xenotransplantation. Fertil Steril. 2002;78(1):77–82.
70. Shea LD, Woodruff TK, Shikanov A. Bioengineering the ovarian follicle environment. Annu Rev Biomed Eng. 2014;16:29–32.

Normal Ultrasound Female Pelvic Anatomy

3

Vincenzo D'Addario, Asim Kurjak,
and Biserka Funduk-Kurjak

Contents

Ultrasound imaging has shown an extremely rapid evolution in the last two decades, thanks to the development of highly sophisticated both two-dimensional (2D) and three-dimensional (3D) technology and blood flow mapping, which render ultrasound the first-line imaging modality for the evaluation of the female pelvis.

The interpretation of the ultrasonographic findings requires knowledge of the uterine and ovarian ultrasound anatomy.

V. D'Addario (✉)
Department of Obstetrics and Gynecology, Medical School University of Bari, Bari, Italy

A. Kurjak
Department of Obstetrics and Gynecology, Medical School University of Zagreb, Zagreb, Croatia

International Academy of Perinatal Medicine, Zagreb, Croatia

Ian Donald Interuniversity School of Ultrasound in Medicine, Zagreb, Croatia

B. Funduk-Kurjak
Department of Obstetrics and Gynecology, Medical School University of Zagreb, Zagreb, Croatia

3.1 Examination Techniques

The ultrasound examination of the pelvis may be performed either with a transabdominal transducer or with a transvaginal high resolution transducer. The transvaginal approach is the best way of pelvic imaging since it offers the advantage of placing a high-frequency endocavitary ultrasound transducer in close proximity to target pelvic organs, thus improving image resolution and obviating the need for patients to have a full bladder before ultrasound examination (Figs. 3.1 and 3.2).

It has the additional advantage of probing pelvic organs to elicit patient's symptoms and thus correlating symptoms with specific pelvic anatomic locations. The practitioner therefore can gain crucial information by adding ultrasound findings with the physical examination [1].

3D technology offers additional advantages to the evaluation of the pelvic organs, such as multiplanar view, tomographic view, rendering view, and volume calculation [2, 3].

A further advantage is offered by the use of Color and Power Doppler technology which allows the examination of the vascular supply of the uterus and ovaries [4].

© Springer Nature Switzerland AG 2020
A. Malvasi, D. Baldini (eds.), *Pick Up and Oocyte Management*, https://doi.org/10.1007/978-3-030-28741-2_3

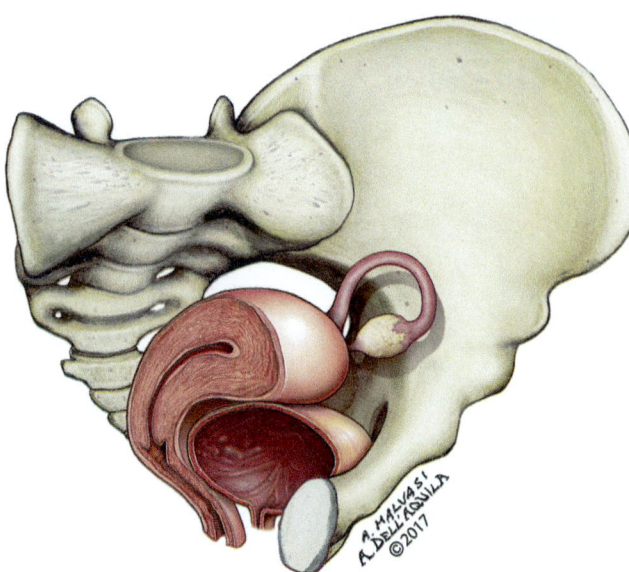

Fig. 3.1 Midsagittal plane of the pelvis

On a sagittal plane, the uterus has a pyriform shape: the superior two thirds correspond to the uterine body and the inferior third to the cervix. The uterine isthmus is identified where the uterine body and cervix meet.

The uterus may lie in the antiverted position (bent forward in relation to the vaginal axis) (Fig. 3.3) or in retroverted position (bent backward in relation to the vaginal axis).

The cervix has an oval conic shape and is approximately 2.5 cm in length. The cervical canal appears as an echogenic line; at the time of ovulation, a hypoechoic or echo-free strip may be seen in the cervical canal due to the fluid mucus production by the cervical glands (Fig. 3.3). Sometimes, cystic structures within the cervix are visualized: they refer to Nabothian cysts, retention cysts of the cervical glands within the vaginal portion of the cervix, which have no clinical value (Fig. 3.4).

The overall uterine length is evaluated in a sagittal view from the fundus to the cervix (to the external os, if it can be identified). When the uterus is markedly anteflexed (the corpus is strongly bent forward in relation to the cervical axis), the total length is obtained by adding the corporal and cervical length (Fig. 3.5). The depth of the uterus (anteroposterior dimension) is measured in the same sagittal view from its anterior to posterior walls, perpendicular to the length (Fig. 3.5). The maximum width is measured in the transverse view (Fig. 3.6).

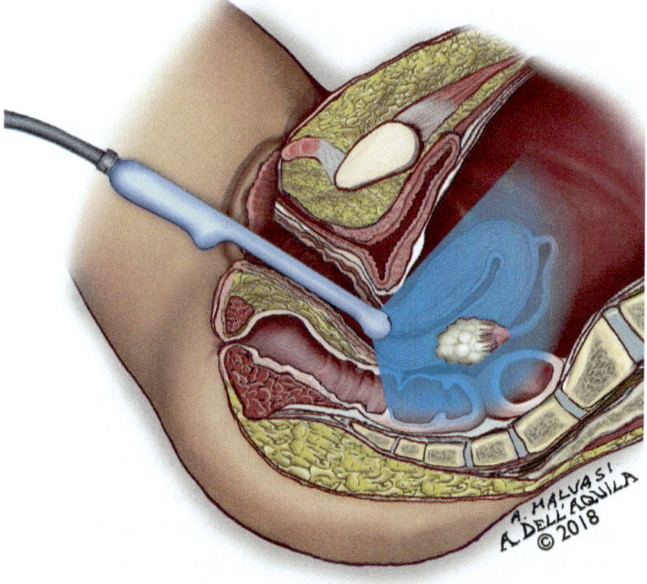

Fig. 3.2 Transvaginal ultrasound scans for the evaluation of the pelvis

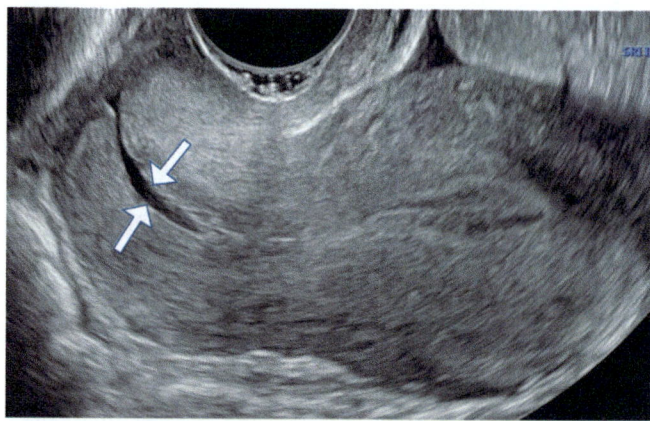

Fig. 3.3 Transvaginal scan of a normal antiverted uterus during the periovulatory phase: an echo-free strip (arrows) may be seen in the cervical canal due to the fluid mucus production by the cervical glands

3.2 Uterus

In examining the uterus, the following should be evaluated: (1) the uterine shape, orientation, and size; (2) the myometrium; (3) the endometrium and (4) the uterine perfusion.

3.2.1 Shape, Orientation, and Size

The uterus represents the essential landmark of pelvic anatomy. It is located in the middle of the pelvis between the urinary bladder lying before and the large bowel lying behind it.

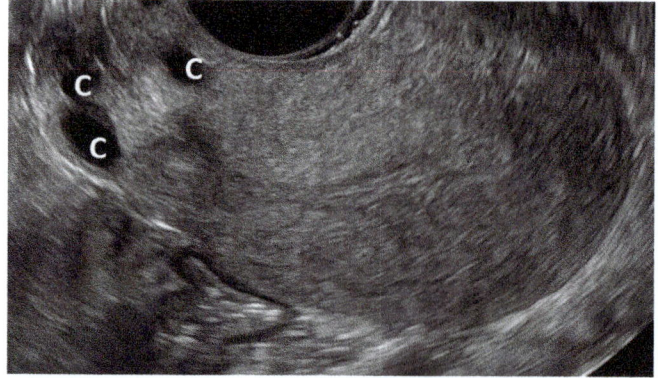

Fig. 3.4 Multiple Nabothian cysts within the cervix

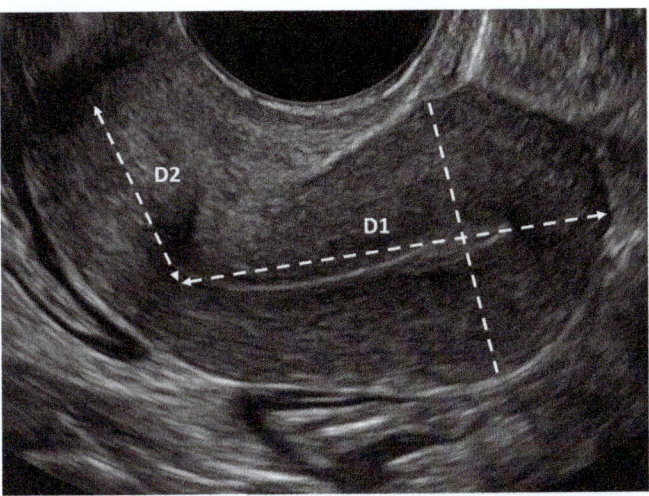

Fig. 3.5 Measurement of the uterine length in an antiflexed uterus, obtained by adding the lengths of the corpus (D1) and the cervix (D2). The depth of the uterus (anteroposterior dimension) is measured in the same sagittal view from its anterior to posterior walls, perpendicular to the longitudinal axis

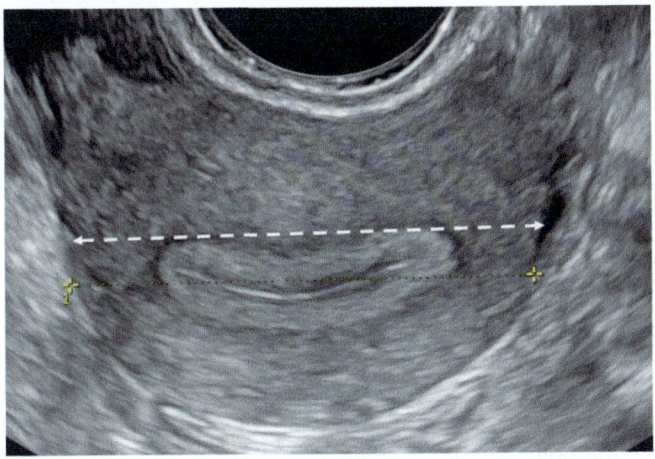

Fig. 3.6 Measurement of the uterine width in the transverse view

The uterine volume may be calculated by the formula of the ellipsoid prolate: Volume = length (cm) × anteroposterior diameter (cm) × transverse diameter (cm) × 0.523 or can be automatically measured by using the VOCAL (virtual organ computer-aided analysis) function offered by the 3D technology. This measurement, however, is not used routinely in the daily clinical setting. The size of the uterus changes according to age and parity. In the reproductive age, the normal uterus is 7.5–9 cm long, 3–4.5 cm deep, and 4.5–6 cm wide. The volume ranges from 50 to 70 cm³ [5].

3.2.2 Myometrium

The myometrium is the muscular part of the uterus, which is ultrasonically characterized by homogenicity and low echogenicity. The inner part of the myometrium confining with

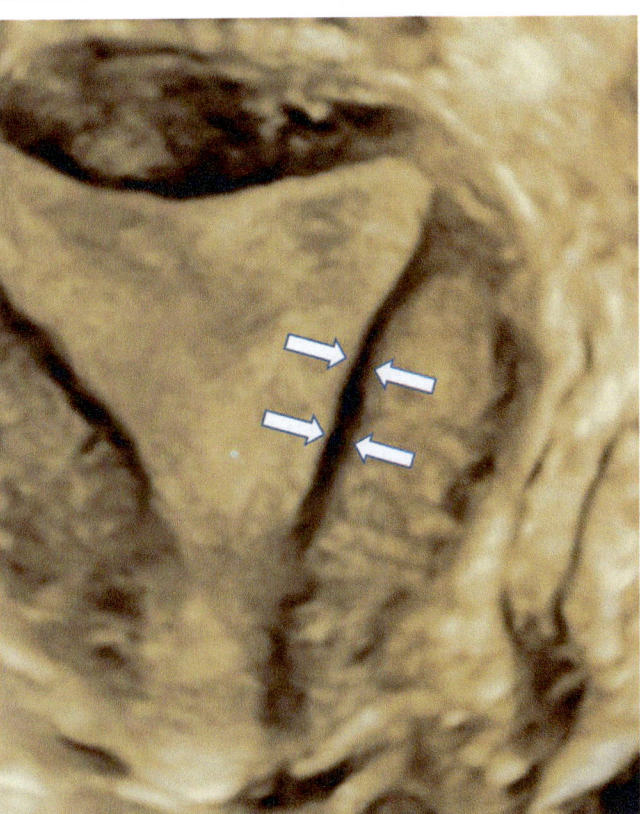

Fig. 3.7 Three-dimensional multiplanar view of the uterus: the Junctional Zone appears as a subendometrial halo in the inner part of the myometrium (arrows)

the endometrium is called Junctional Zone (JZ) or subendometrial halo. It is a thin area of lower echogenicity in comparison with the remaining myometrium. It represents a distinct compartment of the myometrium comprising tightly packed muscle cells with an increased vascularity. Such architecture would increase the density of this tissue layer, altering its acoustic impedance, and account for its echopenic appearance on ultrasound [6]. Although the ZJ may be recognized with the two-dimensional imaging, however the best evaluation is obtained by the three-dimensional multiplanar view, which allows the visualization of the sagittal, transverse, and coronal sections of the uterus [7] (Fig. 3.7).

3.2.3 Endometrium

The sonographic appearance of the endometrium in fertile patients changes with the different phases of the menstrual cycle. Menstruation is characterized by shedding of the functional layer of the endometrium, which is caused by hormonal deprivation and alteration in the spiral arteriolar system. Bleeding is the result of vasoconstriction of the spiral arteries and necrosis of their walls.

During the last menstrual phase, endometrial layers are very thin and ultrasonography shows a single-line with slightly irregular echogenic interphase.

At the beginning of the follicular phase, the endometrium appears as a single hyperechoic line since it is difficult to identify the borders between the two layers (Fig. 3.8).

As the ovulation approaches the endometrial glands increase in number and size and the endometrium shows the typical triple-line appearance. The external hyperechoic lines represent the endometrial-myometrial junction; the middle one is the interface between the two endometrial layers (Fig. 3.9). In the periovulatory phase, the endometrial thickness reaches approximately 12–13 mm (range 10–16) [8, 9]. During a normal menstrual cycle, spontaneous uterine contractions usually occur and can influence the measurement of endometrial thickness [10].

Secretory phase is characterized by progesterone secretion by the corpus luteum following ovulation. Glycoprotein secretion from endometrial glands is increased resulting in disappearance of the three lines present in the late proliferative phase. Sonographically, the endometrium appears as a

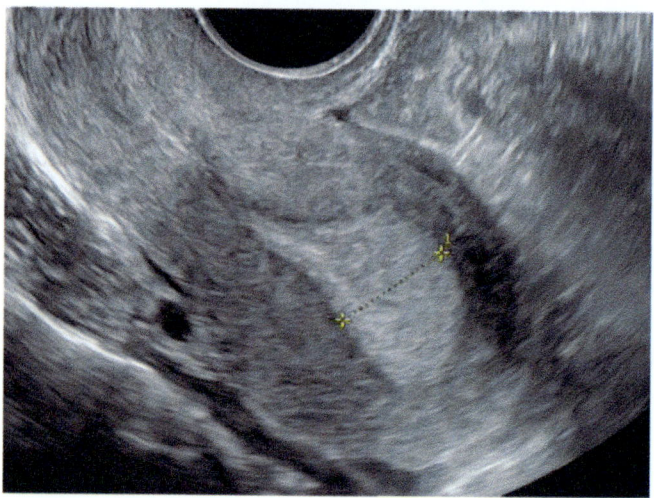

Fig. 3.10 Thickened and hyperechoic endometrium during the secretory phase of the cycle

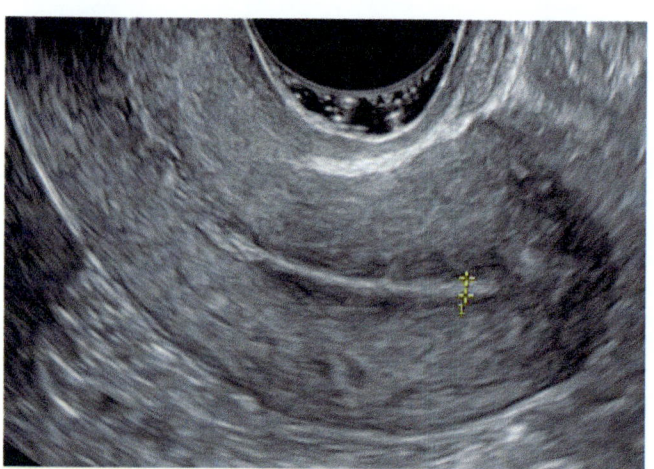

Fig. 3.8 Early proliferative endometrium appearing as a hyperechoic line

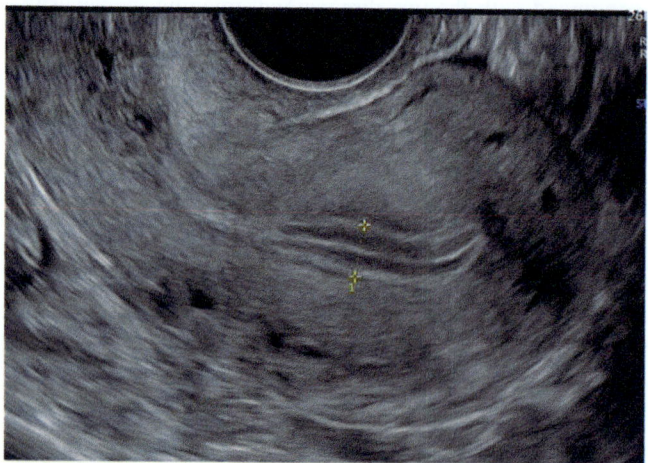

Fig. 3.9 Triple-line endometrium typical of the periovulatory phase

homogeneous and hyperechoic layer measuring 8–14 mm (Fig. 3.10); it has this appearance until the beginning of the menstrual bleeding or pregnancy. In the latter case, echogenicity and thickness are maintained as decidual reaction to implantation.

The hyperechogenic pattern of the endometrium during the secretory phase, acting as a natural contrast agent, is most suitable for determination of the shape of the uterine cavity and diagnosis of congenital uterine malformations [11, 12]. In this field, three-dimensional sonography plays a fundamental and irreplaceable role, thanks to the reconstruction of the coronal plane which allows to visualize the uterine cavity and surrounding myometrium and recognize Mullerian anomalies [13–15] with results comparable with those obtained with MRI [16]. In normal uterus, the endometrial cavity shows a typical triangular shape (Fig. 3.11); in arcuate uterus, the internal border of the fundus is curvilinear; in septate uterus, a complete or partial septum protrudes from the fundus into the uterine cavity; in hemi-uterus, a single small asymmetrical cavity is present; in bi-corporeal uterus, two uterine cavity and two distinct bodies are present (Fig. 3.12).

3.2.4 Uterine Perfusion

Color and Power Doppler allows the visualization of the blood supply to the uterus. This consists of uterine, arcuate, radial, basal, and spiral arteries.

Uterine arteries are branches of the internal iliac arteries and may be recognized running along the cervix and the isthmic part of the uterus (Fig. 3.13). Arcuate arteries create a wreath encircling the uterus and are best seen in the transverse section (Fig. 3.14). Radial arteries arise from the arcuate network and supply the myometrium. The radial arteries

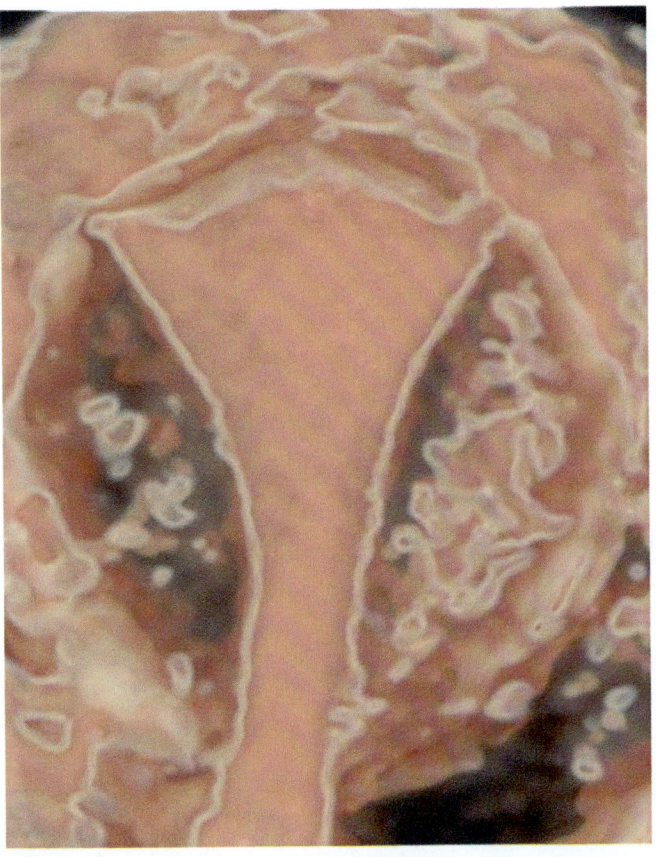

Fig. 3.11 3D multiplanar imaging of the uterus: the coronal view shows the triangular shape of the endometrial cavity

branch into basal and spiral arteries as they pass the myometrial-endometrial border (Fig. 3.15). The relatively short basal arteries terminate in a capillary bed that serves the stratum basalis of the endometrium. Spiral arteries terminate in a vast capillary network that supplies the functional stratum of the endometrium and undergo substantial anatomical changes during the menstrual cycle [17].

A good blood supply to the endometrium is usually considered as an essential requirement for implantation, and therefore assessment of endometrial blood flow in IVF treatment has attracted a lot of attention in recent years. Doppler study of uterine arteries does not reflect the actual blood flow to the endometrium. Endometrial and subendometrial blood flows can be more objectively and reliably measured with three-dimensional power Doppler ultrasound. However, conflicting results are reported with regard to their role in the prediction of pregnancy in IVF treatment [17–21].

3.3 Ovaries

The ovaries (Fig. 3.16) are small paired organ with a complex, constantly changing structure, which have a central role in reproduction being the source of oocytes and the main site of sex steroid hormone production. They continually change in size and activity through life, as an integral part of the changes that the female is going through before, during, and after her reproductive life.

In examining the ovaries, the following should be evaluated: (1) position, shape, and size; (2) changes during the ovarian cycle.

3.3.1 Position, Shape, and Size

Usually, the ovaries are found lateral from the uterus in the ovarian fossa, behind and inside the external iliac vessels (Fig. 3.17).

Sometimes, the ovaries are asymmetrical and mobile and change their position in relation with the degree of urinary bladder repletion, the distension of the bowel, and the presence of adhesions [22]. These fix the position of the ovaries, commonly close to the lateral fornices of the vagina, or posterior to the uterus.

The ovary has an ellipsoid shape with the long axis oriented downward and forward.

The measurements of the ovary are obtained after determining its long axis. Two distances (the length and the width) are measured in this view and a third one (the thickness) is obtained after rotating the transducers with 90°. The mean measurements of the ovary are 3 × 2 × 2 cm. The volume may be calculated by the formula of ellipsoid prolate: Volume (cm^3) = length (cm) × anteroposterior diameter (cm) × transverse diameter (cm) × 0.523 or can be automatically measured by using the VOCAL (virtual organ computer-aided analysis) function offered by the 3D technology. The volume of the ovary changes with female age and with the phase of the cycle. In reproductive age and in the early proliferative phase, the volume is between 6 and 10 cm^3 [23]. 3D volume automatic calculation is slightly more accurate than 2D calculation [24].

3.3.2 Changes During the Ovarian Cycle

The sonographic appearance of the ovary changes widely during the ovarian cycle in relation to the cycling processes of folliculogenesis, ovulation, and corpus luteum formation.

In the early follicular phase, the ovaries are imaged as homogeneous, hypoechogenic ovoid structures with slightly echogenic central part. The developing antral follicles, appearing as small cystic structures, facilitate the identification of the ovaries (Fig. 3.18). The number of antral follicles count (AFC) between day 2 and 4 of a spontaneous cycle is considered a reliable marker of ovarian reserve and good predictor of ovarian response to controlled ovarian stimulation in an ART program. The number of follicles with a

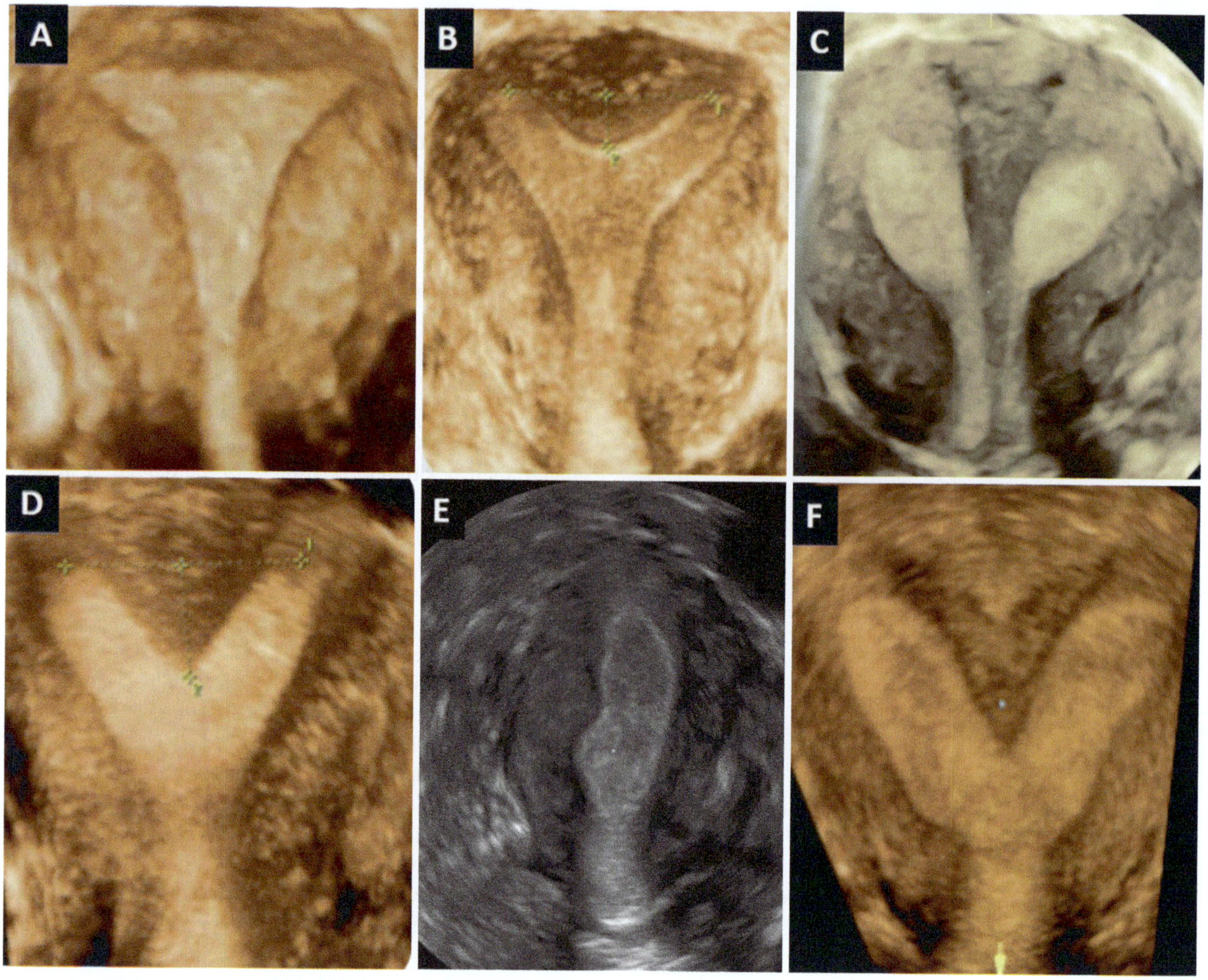

Fig. 3.12 Different shapes of the uterine cavity in case of Mullerian anomalies. (**a**) Normal uterus; (**b**) arcuate uterus: the internal border of the fundus is curvilinear; (**c**) complete septate uterus: the septum arrives at the cervix; (**d**) partial septate uterus: the septum protrudes partially into the uterine cavity; (**e**) hemi-uterus: a single small asymmetrical cavity is present; (**f**) bi-corporeal uterus: two uterine cavity and two distinct bodies are present

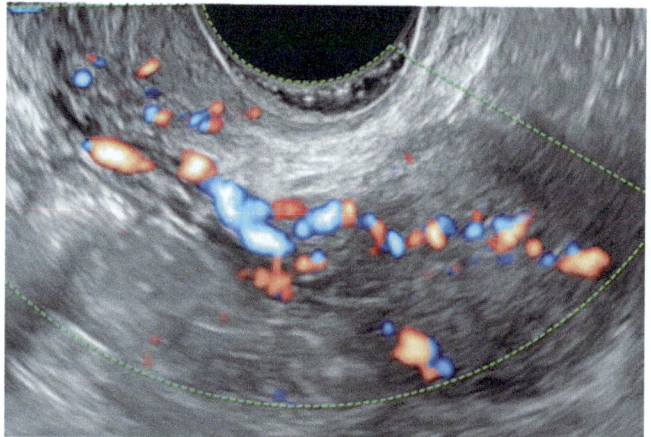

Fig. 3.13 Uterine artery running along the cervix and the isthmic part of the uterus

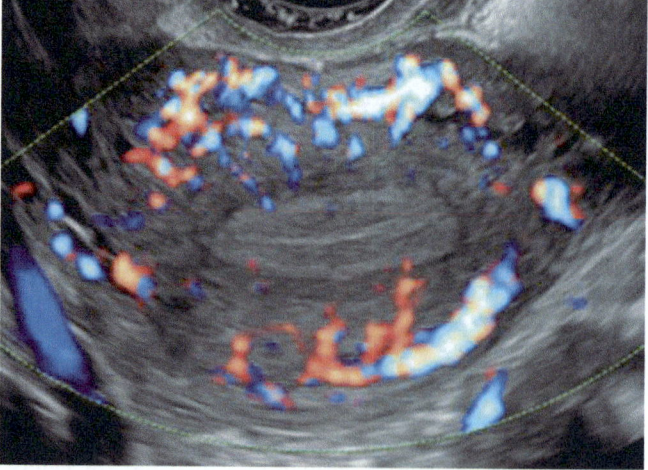

Fig. 3.14 Transverse section of the uterus showing the vascular wreath produced by the arcuate arteries

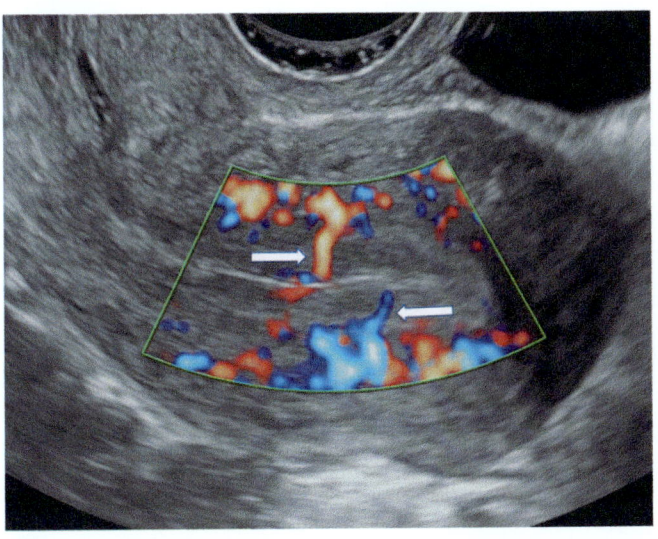

Fig. 3.15 Basal and spiral arteries (arrows) passing the myometrial-endometrial border

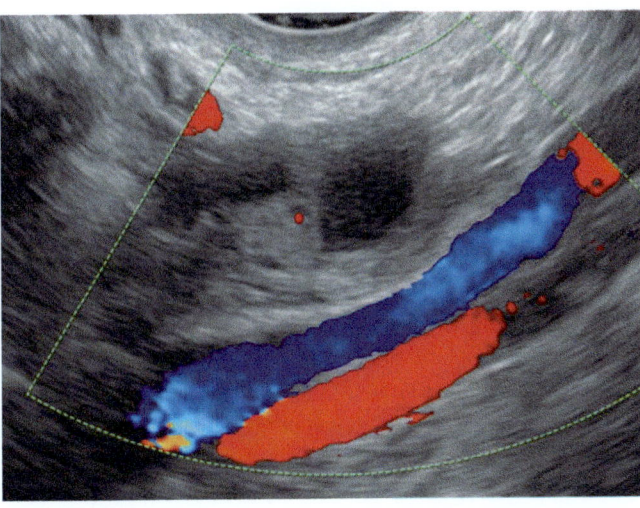

Fig. 3.17 Ovary normally located in the ovarian fossa behind and inside the external iliac vessels

Fig. 3.16 Schematic drawing of the ovary

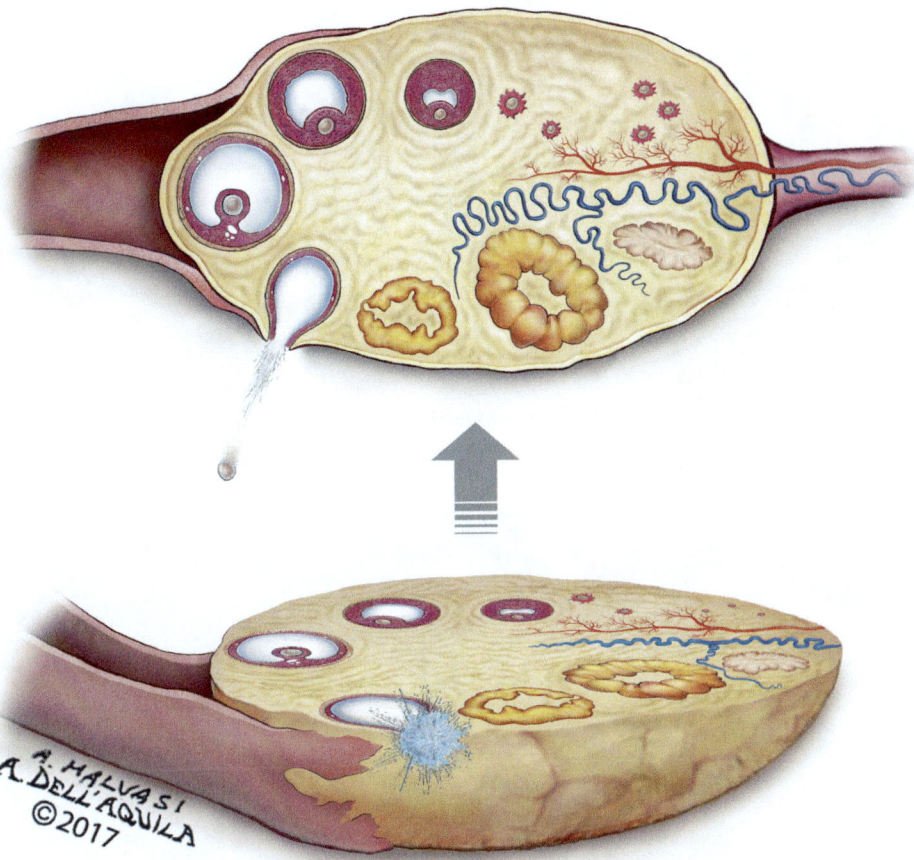

diameter between 2 and 10 mm is counted: if it is less than three, there is a significantly higher chance of cycle cancellation, detection of lower estradiol levels, and use of higher dosage of gonadotropins [25, 26]. Some authors have argued that AFC has higher variability and is less reliable as compared with AMH (Anti-Mullerian Hormone) [27]. The use of a standardized approach in performing AFC could increase the accuracy of the test [28]. To enable lower intra- and interobserver variability, reduce the risk of measurement errors, and improve the predictive capability of AFC, 3D sonography may be useful using the inversion mode, the silhouette mode software (Fig. 3.19), or the Sonography-based Automated Volume Count follicle (SonoAVC™ follicle) software, which automatically calculates the number and volume of anechoic structures (the antral follicles) in a volume sweep of the ovary [29–31] (Fig. 3.20).

With progression of the follicular phase, at the end of the first week, the smaller follicles go to regression with the drop in FSH levels, while the larger ones grow regardless. One becomes dominant, producing substantial amounts of estradiol as it grows. The dominant follicle, also called Graafian follicle, increases in size at a rate of 2–3 mm/day and reaches a diameter ranging from 17 to 27 mm just prior to ovulation (Fig. 3.21).

Dominant follicular development is not always sustained by ovulation, especially in the early reproductive age when

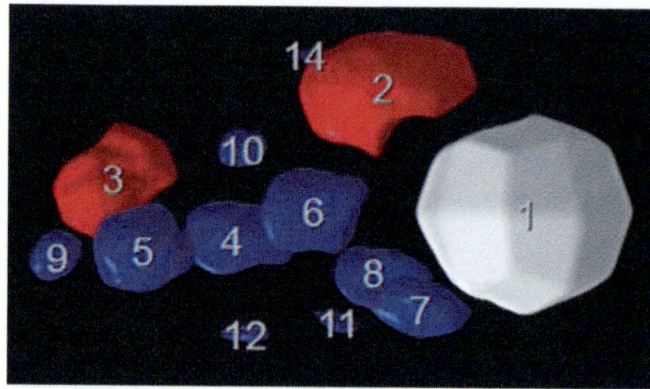

Fig. 3.20 Automatic calculation of the number and volume of the antral follicles with the Sonography-based Automated Volume Count follicle (SonoAVC™ follicle) software

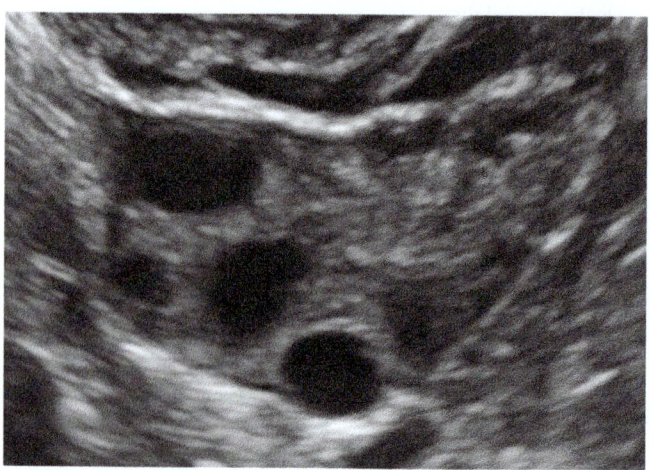

Fig. 3.18 Normal ovary in third day of the cycle. Multiple small developing follicles measuring between 2 and 5 mm are recognized

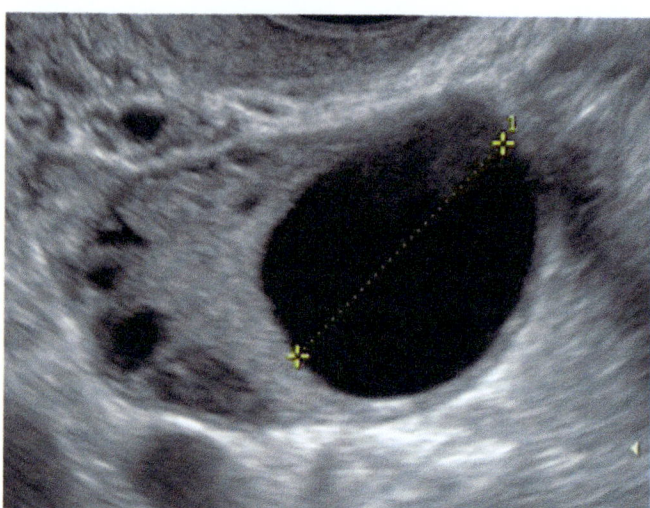

Fig. 3.21 Preovulatory follicle

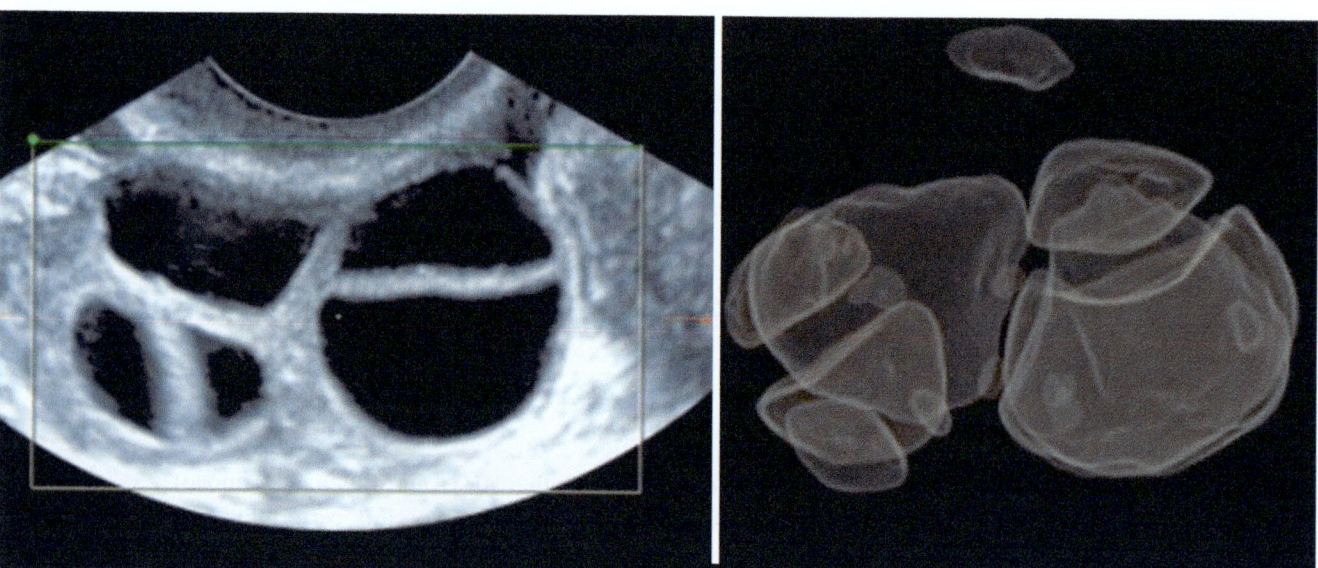

Fig. 3.19 Multiple antral follicles visualized with the 3D silhouette mode

ovulation cannot occur. At this age, the ovaries may sometimes have a multifollicular appearance, explained by persistence of variable sized developing follicles, some of them functioning and some atretic (Fig. 3.22).

Ovulation occurs with segmental dissolution of the follicular wall, liberation of the oocyte, and escape of the follicular fluid into the peritoneal cavity. After ovulation, rapid changes of the dominant collapsed follicle begins: capillaries and fibroblasts from the surrounding stroma proliferate and penetrate the basal lamina; concurrently, the mural granulosa cells undergo morphological changes collectively referred to luteinization. Thus luteinized granulosa cells, surrounding theca-interstitial cells and invading vasculature give origin to the corpus luteum. Sometimes, corpus luteum is hardly seen with ultrasound since it is confused among the stromal ovarian tissue. Commonly, it is visualized as a small structure containing thick irregular hyperechogenic walls surrounding a hypoechoic center. Color Doppler shows the rich neovascularization of the corpus luteum walls, appearing as a "ring of fire" around the corpus luteum (Fig. 3.23). Sometimes, after follicular rupture, corpus luteum presents as a hemorrhagic cyst which can reach even 5–6 cm in diameter (Fig. 3.24) and undergoes progressive reabsorption.

3.3.3 Fallopian Tubes

The fallopian tube can be occasionally seen on ultrasound when distended by fluid (hydrosalpinx) or when peritoneal fluid is present surrounding the adnexa (Fig. 3.25). In the coronal view of the uterus, occasionally the interstitial part may be recognized, originating from the lateral uterine angle (Fig. 3.26). The only way to visualize the tubal lumen and patency is by trans-cervical injection of saline fluid: the method is named transvaginal hystero-contrast-salpingography (Hy-Co-Sy). Originally, this was done with

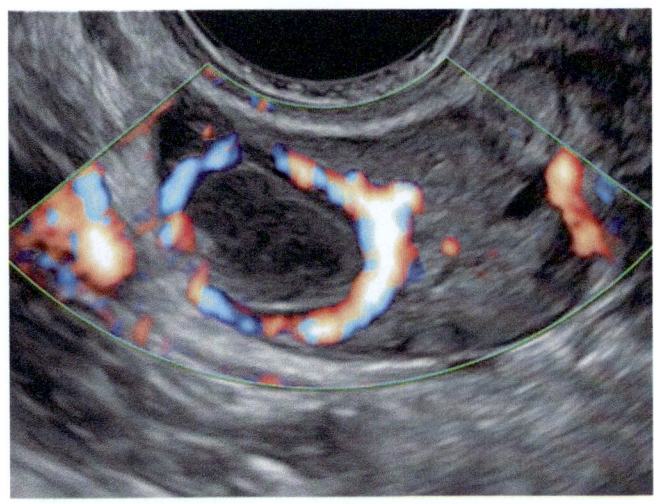

Fig. 3.23 Corpus luteum appearing as a small hypoechoic structure surrounded by the rich neovascularization of its walls ("ring of fire")

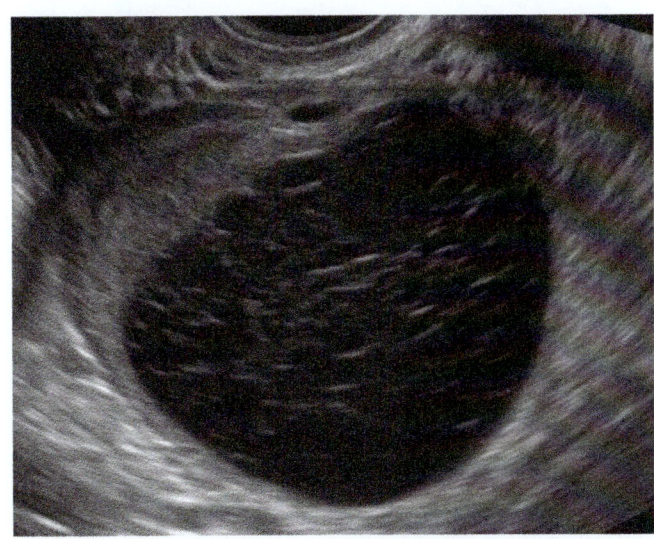

Fig. 3.24 Corpus luteum cyst with blood clots floating inside

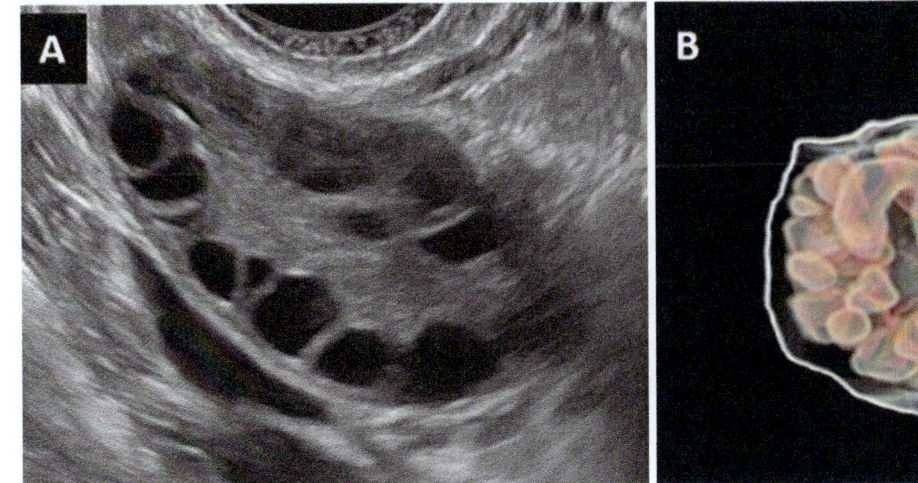
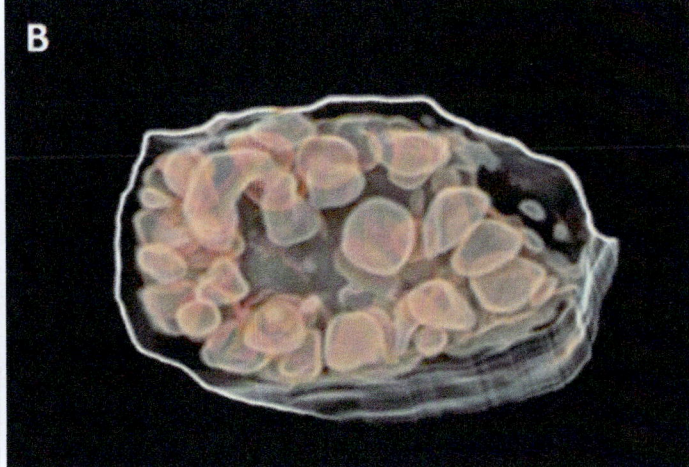

Fig. 3.22 Multifollicular ovary in 2D (a) and 3D silhouette mode (b)

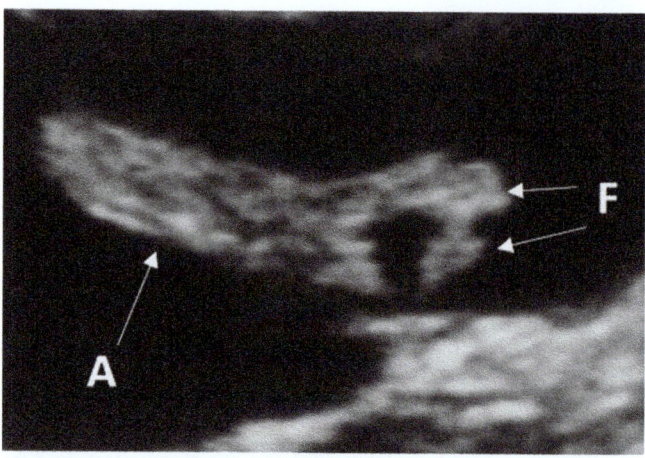

Fig. 3.25 Occasional visualization of tubal ampulla (A) and fimbriae (F) surrounded by free fluid in the pelvis

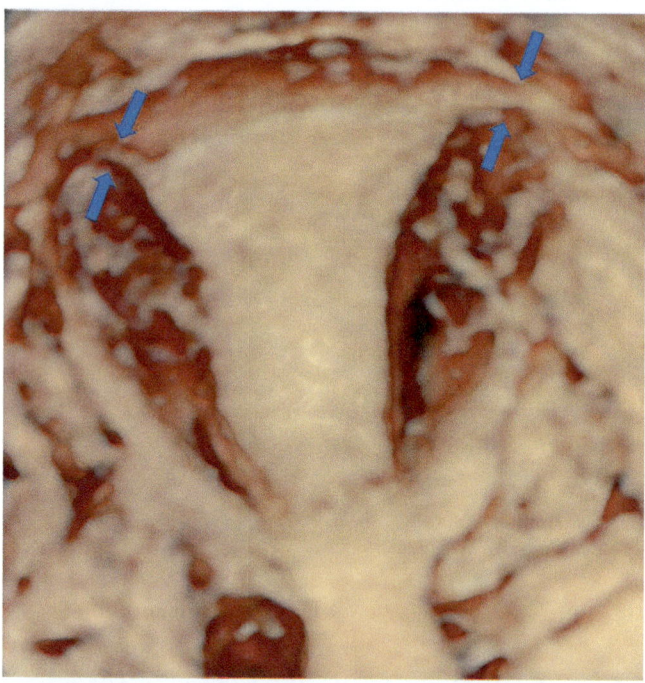

Fig. 3.26 Interstitial portion of the fallopian tube (arrows)

the use of gray scale imaging alone [32] or with the addition of pulsed Doppler [33] or Color Doppler ultrasound [34] in order to recognize in a better and easier way the passage of fluid through the tubal lumen. However, there are several technical difficulties in the visualization of the fallopian tube with 2D Hy-Co-Sy even with the aid of pulsed and Color Doppler: due to their tortuosity, the tubes are rarely seen completely in a single scanning plane; distended bowel may prevent the visualization of the distal part of the tubes and the spillage of fluid in the peritoneal cavity. The use of hyperechogenic contrast media increases the capability to visualize the tubes and the flow

in their lumen. These contrast media consist of suspension of microbubbles made of special galactose microparticles which enhance echo signals [35].

References

1. Benacerraf BR, Abuhamad AZ, Bromley B, Goldstein SR, Groszmann Y, Shipp TD, Timor-Tritsch IE. Consider ultrasound first for imaging the female pelvis. Am J Obstet Gynecol. 2015;212:450–5.
2. Saravelos SH, Jayaprakasan K, Ojha K, Li TC. Assessment of the uterus with three-dimensional ultrasound in women undergoing ART. Hum Reprod Update. 2017;23:188–210.
3. Panchal S, Kurjak A, Nagori C. 3D and 4D studies from human reproduction to perinatal medicine. J Perinat Med. 2017;45:759–72.
4. Kupesic S, Kurjak A. Uterine and ovarian perfusion during the periovulatory period assessed by transvaginal color Doppler. Fertil Steril. 1993;60:439–43.
5. Kelsey TW, Ginbey E, Chowdhury MM, Bath LE, Anderson RA, Wallace HA. A validated normative model for human uterine volume from birth to age 40 years. PLoS One. 2016;11(6):e0157375.
6. Tetlow RL, Richmond I, Manton DJ, Greenman J, Turnbull LW, Killick SR. Histological analysis of the uterine junctional zone as seen by transvaginal ultrasound. Ultrasound Obstet Gynecol. 1999;14:188–93.
7. Abuhamad AZ, Singleton S, Zhao Y, Bocca S. The Z technique: an easy approach to the display of the midcoronal plane of the uterus in volume sonography. J Ultrasound Med. 2006;25:607–12.
8. Bakos O, Lundkvist O, Bergh T. Transvaginal sonographic evaluation of endometrial growth and texture in spontaneous ovulatory menstrual cycles: a descriptive study. Hum Reprod. 1993;8:799–806.
9. Persadie R. Ultrasonographic assessment of endometrial thickness: a review. J Obstet Gynaecol Can. 2002;24:131–6.
10. De Vries K, Lyons EA, Ballard G, et al. Contractions of the inner third of the myometrium. Am J Obstet Gynecol. 1990;162:679–82.
11. Ludwin A, Ludwin I. Comparison of the ESHRE-ESGE and ASRM classifications of Müllerian duct anomalies in everyday practice. Hum Reprod. 2015;303:569–80.
12. Grimbizis GF, Di Spiezio Sardo A, Saravelos SH, Gordts S, Exacoustos C, Van Schoubroeck D, Bermejo C, Amso NN, Nargund G, Timmerman D, Athanasiadis A, Brucker S, De Angelis C, Gergolet M, Li TC, Tanos V, Tarlatzis B, Farquharson R, Gianaroli L, Campo RT. The Thessaloniki ESHRE/ESGE consensus on diagnosis of female genital anomalies. Hum Reprod. 2016;311:2–7.
13. Ludwin A, Ludwin I, Kudla M, Kottner J. Reliability of the European Society of Human Reproduction and Embryology/ European Society for Gynaecological Endoscopy and American Society for Reproductive Medicine classification systems for congenital uterine anomalies detected using three-dimensional ultrasonography. Fertil Steril. 2015;104:688–97.
14. Bocca SM, Abuhamad AZ. Use of 3-dimensional sonography to assess uterine anomalies. J Ultrasound Med. 2013;32:1–6.
15. Moini A, Mohammadi S, Hosseini R, Eslami B, Ahmadi F. Accuracy of 3-dimensional sonography for diagnosis and classification of congenital uterine anomalies. J Ultrasound Med. 2013;32:923–7.
16. Graupera B, Pascual MA, Hereter L, Browne JL, Úbeda B, Rodríguez I, Pedrero C. Accuracy of three-dimensional ultrasound compared with magnetic resonance imaging in diagnosis of Müllerian duct anomalies using ESHRE-ESGE consensus on the classification of congenital anomalies of the female genital tract. Ultrasound Obstet Gynecol. 2015;46:616–22.

17. Kupesic S, Kurjak A, Tripalo A. Normal gynecological anatomy assessed by 2D, 3D Ultrasound and Color Doppler. In: Kupesic S, editor. Color Doppler and 3D ultrasound in gynecology, infertility and obstetrics. New Delhi: Jaypee Eds; 2003. p. 15–28.

18. Kurjak A, Kupesic S, Schulman H, Zalud I. Transvaginal color Doppler in the assessment of ovarian and uterine blood flow in infertile women. Fertil Steril. 1991;56:870–6.

19. Ng EH, Chan CC, Tang OS, Yeung WS, Ho PC. Changes in endometrial and subendometrial blood flow in IVF. Reprod Biomed Online. 2009;18(2):269–75.

20. Ng EH, Chan CC, Tang OS, Yeung WS, Ho PC. The role of endometrial blood flow measured by three-dimensional power Doppler ultrasound in the prediction of pregnancy during in vitro fertilization treatment. Eur J Obstet Gynecol Reprod Biol. 2007;135:8–16.

21. Nandi A, Martins WP, Jayaprakasan K, Clewes JS, Campbell BK, Raine-Fenning NJ. Assessment of endometrial and subendometrial blood flow in women undergoing frozen embryo transfer cycles. Reprod Biomed Online. 2014;28:343–51.

22. Baldini D, Lavopa C, Vizziello G, Sciancalepore AG, Malvasi A. The safe use of the transvaginal ultrasound probe for transabdominal oocyte retrieval in patients with vaginally inaccessible ovaries. Front Womens Health. 2018;3(2):e1–3.

23. Higgins RV, van Nagell JR Jr, Woods CH, Thompson EA, Kryscio RJ. Interobserver variation in ovarian measurements using transvaginal sonography. Gynecol Oncol. 1990;39:69–71.

24. Bozdag G, Salman MC, Mumusoglu S, Yapici Z, Gunalp S. Is ovarian volume estimation reliable when compared with true volume? Am J Obstet Gynecol. 2012;206:44.e1–4.

25. Chang MY, Chiang CH, Hsieh TT, Soong YK, Hsu KH. Use of the antral follicle count to predict the outcome of assisted reproductive technologies. Fertil Steril. 1998;69:505–10.

26. Ng EH, Tang OS, Ho PC. The significance of the number of antral follicles prior to stimulation in predicting ovarian responses in an IVF programme. Hum Reprod. 2000;15:1937–42.

27. Nelson SM, Klein BM, Arce JC. Comparison of antimüllerian hormone levels and antral follicle count as predictor of ovarian response to controlled ovarian stimulation in good-prognosis patients at individual fertility clinics in two multicenter trials. Fertil Steril. 2015;103(4):923–30.

28. Broekmans FJ, de Ziegler D, Howles CM, Gougeon A, Trew G, Olivennes F. The antral follicle count: practical recommendations for better standardization. Fertil Steril. 2010;94(3):1044–51.

29. Raine-Fenning N, Jayaprakasan K, Clewes J, Joergner I, Bonaki SD, Chamberlain S, Devlin L, Priddle H, Johnson I. SonoAVC: a novel method of automatic volume calculation. Ultrasound Obstet Gynecol. 2008;31:691–6.

30. Ata B, Seyhan A, Reinblatt SL, Shalom-Paz E, Krishnamurthy S, Tan SL. Comparison of automated and manual follicle monitoring in an unrestricted population of 100 women undergoing controlled ovarian stimulation for IVF. Hum Reprod. 2011;26: 127–33.

31. Deb S, Batcha M, Campbell BK, Jayaprakasan K, Clewes JS, Hopkisson JF, Sjoblom C, Raine-Fenning NJ. The predictive value of the automated quantification of the number and size of small antral follicles in women undergoing ART. Hum Reprod. 2009;24:2124–32.

32. Deichert U, Schleif R, van de Sandt M, Juhnke I. Transvaginal hysterosalpingo-contrast-sonography (Hy-Co-Sy) compared with conventional tubal diagnostics. Hum Reprod. 1989;4:418–24.

33. Deichert U, Schlief R, van de Sandt M, Daume E. Transvaginal hysterosalpingo-contrast sonography for the assessment of tubal patency with gray scale imaging and additional use of pulsed wave Doppler. Fertil Steril. 1992;57:62–7.

34. Kupesic S, Kurjak A. Gynecological vaginal sonographic interventional procedures: what does color add? Gynecol Perinatol. 1994;3:57–60.

35. Lanzani C, Savasi V, Leone FP, Ratti M, Ferrazzi E. Two-dimensional HyCoSy with contrast tuned imaging technology and a second-generation contrast media for the assessment of tubal patency in an infertility program. Fertil Steril. 2009;92:1158–61.

Ultrasound and Probe Setting

4

Edoardo Di Naro, Luigi Raio, Annachiara Basso, and Mariana Rita Catalano

Contents

E. Di Naro (✉) · A. Basso · M. R. Catalano
Faculty of Medicine, Department of Obstetrics and Gynecology,
University of Bari, Bari, Italy

L. Raio
Department of Obstetrics and Gynecology, Inselspital,
Universitatsspital Bern, Bern, Switzerland

© Springer Nature Switzerland AG 2020
A. Malvasi, D. Baldini (eds.), *Pick Up and Oocyte Management*, https://doi.org/10.1007/978-3-030-28741-2_4

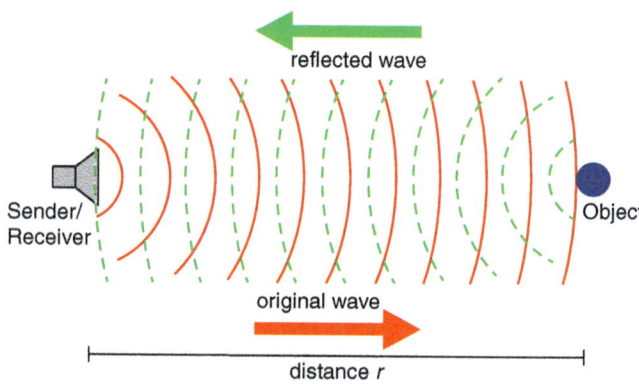

Fig. 4.1 Sound wave

Table 4.1 Different sound frequencies

Infrasonic	<20 Hz
Human audible range	20 Hz–20 KHz
Ultrasonic	>20 kHz

Table 4.2 Characteristics of a sound wave

Length	λ	The distance between two consecutive, identical positions in the pressure wave (e.g., between two compressions or between two rarefactions) It is determined by the frequency of the wave and the speed of propagation in the medium through which it is travelling
Frequency	f	The number of cycles per second performed by the particles of the medium in response to a wave passing through it. Expressed in Hertz, where I Hz = 1 cycle passing a given point each second, therefore 3 MHz = 3 million cycles per second
Period	T	The time taken for a particle in the medium through which the wave is travelling to make one complete oscillation about its test position
Amplitude	A	The maximal displacement of the oscillating particle from the equilibrium position
Velocity of propagation	v	The speed of sound with direction specified. When a sound wave travels through any medium, it is certain that parameters of that medium determine the speed of sound propagation

Ultrasounds are known since about 170 years. Firstly, echo sounding has been used in the First World War to fix the position of submarines, now we apply the echo sounding method in medical imaging to study organs and tissue structures, to learn about the body's function, and to recognize the malfunction. That requires good knowledge about both physical and technological properties in ultrasonic and the tissue interaction with ultrasound waves (Fig. 4.1) [1].

Ultrasound (US) imaging has become an attractive technology for medical diagnosis in a variety of clinical settings, including obstetrics and gynecology, cardiology, and urology. This is due to its noninvasive nature, real-time capability, and cost-effectiveness. Unlike other diagnostic modalities, ultrasound systems do not emit ionizing radiation and scans may be conducted as often as necessary without the risks of repeated exposure to X-rays or radionuclides.

4.1 Basic Physical Principles of Medical Ultrasound

4.1.1 The Sound Wave

In ultrasound diagnosis, we apply the mechanical energy of the sound wave. The wave is physical appearance by which the mechanical energy is propagating through space, by particles oscillation.

Unlike X-rays, sound is not electromagnetic, matter must be present for sound to travel, which explains why sound cannot propagate through a vacuum. Sound propagation is the energy transfer from one place to another within a medium, and some energy is also imparted to the medium [1]. Sound is categorized according to its frequency, number of mechanical variations occurring per unit time, and the terms infrasound and ultrasound are used for frequencies below and above the audible range (Table 4.1):

Ultrasound is sound whose frequency is above the range of human hearing (high frequency sound waves).

The use of high frequencies is limited by their greater attenuation in tissue and thus shorter depth of penetration.

For this reason, different ranges of frequency are used for examination of different parts of the body:

- 3–5 MHz for abdominal areas
- 5–10 MHz for small and superficial parts
- 10–30 MHz for the skin

Although ultrasound images are captured in real time, they can also show movement of the body internal organs as well as blood flowing through the blood vessels.

The characteristics of a sound wave can be described by the following parameters (Table 4.2, Fig. 4.2) [1–4].

The body is elastic medium in which the sound wave longitudinally propagates. The wave frequency is the source oscillation. The sound wave, in reason of the generated mechanical energy, causes the particles oscillation that determines local pressure and medium density regular changes [2].

The relationship between frequency, velocity, and wavelength is given by the following formula:

$$\lambda = c / f$$

The wave propagation velocity is determined by the medium properties: in the air the slowest propagation (344 m/s), increases in liquids and solids (water: 1520 m/s; liver: 1566 m/s; skull bone: 2717–4077 m/s). We can know that ultrasound propagates in soft tissue with an average velocity of around 1540 m/s.

The acoustic impedance, defined as the product of the acoustic velocity in the medium and the density of the medium ($Z = p \times v$), is a parameter that describes how the sound wave differently propagates in tissues.

4.1.2   Generation of Ultrasound

The source of ultrasound waves is a piezoelectric crystal [2–4]. The principle of piezoelectricity is central to the ultrasound generation, it's defined how the ability of some materials produce a voltage when deformed by an applied pressure and produce a pressure when deformed by an applied voltage.

So, when a voltage is applied to the faces of a crystal, it expands or contracts, then it resonates converting electricity to ultrasound. At the same time, when the crystal receives an echo, the sound deforms the crystal and a voltage is produced on its faces. This is analyzed by the system.

Piezoelectric crystal is the source and the detector of ultrasound and, consequently, plays a very important role in transducer technology.

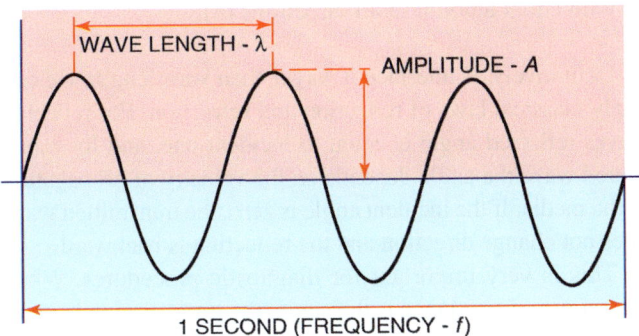

Fig. 4.2 Representation of sound wave characteristics

Ultrasound probes are produced of very thin crystals because the best transformation in both directions by the piezoelectric effect is achieved when the crystal frequency is the same as the frequency of the sound wave. It is realized for thickness of $\lambda/2$.

The most used materials are ferroelectric ceramic, lead zirconate titanate, or plastic, polyvinylidene difluoride. The crystals are sandwiched by silver film electrodes on opposite sides.

The transducer is usually treated as a three-port network including two mechanical ports and one electrical port as shown in Fig. 4.3. The mechanical ports represent the front and back surfaces of the piezoelectric element and the electrical port represents the electrical connection of the piezoelectric element to the electrical source. The front layer is known as an acoustic matching layer, which can improve the transducer performance significantly [1–5].

4.1.3   Interaction of Sound with Tissue

The ultrasound shape beam is important for the image quality. The beam profile is made up of three parts (Fig. 4.4):

1. Near field (Fresnel zone)
2. Far field (Fraunhofer zone)
3. Transition point

The near field or Fresnel zone is the part of the beam useful for imaging; however, this can be quite large in area, depending on the diameter of the crystal. The shape and dimensions of this first trait are determined by the shape and dimensions of the emitter and by the frequencies of the wave. Imaging requires a very narrow beam to produce high-resolution diagnosis. In the far field or Fraunhofer zone, the second trait, the intensity is uniformly decreasing with dis-

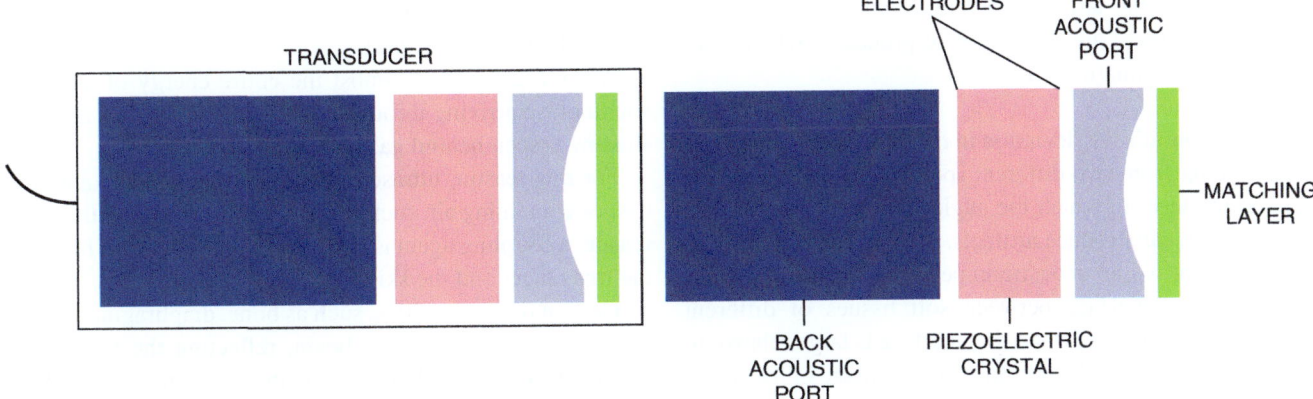

Fig. 4.3 Transducer as a three-port network (in pink: piezoelectric crystal; in glycine and violet: mechanical ports; in green: acoustic matching layer)

Fig. 4.4 The ultrasound shape beam

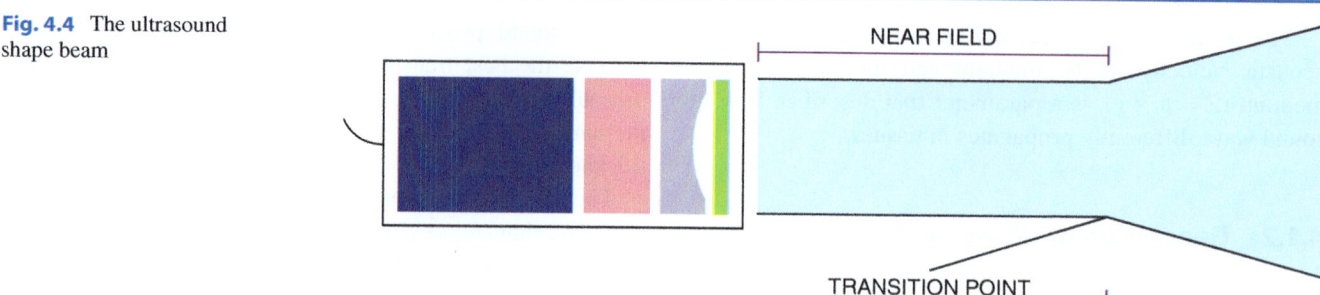

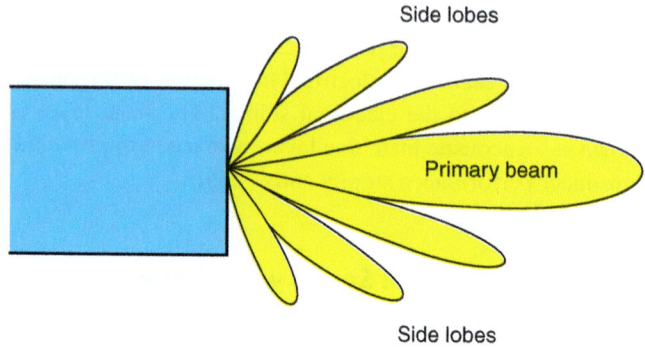

Fig. 4.5 The beam profile with energy divided into primary beam and side-lobes or off-axis areas

tance. Resolution is preserved in a better way if the near field is longer [3–5].

A beam profile of a simple transducer appears as in the diagram below and shows that the energy is not confined to a single lobe, but radiates off at various angles to the transducer face as off-axis energy. These off-axis areas are called side-lobes (Fig. 4.5).

When the ultrasonic wave traverses body's tissues, part of the energy will be transmitted but various factors can cause it to lose energy, decreasing in intensity and amplitude. This phenomenon is called attenuation, and it depends on distance, tissue characteristics, and beam frequency. Approximately, the attenuation rate in soft tissue is 1 Db/MHz/cm, and there are four types of processes which contribute to the attenuation (Fig. 4.6):

- **Refraction**: it's the deviation in the pathway of the beam, generating from two different speeds of sound at the tissues interface, in which the angle of incidence isn't 90°. Refraction can produce artifacts.
- **Reflection**: it's an acoustic impedance mismatch, occurring at the interface between soft tissues of different acoustic impedance, when the interface is large relative to the wavelength. At the interface, a percentage of the sound is reflected, the others are transmitted into the tissue (soft tissue/air interface—99% is reflected, soft tissue/bone—40% is reflected, liver/kidney—2% is reflected).

- **Absorption**: it's a transfer of energy of the beam to the medium in which sound is passing. This kind of attenuation of sounds increases with frequency, so we can understand why high frequency transducers cannot be used for examining deep structures in the body. Absorption increases with the viscosity of the medium. Bone adsorbs ultrasound much more than soft tissue, so that, in general, ultrasound is suitable for only bones surfaces. They can't reach the areas behind bones; therefore, the black zone behind bones is called acoustic shadow.
- **Scattering:** it occurs when interface is equal in size to wavelengths, it's also named non-specular reflection and it's characterized by scattering in many directions not with equal amount in all directions [8].

Definitively, if interface is larger than wavelength, we can apply classical laws of reflection and refraction. For reflected waves reflected angle is equal to incident one, and for transmitted wave the angle depends on the velocity of propagation in the media. If the incident angle is zero, the transmitted wave does not change direction and the reflection is backward.

This is very important for diagnostic procedures. When the acoustic impedance is the same, the transmission is maximal, instead the reflection is maximal with very different acoustic impedance.

The greater the difference in acoustic impedance between two media, the higher the fraction of the ultrasound energy that is reflected at their interface and the higher the attenuation of the transmitted part.

Air and gas reflect almost the entire energy of an ultrasound pulse arriving through a tissue. Therefore, an acoustic shadow is seen behind gas bubbles.

For this reason, ultrasound is not suitable for examining tissues containing air, such as the healthy lungs. For the same reason, a coupling agent is necessary to eliminate air between the transducer and the skin.

Certain tissue densities, such as bone, diaphragm, pericardium, slow the ultrasound beam, reflecting the waves and producing a bright or hyperechoic image. Other tissues allow ultrasound beams to pass and reflect at moderate speeds, creating a gray image on the screen, such as muscle, liver, or kidney.

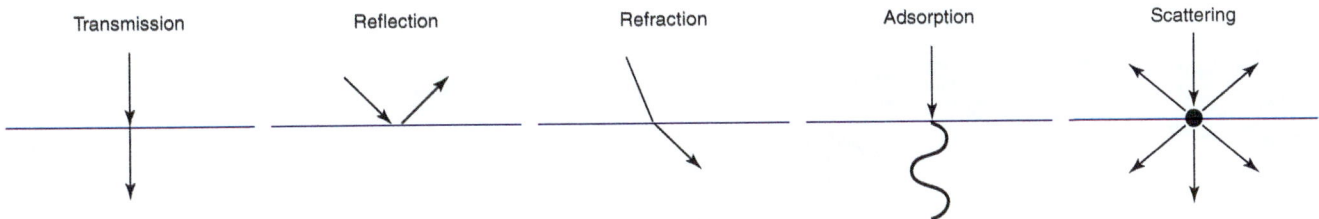

Fig. 4.6 The main processes of attenuation of ultrasonic wave passing through tissues

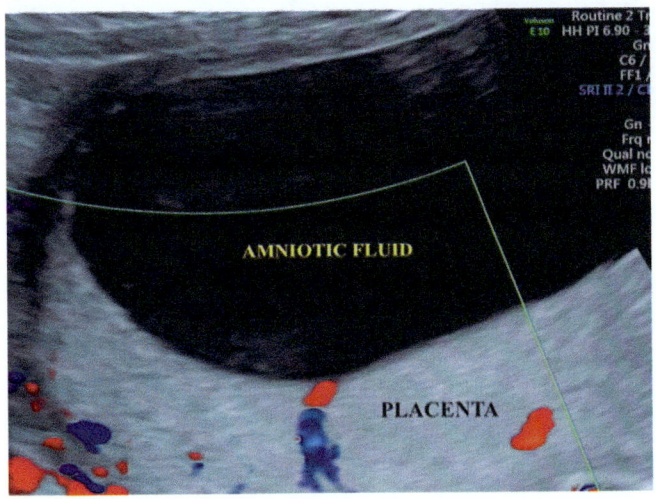

Fig. 4.7 The example of hypoechoic image (amniotic fluid) and hyperechoic image (the placenta)

Some tissue allows ultrasound waves to pass easily and retain their strength, creating dark black or hypoechoic images on the ultrasound screen, such as blood, ascites, amniotic fluid, and urine (Fig. 4.7) [3, 4, 8].

4.1.4   Resolution

Resolution is defined, as the ability to distinguish echoes in terms of space, time, and strength and is critical for the high-quality image resolution.

- **Contrast resolution**: it refers to the ability of an ultrasound system to demonstrate differentiation between different tissues (liver/kidney).
- **Temporal resolution**: it is the ability to show changes over time. This is very important for particular exams, like echocardiography.
- **Spatial resolution**: It is the ability to detect and display structures that are close, together. It is reasonable to consider two different types of spatial resolution: axial and lateral one. Axial resolution is dependent especially upon the length of the pulse used to form the beam (SPL: spatial pulse length), so the shorter the pulse

length, the better the axial resolution. The SPL is determined by the number of cycles in one pulse and the length of each cycle.

We know that the wave length is inversely proportional to the frequency, so higher frequencies generate shorter wavelengths and therefore shorter pulse lengths. In conclusion, we can say that higher frequency transducers will show better axial resolution. On the other hand, the lateral resolution is the ability to distinguish between two separate targets perpendicular to the beam [3, 4, 8].

4.1.5   Artifacts

The term artifact is used to describe part of image that does not accurately represent the anatomic structures present in the subject evaluated. Consequently, features that result from incorrect adjustment of instrument settings, are not true artifacts.

Artifacts may variously affect the image quality, but, in the majority of cases, they are easy to recognize. Sometimes, they hinder the correct diagnosis or lead to false diagnosis of a pathological condition where none exists (Fig. 4.8a–b) [10].

We know that ultrasound systems operate on the basis of described assumptions relating to the interaction of the sound beam with soft tissue interfaces, such as:

- A constant speed of sound in the body (assumed 1540 m/s).
- All echoes detected by the transducer originate from the central axis of the beam.
- The ultrasound beam travels in straight lines.
- The time taken for an echo from a given interfaces to return to the transducer is directly related to its distance from the transducer.
- The rate of attenuation of the beam is constant with depth and throughout the field of view.

If these assumptions are incorrect, the result is the image that does not accurately reflect scan plane anatomy. The list below describes some of the common artifacts, some of which offer useful diagnostic information.

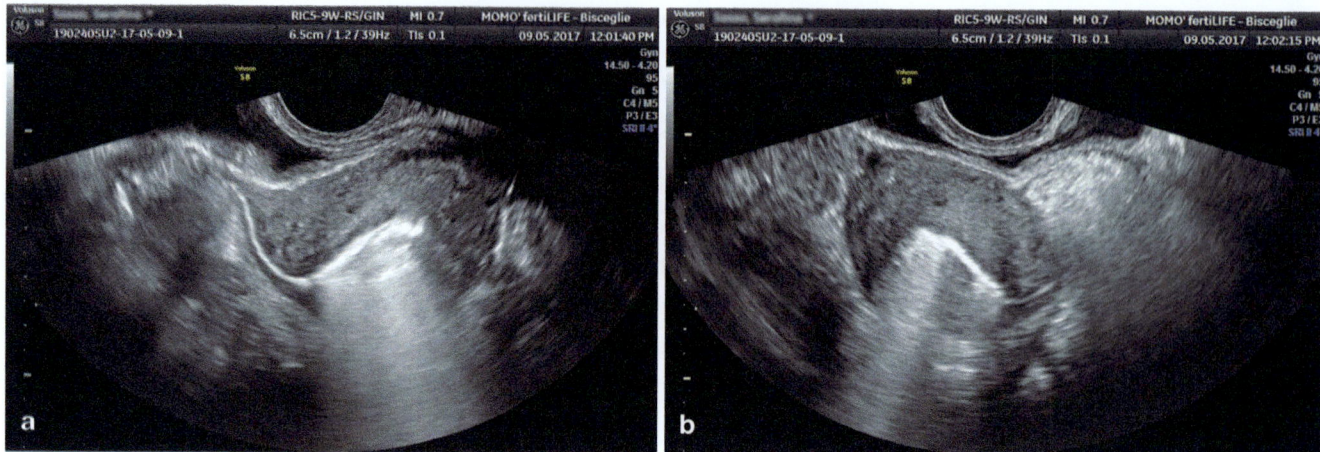

Fig. 4.8 (a–b) Artifact linked to the ultrasound contrast medium

Acoustic Shadowing is a total reflection on a strong reflector, such as gas or foreign body, or extensive absorption (bone), of the ultrasound wave. The shadow is seen underneath the bright object due to US waves reflection towards the probe. However, from a diagnostic point of view, it may limit the examination of body regions behind the gas or the bone, but on the other hand it is useful for diagnosing stones, calcifications, or foreign bodies [9, 10].

Some interfaces causing such effects are:

- **Soft tissue/gas** (bowel, lung)
- **Soft tissue/bone,** calcium (ribs, calculi)
- **Normal tissue/fibrous tissue** (scars, ligaments)

Mirror image artifact is a multiple reflection of the ultrasound beam. Consequently, on the screen there is false representation showing two images of a single object. However, it is possible to distinguish the "mirrored" object from the real image because it appears deeper and will disappear if the probe position is changed.

Examples of these are:

- **Diaphragm/lung interface** (show mirroring of the liver texture, above the diaphragm)
- **Bladder/rectum interface**, when the rectum is gas filled (bladder wall is mirrored together with any bladder contents, such as ureterocele, catheter balloon, and mass)

Posterior acoustic enhancement occurs if ultrasound waves reach quickly a low density medium, such as urine in the bladder, and then reflect back quickly from the next structure encountered, higher in density, such as the posterior bladder wall. In this case, the deepest structure appears falsely hyperechoic, and the gain adjustment may be needed.

The basis for this artifact is that fluid-filled structures (cysts, gall bladder, etc.) attenuate sound to a much lesser degree than solid organs (liver, spleen, etc.). Therefore, there is more sound transmitted to structures deep to the fluid-filled structure and the resulting echoes from this deeper tissue are brighter than those from a similar depth in adjacent solid tissue [5, 10].

4.1.6 Ultrasound Techniques

The echo principle forms represent the basis of all common ultrasound techniques. The distance between the transducer and the reflector in the tissue is measured by the time between the emission of a pulse and reception of its echo. Additionally, the intensity of the echo can be measured. With Doppler techniques, comparison of the Doppler shift of the echo with the emitted frequency gives information about any movement of the reflector. The various ultrasound techniques used are described below [1, 3, 8].

4.1.6.1 A-Mode
A-mode (amplitude modulation, A-scan) is a one-dimensional examination technique in which a single crystal transducer is used. This mode presents amplitudes of reflected ultrasound in dependence of time. The echoes are displayed on the screen along a time axis (distance) as peaks proportional to the intensity of each signal (amplitude) (Fig. 4.9). The use of this technique today is very limited [8].

4.1.6.2 B-Mode
B-mode (brightness modulation) is similar to the precedent technique, but in this case echoes are displayed as points of different gray-scale brightness corresponding to the intensity of each signal (Fig. 4.10). The brightness of the spot is a semi-quantitative measure of impedance relationship for the media building the reflecting interface [8].

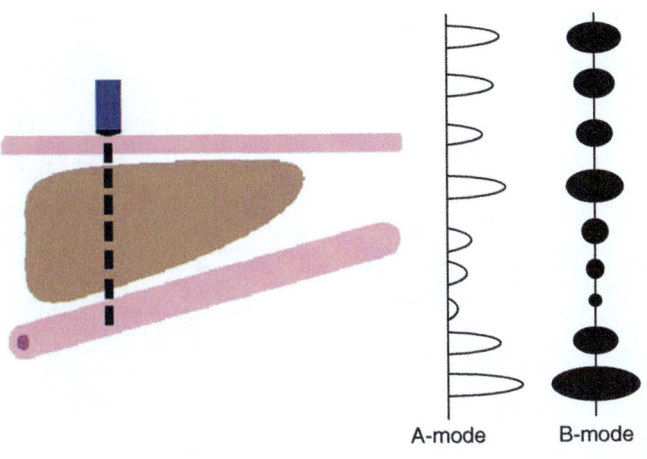

Fig. 4.9 Schematic representation of A-mode and B-mode

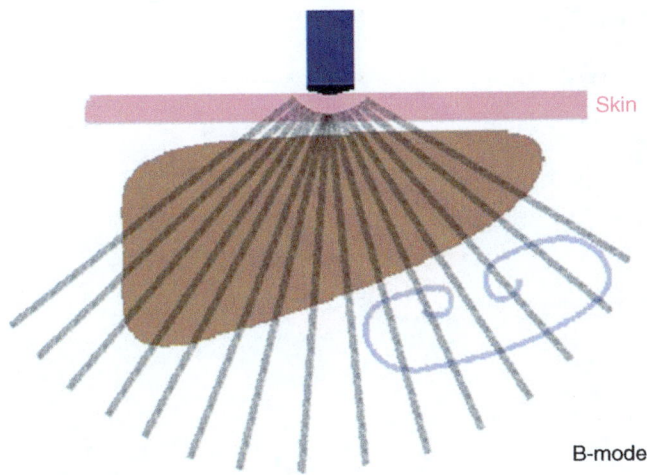

Fig. 4.10 B-mode or brightness mode technique

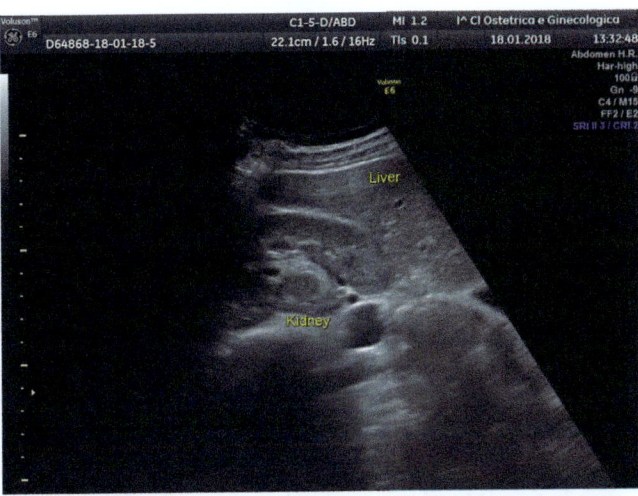

Fig. 4.11 Hepatorenal recess or Morison's pouch, the space that separates the liver from the right kidney

This presentation has a good resolution, but it can't give a lot of data about interfaces nature, presenting only the interfaces of great difference. By adding the gray-scale the image provides more information about the structures. Indeed, in gray scale we have different echo intensities presenting in shades of gray.

While the A-scan is a single line investigation, B-scan is a 2D image and is most commonly used in practice. A probe with more than one crystal is used, and the images are produced by groups of piezoelectric elements. Another aspect is that B-mode images are presented in real time and can even follow the movement inside the tissues (blood flow, heart).

The images we use in diagnostic ultrasound are produced with B-Mode or brightness mode techniques. As a result of the signals caused by returning echoes, we obtain a pattern of dots on the screen. The strength of the echo received determines the brightness of each dot proportionally. For each pulse emitted, there is a line of sight as a result of the echoes derived from the tissue interaction. The image, known as a "frame" on the monitor, is composed of multiple lines of

sights and, consequently, of multiple thousands of dots. Finally, the real-time image is a succession of several frames, generally 10–30 per second (Figs. 4.11 and 4.12).

4.1.6.3 M-Mode (TM-Mode)

This technique analyzes moving structures, such as heart valves. It consists of a continuous recording over time of the echoes generated by the transducer. On the ultrasound screen, there will be shown motion towards and away from the ultrasound probe at any depth along that line [8].

4.1.7 Doppler

In medical ultrasounds, the Doppler effect is used to measure the velocity of organs or fluids in the body, for example, time motion of heart muscle or the speed of blood in arteries. It was initially discovered by Austrian Mathematician Christian Doppler, who hypothesized that the pitch of the sound would change if the source was moving [7].

The practical description of the Doppler effect is that of the change in pitch of a train or siren as they come towards or away from you when you are standing still. The pitch increases as the train is coming towards you and decreases as it is moving away. In medical application, the Doppler effect is applied mostly for detecting the blood flow. In particular, as the blood is moving towards the transducer, the received frequency will be higher than the initial frequency; on the other hand, as the blood is moving away from the transducer, the received frequency will be lower. The Doppler shift frequency is the difference between transmitted and received frequencies. It depends on the insonating frequency ( ), velocity of moving blood (V), speed of sound in tissue (c), and the angle between the ultrasound beam and the flow direction (φ) as shown in the formula below:

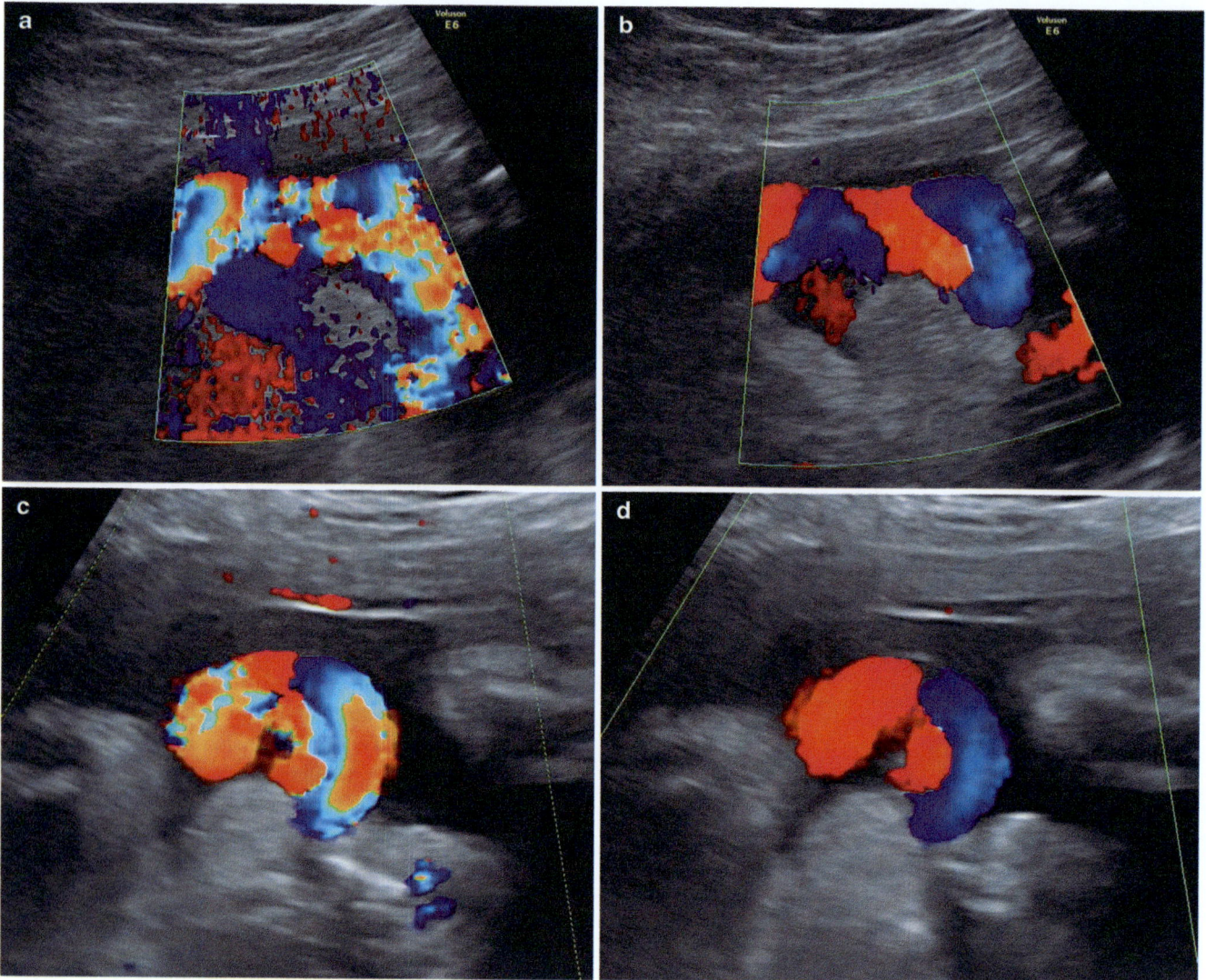

Fig. 4.12 Two examples of optimization of scan image, modifying PRF in the study of umbilical cord. Note the aliasing in (**a–c**), and the absence of that phenomenon in (**b–d**)

$$\cos \varphi$$

Flow speed calculations based on the Doppler shift measurements can only be accomplished correctly with knowledge of the Doppler angle which is in the form of a cosine. For a given flow, the greater the Doppler angle is, the lesser the Doppler shift is. Consequently, a zero degree angle gives the greater Doppler shift and at 90° the Doppler shift is reduced to nil [6, 7].

There are three different types of Doppler equipment used for the detection of flow: Continuous Wave and Pulsed Wave spectral instruments and Color Mapping instruments.

- **Continuous Wave:** the transducer consists of two crystals, one permanently emitting ultrasound and the

Table 4.3 Advantages and disadvantages of continuous wave

Advantages	Disadvantages
Excellent detection of high velocity flows	No range gate location
No aliasing limits	Spectral broadening

other receiving all the echoes. It is possible to measure high flow velocities. Because there is no depth range gate, the signals can be very confusing and include a broad range of frequency shifts (Table 4.3).

- **Pulsed Wave:** pulsed wave as well as for the continuous wave, the transducer works both as a transmitter and a receiver. Moreover, ultrasound is emitted in short pulses, thus the echoes arrive to the transducer between pulses, in an interval named gate. The receiver gate, setting by the operator at a given depth, reproduces only echoes arising from moving reflectors at that depth. A common problem with all pulsed Doppler techniques is the analysis of high velocities: the range for the measurement of Doppler frequencies is limited by the pulse repetition frequency (PRF). Other terms describing PRF are flow rate or scale. This determines the sampling time that is required to process the Doppler information. Since low flow must be sampled for a longer period of time to accurately analyze the information, low PRF must be selected. Higher flows can be sampled more quickly so high PRF can be selected. The preset will be adequate during the exam.

Thus, when the Doppler frequency is higher than the pulse repetition frequency, high velocities are displayed as low velocities in the opposite direction (spectral Doppler) or in the wrong color (Color Doppler). This phenomenon is known as "aliasing" (Fig. 4.10), and is directly comparable to the effect seen in movies where car wheels rotating above a certain speed appear to be turning backward.

This is probably the most common artifact occurring in Doppler studies. It simply means that the speed of the flow being examined is faster than half of the PRF set. Color aliasing can be useful in certain applications to map changes in frequency shift in a vessel with blood flowing at a constant angle with respect to the transducer. The aliasing will be displayed as the wrong color. Color changing from red, through yellow and green, to blue, as a result of changing in direction.

A correct display is possible only for Doppler frequencies within the range ± one half of the pulse repetition frequency, known as the Nyquist limit, as a consequence, increasing the PRF will unwrap the spectrum and display it in the correct direction, above or below the baseline. Doppler examination of higher velocities requires lower ultrasound frequencies and a high pulse repetition frequency, whereas low velocities can be analyzed with higher frequencies, which allow better resolution (Table 4.4).

- **Color Doppler**: data from multiple sample volumes is processed for mean frequency, amplitude, and turbulence, using a system called autocorrelation. Color Doppler is, indeed, a display of mean frequency, which

Table 4.4 Advantages and disadvantages of pulsed wave

Advantages	Disadvantages
Single sample volume	Aliasing-dependent on the PRF
Accurate range location	
Quantitative spectral analysis	

Table 4.5 Color

Color Doppler features
Color Display: a color bar that indicates the direction (red or blue, depending on the allocation or encoding by the operator), amplitude (proportionally to the brightness), and turbulence (green) data in a Color Doppler signal
Region of Interest Box: a suitable area of the field of view adjusted in width, height, and depth into the patient to optimize the frame rate Thus, by reducing
(a) the width: the frame rate increases because fewer color line of sight are required
(b) the height: maintaining the width, the frame rate is the same because the same number of beam paths is still required
(c) the depth: the frame rate increases because for each pulse sent into the patient, the computer receives the echoes faster and may complete the elaboration of each line of sight in a shorter period of time
Angle of Incidence: for a correct use and interpretation of Doppler, it's useful to remember the importance of correction of angle of incidence during the scan
A vessel curving through the color ROI makes it possible for the Doppler to interrogate unidirectional flow in two different directions, towards the transducer and away. This commonly occurs when curving vessels are interrogated at or near 90°. A vessel curving through the color ROI may visualize the unidirectional flow in two different directions by using the Doppler, towards the probe or far away from it. Usually, it occurs when the curving vessels are analyzed at or around 90°, displaying artifacts such as acceleration and aliasing. Correcting the angle of incidence towards 0° may avoid these artifacts. Understanding of the physics of the effect of the angle of incidence on color display will eliminate misinterpretation of this artifact

allows us to easily evaluate hemodynamic events occurring in the region of interest from a quality point of view, such as existence, direction of flow, and existence of turbulent flow. This kind of information provides a road map for pulsed Doppler spectral analysis (Table 4.5) [6, 7].

4.2 Doppler Features

4.2.1 Three/Four-Dimensional Ultrasound

In 1974 Szilard developed a mechanical three-dimensional (3D) display system to see a fetus three dimensionally. Then, in 1982, Brinkley and colleagues [12] invented a 3D position sensor for a probe by taking several tomographic images of a stillborn baby underwater, tracing its outline manually and showing its wire-frame 3D images. However, a modern 3D ultrasound system was introduced for the first time in 1986 by Baba [17, 18], who developed a system for 3D reconstruction of the ultrasonic fetal image in order to facilitate the understanding of the fetal structures in utero and also to make recordings of this image. Later, in the early 1990s, clinical applications of the three-orthogonal-plane display in obstetrics were reported. Thus, since 1994, the number of reports on fetal 3D images has been increasing rapidly in reason of the commercial availability [11–14].

Generally, a 3D ultrasound examination consists of four main steps: data acquisition, 3D visualization, volume/image processing, and storing of volumes, rendered images or image/volume sequences. Three-dimensional data may be acquired in only few seconds in the following ways:

1. with a conventional 2D ultrasound probe: as a large number of consecutive tomographic images (slices), by sweeping the probe over the volume of interest and rotating it at the spot
2. with a 3D probe: the most popular way because of its easiness for scanning

A 3D data set is composed by a set of voxels (volume elements) and each voxel has a gray value. Each 3D data should be processed by a computer to be displayed on a 2D screen to obtain a "volume visualization" [11–19].

There are three methods for volume visualization in 3D ultrasound:

1. Section reconstruction
2. Surface rendering
3. Volume rendering

4.2.1.1 Section Reconstruction

– An arbitrary section is displayed by translating and rotating the 3D data set.

– Three-orthogonal sections or parallel sections displayed on the screen simultaneously [11, 28–32].

4.2.1.2 Surface Rendering

A 3D surface image (Fig. 4.13) of the object is obtained in surface rendering by extracting the data and eliminating unnecessary elements as much as possible. In this way, the object is transformed to a set of intermediate geometrical data, composed of small cubes or small polygons, and displayed on a 2D screen. Moreover, this "extraction" process is performed either by setting an appropriate threshold or by manual tracing [12–19, 33, 34].

4.2.1.3 Volume Rendering

A 3D data set for rendering is projected directly on a projection plane. This method is useful to study, for example, fetal skeleton (Fig. 4.13) (if only the maximal gray values on each ray are displayed on the projection plane) or cystic parts and blood vessels (if only the minimal gray values on each ray are displayed on the projection plane). However, volume rendering is a good rendering method for observation but not for volume measurement [13–19].

Three-dimensional ultrasonography benefits are as follows:

– elevate accuracy in volume measuring
– good measurement reproducibility
– reduction of scanning time and improvement of workflow
– facilitation of telemedicine
– provision of some specific display modes, such as 3D cine, 4D, TUI (Tomography Ultrasound Imaging), VCI (Volume Contrasting Image), Omniview, VCAD (Volume Computed-Aided Diagnosis), and STIC (Spatio-Temporal Image Correlation) (Table 4.6) [19, 29, 32–49].

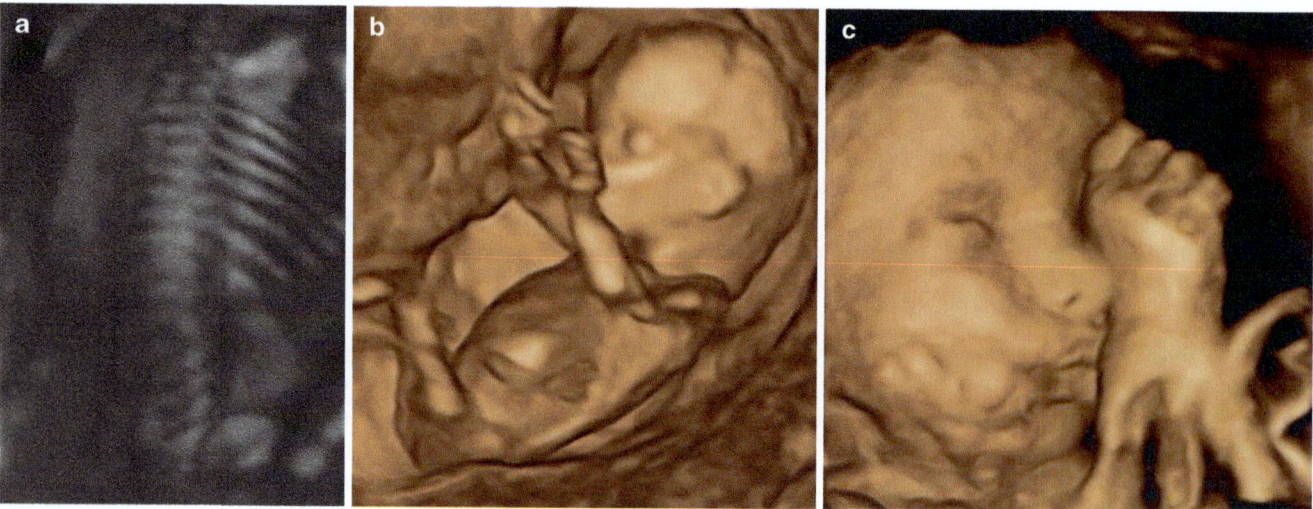

Fig. 4.13 In (**a**) image of volume rendering of fetal skeleton, in (**b**, **c**) image of surface rendering

Table 4.6 Different specific display mode far three-dimensional ultrasonography

Display mode 3D
3D-CINE
A static 3D volume data set, previously recorded by a moving camera, can be moved from one point to the other. Rotation in *x* or *y* axis provides different angle views and a better depth perception. Starring and ending rotation positions can be defined in 360°, but 45–60° are optimal. Both rotation velocity and type of movement can also be defined
4D
The addition of "time dimension" enables real-time observation for both obstetrics and gynecologic exams, even though each volume data set has less quality then a 3D volume
TUI
Three-dimensional image are presented in sequential plans, similarly to a computed tomography (CT) exam. Although the image size is reduced, several parallel planes may be visualized in only one image
VCI
A render mode that improves image contrast, reducing artifacts between tissues. Each image represents a thick slice from volume data set, viewed from longitudinal, coronal, transversal planes simultaneously. Transparency and slice thickness can be adjusted. This method is extremely useful to improve the delineation between myometrium and endometrium or placenta, fetal bones, and soft tissue, and to improve the definition of the fetal central nervous system, fetal thorax, and pelvic floor assessment
OMNIVIEW
A 3D resource that allows rectifies and view curvilinear structures in the same plane. This method, for example, enables to identify both uterine body and cervix at the same coronal plane
VCAD
VCAD aims to minimize operator dependence through image acquisition standardization. This method is useful in the fetal heart evaluation (SonoVCADheart), providing an immediate view of the six recommended volumetric fetal echocardiographic images, and the assessment of fetal head progression during the second stage of labor (SonoVCADlabor)
STIC
A 3D acquisition of moving structures through a post processing volume set, using either color Doppler or B-mode pulsatility to determine heart rate and organize the acquired frames into several 3D data sets. The main clinical employ of this method is the fetal heart. The reconstructed volumes will represent different moments of one cardiac cycle, resembling a real-time scan, in which four chambers, long axes and all the different scanning planes, can be visualized both as clips and as still images

Table 4.7 Probes for 2D imaging

Probe type	Feature	Application	Central frequency
Linear type	Wide footprint and keep same field of view at deep part	– Vascular – Breast – Thyroid – Tendon – Body fat and muscle mass	2.5–12 MHz
Curved type	Wide footprint, field of view will be spread at deep part	– Abdominal application	2.5–7.5 MHz
Phased	Small footprint, field of view will be spread widely at deep part	– Cardiac, transesophageal, and abdominal – Brain diagnosis – Brain, cardiac, transesophageal, and abdominal – Brain diagnosis	2–7.5 MHz

(c) Transducer Pulse Controls
(d) Display
(e) Keyboard/Cursor
(f) Disk storage device (hard disks, floppy disks, compact disks, or digital video disks)
(g) Printer

The transducer probe is the main part of the ultrasound machine. By using the piezoelectric effect, this wand-like instrument produces sound waves and receives the echoes as they bounce off the organs. The performance and imaging quality of ultrasonic scanner are highly affected by the characteristic and the structure of the probe. There are, indeed, different types of transducers: cardiac, vascular, abdominal, transvaginal, endorectal, and transesophageal echocardiography (TEE) (Tables 4.7 and 4.8). The shape of the probe determines its field of view. Cardiac is typically the smallest; vascular ranges in size from 25 to 50 mm; abdominal/curved shape has a larger footprint, and transvaginal transducers are long and skinny with a small head [1, 3, 5, 8].

The CPU is the "brain" of the ultrasound machine that contains the microprocessor, memory, amplifiers, and power supplies. The CPU functions are as follows:

– sending electrical currents to the transducer probe to emit sound waves
– receiving the electrical pulses from the probes, generating from the returning echoes
– processing data
– forming image on the monitor
– storing the processed data and/or image on the disk

The transducer pulse controls allow the sonographer to set and change the frequency and duration of the ultrasound

4.3 Basic Characteristics of the Ultrasound Equipment

4.3.1 The Ultrasound Machine

Generally, a basic ultrasound machine is composed by the following components:

(a) Transducer probe
(b) Central Processing Unit (CPU)

Table 4.8 Probe for 3D scanning

Probe type	Feature	Application	Central frequency
Linear type	Real-time 3D probe with the linear scanning type. The wide footprint probe head is beneficial at near part with the wide field of view	– Breast – Thyroid – Vascular	2.5-12 MHz
Curved type	Real-time 3D probe with the field of view. The wide footprint probe head is beneficial at deep part scanning	– Abdominal application	3.5–6.5 MHz
Transvaginal type	Real-time 3D probe with the wide field of view. The long and small probe head shape is beneficial for endocavitary application	– Transvaginal – Transrectal cardiac, transesophageal, and abdominal – Brain diagnosis	6 MHz

pulses applied to the piezoelectric crystals in the transducer probe, according to the scan mode of the machine [2].

The display, black-and-white or color, is a computer monitor that shows the processed data from the CPU.

Finally, the most common keyboard/cursor is a trackball, which allows the sonographer to add notes and take measurements from the data.

All the images can be stored in disk and after archived, and printed by thermal printers [52–56].

4.3.2 The Different Probes

We have the possibility to use different types of probes, according to the structures analyzing. Ultrasonic probe is a very important sensor, and the performance and imaging quality of exam are high and firstly affected by the characteristics of probe used [56, 57].

The mainly known probes are:

- Flat linear
- Curved linear
- Phased array

These terms refer to the arrangement of the crystals and the shape of the probe.

Flat linear: this kind of probe crystal is in a single row and in a straight line. For this reason, a linear probe will send out the sound signals all parallel to each other, travelling at 90°

to the transducer face, with an uniform density from the top to the bottom of the image, and the field of view is rectangular on the screen. The linear transducer for 2D imaging has a wide footprint and its central frequency is 2.5–12 MHz. The main uses of this probe are for the study of superficial tissues as tendon, fat, muscular, breast, thyroid, and vessels.

The linear transducer for 3D imaging has a wide footprint and a central frequency of 7.5–11 MHz, and it can be used for breast, thyroid, and carotid, or other vascular applications.

Curved linear: in this probe, the crystals are arranged along a curve, but are still in a single line. The sound signals remain at 90° to the transducer face, so they are sent in an arc and this creates a triangle shape or arc shaped imaged on the screen. This transducer is good for in depth examinations, even though the image resolution decreases when the depth increases. This is the most common probe used for the study of the abdomen. The frequency and applications also depend on whether the probe is for 2D or 3D imaging. In fact, the curved linear transducer for 2D imaging has a central frequency of 2.5–7.5 MHz, for 3D imaging has a frequency of 3.5–6.5 MHz (Fig. 4.12).

Phased array: this probe has a flat surface, but the crystals are arranged in a grid or network and are charged with electricity at different times. These probes are a little more complicated because some of crystals are vibrating in-phase with, and some others are vibrating out-of-phase with other crystals. The result is that this probe produces an arc-shaped image despite the fact that the probe is flat. This is the most common probe used for cardiac ultrasound (Fig. 4.14a-b).

Another ultrasound transducer type commonly used is the endocavitary. These probes have the opportunity to perform internal examinations of the patient. Therefore, they are designed to fit in specific body orifices. The endocavitary transducers include endovaginal and endorectal. Typically, they have the smaller footprints and the frequencies vary in the range of 3.5–11.5 MHz (Fig. 4.15a-c) [57–60].

4.3.3 Adjustment of the Equipment: Image Optimization

Only 1% of the operating time is spent by the transducer transmitting sound, whereas 99% of the time is spent listening to echoes. Correct adjustment of an ultrasound scanner is essential for an appropriate exam. The instruments offer a large variety of possible standard setting for each transducer and each body region, which may be adapted to the needs of the sonographer [8].

Throughout any ultrasound examination the operator should be constantly monitoring the image quality with a

a
b
ALOKA
ALOKA

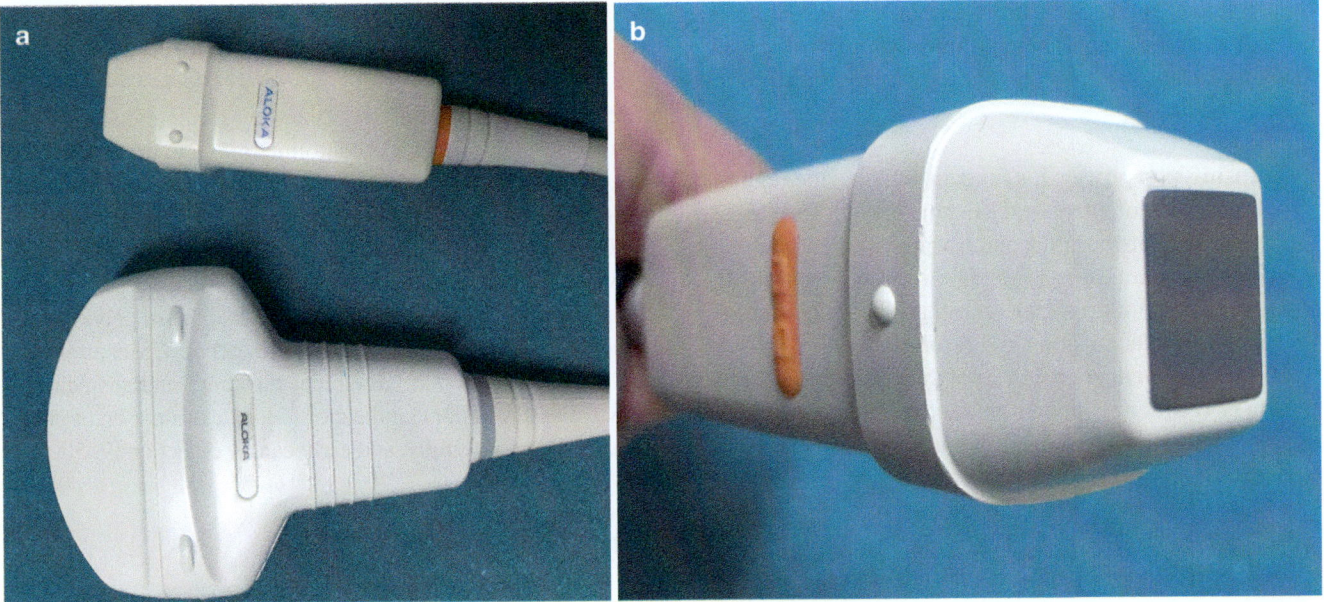

Fig. 4.14 (**a–b**) On the left a phased array linear and curved probe, on the right phased linear probe

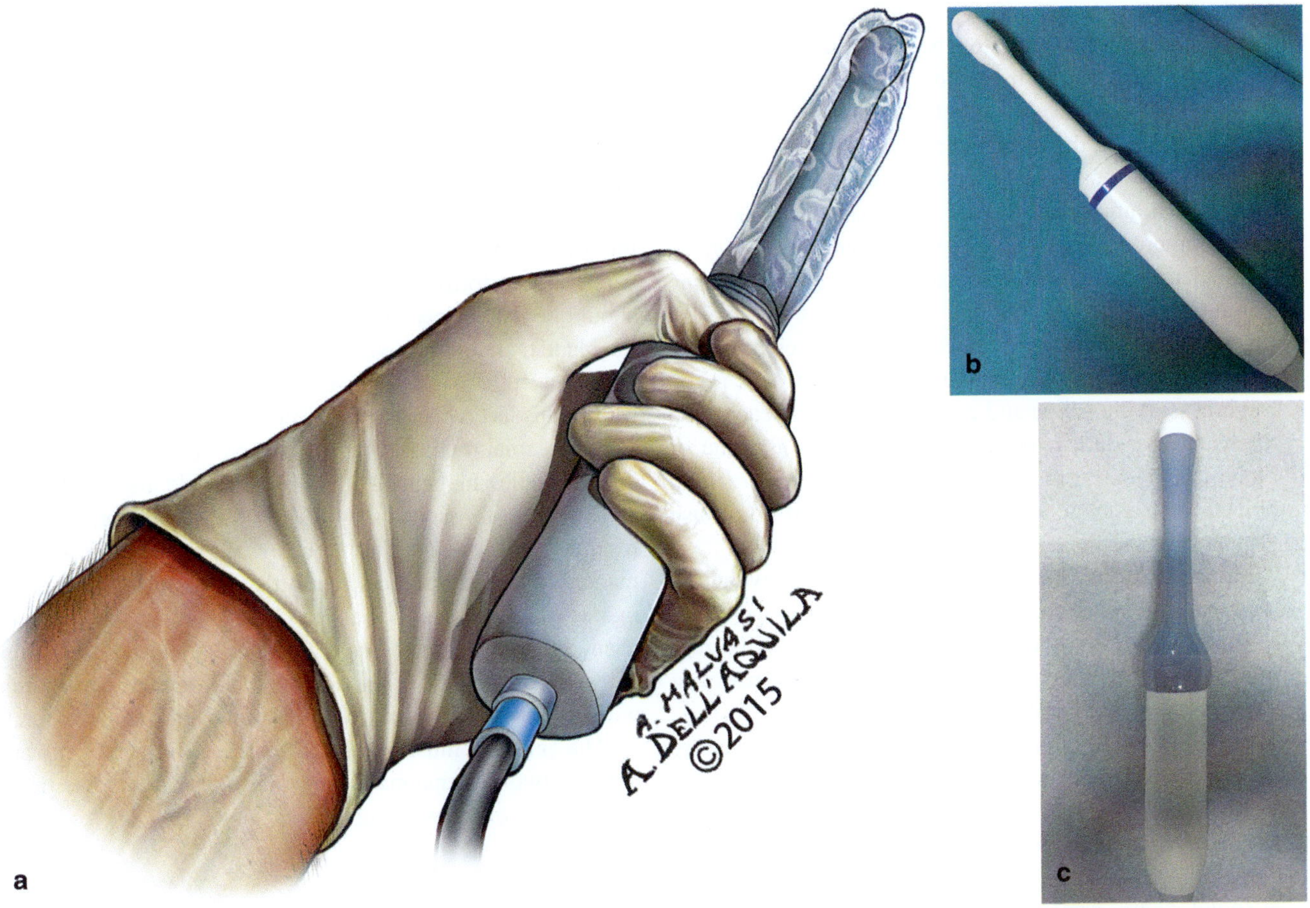

A. MALVASI
A. DELL'AQUILA
©2015
a
b
c

Fig. 4.15 (**a–c**) Two models of endocavitary probe

view to improving it. Sometimes better scanning techniques are required and sometimes optimization of the image by changing system controls can cause the necessary improvement in the image.

- **Transmission power**: it's fundamental that the regulation of the amount of energy exciting the crystal, and therefore the strength of the ultrasound beam. The choice of frequency (and transducer) relies on the penetration depth needed. It's important to note that changing frequency affects image acquisition and resolution.
- **Higher frequency**: greater resolution, poorer penetration.
- **Lower frequency**: poorer resolution, greater penetration. For the abdomen, for example, it may be useful starting with a lower frequency (curved array, 3.5 MHz) and using a higher frequency when the region of interest is close to the probe.
- **Depth:** it should be adjusted to improve the quality of the image by putting the object of interest in the center of the screen. Use small depth of field for superficial structures and large depth of field for deeper ones. On the right side of the screen, markings show depth in centimeters.
- **Focus**: The focus, or zone of the best resolution, should always be adjusted to the point of interest. Ultrasound systems normally have user controlled focal zones, giving best definition at the designated depth of focus. Modern transducers use excellent focusing technology achieving the best resolution. It is possible to expand the focal zone by adding more than one focal point, over a larger portion of the depth of field. In this case, there is slowing of the frame rate.
- **Overall Gain**: it's an amplification of the received signal but doesn't increase the exposure. In other words is the brightness of the image and can be adjusted for each scan to ensure that dark hypoechoic objects such as urine or blood are black on the screen, while bright hyperechoic objects such as bone appear white. Be careful not to use too much or too little gain.
- **Time gain compensation** (TGC): it's a way to overcome ultrasound attenuation, in which signal gain is increased as time passes from the emitted wave pulse. This correction makes equally echogenic tissues look the same even if they are located in different depths.
- **Zoom**: it is used to magnify structures of interest mainly for the final investigation of detail and for preparing the documentation.
- **Angle of incidence**: the largest reflection of sound occurs at 90° to an interface, so the best images will result from a sound beam projected at 90° to the main area of interest.

If there are problems, use of the image optimizer knob and returning to the standard settings may help [1, 4, 8].

4.4 Technical Aspects of the Ultrasound Examination of Female Pelvis

The following standards describe the examination to be performed for each organ and anatomic region in the female pelvis. All structures should be identified by the transabdominal or transvaginal approach. In many cases, both will be needed.

Ultrasound plays the primary role in imaging of the female pelvis. CT and MR are supplemental techniques used when the US examination is equivocal and in the staging of pelvic malignancy. Primary indications for female pelvic US examination are pelvic pain, abnormal vaginal bleeding, and suspicion of pelvic mass. Additional indications include evaluation of precocious puberty, infertility, and early cancer detection [9, 50, 51].

4.4.1 Preparation

Basically, no special preparation is needed for an ultrasound examination, except for the examination of the abdomen, in which a period of fasting is recommended. A coupling agent is necessary to ensure good contact between the transducer and the skin and to avoid artifacts caused by the presence of air between them. The best coupling agents are water-soluble gels, generally composed by 10 g carbomer, 0.25 g ethylenediaminetetraacetic acid (EDTA), 75 g propylene glycol, 12.5 g trolamine, and up to 500 mL demineralized water. A common mistake is to use insufficient gel, making poor contact with the skin surface, reducing the mobility of the transducer face over the skin and producing artifacts and poor imaging. For a pelvic sonogram performed transabdominally, the patient's bladder should be adequately distended. For a transvaginal approach, the bladder should be usually empty [2].

It is useful also to recognize the orientation of the transducer. Most transducer manufacturers provide an orientation mark, usually a small raised bump or light on one side of the transducer handle. In general, this mark should be towards the patient's head for sagittal sections and towards the patient's right for transverse sections. This probe marker corresponds a screen marker on the left of the screen. It's important that the probe marker is on the same side as the screen marker, and it possibly changes its orientation. The transducer should be used as an extension of the hand of the examiner and visualized as a torch, with the ultrasound beam as the light emanating from the torch.

The anatomy must be visualized three-dimensionally and not just two-dimensionally on the monitor; point the transducer at the organ wishing to view.

4.4.2 Uterus

The vagina and uterus provide an anatomic landmark that can be used as a reference point for the remaining normal and abnormal pelvic structures.

In evaluating the uterus, the following should be documented (Fig. 4.16a-b):

- Uterine size
- Uterine shape and orientation
- Endometrium
- Myometrium
- Cervix

The vagina should be imaged as a landmark for the cervix and lower uterine segment. Uterine length is evaluated in the long axis from the fundus to the cervix; the anteroposterior dimension is measured in the same long-axis view from its anterior to posterior wall, perpendicular to the length. The width is measured in transverse view or coronal view. Cervical diameters can be similarly detected. It's necessary to document the cervix relationship with vagina (anteverted/retroverted uterus), and uterus relationship with cervix (anteflexed/retroflexed uterus) [62]. Any anomalies in morphology must be reported by using 2D as well as 3D mode, if possible.

The endometrium should be analyzed for thickness, measuring the thickest part of it perpendicular to its longitudinal plane in the AP diameter from echogenic to echogenic border (adjacent hypoechoic myometrium and fluid in the cavity should be excluded), and echogenicity (Fig. 4.17). If any abnormality is detected, it should be detected the presence of flow (Color Doppler). The myometrium and cervix should be evaluated for contour changes, echogenicity, and masses [63–68, 72].

4.4.3 Adnexa (Ovaries and Fallopian Tubes)

When evaluating the adnexa, an attempt should be made to identify the ovaries first because they can serve as the major

point of reference for adnexal structures. Frequently, the ovaries are situated anterior to the internal iliac (hypogastric) vessels, which serve as a landmark for their identification. The following ovarian findings should be documented as follows:

- Size, shape, contour, echogenicity
- Position relative to the uterus

The ovarian size can be obtained by measuring the length in the long axis with the anteroposterior dimension measured perpendicular to the length. The ovarian width is measured

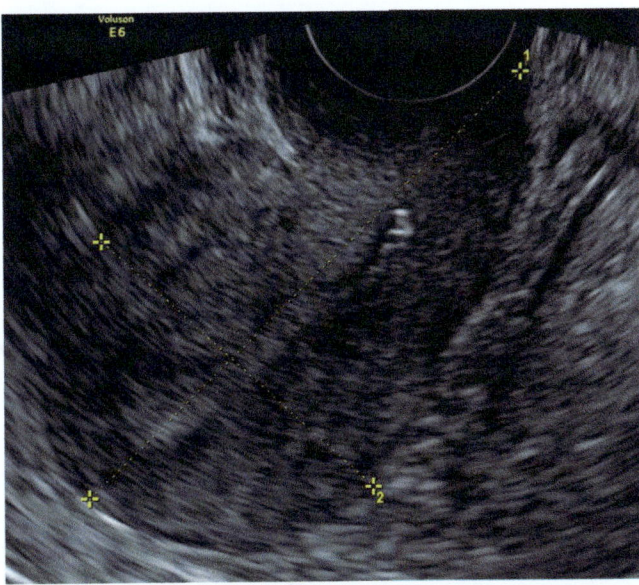

Fig. 4.17 Imagine of a correct way to measure thickness of endometrium and uterine length and anteroposterior dimension

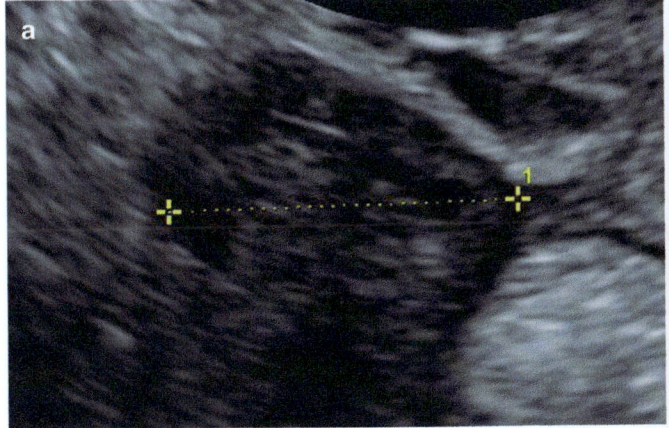
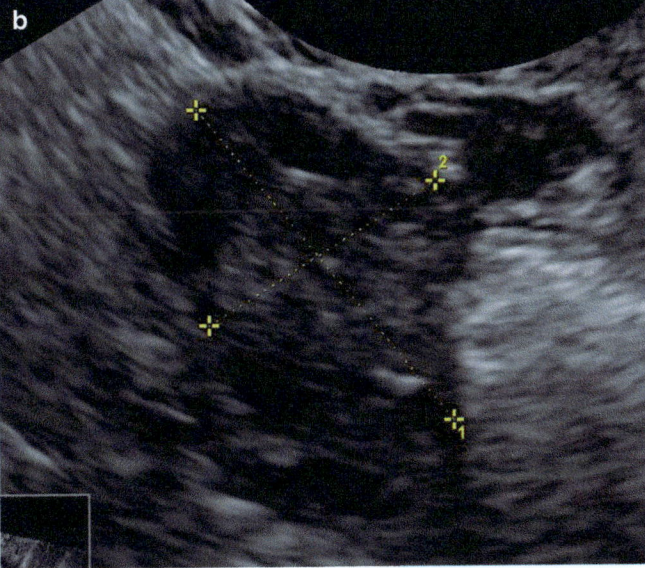

Fig. 4.16 (**a–b**) Upper and down an example of a correct technique to detect ovarian volume

in trans-axial or coronal view, so that it is possible to calculate the volume (Fig. 4.18) [69].

The normal Fallopian tubes are not commonly identified. This region should be surveyed for abnormalities, in particular dilated tubular structures.

If an adnexal mass is noted, its relation to the ovaries and uterus should be documented. Its size and echo pattern should be determined according to actual guidelines [61, 62, 70].

Doppler ultrasound may be useful in selected cases and can identify the vascular nature of pelvic structures [61, 62].

4.4.4 Cul-De-Sac

The cul-de-sac and bowel posterior to the uterus may not be clearly defined. This area should be evaluated for the presence of free fluid or mass (Fig. 4.19). Differentiation of normal loops of bowel from a mass may be difficult if only an abdominal examination is performed. A trans-

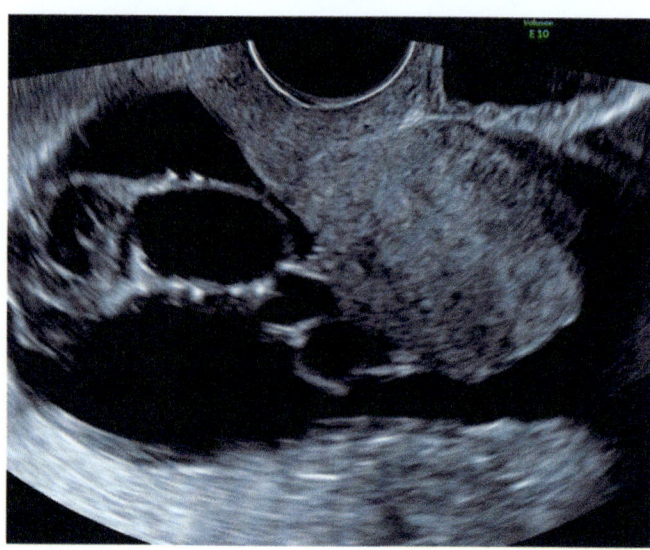

Fig. 4.19 Imagine of free fluid in cul-de-sac, posterior to the uterus and a typical sactosalpinx

Fig. 4.18 Ultrasound evaluation of ovaries

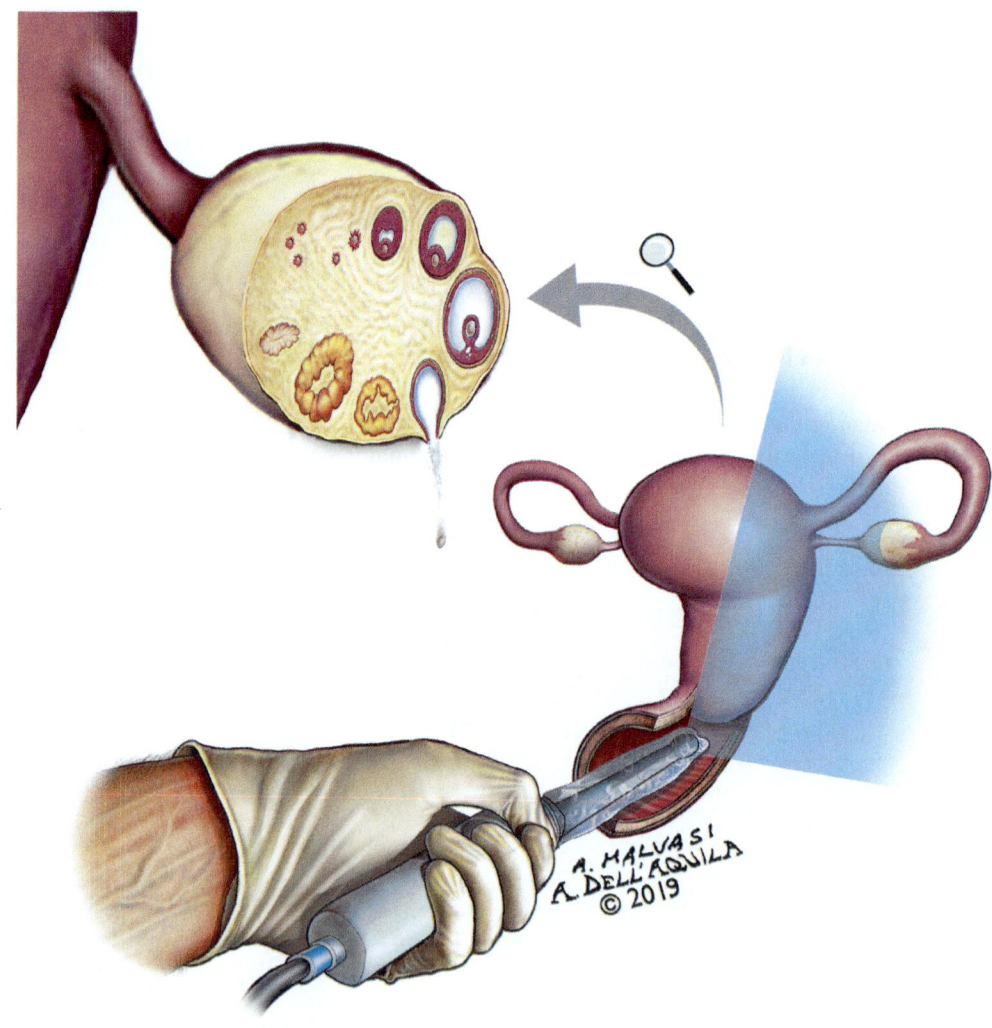

vaginal examination may be helpful to distinguish a suspected mass from fluid and feces within the normal rectosigmoid [61].

4.5   Ultrasound in Human Reproduction

Specific to gynecology, the introduction of high-resolution transvaginal ultrasonography has substantially changed the approach to diagnostic of gynecologic conditions. Today, it is an essential tool in patients suffering from reproductive disorders for assessment of follicular growth pattern, the structure of perifollicular vascular network and endometrium enable close to monitoring and prediction of success of medically assisted reproduction [66, 68, 72].

4.6   Ultrasound and Follicular Growth

Antral follicles of different sizes are present during all phase of menstrual cycle. Commonly, a diameter of 2 mm is considered as the lower limit at which antral follicles can be visualized although with improvement of ultrasound machines even smaller follicles can be visualized today. Visible characteristics of antral follicles which may be used for prediction of the ultimate fate of a follicle are: size (the largest diameter), shape, echogenicity, and antral edge quality [71].

In natural cycle (Fig. 4.20), throughout the follicular phase, antral follicle which will gain dominance is usually regularly shaped with regular antral edge and larger than follicles undergoing atresia. Dominant follicle has echo-

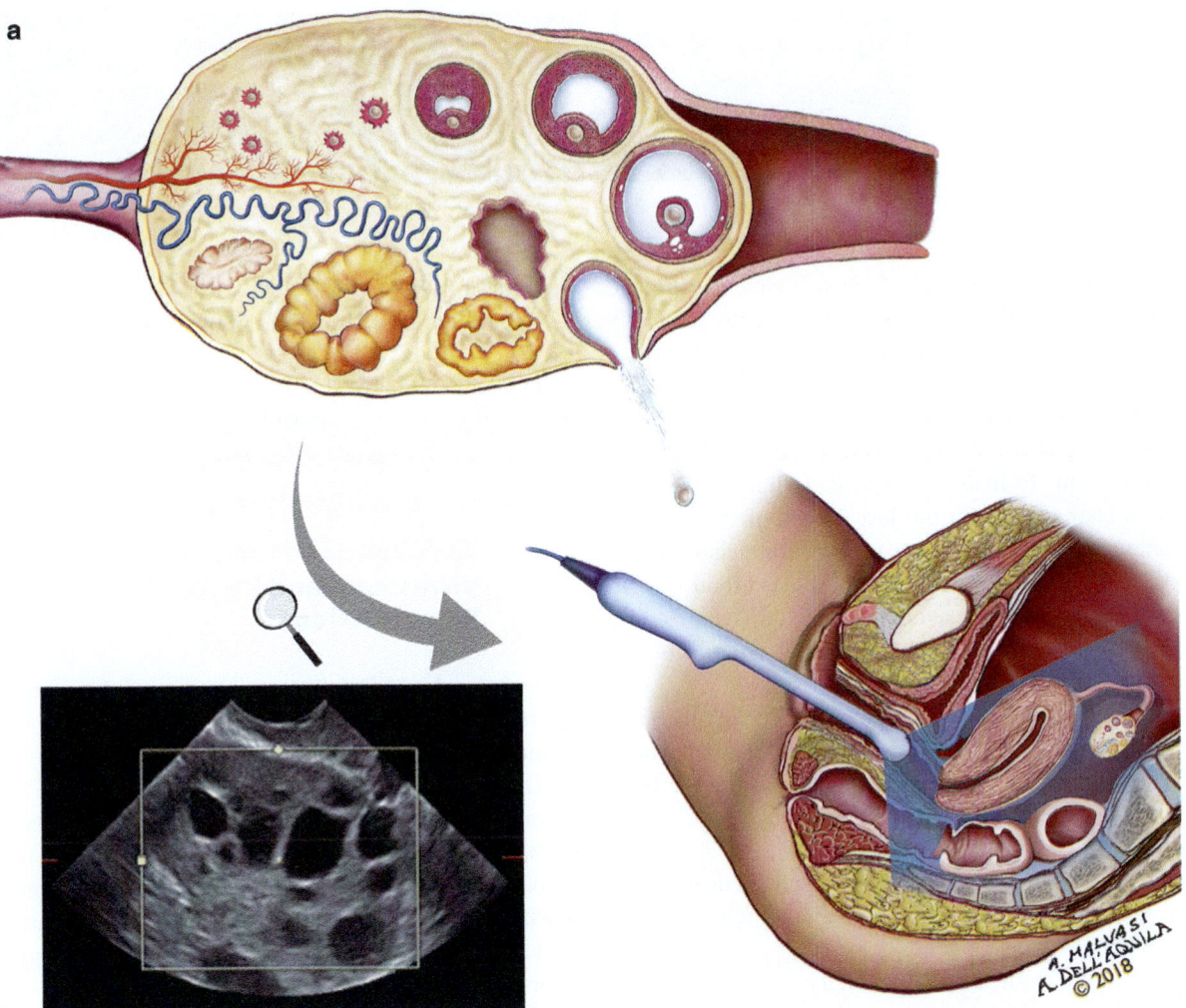

Fig. 4.20 (a) In natural cycle, throughout the follicular phase, antral follicle which will gain dominance is usually regularly shaped with regular antral edge and larger than follicles undergoing atresia. (b) Recently introduced sonography based automated volume count (SonoAVC) algorithm allows for automatic follicle count on ovaries recorded by ultrasound

Fig. 4.20 (continued)

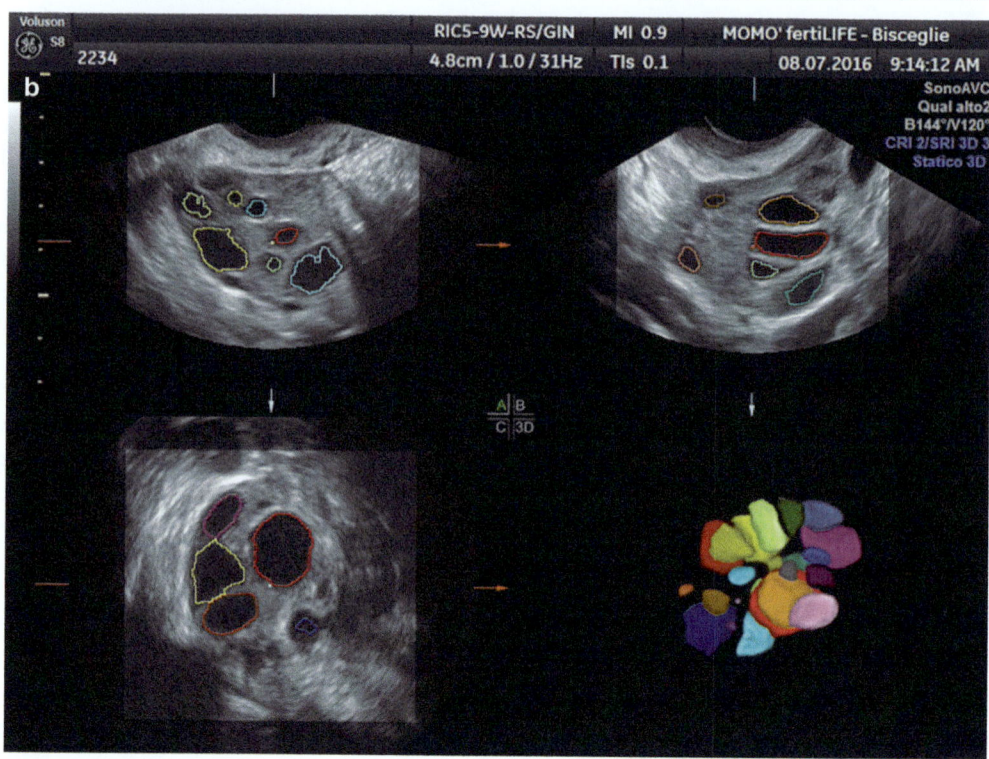

genicity in the middle range, while follicles destined to become atretic generally display higher echogenicity. Early angiographic studies in natural cycle showed that the main characteristics of blood flow in perifollicular tissue of non-dominant growing antral follicles were lower velocity and higher resistance in comparison to perifollicular blood flow of the dominant follicle. Dominant follicle undergoes remarkable changes during the last 7 days of its development. There is a marked increase of number and size of granulosa cells and increase in perifollicular blood flow in the vessels of the teca. These changes can be visualized by ultrasound as an increase in diameter and volume of the follicle [3, 71].

At the time of ovulation, the dominant follicle which has reached its maximal size ruptures, and shortly after, luteogenesis begins. Several sonographic parameters have been investigated as potential markers of ovulation:

- Disappearance of dominant follicle or sudden decrease of its size (the most frequent sign of ovulation with sensitivity of 84%)
- Increase of intrafollicular echogenicity

- Loss of follicular wall regularity
- Accumulation of free fluid in the pouch of Douglas

Doppler studies of dominant follicle in natural cycle have showed that there is a marked increase of blood flow velocity in perifollicular vessels around the time of ovulation.

4.7 Ultrasound and Medically Assisted Reproduction

Early follicular FSH is the most widely used marker of ovarian reserve although it is well-known that it has a relatively limited value in predicting ovarian response. On the other hand, markers such as anti-mullerian hormone (AMH) and antral follicle count (AFC) are today well established as one of the most reliable predictors of ovarian response to exogenous stimulation. AFC is the most verified sonographic marker, but there are also other sonographic markers that have been investigated, such as ovarian volume and ovarian stromal blood flow [72, 73].

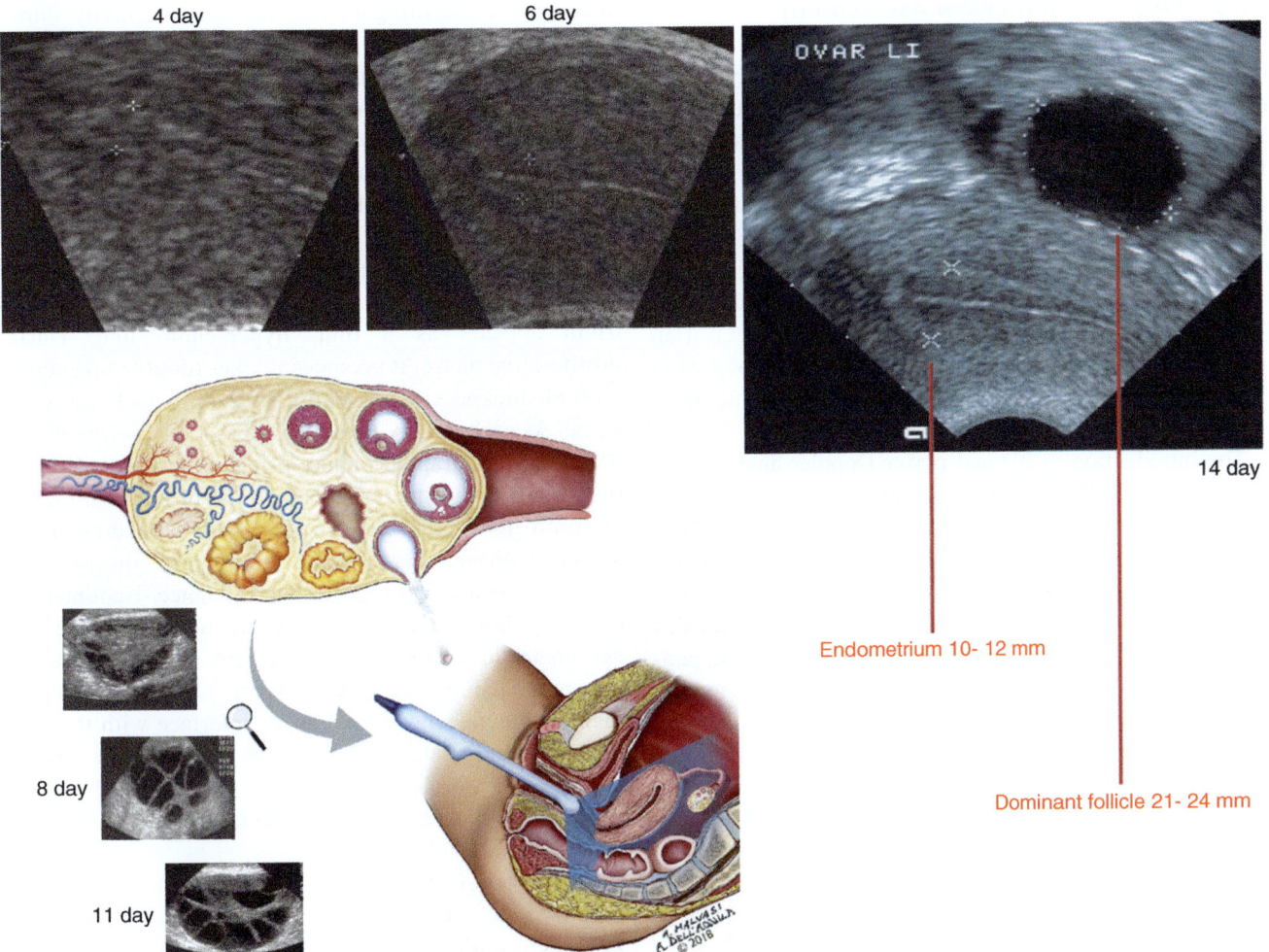

Fig. 4.21 The role of sonographic evaluation of the endometrium-A

4.7.1   Antral Follicle Count

The number of antral follicles (AFC) is a better predictor of ovarian response to controlled ovarian stimulation compared to ovarian volume or age alone: if antral follicle count is less than three, there is a significantly higher chance of cycle cancellation, detection of lower estradiol (E2) levels, and use of higher doses of gonadotropins. Recently introduced sonography-based automated volume count (SonoAVC) (Fig. 4.21) algorithm allows for automatic follicle count on ovaries recorded by ultrasound; this approach enables lower intra- and interobserver variability, reduces the risk of measurement error, and consequently, could further improve the predictive capability of AFC in women undergoing ovarian stimulation [74].

4.7.2   Ovarian Volume

Despite its early promising predictive importance, it is nowadays accepted that ovarian volume has a relatively limited predictive value of ovarian response to stimulation. Evidence of the literature and 3D ultrasound technology has shown that there was no statistically significant difference in ovarian volume between low responders and controls on day 3 of the cycle [70, 73].

4.7.3 Ovarian Blood Flow Assessment

Stromal blood flow is another aspect of ovarian physiology that was made possible to investigate with the introduction of Doppler technique [4, 52]. Commonly used parameters were stromal peak systolic velocity (PSV), pulsatility index (PI), resistance index (RI), and, lately, vascularization index (VI), flow index (FI), and vascularization flow index (VFI). Early investigations have also suggested the value of ovarian stromal blood flow parameters in predicting the success of MAR, but other have failed to prove their predictive ability. Ovarian stromal vessels are thin and torturous, and it is impossible to obtain the angle between the ultrasound beam and the intraovarian vessels accurately.

The introduction of 3D and power Doppler angiography represented significant improvement in terms of ovarian blood flow assessment. In the study using 3D ultrasound, it was demonstrated that the mean ovarian stromal flow index (FI) was an important predictor of ovarian response to controlled stimulation. Similar findings of lower VI, FI, and VFI in poor responders were confirmed in another study. In contrary to these findings, it has been shown that all three indices of vascularity (VI, FI, VFI) were significantly increased during gonadotropin stimulation in the group of normal responders compared to the low ovarian reserve group. However, only AFC and none of the blood flow indices is identified as independent predictor of ovarian response and IVF outcome [73].

4.7.4 Ultrasound Monitoring in Controlled Ovarian Stimulation

Sonographic evaluation of follicle growth and the number of follicles can influence the dose of gonadotropins as well as the timing of hCG administration for triggering final oocyte maturation.

Maturity of oocyte is closely associated with the follicle size and the serum estradiol levels. Common approaches to controlled ovarian stimulation monitoring involve baseline ultrasound and estradiol measurements. Afterwards, the approaches vary and usually combine ultrasound ultrasound and estradiol monitoring, but the target remain the same: obtaining an adequate number of follicles with the estradiol levels that are consistent with the follicle cohort (serum E2 of at least 200 pg/mL per follicle measuring ≥14 mm) [73].

4.7.5 Ultrasound Evaluation of the Endometrium

For any assisted procedure, optimally primed endometrium is essential for successful implantation. Endometrial development resulting in endometrial receptivity during the window implantation requires the subtle collaboration of an extremely large number of factors. Morphological characteristics of endometrium depend on the circulating levels of estrogen and progesterone. Transvaginal ultrasonography can provide insight to the state and development of the endometrium and the capability to be receptive for embryos. Anterior and posterior myometrial-endometrial interfaces are easily recognized in all phases of the menstrual cycle, at the end of menstrual phase, the endometrium appears as a thin, hyperechoic line. During proliferative phase, it becomes thicker (double layer endometrial thickness is normally 5–12 mm) and less echogenic. As early as day 6 and as late as 1 day before the LH peak, the sonographic picture of endometrium changes to the "triple stripe" pattern. At the time of ovulation, endometrium thickness is 10–16 mm. After ovulation, in the secretory phase, characteristic "triple strip" disappears as the consequence of progesterone influence. Endometrium becomes homogenous and hyperechoic. Thickness of endometrium increases only slightly. As a contrast to hyperechogenicity of endometrium, observer could also identify a hypoechoic band at the interface with the myometrium. Endometrial thickness is defined as the distance between the anterior and posterior stratum basalis layers. Its measurement should be performed in the sagittal plane (Fig. 4.22) [72, 73].

Endometrial thickness measurement is an essential part of evaluation of patients with fertility problems. Although multiple studies investigated the predictive value of endometrial thickness and sonographic appearance in IVF cycles, conclusions remain controversial. A recent review has shown that although frequently used cut-off of 7 mm is related to lower chance of pregnancy, the discriminatory capacity of this value in the prediction of pregnancy is virtually absent. There are also other echographic aspects of endometrium, such as homogenous appearance on the day of hCG administration and uterine artery pulsatility index higher than 3.0 that were associated with poor results of stimulated IVF/ICSI cycles. While some investigators suggested that excessive endometrial growth (greater than 14 mm) was also shown to be poor prognostic indicator, others refused this conclusion [75].

The importance of Doppler angiographic indices as tools for evaluation of endometrium has also been studied: cycle-dependent changes in uterine blood flow (VI and PI of uterine artery) are evident, but their predictive value is limited due to diurnal variations and difference between the two uterine arteries (ipsilateral or contralateral to the dominant follicle) (Fig. 4.23) [73].

Fig. 4.22 The role of
sonographic evaluation of the
endometrium-B

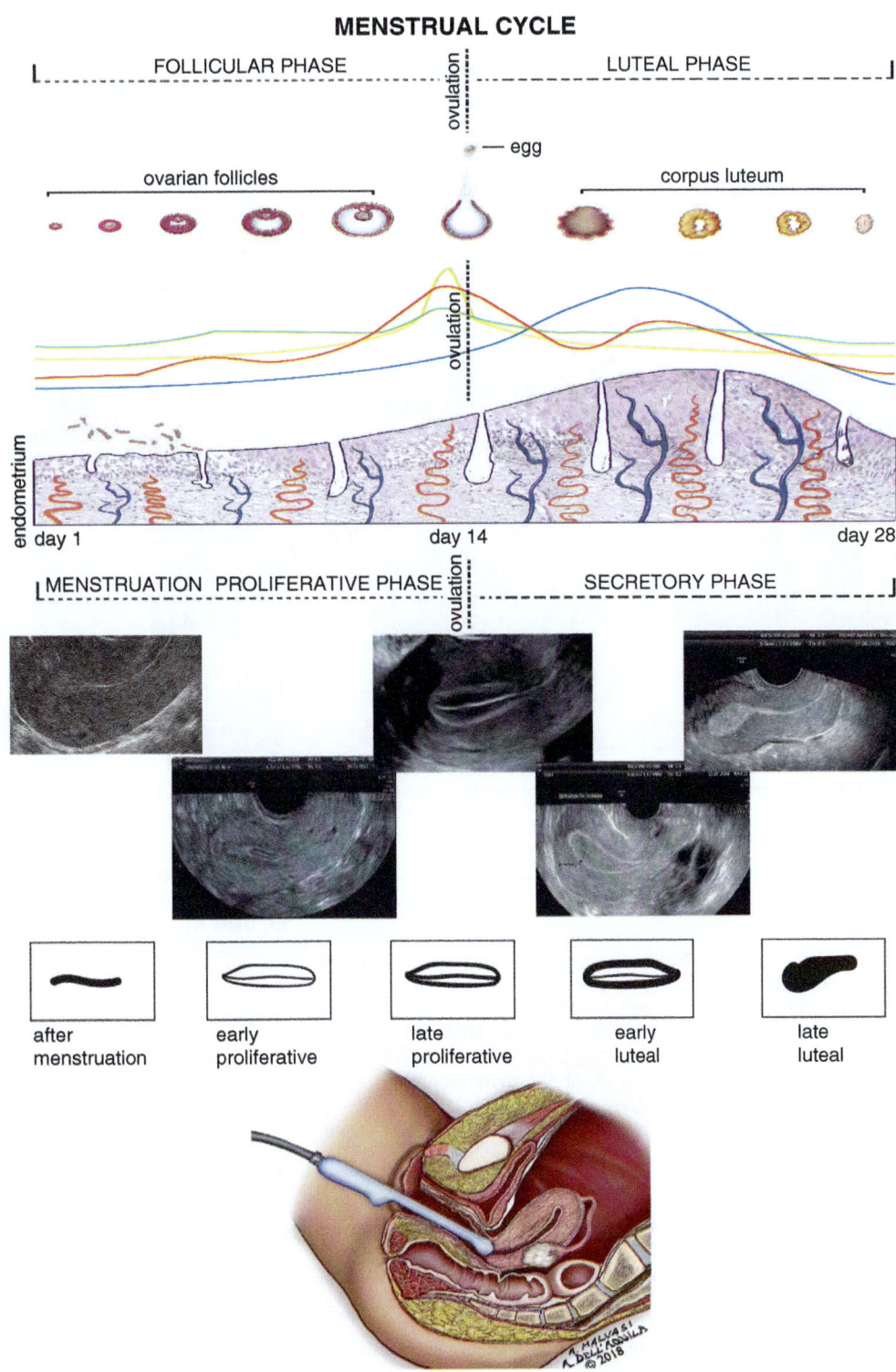

Fig. 4.22 The role of sonographic evaluation of the endometrium-B

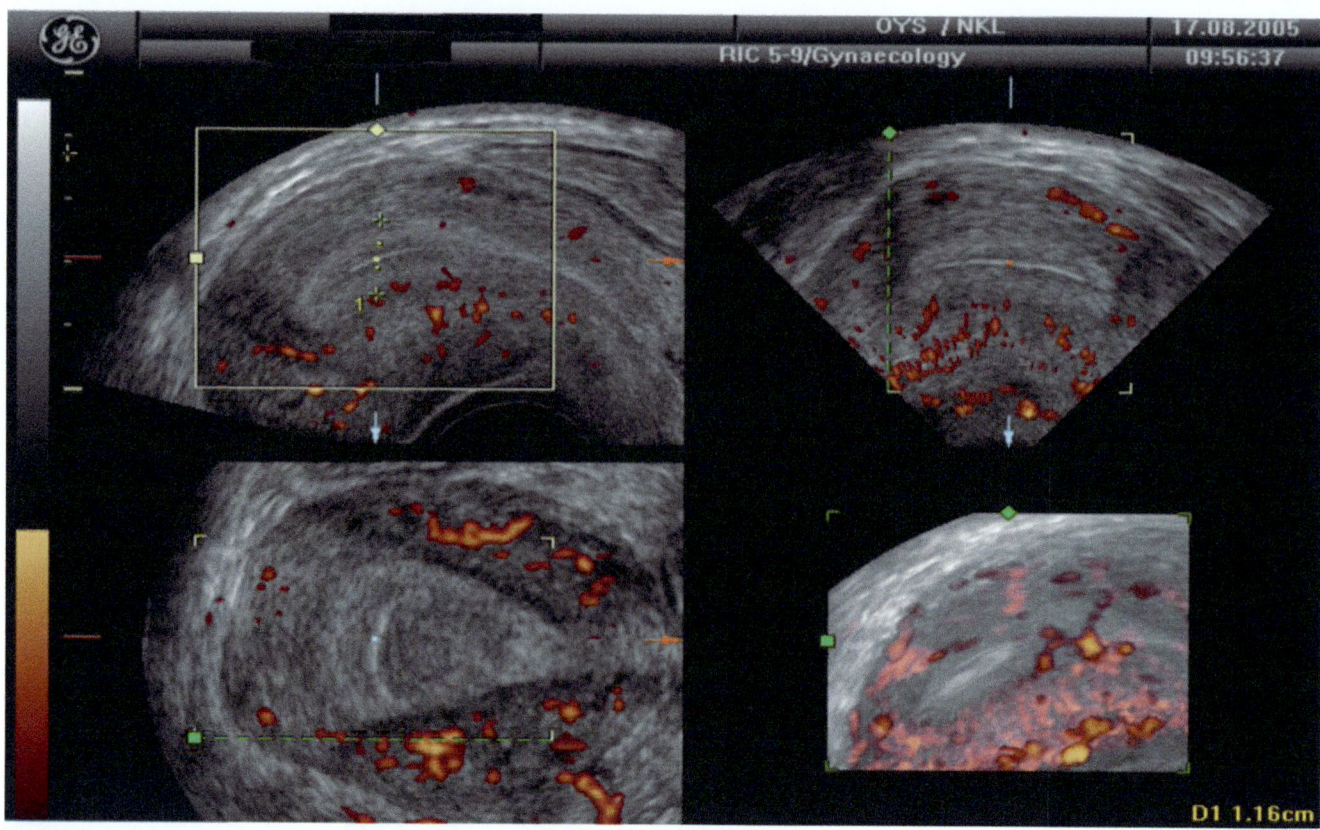

Fig. 4.23 Endometrial and subendometrial blood flows measured by 3D Power Doppler Ultrasound

References

1. Lymphol Z. Ultrasound diagnosis (sonography). Historical development, physical, principles, clinical use. Z Lymphol. 1991;15(1):26–32.
2. Zhou Q, et al. Piezoelectric single crystals for ultrasonic transducers in biomedical applications. Prog Mater Sci. 2014;66:87–111.
3. D'Addario, et al. Basic textbook of ultrasound in obstetrics and gynecology. Basic School. Jaypee; 2015.
4. Manual of diagnostic ultrasound. 2nd ed. World Health Organization.
5. Shah S, et al. Manual of ultrasound for resource-limited settings. Partners in Health.
6. Uppal T, Mogra R. RBC motion and the basis of ultrasound Doppler instrumentation. Australas J Ultrasound Med. 2010;13(1):32–4.
7. Schwippel J. The phenomenon of Doppler. Prague: Christian Doppler and the Royal Bohemian Society of Sciences; 1992. p. 46–54.
8. Zagzebski J. Essentials of ultrasound physics. Amsterdam: Mosby; 1996.
9. Carovac A, Smajlovic F, Junuzovic D. Application of ultrasound in medicine. Review. Acta Inform Med. 2011;19(3):168–71.
10. Myra K, Feldman MD, et al. US artifacts. RadioGraphics. 2009;29:1179–89.
11. Szilard J. An improved three-dimensional display system. Ultrasonics. 1974;12(6):273–6.
12. Brinkley JF, McCallum WD, Muramatsu SK, et al. Fetal weight estimation from ultrasonic three-dimensional head and trunk reconstructions: evaluation in vitro. Am J Obstet Gynecol. 1982;144(6):715–21.
13. Baba K, Satoh K. Development of the system for ultrasonic fetal three-dimensional reconstruction. Acta Obstet Gynecol Jpn. 1986;(39):1385.
14. Kurjak A, Azumendi G, Andonotopo W, Salihagic-Kadic A. Three-and-four-dimensional ultrasonography for the structural and functional evaluation of the fetal face. Am J Obstet Gynecol. 2007;1961:16–28.
15. Merz E, Macchiella D, Bahlmann F, et al. Fetale Fehlbildungs diagnostik mit Hilfeder 3D-Sonographie. Ultraschall Klin Prax. 1991;6:147.
16. Kuo HC, Chang FM, Wu CH, et al. The primary application of the three-dimensional ultrasonography in obstetrics. Am J Obstet Gynecol. 1992;166(3):880–6.
17. Baba K. Development of 3D ultrasound. Donald School J Ultrasound Obstet Gynecol. 2010;4(3):205–2015.
18. Baba K. Basis and principles of the three-dimensional ultrasound. In: Takeuchi H, Baba K, editors. Master three-dimensional ultrasound. Tokyo: Medical View; 2001. p. 12–29.
19. Merz E. 3D ultrasound in prenatal diagnosis. In: Merz E, editor. Ultrasound in obstetrics and gynecology. Vol. 1: obstetrics. Stuttgart: Thieme; 2007.
20. Merz E, Pashaj S. Current role of 3D/4D sonography in obstetrics and gynecology. Donald School J Ultrasound Obstet Gynecol. 2013;7(4):400–8.
21. Sato M, Kanenishi K, Hanaoka U, Noguchi J, Marumo G, Hata T. 4D ultrasound fetal study of fetal facial expressions at 20-24 weeks of gestation. Int J Gynaecol Obstet. 2014;126:275–9.

22. GuimaraesFilho HA, Araujo Junior E, Mello Junior CF, Nardozza LM, Moron AF. Assessment of fetal behavior using four-dimensional ultrasonography: current knowledge and perspectives. Rev Assoc Med Bras. 2013;59:507–13.
23. Albrich S, Shek K, Krahn U, Dietz H. Measurement of the subpubic arch angle by 3D translabial ultrasound and its impact on vaginal delivery. Ultrasound Obstet Gynecol. 2015, 46(4).
24. Devore GR, Polanko B. Tomographic ultrasound imaging of the fetal heart: a new technique for identifying normal and abnormal cardiac anatomy. J Ultrasound Med. 2005;24:1685–96.
25. Yagel S, Cohen SM, Rosenak D, et al. Added value of three/four-dimensional ultrasound in offline analysis and diagnosis of congenital heart disease. Ultrasound Obstet Gynecol. 2011;37:432–7.
26. Paladini D, Vassallo M, Sglavo G, Lapadula C, Martinelli P. The role of spatio-temporal image correlation (STIC) with tomographic ultrasound image (TUI) in the sequential analysis of fetal congenital heart disease. Ultrasound Obstet Gynecol. 2006;27:555–61.
27. Valsky DV, Hamani Y, Verstandig A, Yagel S. The use of 3D rendering, VCI-C, 3D power Doppler and B-flow in the evaluation of interstitial pregnancy with arteriovenous malformation treated by selective uterine artery embolization. Ultrasound Obstet Gynecol. 2007;29:352–5.
28. Vinals F, Munoz M, Naveas R, Shalper J, Giuliano A. The fetal cerebellar vermis: anatomy and biometric assessment using volume contrast imaging in the C-plane (VCI-C). Ultrasound Obstet Gynecol. 2005;26:622–7.
29. Henrich W, Stupin JH. 3D volume contrast imaging (VCI) for the visualization of placenta previa increta and uterine wall thickness in a dichorionic twin pregnancy. Ultraschall Med. 2011;32:406–11.
30. Jantarasaengaram S, Praditphol N, Tansathit T, Vipupinyo C, Vairojanavong K. Three-dimensional ultrasound with volume contrast imaging for preoperative assessment of the myometrial invasion and cervical involvement in women with endometrial cancer. Ultrasound Obstet Gynecol. 2014;43:569–74.
31. Araujo Junior E, Martinez LH, Simioni C, Martins WP, Nardozza LM, Moron AF. Delineation of vertebral area on the coronal plane using three-dimensional ultrasonography advanced volume contrast imaging (VCI) Omni view: intrarater reliability and agreement using standard mouse, high definition mouse, and pen-tablet. J Matern Fetal Neonatal Med. 2012;25:1818–21.
32. Miguelote RF, Vides B, Santos RF, Palha JA, Matias A, Sousa N. The role of the tree-dimensional imaging reconstruction to measure the corpus callosum: comparison with direct mid-sagittal views. Prenat Diagn. 2011;31:875–80.
33. Paladini D, Vassallo M, Sglavo G, Pastore G, Lapadula C, Nappi C. Normal and abnormal development of the fetal anterior fontanelle: a three-dimensional ultrasound study. Ultrasound Obstet Gynecol. 2008;32:755–61.
34. Achiron R, Gindes L, Zalel Y, Lipitz S, Weisz B. Three- and four-dimensional ultrasound: new methods for evaluating fetal thoracic anomalies. Ultrasound Obstet Gynecol. 2008;32:36–43.
35. Youssef A, Montaguti E, Sanlorenzo O, et al. A new simple technique for 3-dimensional sonographic assessment of the pelvic floor muscles. J Ultrasound Med. 2015;34:65–72.
36. Paladini D, Di SpiezioSardo A, Coppola C, Zizolfi B, Pastore G, Nappi C. Ultrasound assessment of the Essure contraceptive devices: is three-dimensional ultrasound really needed? J Minim Invasive Gynecol. 2015;22:115–21.
37. Uitternbogaard LB, Haak MC, van Vugt JM. Feasibility of automated 3-dimensional fetal cardiac screening in routine ultrasound practice. J Ultrasound Med. 2009;28:881–8.
38. Cohen L, Mangers K, Grobman WA, et al. Three-dimensional fast acquisition with sonographically based volume computer-aided analysis for imaging of the fetal heart at 18 to 22 weeks' gestation. J Ultrasound Med. 2010;29:751–7.
39. Ghi T, Contro E, Farina A, Nobile M, Pilu G. Three-dimensional ultrasound in monitoring progression of labour: a reproducibility study. Ultrasound Obstet Gynecol. 2010;36:500–6.
40. DeVore GR, Falkensammer P, Sklansky MS, Platt LD. Spatio-temporal image correlation (STIC): new technology for evaluation of the fetal heart. Ultrasound Obstet Gynecol. 2003;22:380–7.
41. Martins WP, Welsh AW, Falkensammer P, Raine-Fenning NJ. Re: spatio-temporal imaging correlation (STIC): technical notes about STIC triggering and choosing between power Doppler or high-definition color flow. Ultrasound Med Biol. 2013;39:549–50.
42. Martins WP, Welsh AW, Lima JC, Nastri CO, Raine-Fenning NJ. The "volumetric" pulsatility index as evaluated by spatiotemporal imaging correlation (STIC): a preliminary description of a novel technique, its application to the endometrium and an evaluation of its reproducibility. Ultrasound Med Biol. 2011;37:2160–8.
43. Welsh AW, Hou M, Meriki N, Martins WP. Spatiotemporal image correlation-derived volumetric Doppler impedance indices from spherical samples of the placenta: intraobserver reliability and correlation with conventional umbilical artery Doppler indices. Ultrasound Obstet Gynecol. 2012;40:431–6.
44. Miyague AH, Pavan TZ, Grillo FW, Teixeira DM, Nastri CO, Martins WP. Influence of attenuation on three-dimensional power Doppler indices and STIC volumetric pulsatility index: a flow phantom experiment. Ultrasound Obstet Gynecol. 2014;43:103–5.
45. Simioni C, Araujo Junior E, Martins WP, et al. Fetal cardiac output and ejection fraction by spatio-temporal image correlation (STIC): comparison between male and female fetuses. Rev Bras Cir Cardiovasc. 2012;27:275:282.
46. Araujo Junior E, Rolo LC, Simioni C, et al. Comparison between multiplanar and rendering modes in the assessment of fetal atrio-ventricular valve areas by 3D/4D ultrasonography. Rev Bras Cir Cardiovasc. 2012;27:472–6.
47. Abreu Barra D, Martins WP. Specific three-dimensional display modes: 3D Cine, 4D, TUI, VCI, Omniview, SonoVCAD, and STIC. In: Advanced topics on three-dimensional ultrasound in obstetrics and gynecology. 2016. p. 25–34.
48. Gibbs V, Cole D, Sassano A. Ultrasound physics and technology: how, why and when. Edinburgh: Elsevier; 2009.
49. Noble V, Nelson B, Sutingo AN. Fundamentals. Manual of emergency and critical care ultrasound. Cambridge: Cambridge University Press; 2007.
50. Garel L, Dubois J, Grignon A, Filiatrault D, Van Vliet G. US of the pediatric female pelvis: a clinical perspective. Radiographics. 2001;21:1393–407.
51. Brown DL, Zou KH, Tempany CM, et al. Primary versus secondary ovarian malignancy: imaging findings of adnexal masses in the Radiology Diagnostic Oncology Group Study. Radiology. 2001;219:213–8.
52. Fleischer A, et al. Sonography in obstetrics and gynecology, principles and practice. 6th ed. New York: McGraw Hill.
53. Brant WE. Ultrasound: the core curriculum. Philadelphia: Lippincott Williams & Wilkins; 2001.
54. Cosby K, Kendall J. Practical guide to emergency ultrasound. Philadelphia: Lippincott Williams & Wilkins; 2006.
55. Ma OJ, Mateer JR, Blaivas M. Emergency ultrasound. New York: McGraw-Hill; 2007.
56. Rumack CM, Wilson SR, Charboneau JW. Diagnostic ultrasound. 1st ed. St Louis: Mosby; 1991.
57. Mendelson EB, et al. Gynecologic imaging: comparison of transabdominal and transvaginal sonography. Radiology. 1988;166:321.
58. Tessler FN, et al. Transabdominal versus endovaginal pelvic sonography: prospective study. Radiology. 1989;170:553.

59. Council of Scientific Affairs, American Medical Association. Gynecologic sonography. Report of the ultrasonography task force. JAMA. 1991;265(21):2851–5.

60. Doubilet PM. Transvaginal sonography versus transabdominal pelvic sonography. AJR. 1999;173(3):846.

61. Timmerman D, et al. International Ovarian Tumor Analysis group. Terms, definitions, measurements to describe the sonographic features of adnexal tumors: a consensus opinion from the IOTA group. Ultrasound Obstet Gynecol. 2000;16:500–5.

62. Linee Guida SIEOG, Società Italiana di Ecografia Ostetrico Ginecologica, 2010, Editeam Editore.

63. Grunfeld L, et al. The uterus and endometrium. Clin Obstet Gynecol. 1996;39:175–87.

64. Nalaboff KM, et al. Imaging the endometrium: disease and normal variants. Radiographics. 2001;21:1409–24.

65. Leone FP, et al. Terms, definitions, measurements to describe the sonographic features of the endometrium and intrauterine lesions: a consensus opinion from the International Endometrial Tumor Analysis (IETA) group. Ultrasound Obstet Gynecol. 2010;35(1):103–12.

66. Smith-Bindman R, et al. Endovaginal ultrasound to exclude endometrial cancer and other endometrial abnormalities. JAMA. 1998;280:1510–7.

67. Ferrazzi E, et al. Sonographic endometrial thickness: a useful test to predict atrophy in patients with postmenopausal bleeding. Ultrasound Obstet Gynecol. 1996;7:315–21.

68. American college of radiology. ACR appropriateness. Criteria expert panel on women's imaging. 2005.

69. Campbell S, et al. Real time ultrasonography for determination of ovarian morphology and volume: a possible early screening test for ovarian cancer? Lancet. 1982;1:425.

70. Ferrazzi, et al. Differentiation of small adnexal masses based on morphologic characteristics of transvaginal sonographic imaging: a multicenter study. J Ultrasound Med. 2005;24:1467–73.

71. Kurjak A, Chervenak FA. Donald School Textbook of Ultrasound in obstetrics and gynecology. 4th ed. 2017.

72. De Geyter C, Schmitter M, De Geyter M, et al. Prospective evaluation of ultrasound appearance of the endometrium in a cohort of 1186 infertile women. Fertil Steril. 2000;73:106.

73. Guerriero S, Martins W, Alcazar JL, Managing Ultrasonography in Human Reproduction. A Practical Handbook, Springer International Publishing AG, 2017.

74. Raine-Fenning N, Jayaprakasan K, Clewes J, Joergner I, Bonaki SD, Chamberlain S, Devlin L, Priddle H, Johnson I., SonoAVC: a novel method of automatic volume calculation, Ultrasound Obstet Gynecol. 2008;31(6):691–6.

75. Kasius A, Smit JG, Torrance HL, Eijkemans MJC, Willem Mol B, Opmeer BC, Broekmans FMC, Endometrial thickness and pregnancy rates after IVF: a systematic review and meta-analysis, Human Reproduction Update, Vol. 20, No.4 pp. 530–541, 2014.

Oocytes Retrieval Theater

5

Domenico Baldini, Domenico Carone,
Antonino Guglielmino, and Sandro Gerli

Contents

The oocyte retrieval theater is only a small part of a larger structure that is the center of assisted reproduction.

The assisted fertilization center is a complex structure with many areas that serve very specific purposes.

In this structure, the pathways of patients and operators play a fundamental role [1]. The pathway must be studied according to the dictates of ergonomics [2–5] (Fig. 5.1).

Oocyte collection takes place in an environment where all quality and safety standards for human surgery should be guaranteed. This environment is the surgery room [6] (Figs. 5.2 and 5.3).

The surgery room, where the oocyte collection is carried out, is preferably connected to the Embryology Laboratory with an access through a window or a door. It should be located with a direct access to the operating room, in order to minimize the thermal stress of transport to the oocytes.

The dressing room must be a separate area but located within the operational theater complex [7, 8].

The area, surgery room where the egg collection takes place must be adequately equipped and include:

- Surgical bed with the possibility to tilt the patient's head downwards (Fig. 5.4)
- Supply of oxygen and the apparatus to deliver oxygen to the patient (Fig. 5.5)
- Adequate suction equipment (Fig. 5.6)
- Resuscitation equipment and medications
- Availability of the electrocardiography and pulse oximeter
- Availability to specialized equipment necessary for continuous patient care

D. Baldini (✉)
Center for Medically Assisted Procreation, MOMO' fertiLIFE, Bisceglie, Italy

D. Carone
Clinica Eugin, Taranto, Italy

A. Guglielmino
Hera U.M.R. Unit of Reproductive Medicine, Catania, Italy

S. Gerli
Department of Obstetrics and Gynaecology, University of Perugia, Perugia, Italy
e-mail: sandro.gerli@unipg.it

© Springer Nature Switzerland AG 2020
A. Malvasi, D. Baldini (eds.), *Pick Up and Oocyte Management*, https://doi.org/10.1007/978-3-030-28741-2_5

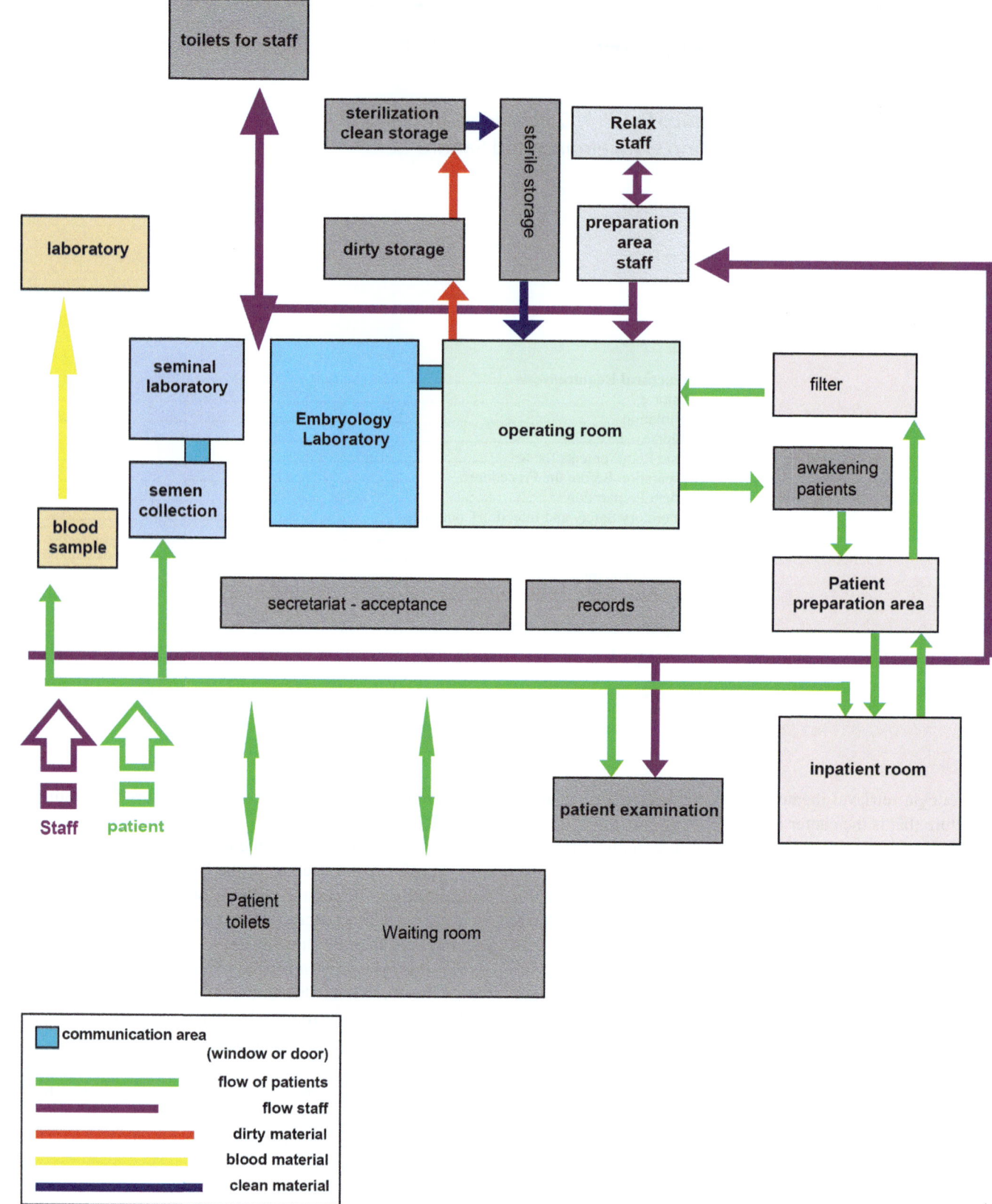

Fig. 5.1 In this drawing is represented an IVF center and the work flows of patients and staff

Fig. 5.2 Schematic representation of the surgery room for oocyte retrieval with gynecologist and anesthesiologist; low ultrasound and aspirator, right respirator, high table servant and sink

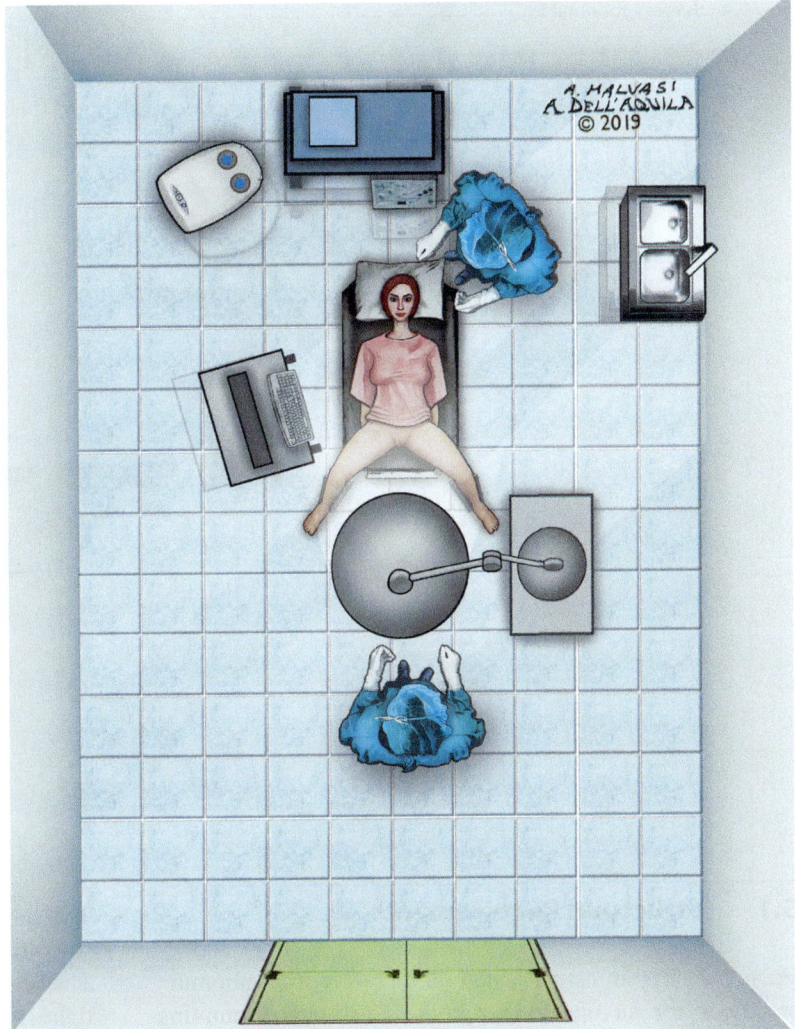

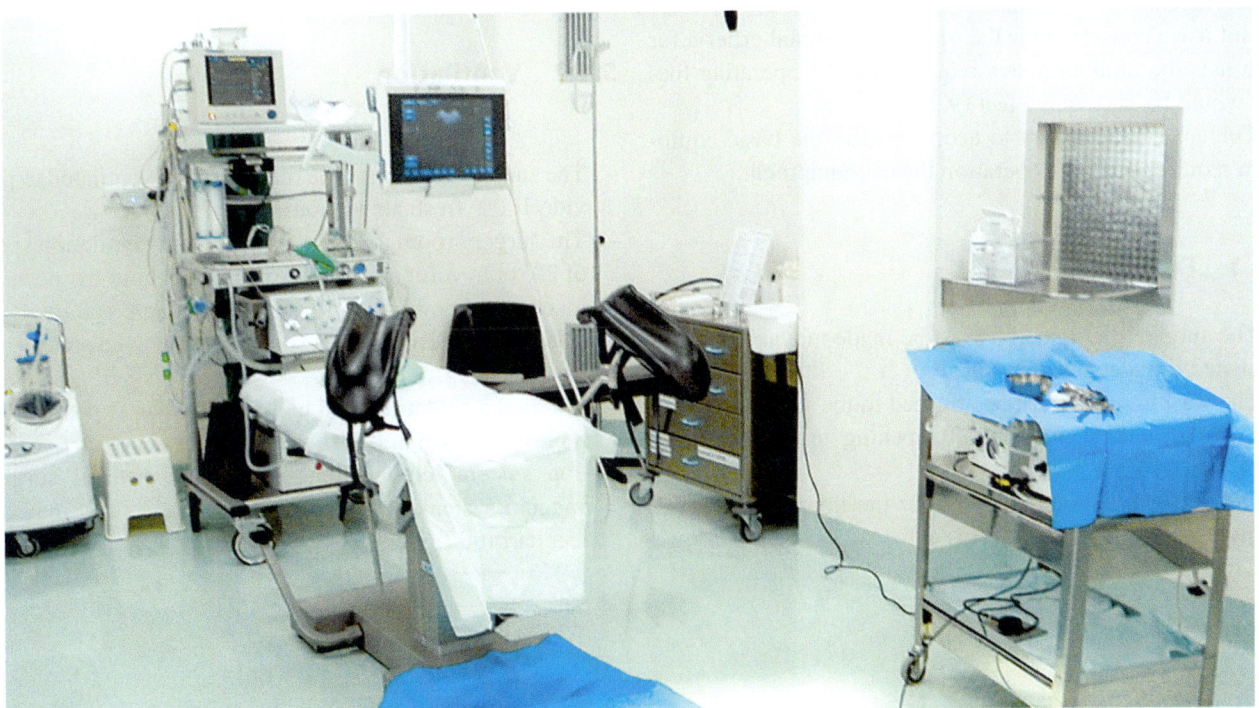

Fig. 5.3 Theater of oocyte retrieval

Fig. 5.4 Surgery room table

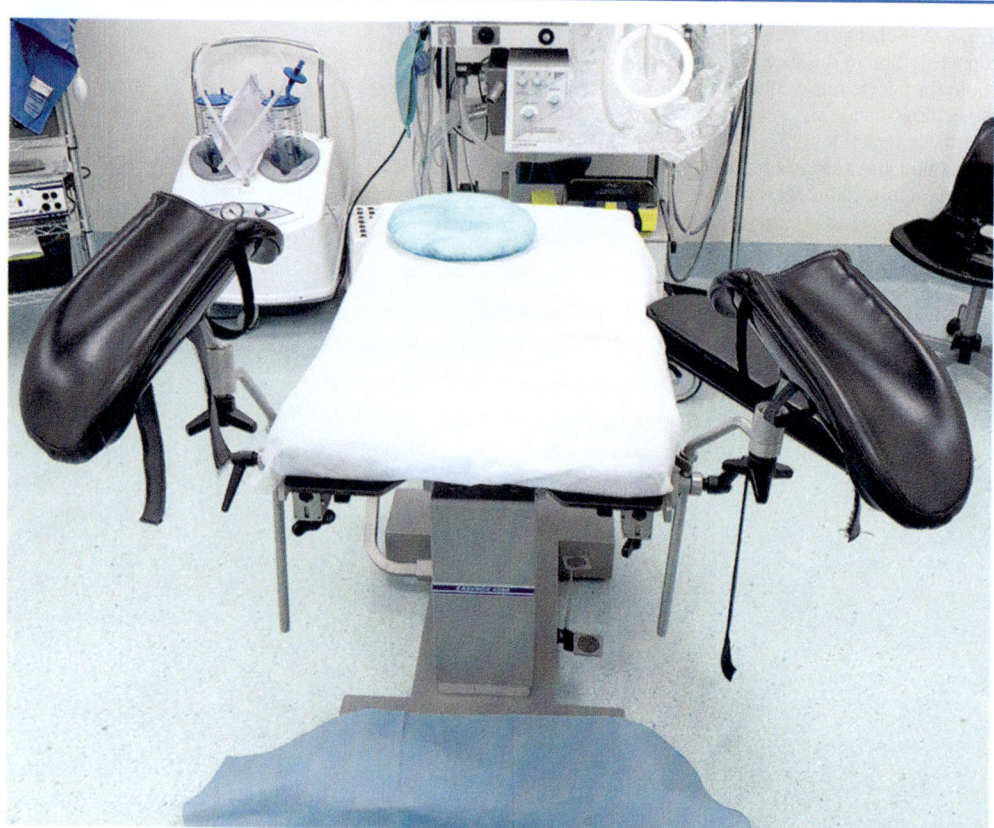

5.1 Structural Requirements

Each state has an own legislation; therefore, the minimum standards for an operating room where oocyte sampling takes place are often different from each other, and, in some cases, there is no constraint.

But if we consider only the minimum optimal criteria for such use, the minimum area required for the operating theater would be 100 square feet (9.29 m²).

This area is necessary to accommodate the basic equipment required for ART operation theater equipment.

5.1.1 Features

– The surgical light source must be made movable or connected for adequate exposure.
– The washing area must be attached to the surgery.
– There should be no sunlight opening in the operating theater.
– Durable vinyl should be used for the floor with a minimum height of 10 in. (10 cm) at the edges.

– The interior finishes of the operating theater should be smooth, seamless, and uninterrupted.
– The operation theater should have a seamless ceiling with lights to prevent particles above the ceiling from having direct access to the area of the operating theater.

5.1.2 Ventilation

– The surgery room must be mechanically ventilated to provide 100% fresh air without recirculation.
– The surgery room must have a minimum ventilation speed of 20 room volumes of air exchange per hour by means of mechanical power supply and air discharge system.
– These characteristics are used to minimize the presence of particles (Fig. 5.7).
– External air inlets should be located as far as possible but no less than 7.6 m (23 ft) from the outlets of any ventilation system, combustion equipment, medical surgical vacuum system, or hydraulic venting areas that may collect harmful fumes.

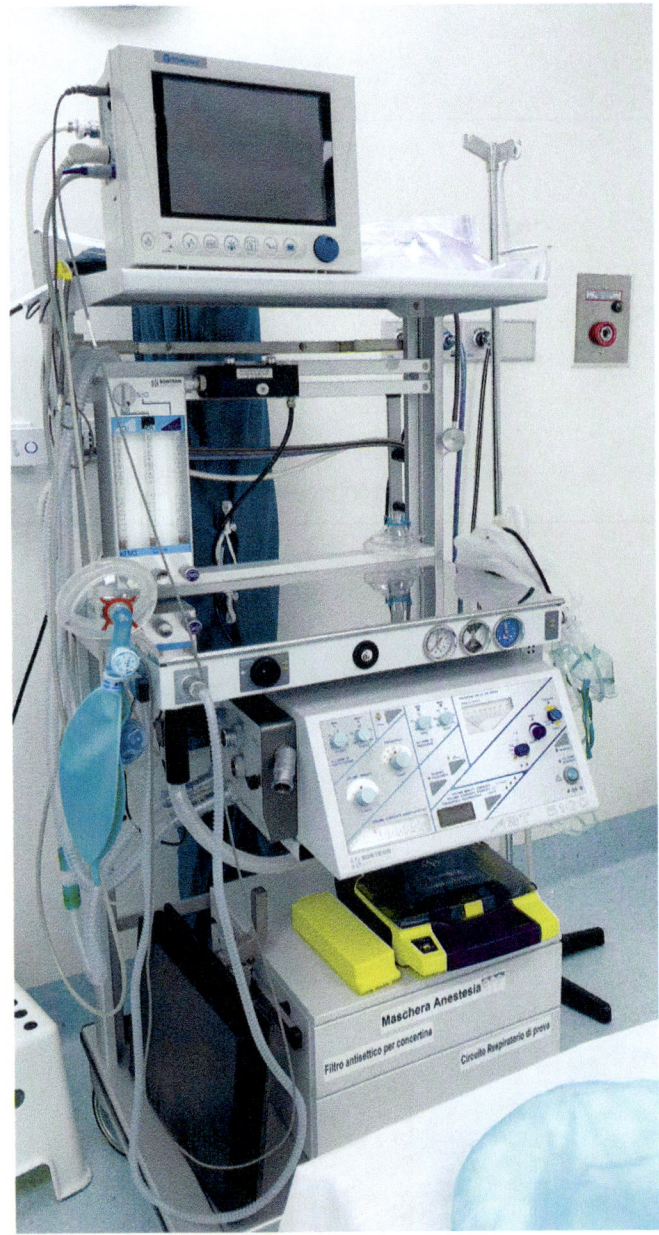

Fig. 5.5 Supply of oxygen and the apparatus to deliver oxygen to the patient

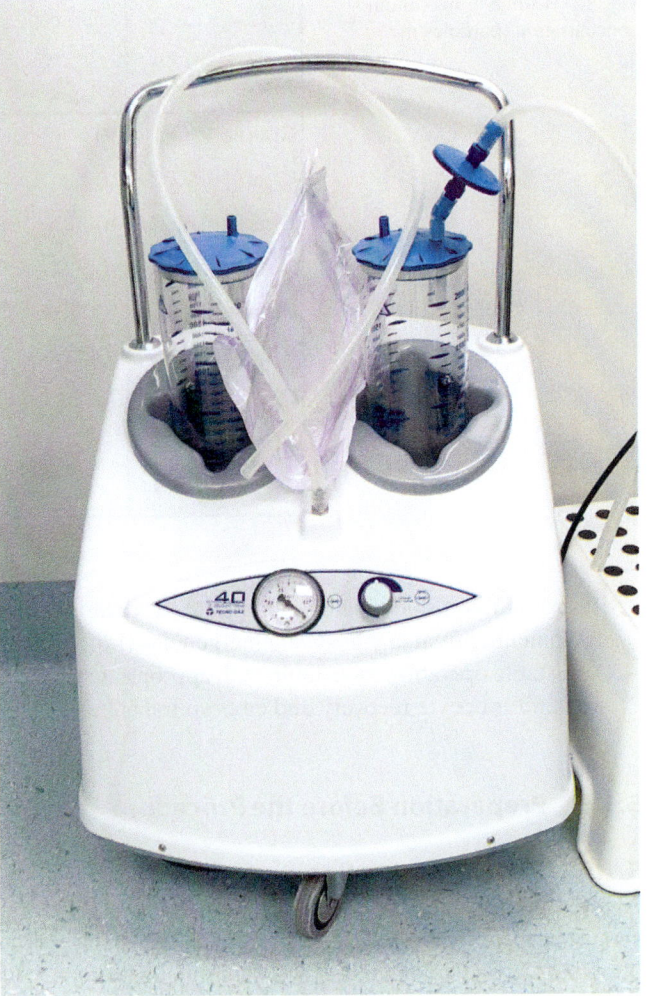

Fig. 5.6 Adequate suction equipment

It must be able to facilitate and resist frequent cleaning and disinfection.

5.1.4 Basic Requirements for Art

– A 2-D ultrasound machine for transvaginal and transabdominal scanning with the availability of a needle biopsy guideline connected to a TV monitor for transvaginal oocyte retrieval.
– Oocyte recovery system with a suction system and tube warmer connected to it to keep the tubes at 37 °C during the procedure.
– Patient monitoring must be present—oximetry monitoring and continuous monitoring of blood pressure (BP) and pulse rate (PR).

– The lower part of the outside air intake should be located high up, but not less than 3 ft (0.9 m) above the ground level or if installed through the roof, not less than 3 ft (0.9 m) above the roof level.

5.1.3 Climate

The temperature of the operating theater must be kept at 24–26 °C.

Fig. 5.7 Limits of maximum concentration (particles/m³ air)

	Limits of maximum concentration (particles / m³ air)					
	0,1 μm	0,2 μm	0,3 μm	0,5 μm	1 μm	5 μm
Classe ISO 1	10	2				
Classe ISO 2	100	24	10	4		
Classe ISO 3	1000	237	102	35	8	
Classe ISO 4	10000	2370	1020	352	83	
Classe ISO 5	100000	23700	10200	3520	832	29
Classe ISO 6	1000000	237000	102000	35200	8320	293
Classe ISO 7				352000	83200	2930
Classe ISO 8				3520000	832000	29300
Classe ISO 9				35200000	8320000	293000

- Resuscitation trolley with appropriate medication and equipment to treat any medical emergencies (Fig. 5.8).
- Adjustable operating room table with appropriate surgical session for oocyte recovery and embryo transfer.

5.1.5 Preparation Before the Procedure

5.1.5.1 Patient Preparation

A consent form must be signed by the patient and a copy should be kept in the patient's records for any ART procedure that the patient and/or the couple are to undergo.

5.1.5.2 Laboratory Safety and Infection Control

- Pairs treated should be subjected to appropriate infectious disease screening and quarantine to ensure that gametes and embryos are free from infectious diseases. The minimum diseases to be screened are HIV1, HIV2, hepatitis B, and syphilis. HIV-positive patients are referred to the appropriate medical specialist for further treatment. Syphilis carriers are treated with the appropriate antibiotic before proceeding with ART.
- HIV and hepatitis carriers should be listed as the last case and the operating room should then be closed and cleaned using the standard hospital procedure for such cases. Laboratory staff should manage all gametes from these patients using the standard double-acting technique in addition to aseptic techniques.
- Gametes should be incubated separately from those of other patients.

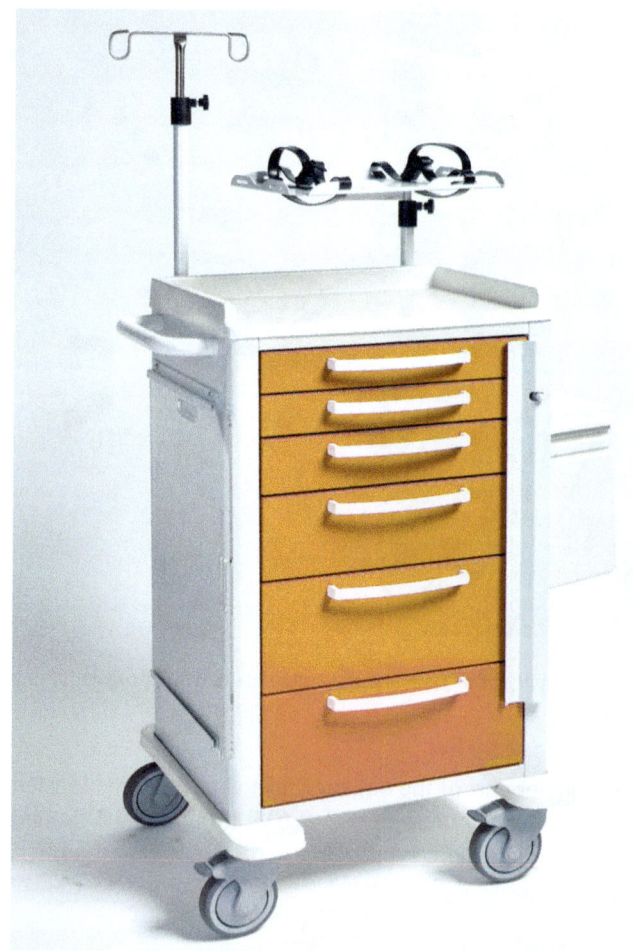

Fig. 5.8 Resuscitation trolley with appropriate medication and equipment to treat any medical emergencies

5.1.6 Biosafety

– To protect the safety of gametes, only authorized personnel may enter the laboratory or storage area. Security measures should be in place to prevent unauthorized access.
– All gametes and embryos containers must be properly labeled and registered.
– All disposable gametes management devices should be used only once.
– All storage containers should be locked and stored in secure facilities.

5.1.7 Outpatient Surgery Room

5.1.7.1 General Principles [9, 10]

• Patient is scheduled for surgery (collecting the egg) and has previously been informed of the procedure to be sure of understanding the instructions on how to prepare for surgery.
• In performing the tasks necessary for outpatient surgery, OR specialists must coordinate their work to provide a safe and efficient environment for the patient.
• Definition of Circulator: The OR team technician who works outside the sterile field during surgery.
• Definition of Scrub: The OR team technician who washes, wears sterile shirts and gloves, and functions within the sterile area.
• Lack of coordination (or teamwork) causes errors, misunderstandings among staff and loss of time. Considering the relevance of the care given to the patient in the operating room, each of these results can have disastrous consequences for the patients.
• Professional staff (circulator and scrub) are responsible for developing a systematic method (work plan) for operational procedures.
• Methods for performing procedures may vary among specialists, but the rules for observing aseptic technique as well as the circulatory and scrub functions are common to each operating procedure. The operating room specialist can be assigned to perform functions such as the circulator or scrub during a surgical procedure.

The surgical team is a group of people in the operating room during a surgical procedure.

This group includes the surgeon (specialist O and G trained in ART), an assistant (the nurse or specialist to exercise the scrub functions), the anesthetist, and the nurse or specialist to exercise the functions in circulation.

All team members work together to provide the best possible care to the patient. Any work done in the operating room, no matter how small, contributes to the patient's wellbeing. No job is so important as to account only for the recovery of the patient.

5.1.8 Circulator Duties

To work efficiently during a surgical procedure, the circulator must be familiar with the routine established in the operating room. He should know the instruments, equipment, and supplies—including the supplies needed to position the patient—to enable them to provide the appropriate items. He should also know their location to avoid wasting time in obtaining them. The functions performed by the circulator are routine. Additional functions can be assigned to him/her by the professional members of the operating team.

The defined routines are established for the preparation of an operating room for surgery:

• The circulator is at a safe distance from the sterile field when adjusting the light on it.
• He should never enter the sterile field to perform tasks and must keep the extra supplies needed or allow the scrub to reach them.
• When moving a sterile table, the circulator grasps the table legs well below the table above and below the sterile curtains.
• The circulator "flips" the sterile material on the rear table.
• He switches on the ceiling light to ensure correct operation.
• He should check that the operating table is working properly, with particular attention to the set of instruments for collecting the eggs.
• Finally, the circulator should check:
  – The vacuum pump (to provide a low flow for general suction) and in particular the control of:
      The correct activation of the vacuum response pedal on the needle tip.
      If the pump maintains a vacuum at its set level.
      If the LED displays the vacuum pressure in mmHg (pressure).
      Pipe pre-heating unit (temperature).
  – Other equipment (such as electrosurgical units, etc.)

Fig. 5.9 Surgical table for oocytes retrieval

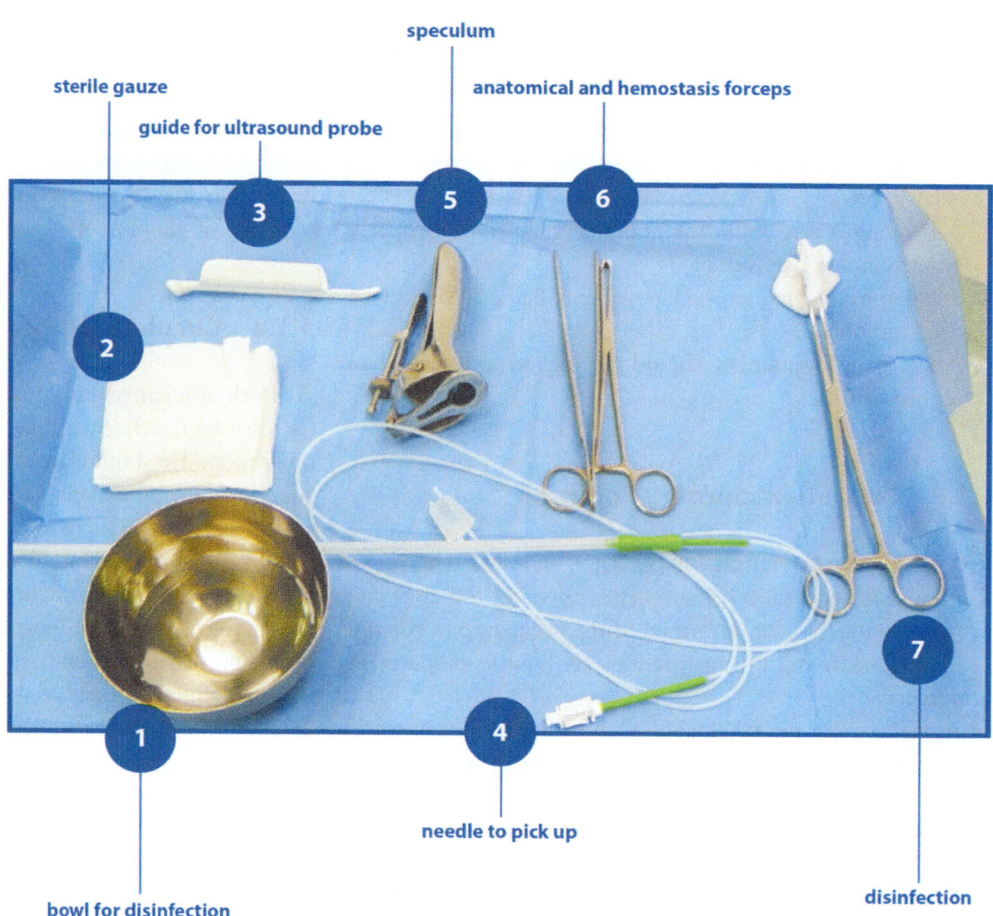

speculum

sterile gauze

guide for ultrasound probe

anatomical and hemostasis forceps

needle to pick up

bowl for disinfection

disinfection

5.2   Preparation of the Prep Set

Most centers use disposable preparation sets.

When disposable ready-made sets are not used, the preparation of the set is the same.

The circulator has opened the preparation set and checked the sterilized indicator for sterilization.

He places the objects on the surgical (Fig. 5.9) preparation table—speculum, sponges, sponge bowl, sponge pliers (Foerster-Ballenger Forceps Sponge), hemostatic pliers and prep cup (metal cup for antiseptic or physiological solution). He places the preparation gloves on the preparation table with a towel resting on them. Once the circulator has poured physiological solution into the sponge bowl, moisten a sponge and clean the dust from the glove.

5.3   Scrub Area

A washing area (Fig. 5.10) should be located between the operating room [11–13] and the laboratory and should be opened directly in an operating room. Sinks should be deep enough, at least one foot, so that water is not sprayed on clothing, floor, hands, and arms during the procedure. Sinks should be equipped with hot and cold water taps which should be controlled by knee levers or levers. If arm or hand levers are to be used, these controls should be adjusted for the flow of water temperature before rubbing. If the hands or arms of the specialist accidentally touch the faucets or sink during any phase after the start of the scrub, it will become contaminated and the washing cycle should resume [14, 15].

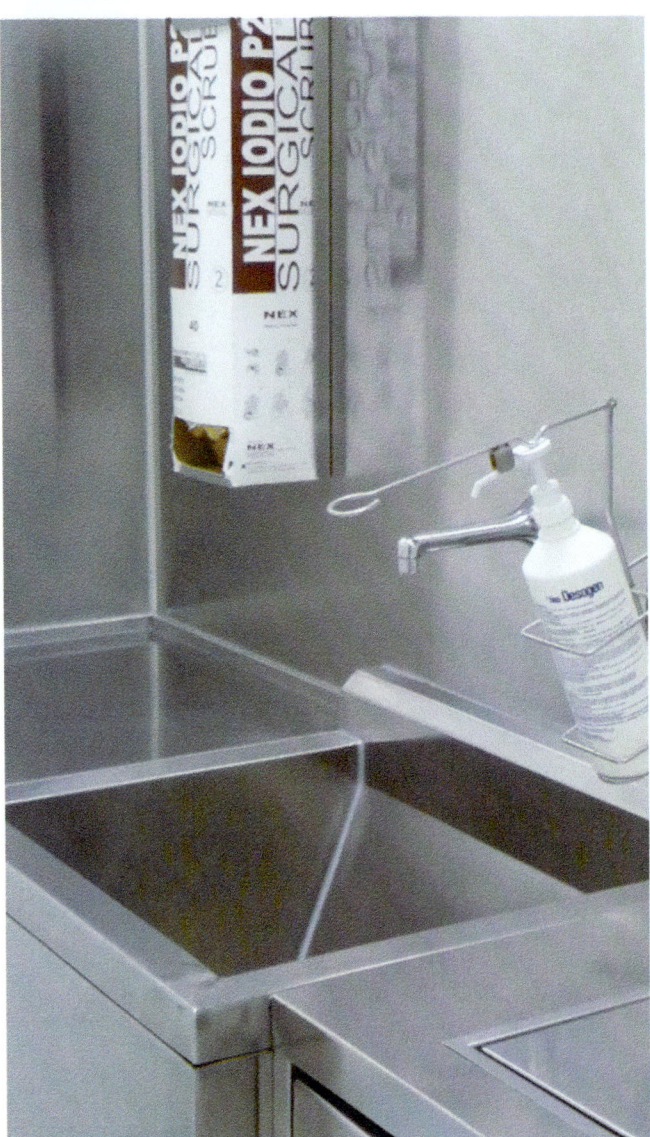

Fig. 5.10 Washing area

The containers for surgical cleaners (disinfectant and MEA IVF-tested detergent) are placed between two sinks. Pedal-operated pedals attached to the containers provide a convenient method of dispensing detergents without contaminating the hands. Brushes (depending on the type used) can be placed in dispensers, one between the two sinks.

References

1. Nielsen K, Cleal B. Predicting flow at work: investigating the activities and job characteristics that predict flow states at work. J Occup Health Psychol. 2010;15(2):180–90.
2. Berguer R. The applications of ergonomics in the work environment of general surgeons. Rev Environ Health. 1997;12(2):99–106.
3. Berguer R, Forkey DL, Smith WD. Ergonomic problems associated with laparoscopic surgery. Surg Endosc. 1999;13:466–8.
4. Berguer R. Surgical technology and the ergonomics of laparoscopic instruments. Surg Endosc. 1998;12:458–62.
5. Berguer R. Ergonomics in the operating room. Am J Surg. 1996;171:385–6.
6. Stahl JE, Egan MT, Goldman JM, Tenney D, Wiklund RA, Sandberg WS, Gazelle S, Rattner DW. Introducing new technology into the operating room: measuring the impact on job performance and satisfaction. Surgery. 2005;137(5):518–26.
7. Ulrich RS. View through a window may influence recovery from surgery. Science. 1994;224:420–1.
8. Ulrich RS. Effects of health cave interior design on wellness: theory and recent scientific research. In: Marberry SO, editor. Innovations in healthcare design. New York: Van Nostrand Reinhold; 1995. p. 88–104.
9. Rosenstein AH. Measuring and managing the economic impact of disruptive behaviors in the hospital. J Healthc Risk Manag. 2010;30(2):20–6.
10. Markovic G, Jaric S. Movement performance and body size: the relationship for different groups of tests. Eur J Appl Physiol. 2004;92(1–2):139–49.
11. AIA. Guidelines for design and construction—hospital and healthcare facilities, 1996/97. Washington, DC; 1997.
12. Burrows M, et al. Management for hospital doctors. Oxford: Butterworth-Heinemann; 1994.
13. Cox A, Groves P. Design for health care. London: Butterworth; 1981.
14. Selmanovic S, Ramic E, Pranjic N, Brekalo-Lazarevic S, Pasic Z, Alic A. Stress at work and burnout syndrome in hospital doctors. Med Arh. 2011;65(4):221–4.
15. Baldini D, Lavopa C, Vizziello G, Sciancalepore AG, Malvasi A. The safe use of the transvaginal ultrasound probe for transabdominal oocyte retrieval in patients with vaginally inaccessible ovaries. Front Womens Health. 2018;3(2):1–3.

Hysteroscopy Before Oocytes Retrieval

Giuseppe Trojano, Vita Caroli Casavola, Antonio Malvasi,
Sergio Haimovich, Alessandro Favilli, and Ettore Cicinelli

Contents

The introduction of in vitro fertilization in the late 1970s resulted in the continuous development of reproductive medicine by innovative techniques to solve the various causes of couples' sterility.

Common causes of infertility and sterility are endometritis, genetic abnormalities, congenital or acquired uterine malformation, endocrine dysfunction, thrombophilic disorders, autoimmune diseases, incompetent cervix, luteal phase defect, certain infections, and sperm DNA abnormalities.

This chapter reviews the structural uterine and endometrial causes of infertility and sterility and highlights the important role of office hysteroscopy in the diagnosis and treatment of uterine pathologies associated with infertility and sterility.

G. Trojano (✉)
Department of Obstetrics and Gynaecology, ASM Matera, Bari, Italy

V. Caroli Casavola
UOSD Gynecologic Oncology—Ente Ecclesiastico Ospedale Generale Regionale "F. Miulli", Bari, Italy

A. Malvasi
Department of Obstetrics and Gynecology, GVM Care and Research Santa Maria Hospital, Bari, Italy

Laboratory of Human Physiology, Phystech BioMed School, Faculty of Biological and Medical Physics, Moscow Institute of Physics and Technology (State University), Dolgoprudny, Russia

S. Haimovich
Hille Yaffe Medical Center Israel, Hadera, Israel

A. Favilli
Department of Obstetrics and Gynaecology, USL 1 Umbria, Alta Valle del Tevere Hospital, Città di Castello, PG, Italy

E. Cicinelli
Department of Obstetrics and Gynaecology, AOU Policlinico University Hospital, Bari, Italy

6.1 Introduction

The introduction of in vitro fertilization in the late 1970s lead to a continuous development of reproductive medicine with the introduction of innovative techniques to solve the various causes of couples' sterility.

Infertility and sterility are caused by several etiopathogenetic factors, such as: genetic abnormalities, endocrine dysfunctions, thrombophilic disorders, autoimmune diseases,

© Springer Nature Switzerland AG 2020
A. Malvasi, D. Baldini (eds.), *Pick Up and Oocyte Management*, https://doi.org/10.1007/978-3-030-28741-2_6

endometriosis, incompetent cervix, luteal phase defect, certain infections, and sperm DNA abnormalities.

The work up of patients affected by infertility and sterility includes congenital malformation (bicornuate, didelphic, septate, and unicornuate uterus) acquired defects (fibroids, adenomas, adhesions, and polyps) and chronic endometrial (CE) infection.

Suspected congenital malformations may emerge during transvaginal ultrasound procedures and are subsequently confirmed by diagnostic hysteroscopy. Acquired defects may also be suspected during transvaginal ultrasound, but their diagnosis is based on histological findings. On the other hand, hysteroscopy rather than ultrasound is needed to suspect CE with subsequent diagnosis being confirmed by histological findings. For this reason, hysteroscopy plays an important diagnostic role in uterine sterility factor [1].

6.2 Hysteroscopic Technique and Instruments

Current hysteroscopic techniques allow both diagnosis and treatment of uterine cavity diseases [2].

Traditional hysteroscopy was only a diagnostic technique considered as a painful procedure due to frequent vasovagal reaction. Often it required analgesia and was performed into operating room (Fig. 6.1) [3].

Technological improvement has resulted in hysteroscopy to become an operative outpatient procedure performed without analgesia.

Diagnostic hysteroscopy is now performed with a vaginoscopic approach, without speculum, using a saline solution at low pressure for distending the uterine cavity and a mini-hysteroscopy (3.5 mm or less in size) ensuring only minimal patients' discomfort [4].

It has been shown that fiberoptic-hysteroscopes offer several advantages over the lens-based instruments (first of all they are more resistant) but they cannot yet match the image quality of a rod-lens-based telescope system [5].

Operative instruments have also been miniaturized (5F forceps and a bipolar coaxial electrode) allowing a "see-and-treat" approach [6] and many uterine cavity diseases (biopsy, polypectomy, synechiae, septum) can be treated by office hysteroscopy immediately after diagnosis using operative hysteroscopes sized 5 mm equipped with a 5F operative canal (Fig. 6.2) [7].

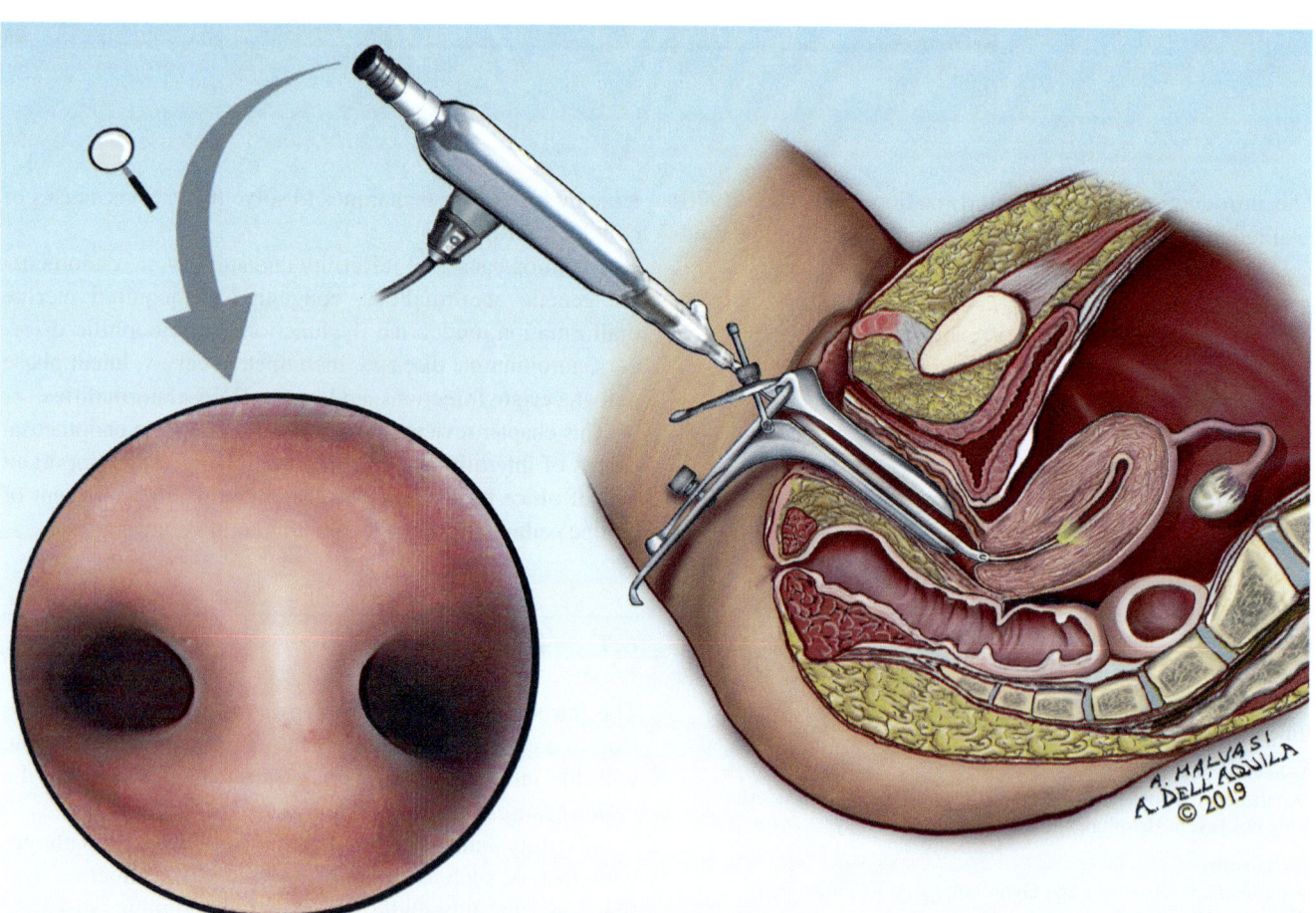

Fig. 6.1 Schematic representation of hysteroscopy in a case of Asherman's syndrome

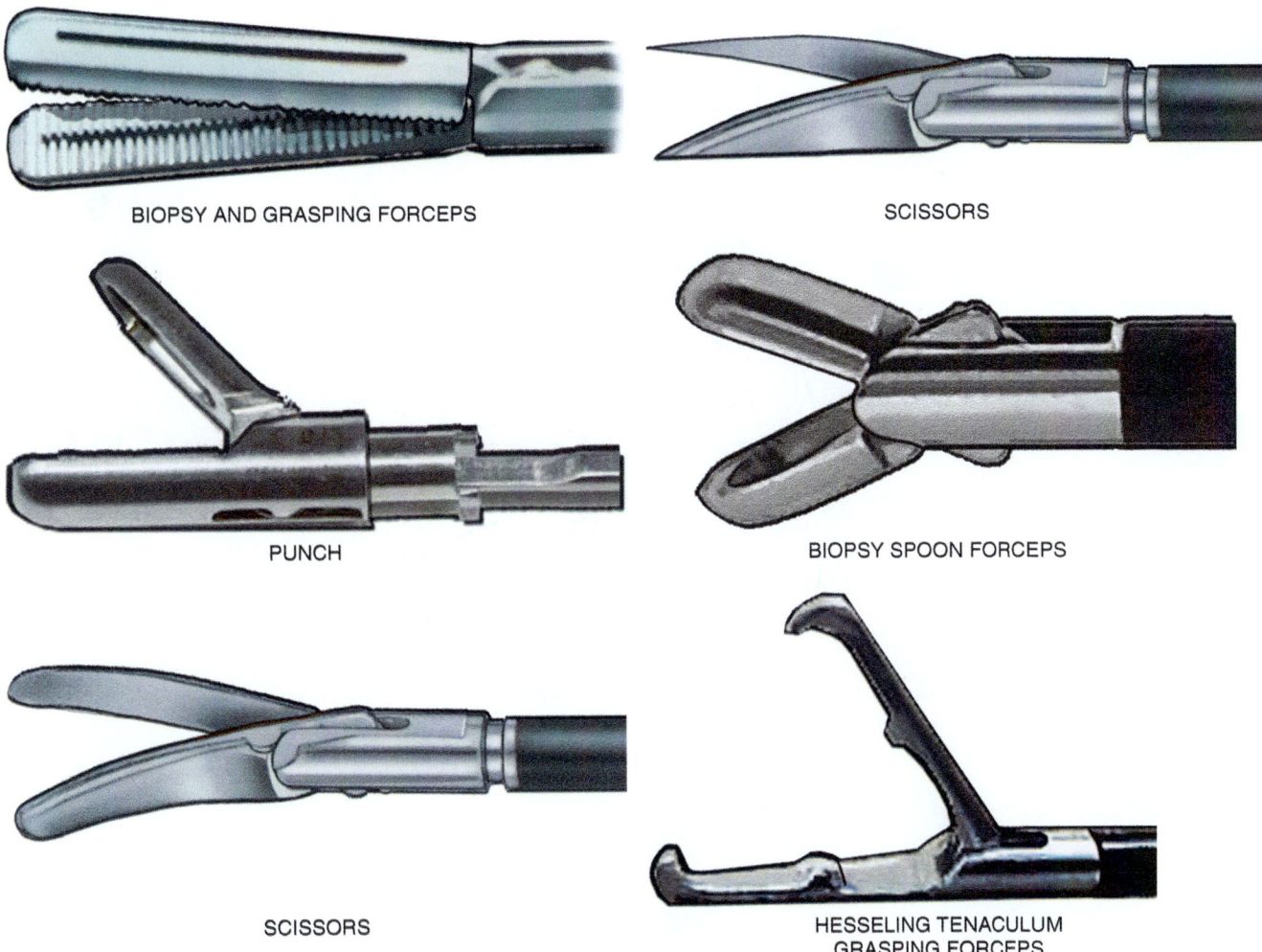

Fig. 6.2 List of surgical instruments that can be used in an operative hysteroscopy

6.3 Asherman's Syndrome

The presence of acquired intrauterine adhesions is known as Asherman's syndrome (Figs. 6.3, 6.4, and 6.5). Potential causes include intrauterine retention of post-abortion or postpartum material and post-abortion curettage or endometrial infections [8].

Asherman's syndrome may be totally asymptomatic or it may cause hypomenorrhea, secondary amenorrhea, pelvic pain, and hematometra. Intrauterine adhesions could cause infertility or pregnancy loss [9].

For the Asherman's syndrome's diagnosis, a combination of ultrasound (2D and 3D) and hysteroscopy is needed. It is mandatory to perform a mapping of synechiae to avoid inadvertent uterus perforation during hysteroscopy. The American Society for Reproductive Medicine (ASRM) identifies three different types of Asherman's syndrome on the basis of: characteristics of

the menstrual flow, type of synechiae, and portion of uterine cavity obliterated.

The gold standard treatment of Asherman's syndrome is office hysteroscopy, which consists of a surgical adhesiolysis performed without general or regional anesthesia [10, 11]. IUD Foley catheter or Cook intrauterine splint can be used to recurrences of synechiae [12].

Approximately 70–90% of patients with hypomenorrhea or amenorrhea return to have a regular menses after hysteroscopic adhesiolysis showing an improvement of pregnancy rate and rate of live births [13].

6.4 Müllerian Anomalies

An impaired median fusion of Müllerian ducts during embryonic life causes anatomical abnormalities of the female genital tract, known as Müllerian anomalies. Müllerian anomalies are more prevalent in infertile than in sterile patients [14] and are associated with recurrent (41%) miscarriages [15].

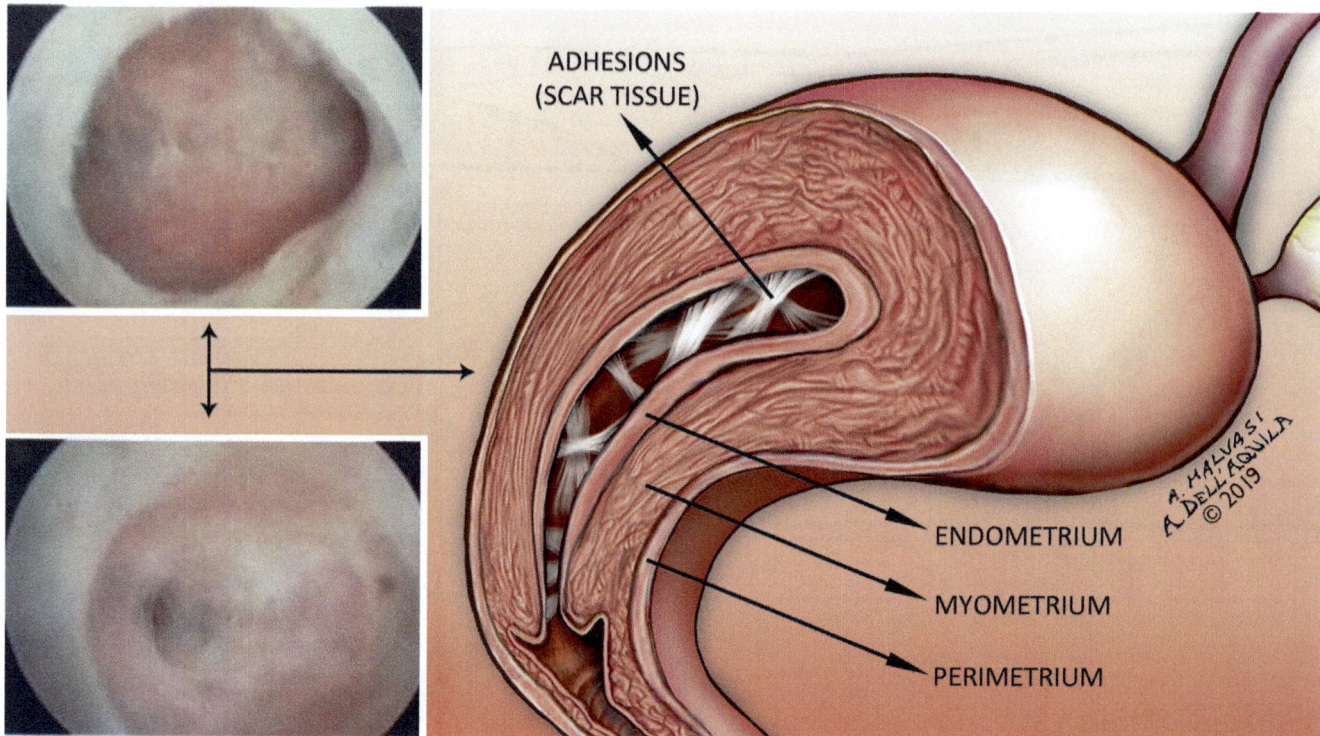

Fig. 6.3 Asherman's syndrome

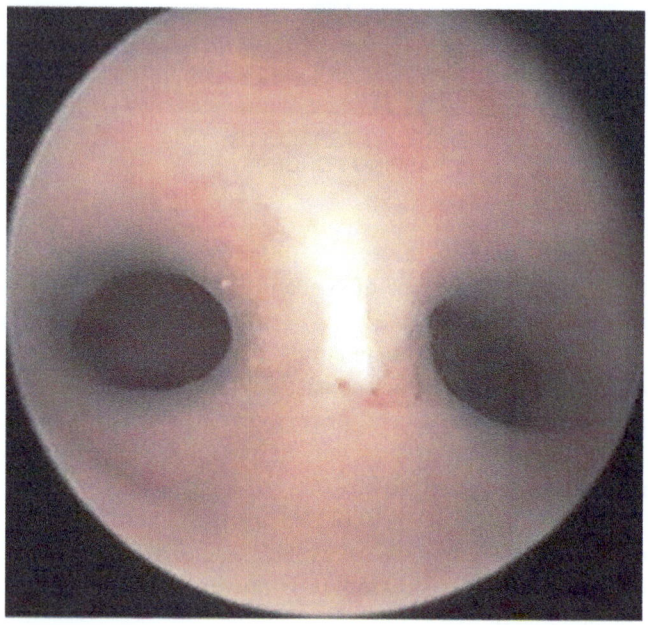

Fig. 6.4 Asherman's syndrome

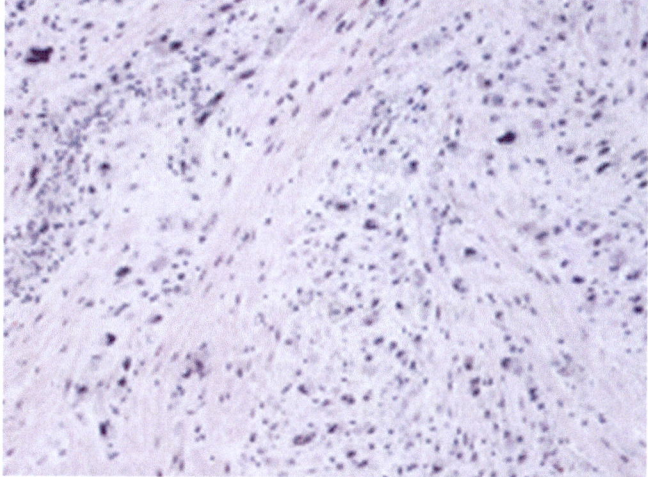

Fig. 6.5 Asherman's syndrome: anatomopathological evaluation

Since 2013 the ESHRE/ESGE classification system has divided Müllerian anomalies into seven main classes (from U0 to U6), describing uterine anatomical deviations of the same embryological origin (Fig. 6.6). Anatomical varieties expressing different clinical significance, within main classes, have been divided into subclasses. Cervical and vag-inal anomalies are classified independently into subclasses having clinical significance [16].

The most common Müllerian anomaly is the septate uterus, with the worse reproductive outcome and poor obstetrical out-comes, including malpresentation, preterm delivery, intrauter-ine growth restriction, placental abruption, and perinatal mortality. This is due to its own histological features present-ing poorly vascularized fibrous tissue and subatrophic endo-metrium [17]. Before any surgical intervention, it is mandatory to perform an accurate differential diagnosis between septate,

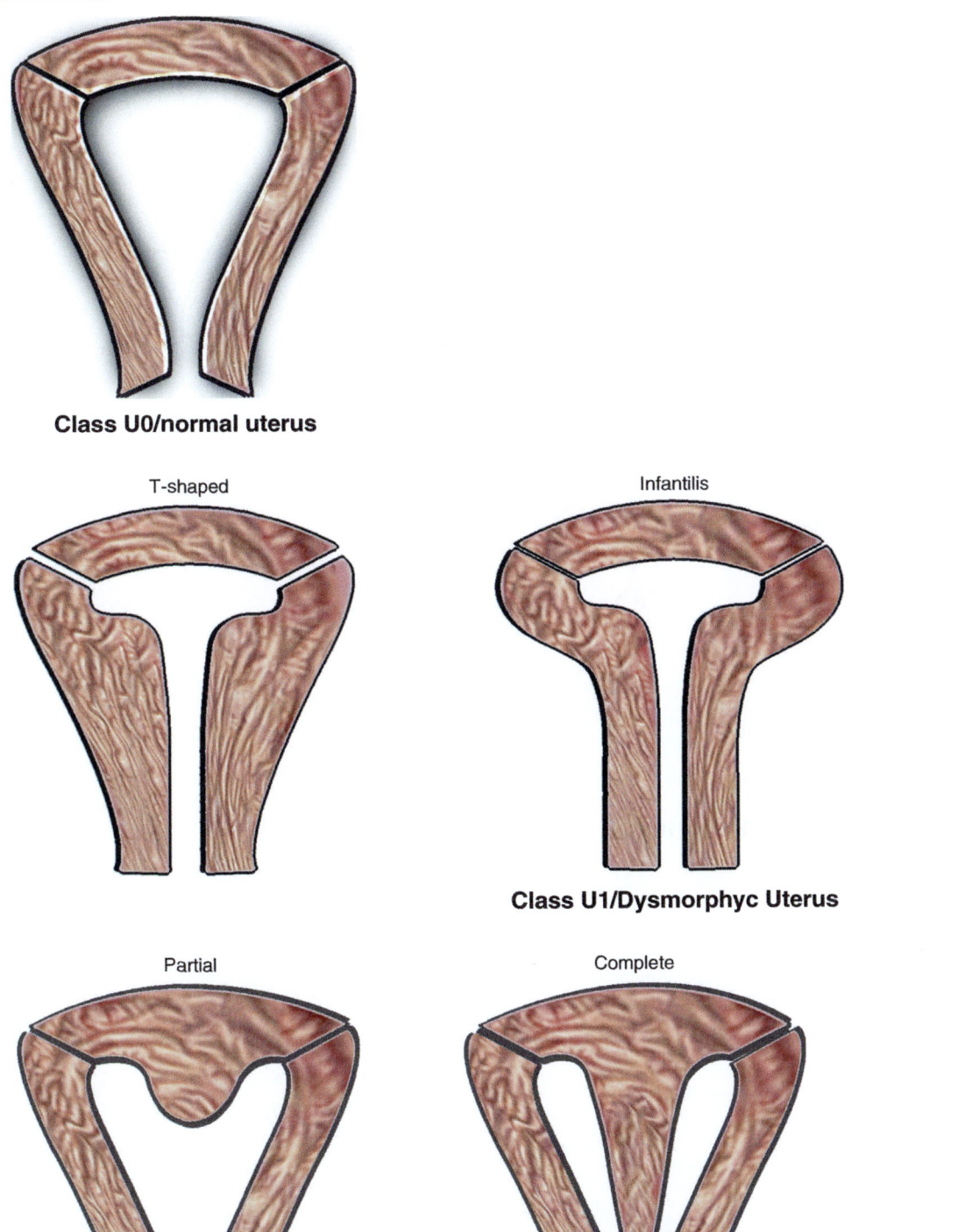

Class U0/normal uterus

T-shaped

Infantilis

Others

Class U1/Dysmorphyc Uterus

Partial

Complete

Class U2/Septate Uterus

Fig. 6.6 Classification of female genital tract congenital anomalies by ESHRE/ESGE consensus

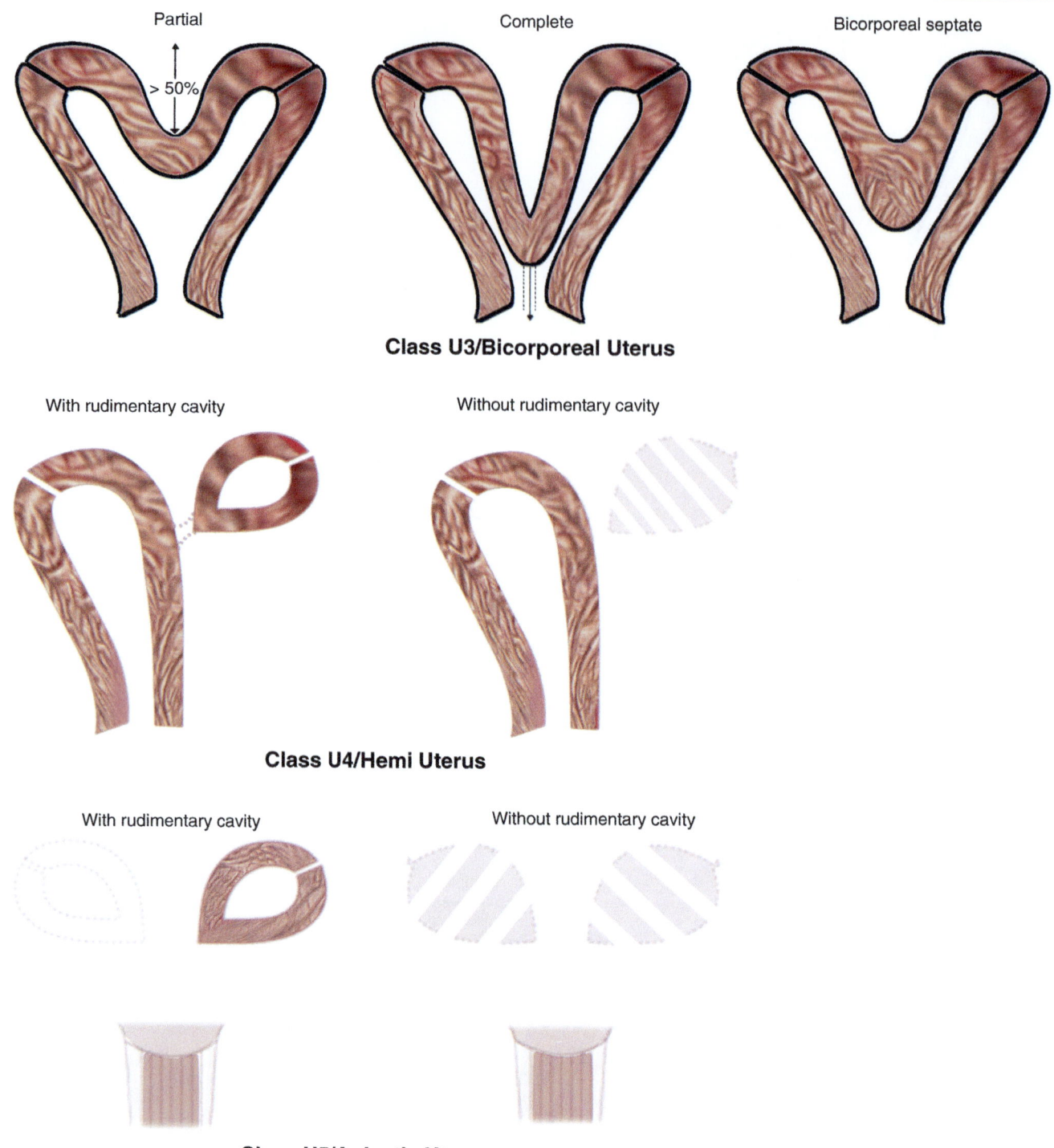

Fig. 6.6 (continued)

arcuate, and bicornuate uterus to avoid inadvertent fundal perforation (Fig. 6.7). The uterus with an abnormal fundal outline is a bicornuate uterus (external fundal indentation >1 cm) while arcuate and septate uterus have regular external profile. Septate, arcuate, and bicornuate uterus, all have a—larger o smaller—inner indentation and angle of the indentation:

arcuate—depth <1 cm angle >90°, septate—depth >1.5 angle of the indentation <90°, bicornuate—endometrial cavity is similar to a partial septate uterus (Fig. 6.8 bis) [18].

To perform an accurate differential diagnosis between septate, arcuate, and bicornuate uterus, it is necessary to visualize both outline and innerline of the uterus. For this

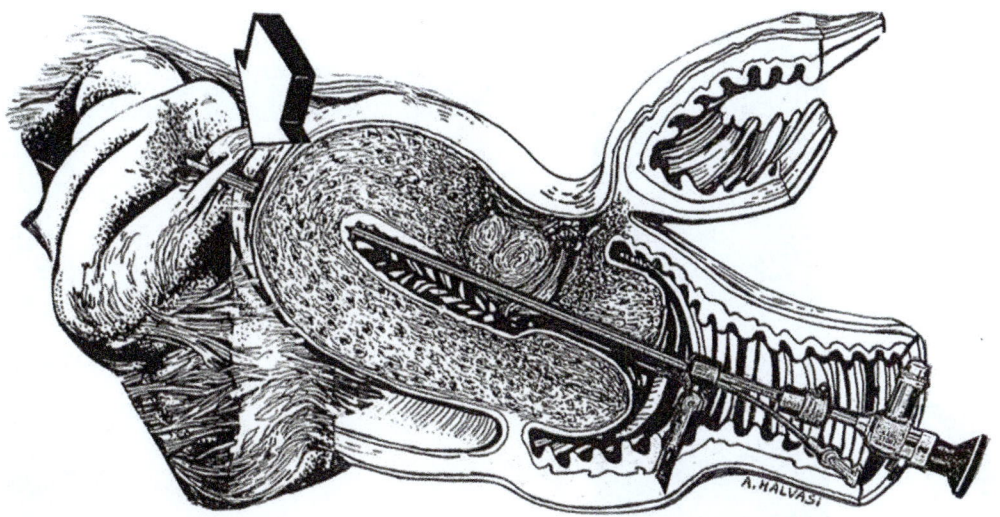

Fig. 6.7 Before any surgical intervention, it is mandatory to perform an accurate differential diagnosis between septate, arcuate, and bicornuate uterus to avoid inadvertent fundal perforation and bowels complication

reason, the gold standard diagnostic technique is 3D ultrasound associated or not with hysteroscopy [19].

The hysteroscopic surgery under ultrasound guidance, performed in the operating room or in an office setting, is the gold standard technique to treat the septate uterus [20]. Proceeding from both sides, the septum is cut from the apex to the fund by cold scissors, unipolar or bipolar cautery, laser, or resectoscope until the cavity is flush with the fundic portion. Then hysteroscope/resectoscope can visualize both tubal ostia without colliding with the residue of the septum [21]. After septum incision, there is a risk of subsequent pregnancy-related uterine rupture, which may be due to an extreme septal excision, penetration of the myometrium, uterine perforation, or excessive use of cautery or laser energy [22]. Several studies compared resectoscopic and hysteroscopic technique [23–26]. The Versapoint technique is a safe and effective alternative to the resectoscope avoiding cervical dilation and cervical incompetence and lacerations, and lowering the risk of uterine perforation [27]. Some have expressed a preference for the use of cold scissors rather than bipolar Versapoint to avoid thermal and cautery damage to the cut edges [26].

Many IVF centers recommend removal of the septum before assisted reproductive treatment to reduce the risk of miscarriage.

6.5 Myomas

Common benign uterine findings during women's fertile life are myomas, which consist of muscle cells circumscribed by a capsule. Macroscopically, they present the characteristic vortex appearance. According to their histological composition (fibrous or muscular), their consistency may vary from soft to hard and may present colliquated or calcified areas. Their growth is influenced by local growth factors, cytokines, estrogen, and progesterone [28].

Myomas may be totally asymptomatic or they may cause menorrhagia, pelvic pain, dysmenorrhea, bladder and bowel dysfunction (due to mass-effect), and infertility. Symptoms depend on number, size, and localization. Myomas are classified in submucosal, intramural, and subserosal according to their relationship with endometrium, myometrium, and uterine surface. The leiomyoma subclassification system of the Federation of Gynecology and Obstetrics (FIGO) classifies myoma into eight classes (from 0 to 7) according to their localization (Fig. 6.9). Submucosal myomas are classified in type 0 (Fig. 6.10) (100% intracavity), type 1 (>50% intracavity), and type 2 (<50% intracavity). Intramural myomas are classified into type 3 (in contact with endometrium) and type 4 (100% intramural). Type 5 includes intramural but <50% subserosal myomas, type 6 subserosal but <50% intramural. Subserosal peduncolate myomas are classified as type 7 [29].

Submucosal and intramural myomas could cause sterility and infertility by several mechanisms. For instance, irregular uterine contractility and abnormal local endocrine patterns may interfere with sperm transport, while endometrial inflammation and abnormal vascularization may cause embryo-implantation failure [30, 31].

Office hysteroscopy allows to classify submucous myomas from FIGO class 0 to FIGO class 2 according to their development into uterine cavity or into uterine wall: different inflow pressure of the distension medium can show the angle between endometrium and myoma (type 1 < 90°, type 2 > 90°) (Figs. 6.7, 6.11).

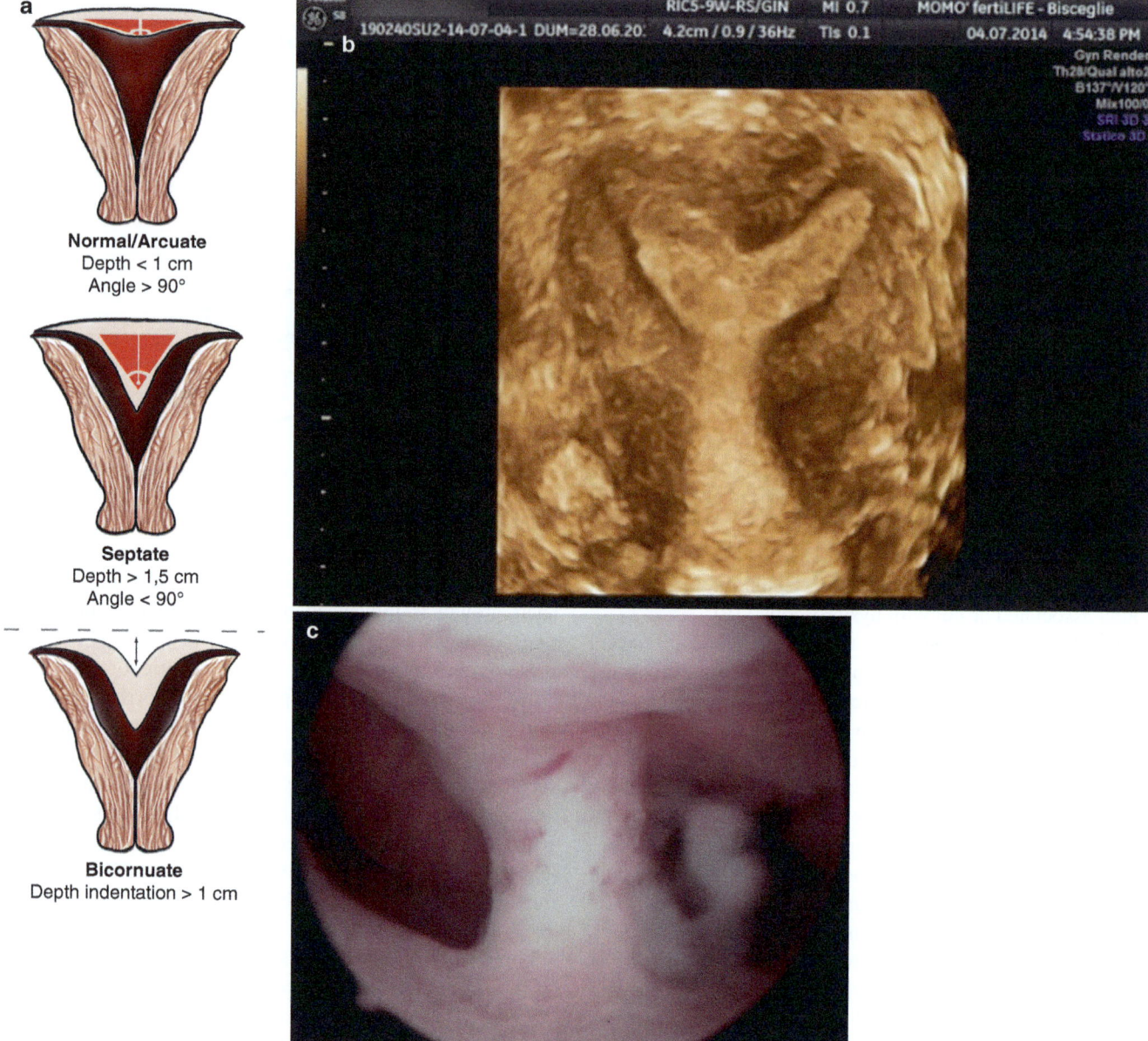

Fig. 6.8 (**a**) ASRM. Uterine septum. Fertil Steril 2016. (**b**) The 3D ultrasonography represents ancillary techniques with hysteroscopy for septate uterus diagnosis, and evaluation before the operative hysteros-copy. (**c**) Hysteroscopic finding of upper ultrasound image (courtesy of Dr. Domenico Silletti, Bari)

The hysteroscopic surgery is the gold standard technique to treat submucous myomas (Fig. 6.11). It may be performed in the operating room under general or spinal anesthesia after cervical dilatation, or (when myomas are no larger than 2 cm) in an office setting by bipolar hysteroscopic system, bipolar scissors, and a special morcellator [32, 33].

6.6 Endometrial Polyps

Other common benign uterine findings are endometrial polyps (EP), overgrowths of endometrium composed by a connective and vascular axis, covered by epithelial tissue (Fig. 6.12). According to their histological composition, EP are defined as adenomatous or fibrous and can be isolated or

Fig. 6.9 Leiomyoma subclassification system of the Federation of Gynecology and Obstetrics (FIGO)

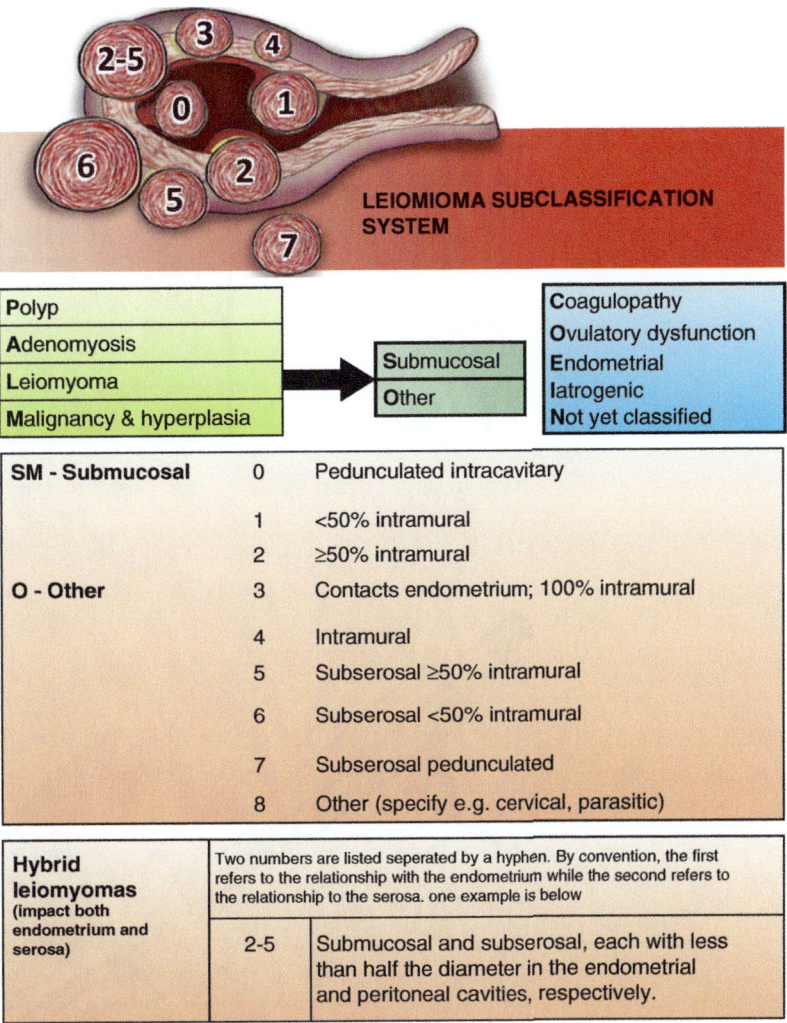

SM - Submucosal	0	Pedunculated intracavitary
	1	<50% intramural
	2	≥50% intramural
O - Other	3	Contacts endometrium; 100% intramural
	4	Intramural
	5	Subserosal ≥50% intramural
	6	Subserosal <50% intramural
	7	Subserosal pedunculated
	8	Other (specify e.g. cervical, parasitic)

Hybrid leiomyomas (impact both endometrium and serosa)	Two numbers are listed seperated by a hyphen. By convention, the first refers to the relationship with the endometrium while the second refers to the relationship to the serosa. one example is below	
	2-5	Submucosal and subserosal, each with less than half the diameter in the endometrial and peritoneal cavities, respectively.

multiple, sessile (anchored to the uterine wall by a large base of plant), or pedunculated (anchored to the uterine wall by a vascular pedicle) (Fig. 6.13).

EP may be totally asymptomatic or they may cause menometrorrhagia, sterility, and infertility due to mechanical and chemical interference with sperm transport and embryo implantation [34]. EP are found in 32% of patients undergoing assisted reproduction (ART) [35].

The gold standard diagnostic technique for EP is hysteroscopy [36].

Hysteroscopy allows diagnosis and treatment (under direct vision) of polyps simultaneously while blind curette procedures cannot ensure that EP are fully removed [37, 38]. Hysteroscopic polypectomy is performed by scissors, electrode loop, electric probe, or morcellator when EP are smaller than 2 cm. No differences in the rate of polyp excision, surgical time, or induced pelvic discomfort were observed between electrosurgical and mechanical techniques [39].

If EP are >2 cm or when they are localized at uterine fundus, polypectomy is performed by resectoscope [40].

Polypectomy (Fig. 6.14) is performed to reduce symptoms in women affected by abnormal uterine bleedings or to improve pregnancy rate during ART. However, the most important reason to perform polypectomy is to exclude atypical and/or malignant endometrial changes.

After hysteroscopic polypectomy, pregnancies are frequently obtained spontaneously [41].

If EP are smaller than 2 cm, hysteroscopic polypectomy offers no advantages in pregnancy rates following IVF treatment [42].

6.7 Chronic Endometritis

Chronic endometritis (CE) is a persistent inflammation of the endometrial lining [43]. Culture analyses indicate that CE are caused by common bacterial pathogens (70%) or are

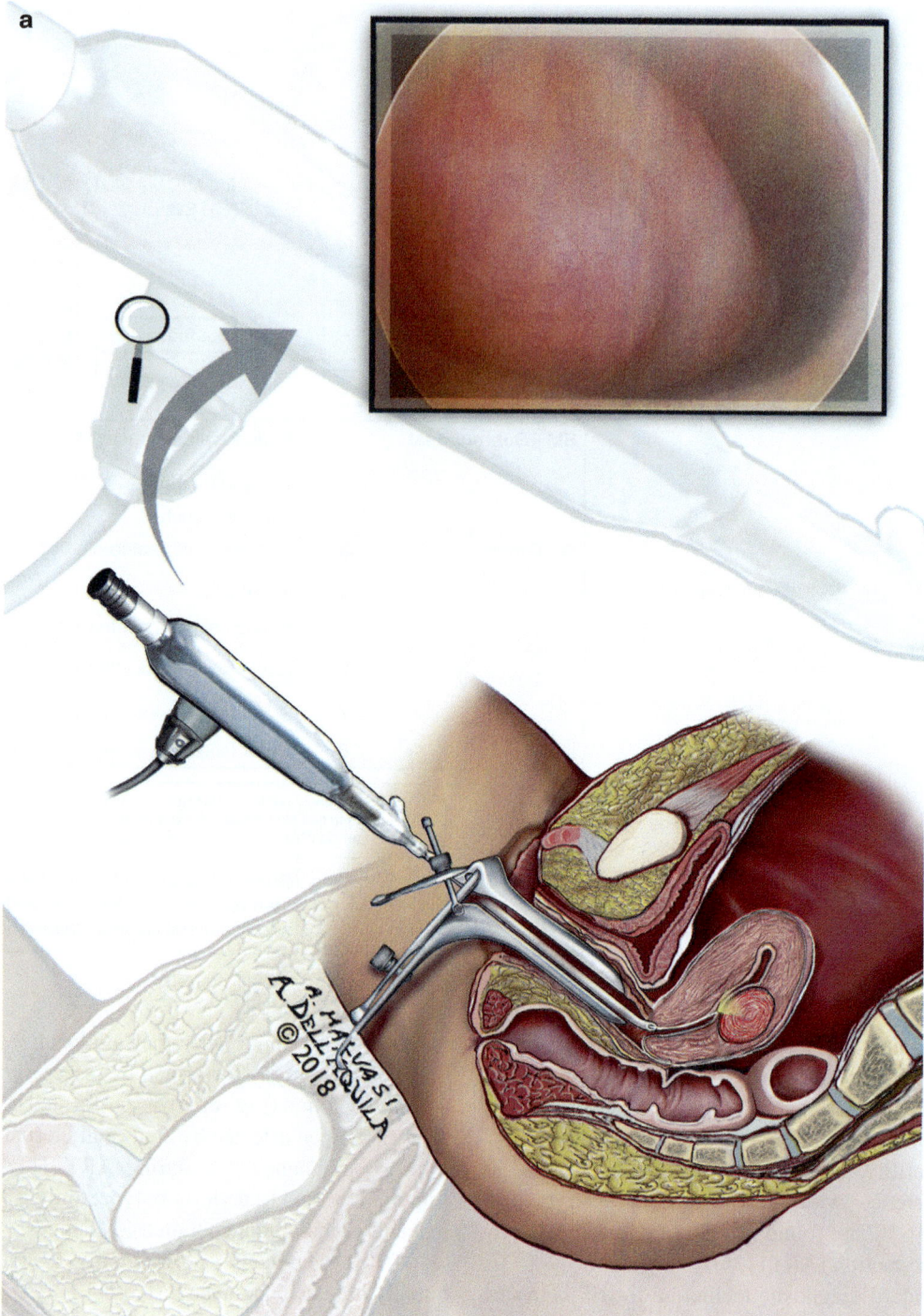

Fig. 6.10 (**a**) Submucous type 0 myoma. (**b**) bis Submucous type 0 myoma

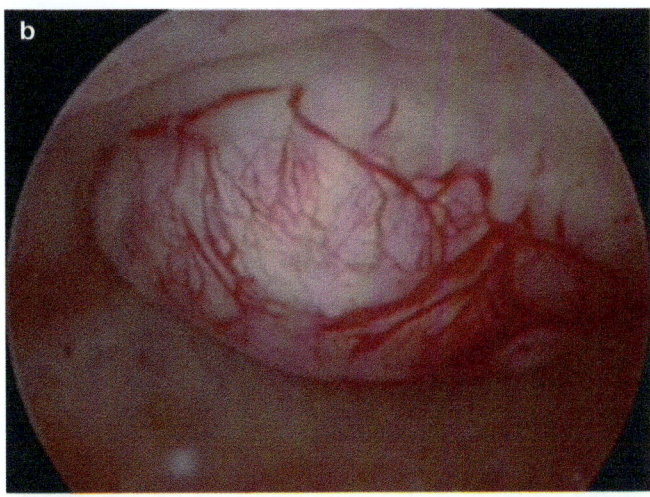

Fig. 6.10 (continued)

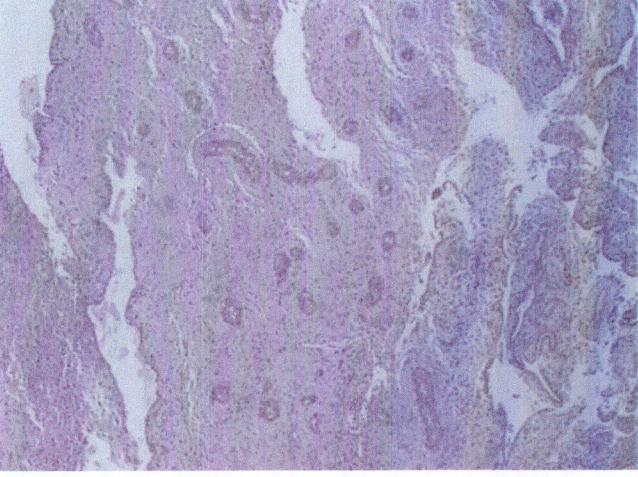

Fig. 6.12 Endometrial polyp: vascular axis

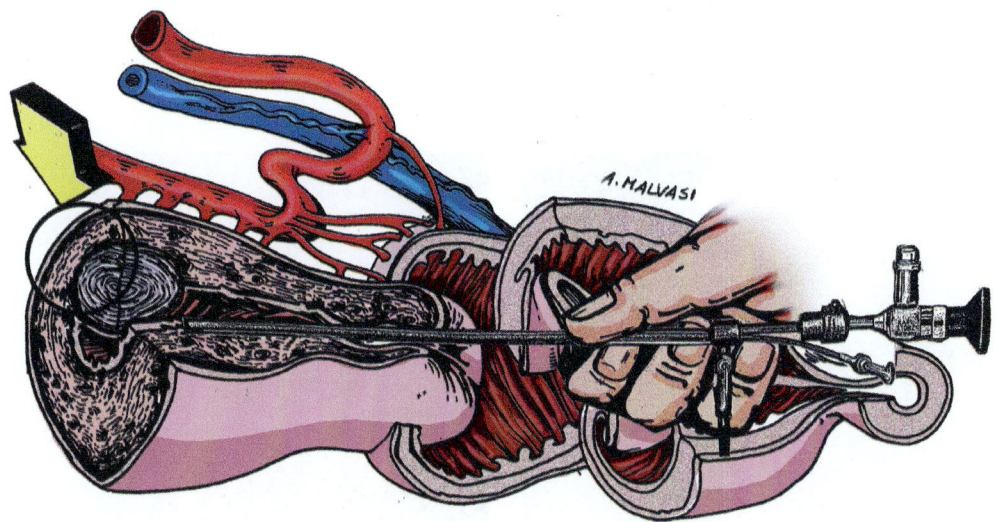

Fig. 6.11 The drawing shows the distance between the outer surface of the submucosal myoma and the uterine wall. Black circle and yellow arrow and uterine vessels. Office hysteroscopy allows to classify submucous myomas from FIGO class 0 to FIGO class 2 according to their development into uterine cavity or into uterine wall: different inflow pressure of the distension medium can show the angle between endometrium and myoma (type 1 < 90°, type 2 > 90°)

associated with sexually transmitted infections such as mycoplasma and ureaplasma (about 20%) and chlamydia (about 10%) [44].

Usually, CE is asymptomatic and there are not specific signs to suspect it. However, patients have reported at times pelvic pain, dysfunctional uterine bleeding, dyspareunia, and leucorrhea [45].

CE is highly prevalent in patients with unexplained infertility and women diagnosed with CE have a low implantation rate (11.5%) after an IVF cycle (Fig. 1.10) [46, 47]. CE is identified in infertile women with repeated implantation failure (RIF), defined as serial negative pregnancy tests following transfer of three or more embryos or blastocysts, (14–31%) and recurrent pregnancy loss (9–13%) [48].

It is still unclear how CE cause those effects. There are many possible mechanisms: an altered lymphocyte, cytokines, growth factors, and apoptotic proteins pattern plus

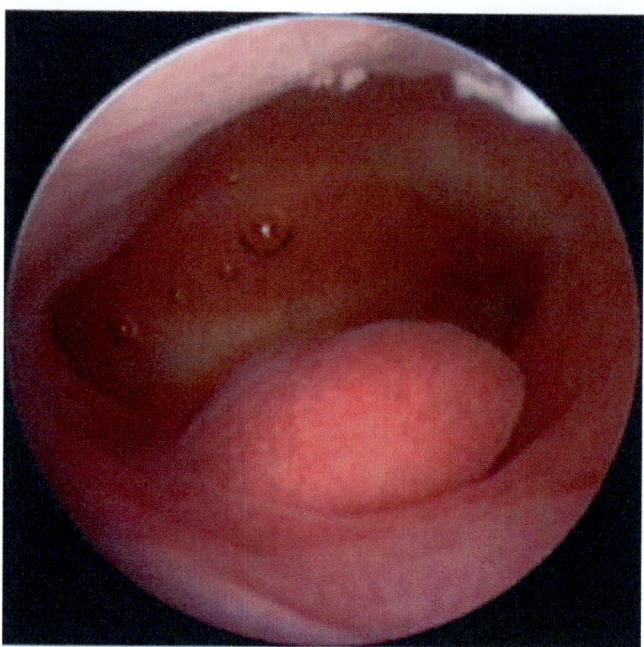

Fig. 6.13 Hysteroscopic view of endometrial polyp located in posterior uterine wall

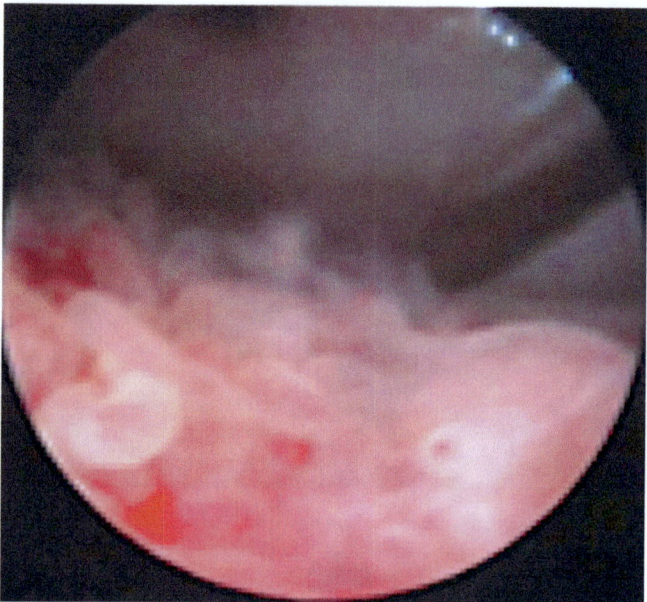

Fig. 6.15 Chronic endometritis: stromal edema and focal hyperemia

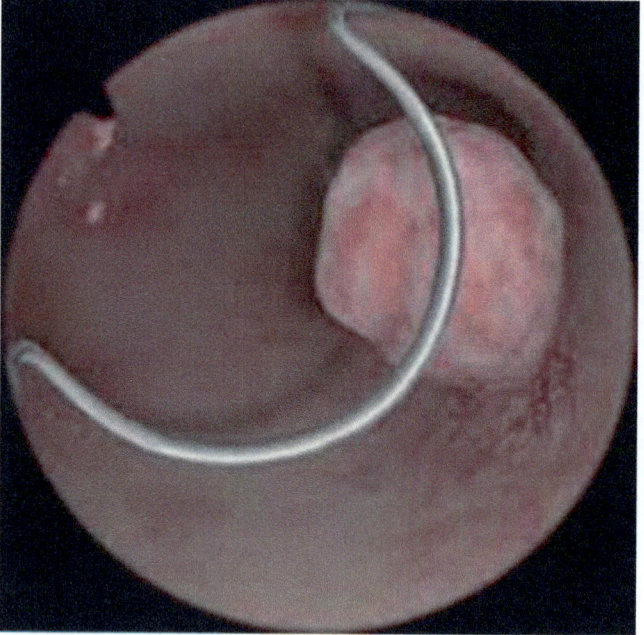

Fig. 6.14 Endometrial polyp during operative hysteroscopy

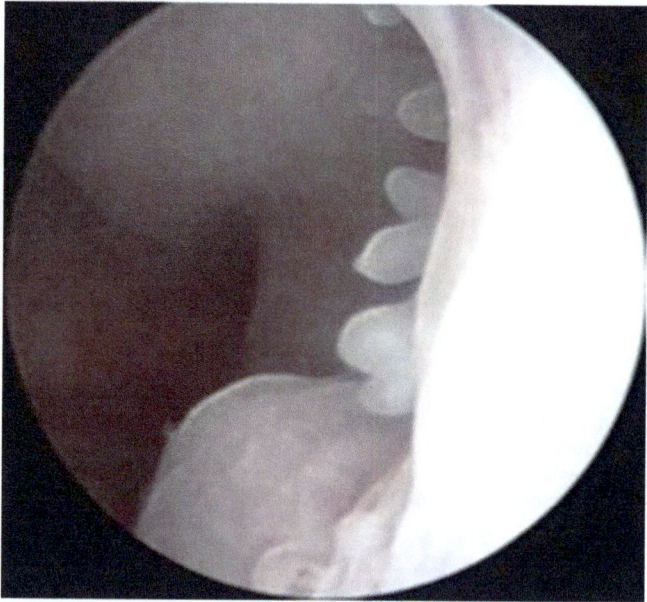

Fig. 6.16 Chronic endometritis: micro-polyps

abnormal contractility are the most important mechanical and chemical interference on endometrial receptivity [49–52].

Hysteroscopy shows CE typical features allowing diagnosis: stromal edema, focal, or diffuse hyperemia (Fig. 6.15) and endometrial micro-polyps: small outgrowths (<1) mm in size with a distinct connective-vascular axis [44, 53]. Micro-polyps, identified floating into the distention medium, are the most specific CE signs (Fig. 6.16). To detect micro-polyps, hysteroscope should be directed parallel to the endometrial wall obtaining a tangential view of the surface.

The gold standard diagnostic techniques of CE rely on the histological identification in the endometrial stroma of

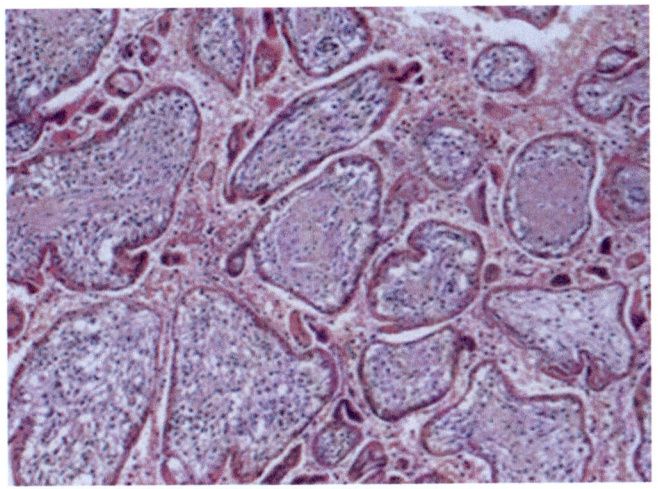

Fig. 6.17 Abortion in chronic endometritis

lymphocytes and plasma cells (presence of 1–5 plasma cells/hpf) characterized by CD 138, an immunohistochemical-specific marker [54, 55]. A limitation of histological diagnosis is the fact that plasma cells are normally present in the endometrium especially before menstruation. Therefore, results may depend on the date of sampling with respect to the menstrual cycle.

Antibiotic therapy of CE allows hysteroscopic, cultural, and histologic findings normalization [56]. Cicinelli et al. demonstrated an improvement of spontaneous pregnancy rate and live birth rate after therapy in women with recurrent miscarriage and RIF, suggesting a causal relationship between CE and defective endometrial receptivity [57] (Fig. 6.17). Kitaya et al. studied clinical pregnancy rate, miscarriage rate, and live birth rate in infertile women with RIF affected by CE following the first-line doxycycline treatment (100 mg tablet, twice per day, 14 days). Their study showed a histopathologic normalization in the subsequent endometrial biopsy (92.3%) and a significant improvement in each of all outcomes. A second-line metronidazole/ciprofloxacin treatment (250 mg, twice per day, 14 days/200 mg, twice per day, 14 days) was administrated to doxycycline-resistant patients to obtain the histopathologic cure rate [58, 59]. Before proceeding with embryo transfer it is necessary to perform a second hysteroscopy with endometrial sampling in the follicular phase of the cycle.

6.8   Conclusion

In conclusion, hysteroscopic procedures performed in office are key to the diagnosis and treatment of several conditions causing infertility and sterility (i.e., congenital malformation, acquired defects, and chronic endometrial infection).

If detailed diagnostic information is required in women in whom there is no clinical or ultrasound evidence of pelvic pathology, hysteroscopy can be considered to be appropriate. This technique allows to confirm the specific characteristics of the endometrium and the risk of infection. Although hysteroscopy remains an invasive technique, the office approach has increased patients' compliance and has significantly reduced the costs.

Acknowledgement The authors of this chapter thanks to Domenico Silletti, MD, for hysteroscopic images made available by him, Department of Obstetrics and Gynecolgy, Santa Maria Hospital, GVM Care and Research, Bari, Italy.

References

1. Trojano G, Malvasi A, Caroli Casavola V, Marinelli E, Resta L, Cicinelli E. Outpatient hysteroscopy in recurrent pregnancy loss. In: Tinelli A, et al., editors. Hysteroscopy: Springer International Publishing AG; 2018.
2. Cicinelli E. Hysteroscopy without anesthesia: review of recent literature. J Minim Invasive Gynecol. 2010;17(6):703–8. https://doi.org/10.1016/j.jmig.2010.07.003.
3. Cicinelli E, Didonna T, Ambrosi G, Schönauer LM, Fiore G, Matteo MG. Topical anaesthesia for diagnostic hysteroscopy and endometrial biopsy in postmenopausal women: a randomised placebo-controlled double-blind study. Br J Obstet Gynaecol. 1997;104:316–9.
4. Cicinelli E, Parisi C, Galantino P, Pinto V, Barba B, Schonauer S. Reliability, feasibility, and safety of minihysteroscopy with a vaginoscopic approach: experience with 6,000 cases. Fertil Steril. 2003;80:199–202.
5. Unfried G, Wieser F, Albrecht A, Kaider A, Nagele F. Flexible versus rigid endoscopes for outpatient hysteroscopy: a prospective randomized clinical trial. Hum Reprod. 2001;16:168–71.
6. Bettocchi S, Ceci O, Di Venere R, et al. Advanced operative office hysteroscopy without anaesthesia: analysis of 501 cases treated with a 5 Fr. bipolar electrode. Hum Reprod. 2002;17:2435–8.
7. Bettocchi S, Ceci O, Nappi L, et al. Operative office hysteroscopy without anesthesia: analysis of 4863 cases performed with mechanical instruments. J Am Assoc Gynecol Laparosc. 2004;11:59–61.
8. Lemmers M, Mol BW. Dilatation and curettage increases the risk of subsequent preterm birth: a systematic review and meta-analysis. Hum Reprod. 2016;31(1):34–45.
9. Gilman AR, Fluker MR. Intrauterine adhesions following miscarriage: look and learn. J Obstet Gynaecol Can. 2016;38(5):453–7.
10. Bougie O, Singh SS. Treatment of Asherman's syndrome in an outpatient hysteroscopy setting. J Minim Invasive Gynecol. 2015;22(3):446–50.
11. Saravelos SH, Li TC. Ultrasound guided treatment of intrauterine adhesions in the outpatient setting. Ultrasound Obstet Gynecol. 2017;50(2):278–80. https://doi.org/10.1002/uog.16218.
12. Cai H, He Y. Oxidized, regenerated cellulose adhesion barrier plus intrauterine device prevents recurrence after adhesiolysis for moderate to severe intrauterine adhesions. J Minim Invasive Gynecol. 2017;24(1):80–8.
13. Lin X, Zhang SA. Comparison of intrauterine balloon, intrauterine contraceptive device and hyaluronic acid gel in the prevention of adhesion reformation following hysteroscopic surgery for Asherman syndrome: a cohort study. Eur J Obstet Gynecol Reprod Biol. 2013;170(2):512–6.
14. Raga F, Pellicer A. Reproductive impact of congenital Mullerian anomalies. Hum Reprod. 1997;12:2277–8.

15. Elmandooh M. Validity of hysteroscopy in detection of uterine cavity abnormalities in women with recurrent pregnancy loss. J Gynecol Res Obstet. 2016;2(1):26–30.

16. Grigoris F, et al. The ESHRE/ESGE consensus on the classification of female genital tract congenital anomalies. Hum Reprod. 2013;28(8):2032–44.

17. Venetis CA, Grimbizis GF. Clinical implications of congenital uterine anomalies: a meta-analysis of comparative studies. Reprod Biomed Online. 2014;29:665–83.

18. Pfeifer S, Butts S, Dumesic D, Gracia C, Vernon M, Fossum G, La Barbera A, Mersereau J, Odem R, Penzias A, Pisarska M, Rebar R, Reindollar R, Rosen M, Sandlow J, Widra E. Uterine septum: a guideline. Fertil Steril. 2016;106(3):530–40. https://doi.org/10.1016/j.fertnstert.2016.05.014. Epub 2016 May 25.

19. Ludwin A, Knafel A. Two- and three-dimensional ultrasonography and sonohysterography versus hysteroscopy with laparoscopy in the differential diagnosis of septate, bicornuate, and arcuate uteri. J Minim Invasive Gynecol. 2013;20:90–9.

20. Coccia ME, Scarselli G. Intraoperative ultrasound guidance for operative hysteroscopy. A prospective study. J Reprod Med. 2000;45(5):413–8.

21. Karande VC, Gleicher N. Resection of uterine septum using gynaecoradiological techniques. Hum Reprod. 1999;14:1226–9.

22. Valle RF, Ekpo GE. Hysteroscopic metroplasty for the septate uterus: review and meta-analysis. J Minim Invasive Gynecol. 2013;20:22–42.

23. Colacurci N, De Placido G. Small-diameter hysteroscopy with Versapoint versus resectoscopy with a unipolar knife for the treatment of septate uterus: a prospective randomized study. J Minim Invasive Gynecol. 2007;14:622–7.

24. Litta P, Cosmi E. Resectoscope or Versapoint for hysteroscopic metroplasty. Int J Gynaecol Obstet. 2008;101:39–42.

25. Bradley L, Falcone T. Hysteroscopy for evaluating and treating recurrent pregnancy loss. In: Bradley L, Falcone T, editors. Hysteroscopy: office evaluation and management of the uterine cavity. Philadelphia: Elsevier Health Sciences; 2008. p. 156–69.

26. Cararach M, Labastida R. Hysteroscopic incision of the septate uterus: scissors versus resectoscope. Hum Reprod. 1994;9(1):87–9.

27. Tomazevic T, Bokal E. Septate, subseptate and arcuate uterus decrease pregnancy and live birth rates in IVF/ICSI. Reprod Biomed Online. 2010;21(5):700.

28. Sozen I, Arici A. Interactions of cytokines, growth factors, and the extracellular matrix in the cellular biology of uterine leiomyomata. Fertil Steril. 2002;78:1–12.

29. Munro MG, Critchley HO, Broder MS, Fraser IS. The FIGO Classification System ("PALM-COEIN") for causes of abnormal uterine bleeding in non-gravid women in the reproductive years, including guidelines for clinical investigation. Int J Gynaecol Obstet. 2011;113:3–13.

30. Donnez J, Jadoul P. What are the implications of myomas on fertility? A need for a debate? Hum Reprod. 2002;17:1424–30.

31. Farhi J, Ashkenazi J, Feldberg D, Dicker D, Orvieto R, Ben RZ. The effects of uterine leiomyomata on in-vitro fertilization treatment. Hum Reprod. 1995;10:2576–8.

32. Pakrashi T. New hysteroscopic techniques for submucosal uterine fibroids. Curr Opin Obstet Gynecol. 2014;26(4):308–13.

33. Bettocchi S, Ceci O, Nappi L, et al. Treatment of intramural myomas in an office setting. Can we do it? J Am Assoc Gynecol Laparosc. 2005;12(Suppl):77.

34. Richlin S, Parthasarathy S. Glycodelin levels in uterine flushings and in plasma of patients with leiomyomas and polyps: implications and implantation. Hum Reprod. 2002;17:2742–7.

35. Hinckley MD, Milki AA. 1000 office-based hysteroscopies prior to in vitro fertilization: feasibility and findings. JSLS. 2004;8:103–7.

36. Rosa DS, Ferriani RA. Routine office hysteroscopy in the investigation of infertile couples before assisted reproduction. J Reprod Med. 2005;50:501–6.

37. Loiacono RM, Trojano G, Del Gaudio N, Kardhashi A, Deliso MA, Falco G, Sforza R, Laera AF, Galise I, Trojano V. Hysteroscopy as a valid tool for endometrial pathology in patients with postmenopausal bleeding or asymptomatic patients with a thickened endometrium: hysteroscopic and histological results. Gynecol Obstet Investig. 2015;79(3):210–6.

38. Trojano G, Damiani GR, Caroli Casavola V, et al. The role of hysteroscopy in evaluating postmenopausal asymptomatic women with thickened endometrium. Gynecol Minim Invasive Ther. 2018;7(1):6–9.

39. Garuti G, Centinaio G, Luerti M. Outpatient hysteroscopic polypectomy in postmenopausal women: a comparison between mechanical and electrosurgical resection. J Minim Invasive Gynecol. 2008;15:595–600.

40. Muzii L, Benedetti Panici P. Resectoscopic versus bipolar electrode excision of endometrial polyps: a randomized study. Fertil Steril. 2007;87(4):909–17.

41. Perez-Medina AP. Endometrial polyps and their implication in the pregnancy rates of patients undergoing intrauterine insemination: prospective, randomized study. Hum Reprod. 2005;20:1632–5.

42. Lass A, Brinsden P. The effect of endometrial polyps on outcomes of in vitro fertilization (IVF) cycles. J Assist Reprod Genet. 1999;16:410–5.

43. Farooki MA. Epidemiology and pathology of chronic endometritis. Int Surg. 1967;48:566–73.

44. Cicinelli E, De Ziegler D, Nicoletti R, Colafiglio G, Saliani N, Resta L, Rizzi D, De Vito D. Chronic endometritis: correlation among hysteroscopic, histologic, and bacteriologic findings in a prospective trial with 2190 consecutive office hysteroscopies. Fertil Steril. 2008;89(3):677–84. Epub 2007 May 25.

45. Smith M, Bocklage T. Chronic endometritis: a combined histopathologic and clinical review of cases from 2002 to 2007. Int J Gynecol Pathol. 2010;29:44–50.

46. Quaas A, Dokras A. Diagnosis and treatment of unexplained infertility. Rev Obstet Gynecol. 2008;1:69–76.

47. Park HJ, Kim YS, Yoon TK, Lee WS. Chronic endometritis and infertility. Clin Exp Reprod Med. 2016;43:185–92.

48. Cicinelli E, Matteo M, Tinelli R, et al. Chronic endometritis due to common bacteria is prevalent in women with recurrent miscarriage as confirmed by improved pregnancy outcome after antibiotic treatment. Reprod Sci. 2014;21:640–7.

49. Pinto V, Matteo M, Tinelli R, Mitola PC, De Ziegler D, Cicinelli E. Altered uterine contractility in women with chronic endometritis. Fertil Steril. 2015;103:1049–52.

50. Kitaya K, Yasuo T. Aberrant expression of selectin E, CXCL1, and CXCL13 in chronic endometritis. Mod Pathol. 2010;23:1136–46.

51. Di Pietro C, Cicinelli E, Guglielmino MR, et al. Altered transcriptional regulation of cytokines, growth factors, and apoptotic proteins in the endometrium of infertile women with chronic endometritis. Am J Reprod Immunol. 2013;69:509–17.

52. Kitaya K, Tada Y, Hayashi T, Taguchi S, Funabiki M, Nakamura Y. Comprehensive endometrial immunoglobulin subclass analysis in infertile women suffering from repeated implantation failure with or without chronic endometritis. Am J Reprod Immunol. 2014;72:386–91.

53. Cicinelli E, Resta L, Nicoletti R, Zappimbulso V, Tartagni M, Saliani N. Endometrial micropolyps at fluid hysteroscopy suggest the existence of chronic endometritis. Hum Reprod. 2005;20(5):1386–9. Epub 2005 Feb 25.

54. Resta L, Palumbo M, Rossi R, Piscitelli D, Grazia Fiore M, Cicinelli E. Histology of micro polyps in chronic endometritis.

Histopathology. 2012;60(4):670–4. https://doi.org/10.1111/j.1365-2559.2011.04099.x. Epub 2012 Jan 17.

55. Moreno I, Cicinelli E, Garcia-Grau I, et al. The diagnosis of chronic endometritis in infertile asymptomatic women: a comparative study of histology, microbial cultures, hysteroscopy, and molecular microbiology. Am J Obstet Gynecol. 2018;218(6):602.e1–602.e16.

56. Cicinelli E, Matteo M, Trojano G, Mitola PC, Tinelli R, Vitagliano A, Crupano FM, Lepera A, Miragliotta G, Resta L. Chronic endometritis in patients with unexplained infertility: prevalence and effects of antibiotic treatment on spontaneous conception. Am J Reprod Immunol. 2018;79(1). https://doi.org/10.1111/aji.12782. Epub 2017 Nov 14.

57. Cicinelli E, Matteo M, Tinelli R, et al. Prevalence of chronic endometritis in repeated unexplained implantation failure and the IVF success rate after antibiotic therapy. Hum Reprod. 2015;30:323–30.

58. Kitaya K, Matsubayashi H, Takaya Y, et al. Live birth rate following oral antibiotic treatment for chronic endometritis in infertile women with repeated implantation failure. Am J Reprod Immunol. 2017;78(5):e12719.

59. Cicinelli E, Bettocchi S, de Ziegler D. Chronic endometritis, a common disease hidden behind endometrial polyps in premenopausal women: first evidence from a case-control study. J Minim Invasive Gynecol. 2019 Jan 29.

Anesthesia and Analgesia for Women Undergoing Oocyte Retrieval

7

Renata Beck, Agostino Brizzi, Gilda Cinnella,
Pasquale Raimondo, and Krzysztof M. Kuczkowski

Contents

R. Beck (✉) · A. Brizzi
Department of Anesthesia, Santa Maria Hospital, GVM Care and Research, Bari, Italy

G. Cinnella
Unit of Anesthesia and Intensive Care, Department of Surgical and Medical Sciences, University of Foggia, Foggia, Italy
e-mail: gilda.cinnella@unifg.it

P. Raimondo
Pediatric Department of Anesthesia and Intensive Care Unit (General and Post Cardiac Surgery), Giovanni XXIII—Policlinico di Bari, Bari, Italy

K. M. Kuczkowski
Department of Anesthesia for Obstetrics and Maternal Fetal & Neonatal Medicine, La Jolla, CA, USA

7.1 History of General Anesthesia

Attempts at producing a state of general anesthesia can be traced throughout history in the writings of the ancient Sumerians, Babylonians, Assyrians, Egyptians, Greeks, Romans, Indians, and Chinese. The Renaissance made significant advances in anatomy and surgical techniques, despite all this progress only with the discovery and introduction of general anesthesia in late eighteenth century permitted development of modern surgery.

Humphry Davy (1778–1829) discovered the anesthetic properties of nitrous oxide, call it laughing gas and published his findings in the systematic written scientific work. He was the first to document the analgesic effects of nitrous oxide, as well as its benefits in relieving pain during surgery. Horace Wells (1815–1848) was an American dentist who pioneered the use of anesthesia in dentistry, specifically he studied nitrous oxide during painless tooth

© Springer Nature Switzerland AG 2020
A. Malvasi, D. Baldini (eds.), *Pick Up and Oocyte Management*, https://doi.org/10.1007/978-3-030-28741-2_7

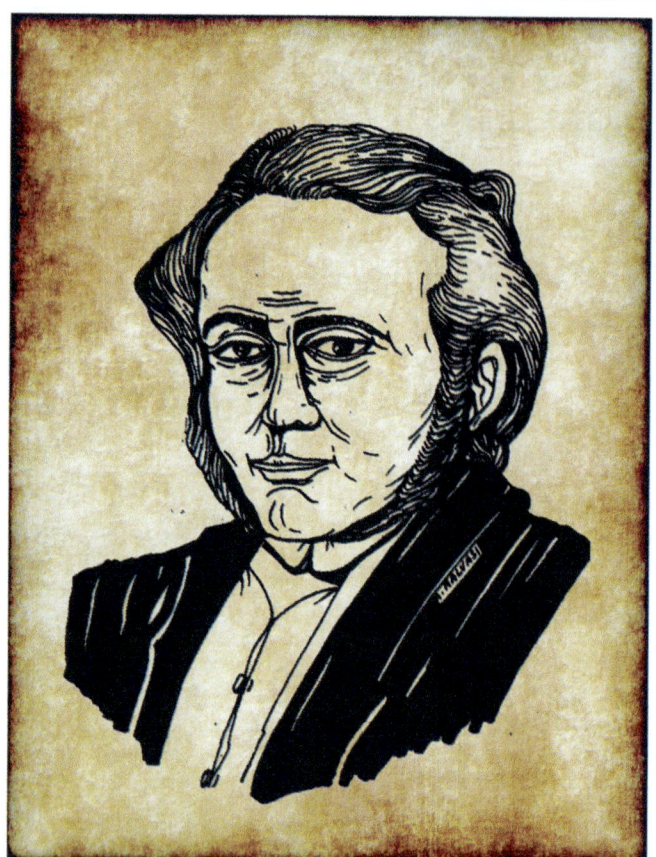

Fig. 7.1 Horace Wells (1815–1848) was an American dentist who pioneered the use of anesthesia in dentistry, specifically he studied nitrous oxide during painless tooth extraction

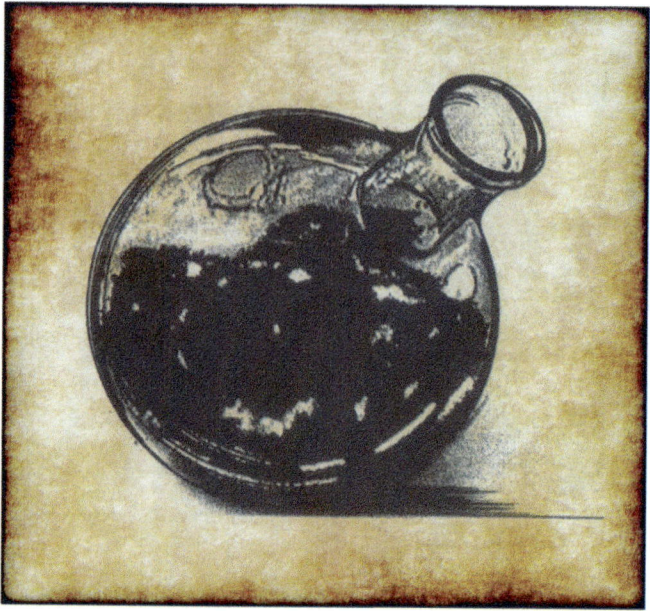

Fig. 7.2 William Thomas Green Morton (1819–1868) used a glass sphere containing a sponge soaked in ether which evaporated and brought the patient to sleep

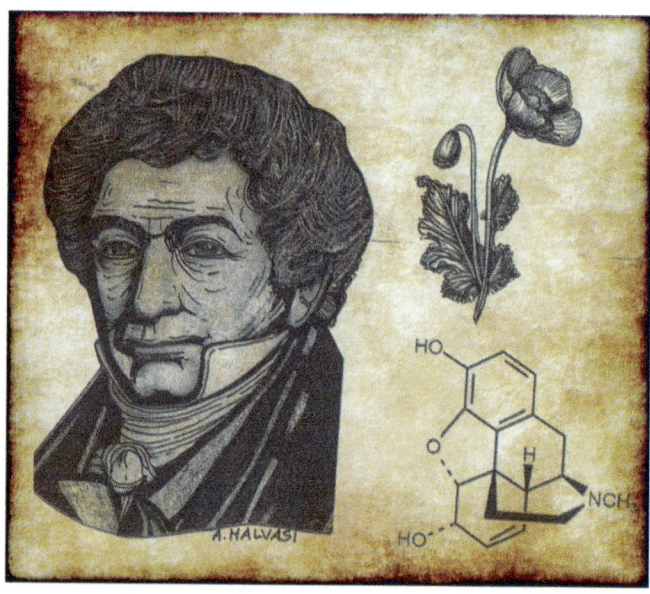

Fig. 7.3 Friedrich Wilhelm Adam Sertürner (1783–1841) was the German pharmacist and a pioneer of alkaloid chemistry. He was the first to isolate the extract of morphine crystals from the opium poppy (Papaver somniferum)

extraction (Fig. 7.1). Subsequently, his apprentices William Morton (1819–1868) in Boston made first public demonstration on the use of ethereal general anesthesia for surgical operation on the neck without pain. He used a glass sphere (Fig. 7.2) containing a sponge soaked in ether which evaporated and brought the patient to sleep. Friedrich Wilhelm Adam Sertürner (1783–1841) was a German pharmacist and a pioneer of alkaloid chemistry. Sertürner in 1805 isolated successfully morphine extract crystals from the opium poppy (Papaver somniferum) (Fig. 7.3). After a series of experiments on rats and stray dogs, he reported his discovery of a sleep-inducing molecule. Since his discovery occurred almost 50 years before the invention of the hypodermic syringe, the drug had to be administered orally. He was a pioneer and promoted a new branch of science that came to be known as alkaloid chemistry. John Snow (1813–1858) conducted translational research that permitted him to understand the mechanisms of vaporizing volatile anesthetic agents, ether and chloroform, so that safe delivery systems of anesthesia could be designed. He made about 4000 anesthesia and treated 77 obstetric patients with chloroform using chloroform as an anesthetic for childbirth and brought obstetric anesthesia

to be accepted against religious, ethical, and medical beliefs by administering chloroform to Queen Victoria for the births of Prince Leopold and Princess Beatrice (Figs. 7.4 and 7.5) [1]. Robert Macintosh (1897–1989) designed laryngoscope, endobronchial tube, and anesthetic vaporizer. He travelled widely, giving demonstrations of safe and simple anesthesia.

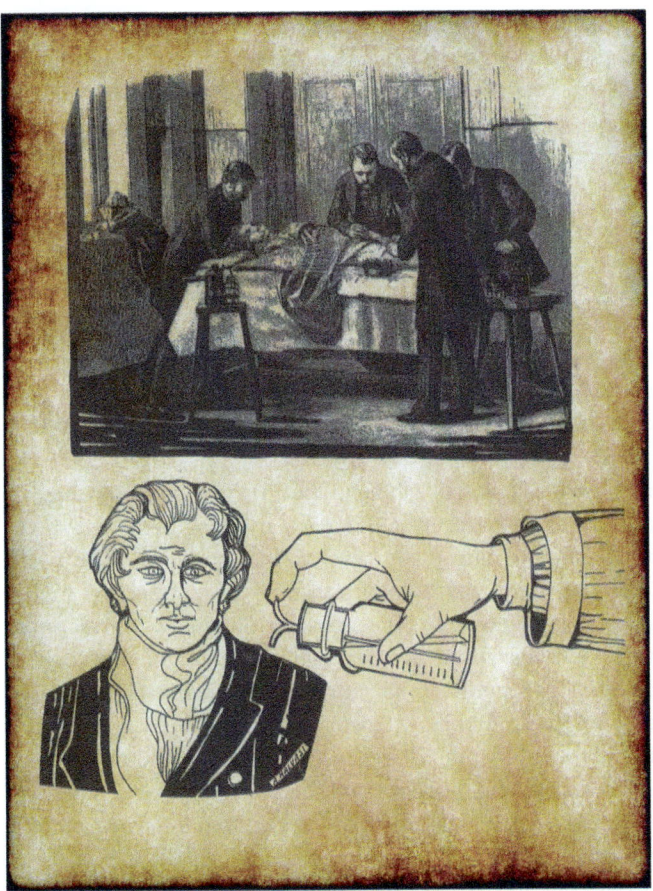

Fig. 7.4 John Snow (1813–1858) studied and calculated dosages for the use of ether and chloroform as surgical anesthetics. He made about 4000 anesthesia and treated 77 obstetric patients using chloroform as an anesthetic for childbirth

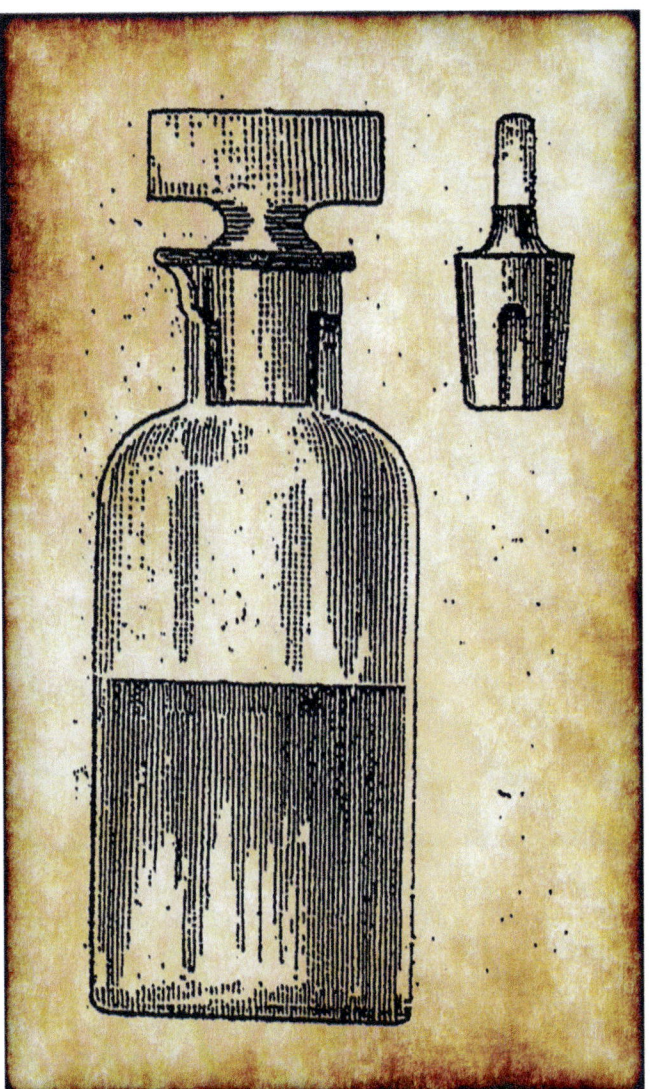

Fig. 7.5 Ancient bottle of chloroform

7.2   Introduction

The history of in vitro fertilization (IVF) and embryo transfer (ET) dates back as early as the 1890s when Walter Heape, a professor at the Cambridge University, United Kingdom, reported the first known case of embryo transplantation in rabbits. In vitro fertilization and ET technology developed rapidly in humans since the first successful birth of a child (Louise Brown) occurred in 1978 as a result of a scientist Robert Edwards and his gynecologist Patrick Steptoe's IVF techniques [2] (Fig. 7.6).

The assisted reproductive technologies have evolved tremendously since the emergence of IVF techniques and today anesthesiologists play an important role in the process of oocyte retrieval and other IVF-related procedures [3]. A variety of anesthetic techniques like conscious sedation, general anesthesia, and regional anesthesia have been tried with none being superior to the other. However; irrespective of the techniques the key point of anesthesia for IVF is to provide the anesthetic exposure for least duration so as to avoid its detrimental effects on the embryo cleavage and fertilization.

In vitro fertilization treatment is most commonly conducted using exogenous FSH to induce follicular growth and human chorionic gonadotropin (hCG) to induce final oocyte maturation. It is very important for the gynecologists that the harvesting of oocytes takes place within a defined period of time to ensure the best fertility outcomes. These oocytes are subsequently fertilized in vitro and allowed to develop into embryos that are finally transferred into the uteri of patients.

In the beginning, oocyte harvesting was performed by laparoscopy, a process that required the administration of general anesthesia in the hospital setting. The technological progress and development of transvaginal ultrasounds allowed oocyte retrieval from the ovary through the puncture of the vaginal wall under the ultrasound guide and under conscius sedation (Fig. 7.7).

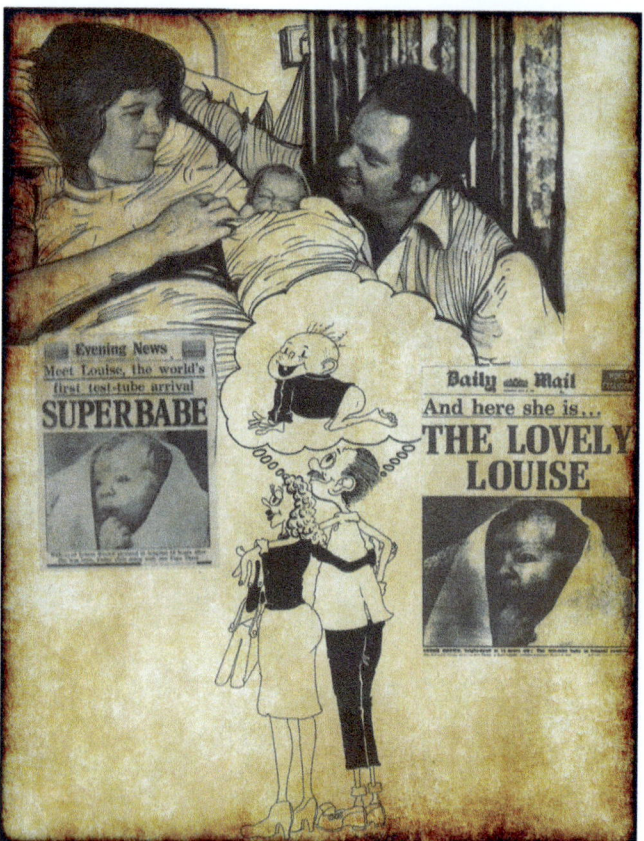

Fig. 7.6 The first successful birth of a child (Louise Brown) occurred in 1978 as a result of a scientist Robert Edwards and his gynecologist Patrick Steptoe's IVF techniques

Oocyte (egg) retrieval for in vitro fertilization is a relatively short procedure, usually performed as an outpatient. The duration of oocyte retrieval is on average several minutes (maximum a half an hour), depending on the amount of follicles to be aspirated and the anatomical position of the ovaries. It is a common belief that when the duration of oocyte retrieval procedure is >10–15 min, immediate post-procedure pain score is significantly higher compared to those patients whose procedure where for <10–15 min.

Conscious sedation is the most commonly used technique in IVF because it is relatively safe. Target-controlled infusion (e.g., propofol) is a suitable anesthetic technique. Propofol is the preferred anesthetic agent for oocyte retrieval, but should be used by specially trained personnel (Figs. 7.8, 7.9, and 7.10). After the oocyte retrieval, women are kept under observation for a few hours to make sure that there are no complications and they have regained the level of consciousness. Usually, the discharge from the IVF center takes place for a few hours (e.g., 2–4 h) after the oocyte retrieval.

Furthermore, an increased attention has also developed the potential adverse effects of different types of anesthesia, not only on the patients undergoing oocyte retrieval but also on the quality of the oocytes that may eventually effect embryo development and pregnancy success [4, 5].

7.3 Oocyte Retrieval: Pre-procedure Considerations

Oocyte retrieval for in vitro fertilization is one of the most common minor surgical procedures. As in any surgical procedure, there are some common basic requirements that should be fulfilled before any technique can be used in the treatment of patients. The anesthetic agent should be easy to administer, its effects should be easily monitored, and short-acting agents with ready reversible effects should be used. Adequate pain control is of paramount importance. A multi-disciplinary approach is necessary to obtain a better diagnostic classification of women who present themselves for assisted conception, and subsequently better reproductive technologies outcomes. Obstetric anesthesia is considered a high-risk subspecialty of anesthesia [6, 7]. A long series of evidence-based guidelines and reviews of mortality and morbidity have been used to adopt constant improvement in maternal safety and perioperative outcomes [8–11].

Usually, this population of patients is healthy and in their 30–40 years, however some women might present with various comorbidities (e.g., hypertension, diabetes mellitus, obesity) [3]. The development of the transvaginal approach for oocyte retrieval has allowed the possibility of using sedation for most cases and regional anesthesia and/or general anesthesia only with more complex cases where sedation might not be adequate.

The American Society of Anesthesiologists classification of physical status (ASA PS) is a widely used system for categorizing the preoperative status of patients [12]. The ASA class is a good independent predictor of perioperative morbidity and mortality. However; the definitions of the ASA classes have been amended several times since 1941, resulting in inconsistent and confusing usage in the current literature.

Since most of the anesthetic agents, either inhalational and/or intravenous, reach the follicular fluid within minutes after administration [13], they should be devoid of any toxic effects on the oocyte.

Guasch et al. [14] designed a clinical trial to determine the plasma and follicular levels of prolactin and cortisol in patients in an assisted reproduction program. Women were randomized to three anesthetic groups: (1) general anesthesia, (2) spinal anesthesia, or (3) sedation with alfentanil and mid-

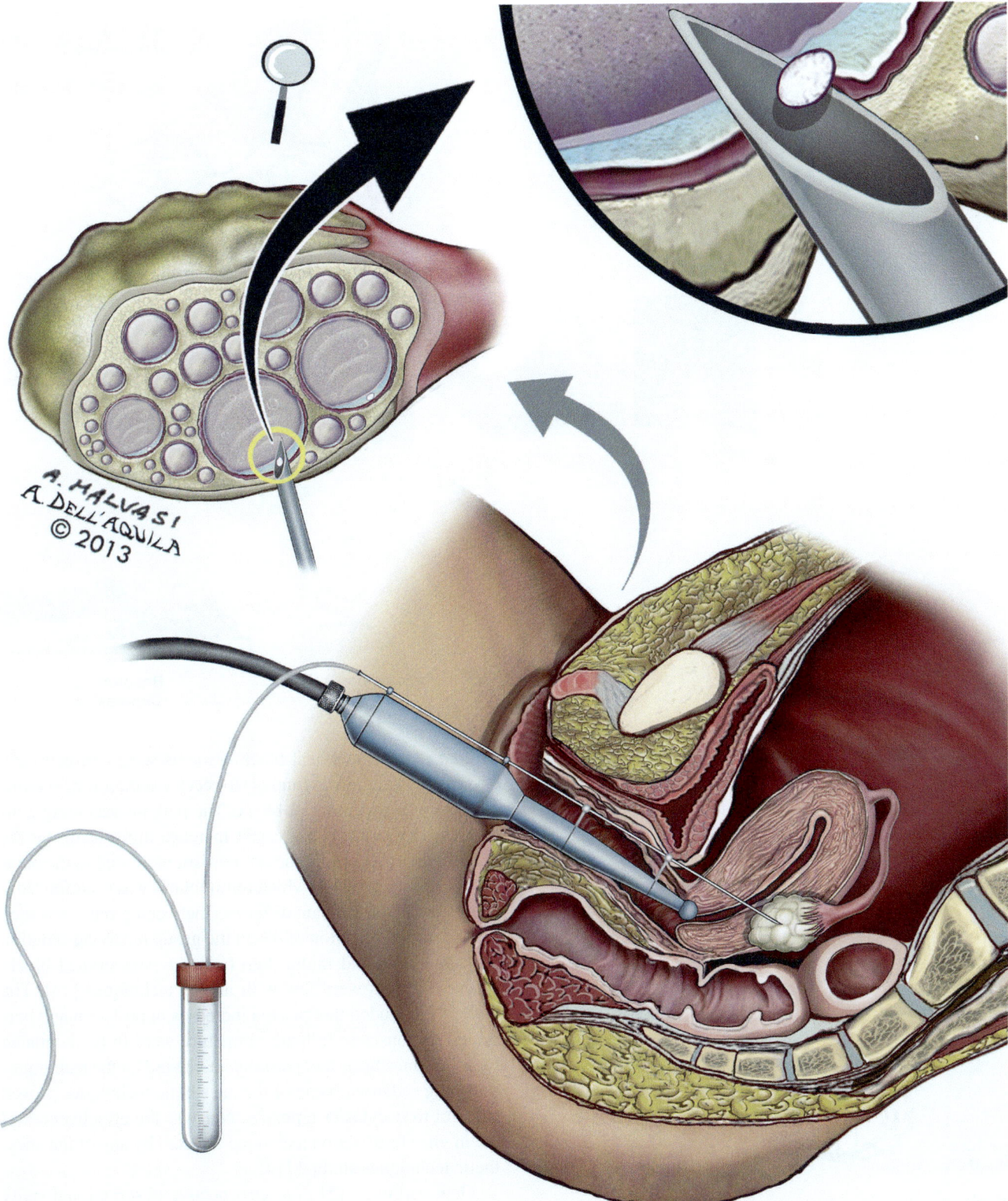

Fig. 7.7 The transvaginal ultrasound technique permitted the puncture and aspiration of the follicles through the vaginal wall under direct sonographic visualization

Fig. 7.8 Flow chart on side-effects of IV anesthetic propofol

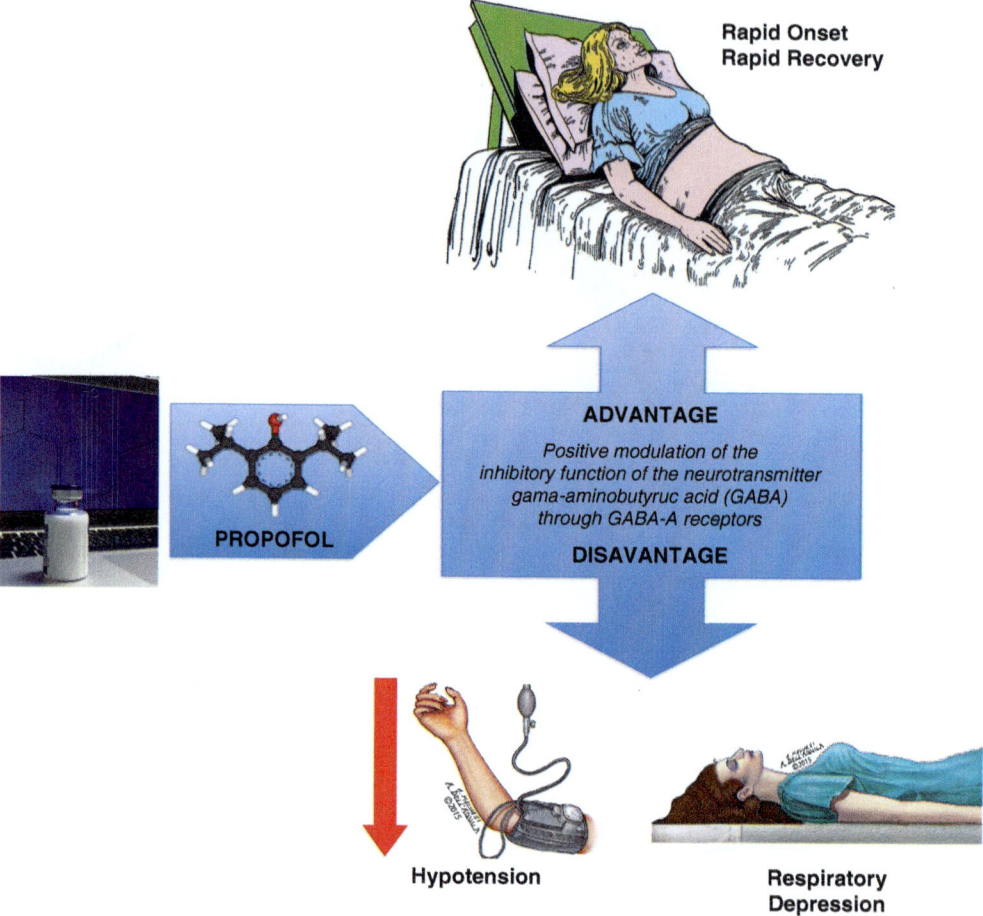

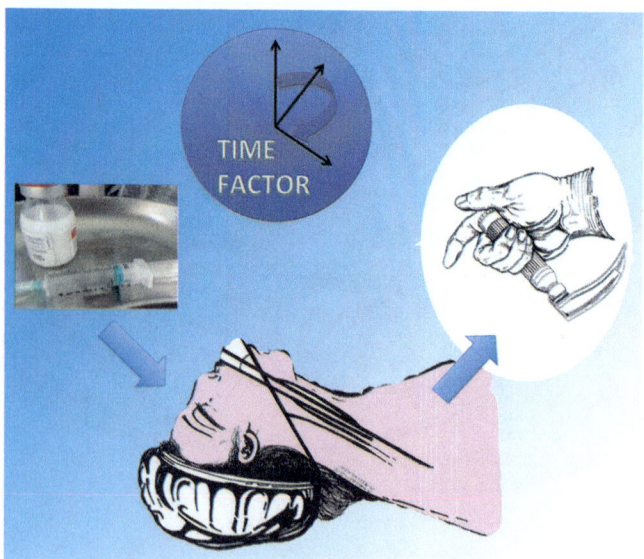

Fig. 7.9 Rapid sequence intubation

azolam plus paracervical block. Patients were consecutively assigned to the fourth group (4) to receive sedation with remifentanil plus paracervical block. The patients receiving general anesthesia had the greatest increase in prolactin by the end of the procedure. Follicular cortisol increased in the paracervical block group in which remifentanil was used for sedation. The only significant difference between groups was seen for the rate of gestation of 0% in the group receiving sedation with alfentanil and midazolam before a paracervical block. Adverse effects were few with all the techniques [14]. The authors concluded that plasma increases in prolactin and hormonal responses to follicular puncture were fully attenuated by spinal anesthesia and partially attenuated by the techniques requiring sedation. None of the anesthetic techniques proved harmful to oocytes or embryos. Nor was the effectiveness of the in vitro fertilization technique affected by any of the anesthetic techniques studied [14].

Gejervall et al. [5] in a retrospective observational study compared the effect of different doses of alfentanil (Fig. 7.11)

Fig. 7.10 Side-effects of
propofol general anesthesia

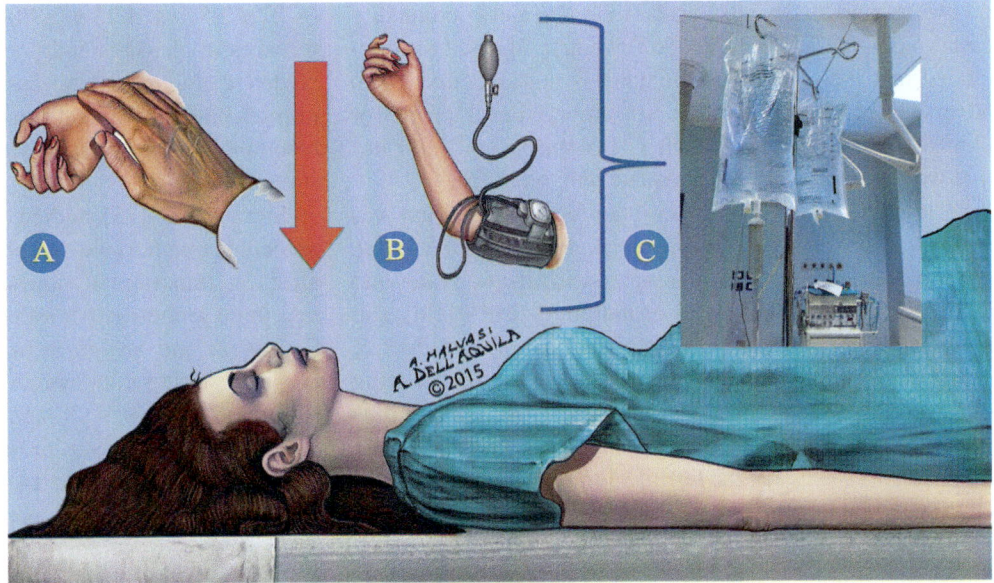

Fig. 7.11 Flow chart on the
side-effects of opioid
alfentanil

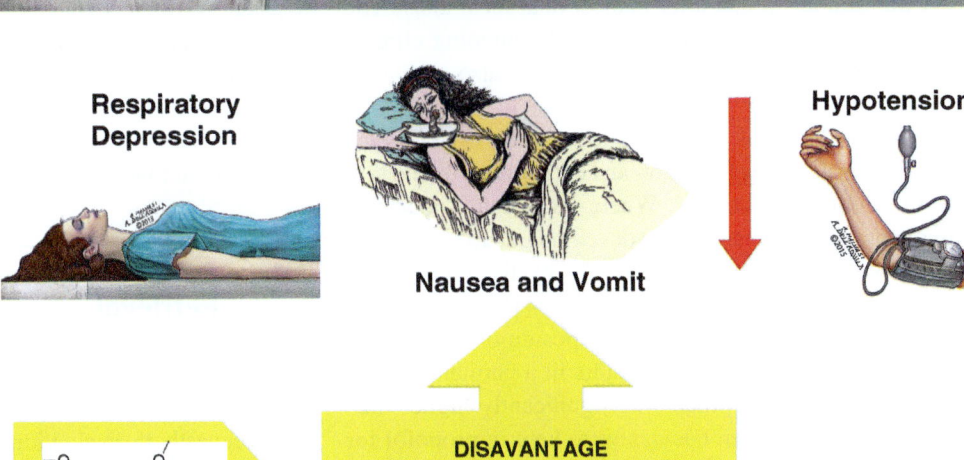

**Respiratory
Depression**

Nausea and Vomit

Hypotension

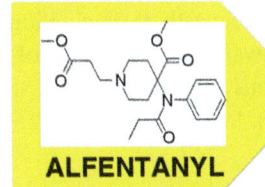

ALFENTANYL

DISAVANTAGE

*Alfentanil primarily binds to mu-opioid
receptor, mimicking the actions of morphine,
the prototypical mu receptor agonist*

ADVANTAGE

**Rapid Onset
Rapid Recovery**

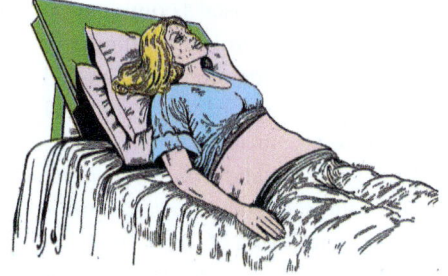

on two primary endpoints, fertilization rate and good quality embryo (GQE) rate 663 (N = 663) women. The authors concluded that the amount of alfentanil is not associated with adverse effects on fertilization rate, embryo development, or clinical pregnancy rate, which is reassuring and indicates that women can be offered adequate pain relief [5].

A total of 202 patients undergoing fertility treatment was included in a prospective, matched, controlled study, in which Christiaens et al. [15] compared fertilization rates and embryo development in terms of morphological quality and speed of development and the implications for reproductive outcome and pregnancy following general anesthesia using either propofol or a paracervical local anesthetic block during oocyte collection. The authors concluded that there were no differences between the fertilization rates and the embryo cleavage characteristics for the two groups. The initial implantation rate per transferred embryo after general anesthesia was similar to that after paracervical local anesthetic block (13.4 versus 18.6%; P = 0.10). The ongoing clinical implantation rates per embryo transfer were also similar in the two groups [15].

Janssenswillen et al. [16] designed a study to assess the effect of propofol on fertilization and early embryo development in a mouse IVF model. Where fertilization occurred, subsequent embryo cleavage and development up to the blastocyst stage was affected significantly by the presence of propofol solution in the medium, (i.e., 3–41%) in comparison with the control group (76%). Exposure of unfertilized oocytes for 30 min to propofol results in a parthenogenetic activation of 33–60%, which was significantly higher than the control (10%). When oocytes were kept in propofol for 24 h, a mean of 30% of activation was observed as compared with 0.5% for the control. The authors concluded from these experiments that even a brief exposure of cumulus-enclosed oocytes to a low concentration of propofol is deleterious to subsequent cleavage. Exposure of unfertilized oocytes to propofol results in a high degree of parthenogenetic activation [16].

Hammadeh et al. [17] conducted a study to compare the effects of two different anesthetic techniques (general anesthesia versus sedation) used for oocyte retrieval on IVF outcome. For general anesthesia, the authors used a combination of remifentanil (Ultiva) with either propofol or isoflurane in hypnotic concentrations. For sedation, the protocol included midazolam, diazepam, or propofol according to clinical needs. In total, 202 women were enrolled in the study. Ninety-six women opted for sedation and 106 for general anesthesia. The number of collected oocytes was significantly higher with general anesthesia (10.54 ± 5.43 [mean ± SD]) than with sedation (6.25 ± 3.65, P < 0.0001), whereas the number of fertilized oocytes was not different

(4.70 ± 3.57 vs. 4.23 ± 2.90). There were no significant differences in cleavage and pregnancy rates. The authors concluded that remifentanil-based general anesthesia without nitrous oxide is a suitable alternative to sedation and may be recommended for IVF oocyte retrieval if general anesthesia is requested [17].

Sterzik et al. [18] studied the effect of different anesthetic procedures on hormone levels in women. Fifty-four patients awaiting transvaginal oocyte aspiration were randomized into three groups: (1) anesthesia with ketamine as an induction agent and analgesic (n = 20); (2) general intubation anesthesia using thiopentone for induction and enflurane for maintenance (n = 18); and (3) no anesthesia (n = 16). Estradiol, progesterone, prolactin, and beta-endorphin were measured from day 3 to 14 referring to follicle aspiration. Differences between preoperative hormone levels and their intra- and postoperative peaks were analyzed using the Kruskal-Wallis test (P < 0.03). The authors concluded that the increased prolactin and beta-endorphin plasma levels associated with ketamine and general anesthesia reflect a significant alteration of the observed hormone levels. When anesthesia is indicated, they try to avoid general intubation anesthesia in favor of ketamine [18].

7.4 Principles of Anesthesia for Oocyte Retrieval

7.4.1 Preanesthetic Evaluation

The preanesthetic evaluation of patients scheduled for oocyte retrieval is similar to that of other preoperative patients, with a focus on assessment of the airway (Figs. 7.12, 7.13, and 7.14), lower back (Fig. 7.15), and coexisting patient's medi-

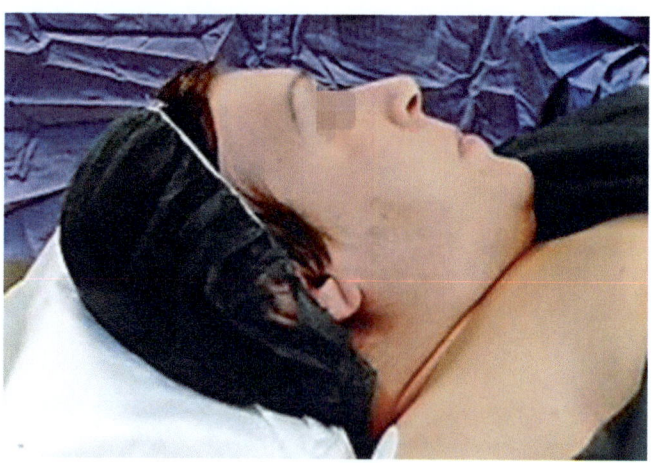

Fig. 7.12 Obesity patient with difficult airway management

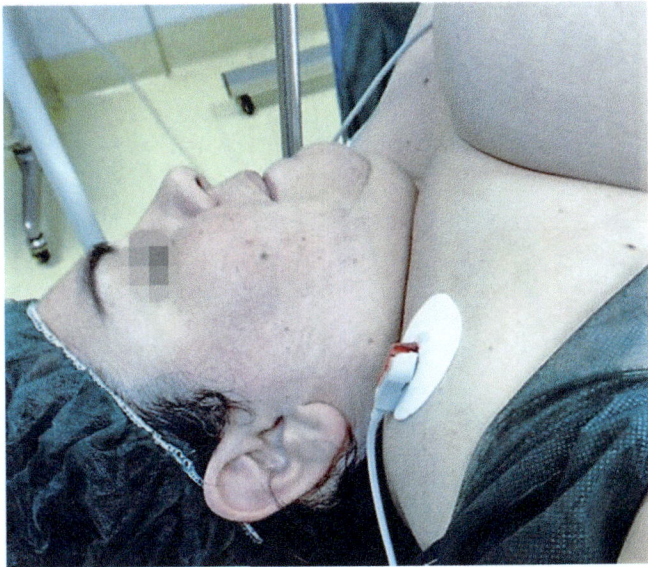

Fig. 7.13 Obesity patient and large breast

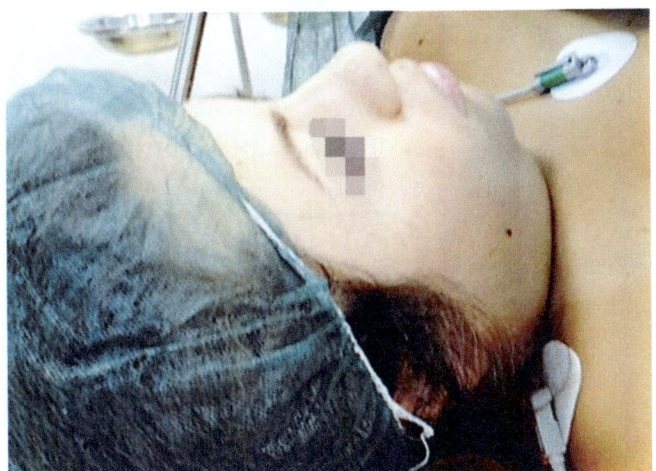

Fig. 7.14 Lower jaw with receding chin

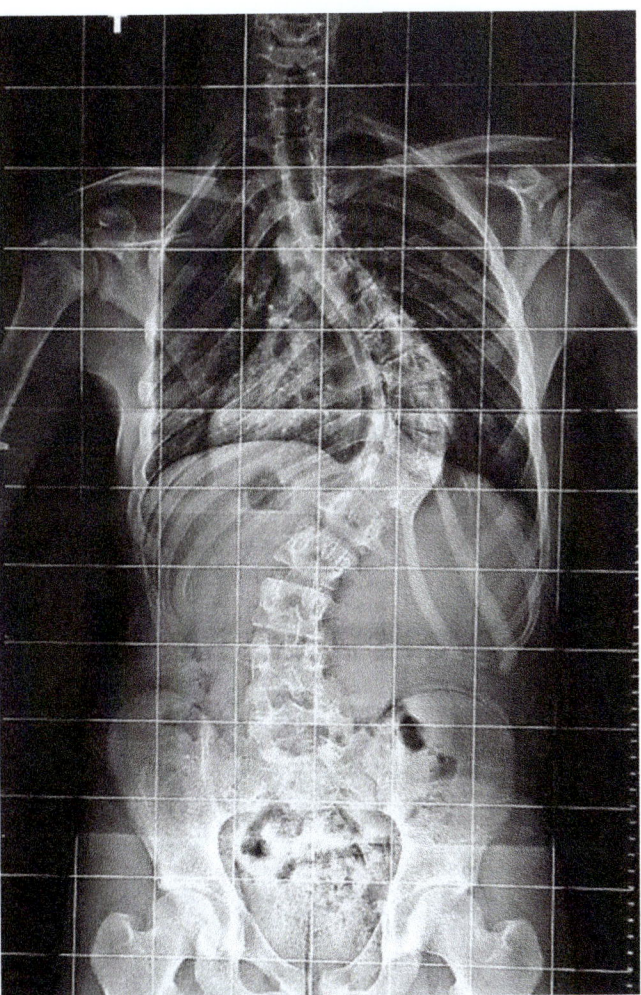

Fig. 7.15 Severe thoracic and lumbar scoliosis and difficult execution of neuraxial anesthesia

cal conditions. Challenges and complications related to anesthesia are more common in obese patients (see Figs. 7.12, 7.13, and 7.14) and include difficulty with monitoring, positioning, airway management (Figs. 7.16, 7.17, 7.18, 7.19, 7.20, 7.21, and 7.22), and neuraxial techniques (Figs. 7.23, 7.24, and 7.25) [19]. In patients with specific medical issues, such as predicted difficult airway (see Figs. 7.12, 7.13, and 7.14) or (rarely) malignant hyperthermia susceptibility, there are additional reasons to avoid general anesthesia. Therefore, anesthesiology consultation is always recommended.

IVF procedures can be conducted with local infiltration, neuraxial anesthesia, and conscious sedation and under general anesthesia.

7.5 Sedation

The American Society of Anesthesiologists (ASA) House of Delegates approved the definition of General Anesthesia, Depth of Sedation, Levels of Sedation/Analgesia [20]. Minimal Sedation (Anxiolysis) is drug-induced state during which patients respond normally to verbal commands. Citations from the ASA document are listed below:

Their definition:

Minimal Sedation (Anxiolysis) is a drug-induced state during which patients respond normally to verbal commands. Although cognitive function and physical coordination may be impaired, airway reflexes, and ventilatory and cardiovascular functions are unaffected.

Moderate Sedation/Analgesia (Conscious Sedation) is a drug-induced depression of consciousness during which

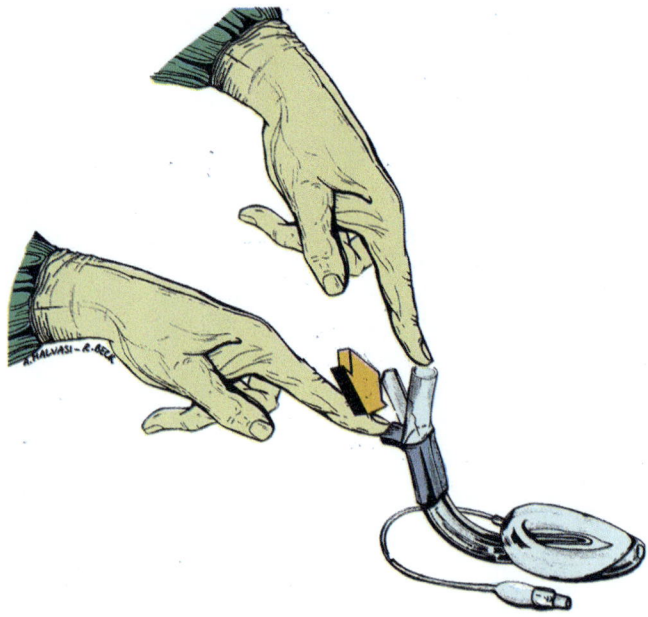

Fig. 7.16 Laryngeal mask airway (LMA) a supraglottic management device

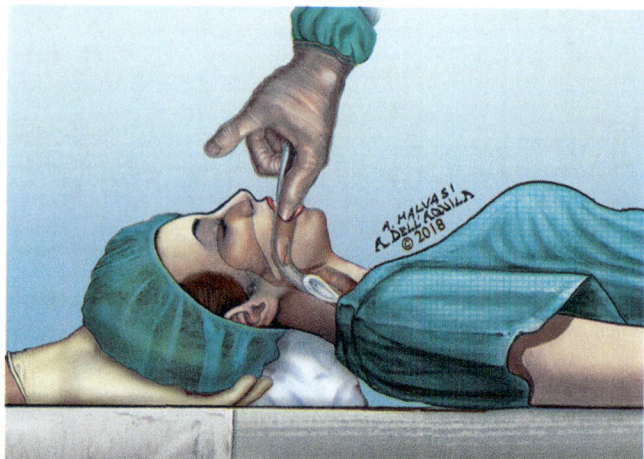

Fig. 7.17 Insertion of the LMA holding the LMA with the index finger of the dominant hand at the junction of the mask and pushing it back against the hard palate

patients respond purposefully[1, 2] to verbal commands, either alone or accompanied by light tactile stimulation. No interventions are required to maintain a patent airway, and spontaneous ventilation is adequate. Cardiovascular function is usually maintained.

---

[1]Monitored Anesthesia Care ("MAC") does not describe the continuum of depth of sedation, rather it describes "a specific anesthesia service in which an anesthesiologist has been requested to participate in the care of a patient undergoing a diagnostic or therapeutic procedure."

[2]Reflex withdrawal from a painful stimulus is NOT considered a purposeful response.

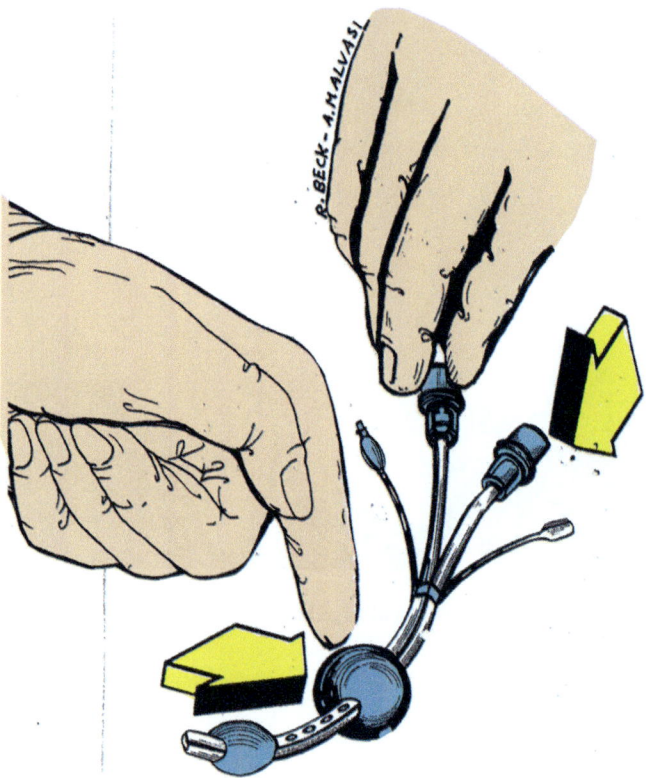

Fig. 7.18 Esophageal tracheal combitube (ETC)

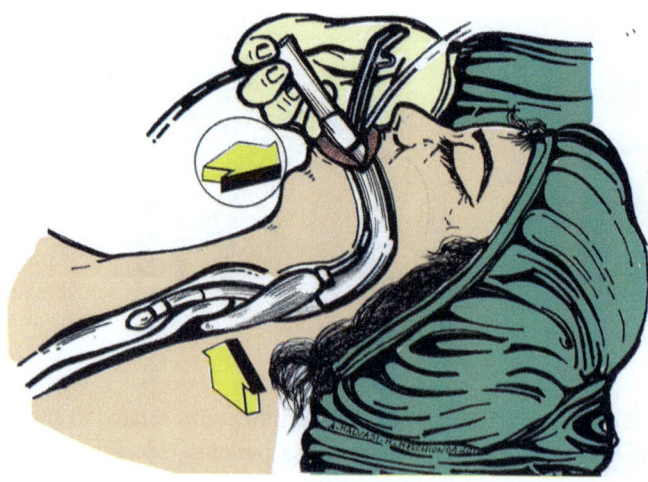

Fig. 7.19 Insertion of the intubating laryngeal mask airway (ILMA)

Deep Sedation/Analgesia is a drug-induced depression of consciousness during which patients cannot be easily aroused but respond purposefully[2] following repeated or painful stimulation. The ability to independently maintain ventilatory function may be impaired. Patients may require assistance in maintaining a patent airway, and spontaneous ventilation may be inadequate. Cardiovascular function is usually maintained.

Conscious sedation, defined as a "minimally depressed level of consciousness that retains the ability of the patient to maintain a patent airway independently and continuously

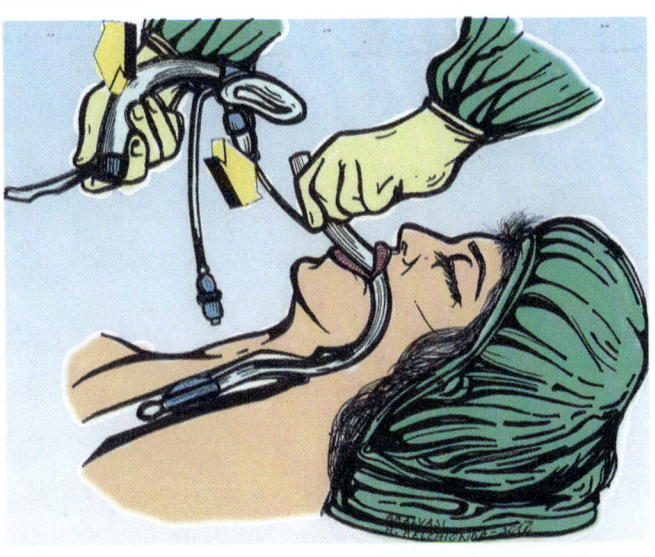

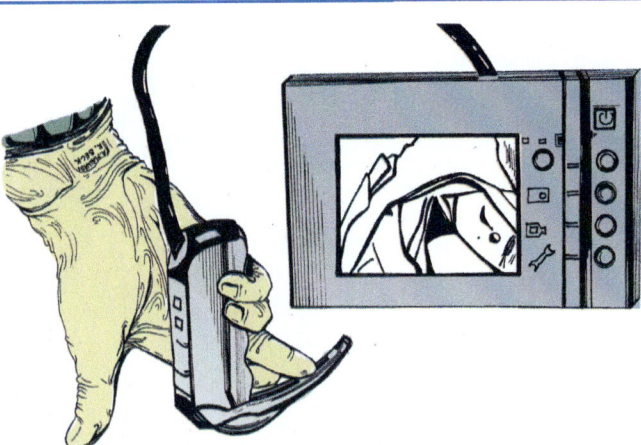

Fig. 7.21 Videolaryngoscopy for difficult airway management

Fig. 7.20 Intubating through the ILMA. Once the patient is intubated, the LMA can be removed by deflating the cuff and passing it over the tube using a stabilizer rod

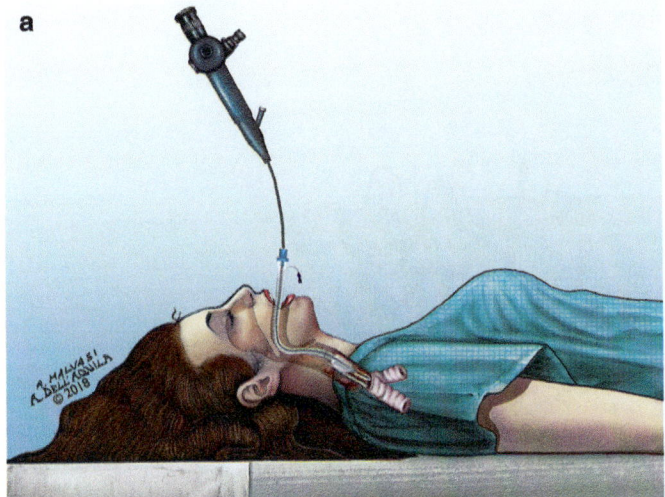

Fig. 7.22 (**a**) Fibrobrochoscopy for difficult airway management. (**b**) Insertion of the endotracheal tube through the fibrobronchoscopic vision into the trachea

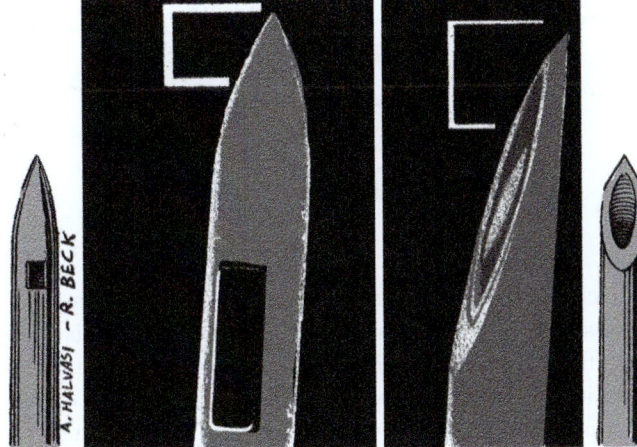

Fig. 7.23 Types of spinal needles: left atraumatic Sprotte needle, right cutting Quincke needle

and to respond appropriately to verbal commands" [21], is currently the most common form of anesthesia used during oocyte retrieval in the United States [22]. Conscious sedation can be achieved either with inhalation or intravenous agents. Intravenous agents are more popular because they cause less postoperative nausea and vomiting and are easier to administer.

7.5.1 Agents Used for Conscious Sedation

Opioids (morphine, meperidine, fentanyl, alfentanil) (see Figs. 7.3, 7.11, and 7.26) are used in conscious sedation primarily for their analgesic effects. Opioids act on the hypothalamus to decrease the body's response to the stressful

Fig. 7.24 Insertion of the epidural catheter into the epidural space

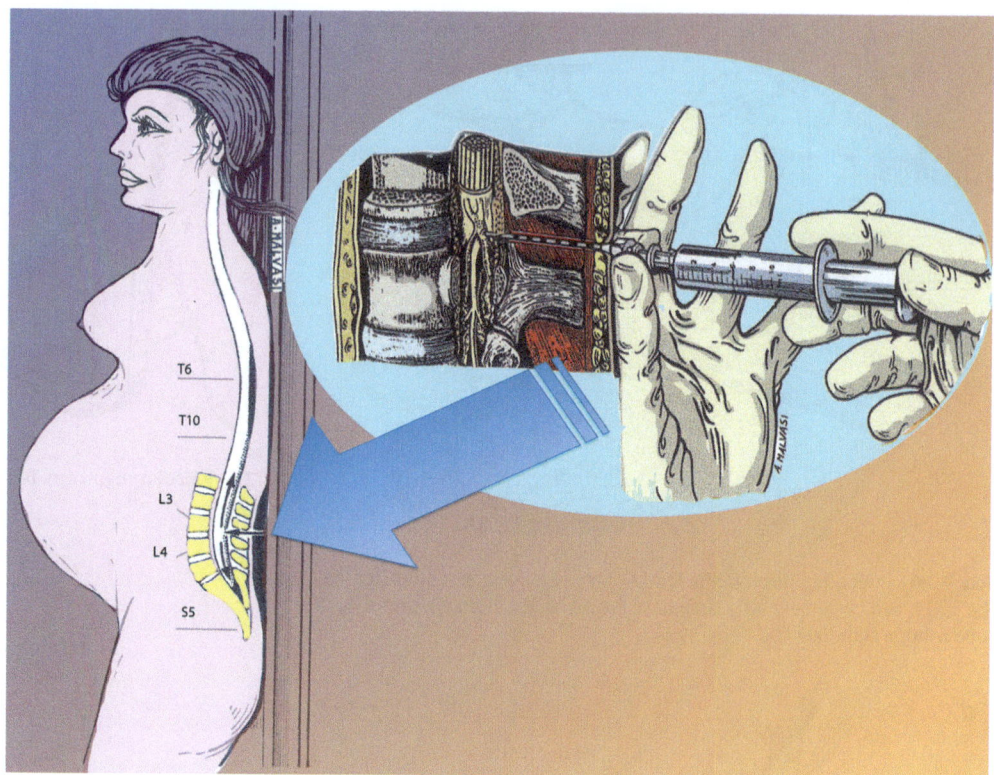

Fig. 7.25 Neuraxial technique: midline insertion of the spinal needle (left) and lateral insertion of the spinal needle with an angle of 30° in the caudal direction (right)

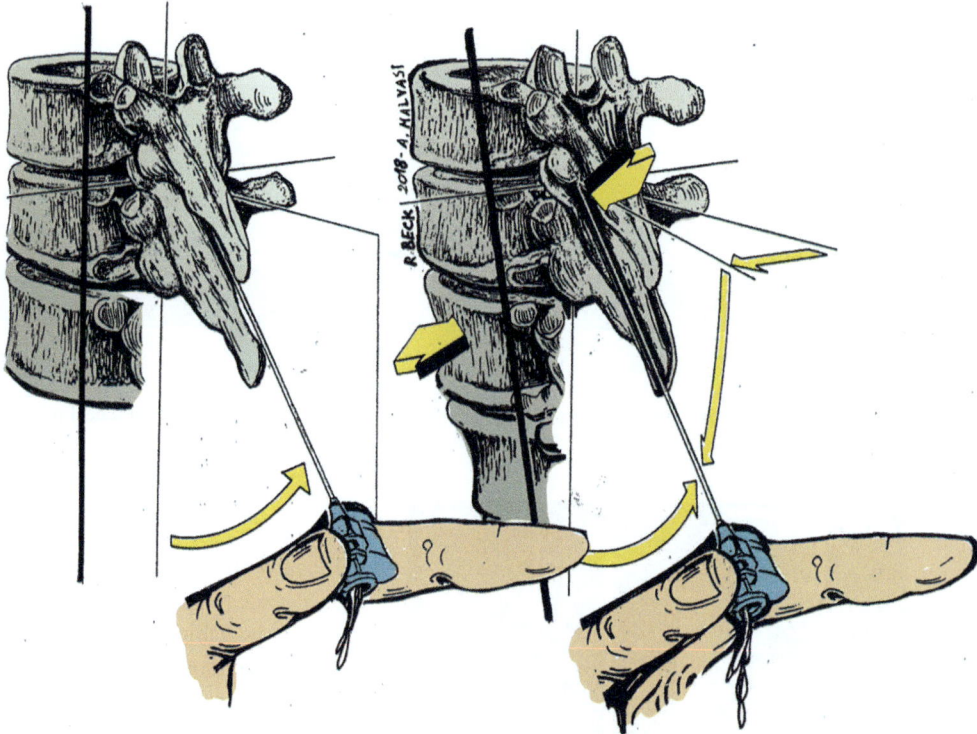

stimuli. Opioids have a direct effect on the medulla, producing a dose-dependent depression of respiration in response to hypercapnia. Opioid administration decreases minute ventilation by decreasing respiratory rate and may lead to apnea. Rapid administration of opioids can induce rigidity of the thoracic muscles (stiff chest syndrome), which can also involve the laryngeal and pharyngeal muscles. This is a potential life-threatening complication that may result in the inability to ventilate the patient. Administration of an opioid antagonist such as naloxone or a muscle relaxant such as

Fig. 7.26 Flow chart on the side-effects of opioid fentanyl

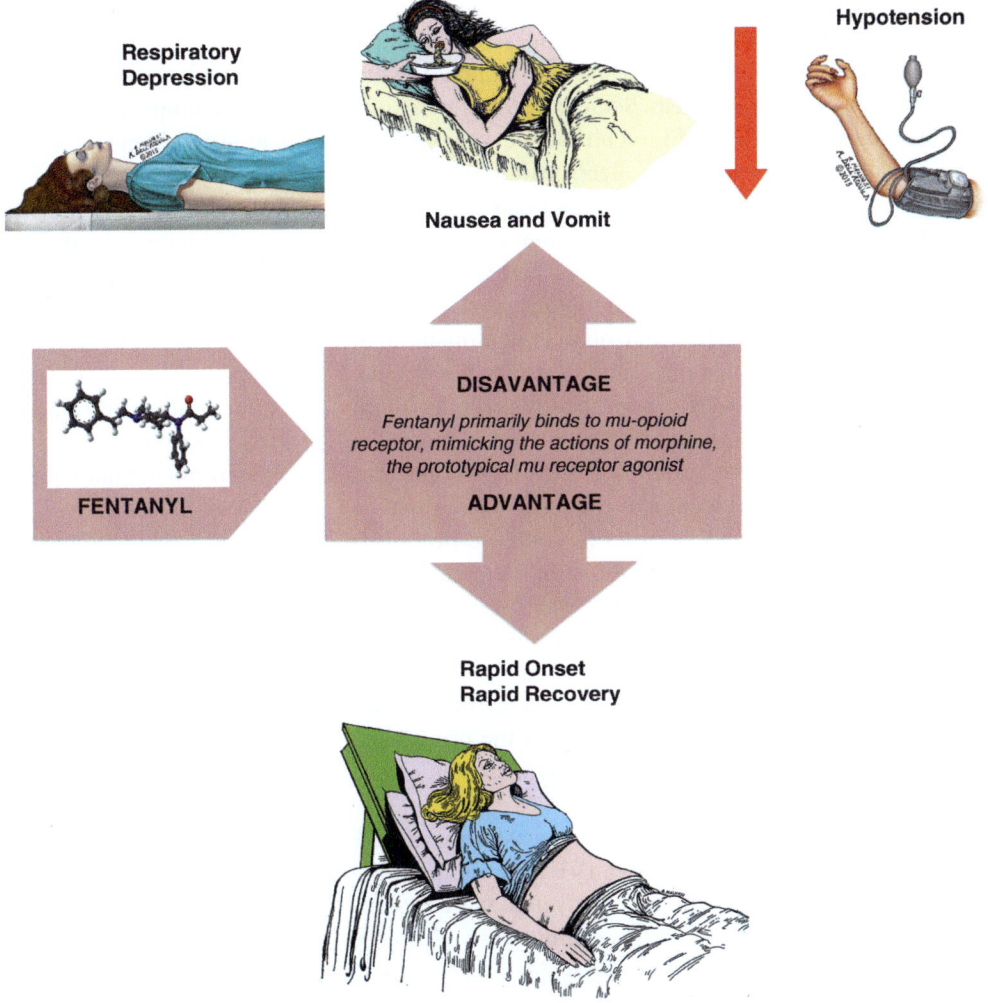

Respiratory Depression

Nausea and Vomit

Hypotension

DISAVANTAGE

Fentanyl primarily binds to mu-opioid receptor, mimicking the actions of morphine, the prototypical mu receptor agonist

FENTANYL

ADVANTAGE

Rapid Onset Rapid Recovery

succinylcholine followed by immediate intubation may be required. Opioids can also cause sedation and have a synergistic effect when given in combination with benzodiazepines. Fortunately, all the effects of opioids, including respiratory depression and pruritus, can be readily reversed with the administration of opioid antagonists, with the exception of the stiff chest syndrome that may require the additional administration of muscle relaxants.

Benzodiazepines (midazolam, diazepam, lorazepam) are used mainly because of their sedative, anxiolytic, and amnesic effects. Their analgesic effect is minimal. Additional properties of benzodiazepines include muscle relaxation through their action on spinal internuncial neurons and anticonvulsive effects. In combination with opioids, their sedative effects are enhanced, therefore allowing the use of reduced doses of both medications. However, the concurrent use of benzodiazepines and opioids may increase the incidence of apnea and respiratory depression. This effect is more prominent in patients with chronic obstructive pulmonary disease. Benzodiazepines offer only antegrade amnesia (patients do not have any recollection of the events following administration) so it is important to ensure that they are given early enough in the procedure.

Propofol, a relatively new agent, has been widely used either alone or in combination with other agents for oocyte retrieval. It provides rapid onset of analgesia and anesthesia, short duration of action, and rapid recovery with minimal drug accumulation. The mechanism of action of propofol is poorly understood. It has been reported that it may inhibit excitatory stimuli in the olfactory cortex and spinal cord through inhibition of the N-methyl-D-aspartate receptor (NMDA) channels. In addition, propofol seems to potentiate gamma-aminobutyric acid (GABA)-mediated synaptic inhibition in a variety of systems [23, 24] (see Figs. 7.8, 7.9, and 7.10). Propofol administration has been associated with a dose-dependent decrease in systemic blood pressure due to a decrease in systemic vascular resistance and suppression of myocardial contractility. These effects, in combination with a dose-dependent respiratory depression that ultimately results in apnea requiring assistance of ventilation, make propofol use appropriate only by personnel skilled in airway management (see Figs. 7.16, 7.17, 7.18, 7.19, 7.20, 7.21, and 7.22).

Most often a combination of propofol, fentanyl, and midazolam is used for conscious sedation. After an intravenous access has been established, the patient is connected to the standard American Society of Anesthesiology (ASA) monitors that record blood pressure every 3–5 min, oxygen saturation, continuous electrocardiogram, heart rate, percentage of inspired oxygen, and end tidal carbon dioxide. A precordial stethoscope to monitor respiratory rate and the quality of breath sounds is highly advisable. Oxygen 2–4 L/min is administered by face mask throughout the procedure. Initially, midazolam is administered at a dose of 1–2.5 mg to induce anxiolysis and amnesia. Propofol boluses of 10–20 mg are given every 1–2 min until the patient has been adequately sedated. Alternatively, a continuous propofol infusion of 80–150 µg/kg/min can be used. An intravenous local anesthetic such as lidocaine at a dose of 1 mg/kg may be used to decrease propofol-related burning at the site of the infusion. Fentanyl 25 µg titrated slowly to a total of 50–100 µg can also be added to the regimen for postoperative analgesia. For better pain control, the analgesic agent (i.e., fentanyl) should be administered prior to any painful stimuli, a method known as preemptive analgesia. At completion of the procedure, discontinuation of the infusion results in the patient awakening within 3–5 min [25].

Conscious sedation as a method of anesthesia gained its popularity for oocyte retrieval in IVF because it is easy to administer in patients who are motivated and cooperative. In addition, it is very safe to administer in relatively healthy individuals. The majority of women who participate in an IVF program are relatively young, healthy, and motivated. For patients with underlying cardiovascular or respiratory conditions, or for very obese patients, conscious sedation may not be appropriate. There is a fine line between conscious sedation with good pain control and general anesthesia with respiratory suppression that requires assisted ventilation or even intubation. Careful monitoring of the patients by an experienced individual such a registered nurse or an anesthesiologist, and with the use of a pulse oximeter and continuous electrocardiographic monitoring is very important to assure patient safety.

Young couples presenting for infertility treatment at medical attention are commonly anxious, so subsequently of sedation has a positive impact on women undergoing oocyte retrieval: reducing stress, panic, and anxiety. Unfavorable and untoward events can be prevented by accurate, preoperative assessment and proper monitoring in the perioperative period as well as during the emergency [26].

The management of any medical urgency should be conducted with assessment of the airway, breathing and circulation, as outlined in the Basic Life Support Guidelines (IRC—2015).

7.5.2 Complications During Sedation

- Nausea and Vomiting: Nausea and vomiting may be side-effects of opioids administration. Reduced dose of opioid and use anti-emetic agents as metoclopramide or ondansetron are helpful (see Figs. 7.11 and 7.26).
- Pulmonary Aspiration: The aspiration of gastric contents into the lungs usually occurs when the patient is unconscious. This complication may lead to pneumonia, pulmonary distress, and death.
- Respiratory Depression: Respiratory depression is defined as apnea, hypopnea, and oxyhemoglobin desaturations. It is important to distinguish the opioid or benzodiazepine-related respiratory depression from airway obstruction. Flumazenil or Naloxone is used for reversal of respiratory depression (see Figs. 7.11 and 7.26).
- Airway Obstruction: The airway obstruction can result from pathological condition of anatomical structures or the presence of foreign body (e.g., false teeth). Other causes of airway obstruction include exposure to smoke, asthma (e.g., bronchospasm, laryngospasm), anaphylactoid reaction or hyper-reactive airway. The management depends on the cause and severity of the case.
- Hypoxia: It is relatively the most common cardiorespiratory complication during sedation. It is a consequence of respiratory depression or airway obstruction.
- Hypotension: Cardiovascular effects of propofol, opioid, or benzodiazepine include decreased cardiac output, systemic vascular resistance, and arterial blood pressure. The literature defines hypotension as declined in blood pressure of less than 90 mmHg which is due to a fall in either cardiac output or total peripheral resistance (leading to drop in the patient's mean arterial pressure). The use of intravascular fluid supplementation or administration of vasopressor might be beneficial (see Figs. 7.8, 7.10, 7.11, and 7.26).
- Hypertension: Causes include systemic hypertension, anxiety, pain, and reflex pressure in response from intubation. Proper preoperative assessment of patients with pre-existing condition/s is necessary.
- Arrhythmias, Myocardial ischemia/infarction, and Cardiac arrest: The use of ECG during sedation is mandatory. Sinus tachycardia can be related to pain or hypotension. It is rarely that we can observe myocardical ischemia/infarction and cardiac arrest in these populations of patients.

7.6 General Anesthesia

The definition of general anesthesia by the American Society of Anesthesiologists. Continuum of Depth of Sedation: Definition of General Anesthesia and Levels of Sedation/Analgesia [20] is provided below:

General anesthesia is a drug-induced loss of consciousness during which patients are not arousable, even by painful stimulation. The ability to independently maintain ventilatory function is often impaired. Patients often require assistance in maintaining a patent airway, and positive pressure ventilation may be required because of depressed spontaneous ventilation or drug-induced depression of neuromuscular function. Cardiovascular function may be impaired.

Because sedation is a continuum, it is not always possible to predict how an individual patient will respond. Hence, practitioners intending to produce a given level of sedation should be able to rescue[2,3] patients whose level of sedation becomes deeper than initially intended. Individuals administering Moderate Sedation/Analgesia (Conscious Sedation) should be able to rescue[2,3] patients who enter a state of Deep Sedation/Analgesia, while those administering Deep Sedation/Analgesia should be able to rescue[2,3] patients who enter a state of General Anesthesia.

General anesthesia should be administered invariably by specially trained personnel in a hospital-based environment. General anesthesia may preserve spontaneous ventilation or may require mechanical ventilation through an endotracheal tube or a laryngeal mask airway. General anesthesia, accomplished either by inhalational or intravenous agents, is frequently associated with prolonged recovery time and increased postanesthesia adverse effects. Other adverse systemic effects of general anesthesia that may have a potential detrimental effect on reproductive outcome include transient elevation of serum prolactin levels and suppression of progesterone production by corpus luteum [27].

Gottschalk et al. [28] conducted the selective review of the literature with focus on anesthesia-related mortality. Anesthesia-related mortality has fallen from 6.4/10,000 in the 1940s to 0.4/100,000 at present, largely because of the introduction of safety standards and improved training. The current figure of 0.4/100,000 applies to patients without major systemic disease; mortality is higher among patients with severe accompanying illnesses, yet in this group, too, perioperative mortality can be reduced by appropriate anesthetic management. Moreover, the use of regional anesthesia can also improve the outcome of major surgery [28]. The authors concluded that a recent increase in the percentage of older and multimorbid patients among persons undergoing surgery, along with the advent of newer types of operation that would have been unthinkable in the past, has led to an apparent rise in anesthesia-associated mortality, even though the quality of anesthesiological care is no worse now than in the past. On the contrary, in recent years, better anesthetic management has evidently played an important role in improving surgical outcomes [28].

As previously indicated [26], the risk for complications while providing moderate and deep sedation is greatest when caring for patients already medically compromised. It is reassuring that significant untoward events can generally be prevented by careful preoperative assessment, along with attentive intraoperative monitoring and support. Nevertheless, we must be prepared to manage untoward events should they arise. This continuing education article will review critical aspects of patient management of respiratory and cardiovascular complications.

7.7 Regional Anesthesia

"Regional anesthesia makes a specific part of the body numb to relieve pain or allows surgical procedures to be done" (JAMA, 2011) [29].

Regional anesthesia for oocyte retrieval can be provided in the form of spinal or epidural anesthesia collectively known as neuraxial anesthesia. Epidural anesthesia is achieved by the injection of local anesthetics in the epidural space whereas spinal anesthesia is achieved by the injection of local anesthetic into the subarachnoid space. By using different types and doses of local anesthetics, we can achieve various degrees of motor and sensory block within a specific area of the lower abdomen. Segmental block of specific neurotomes that innervate the lower abdominal area, sparing the lower extremities, allow the patient to remain comfortable and pain free during the procedure and still able to move the lower extremities and ambulate [30]. In addition, by using different local anesthetics, the onset of action and duration of anesthesia can be controlled easily and for this reason spinal anesthesia can provide an excellent operating condition for IVF. The anesthetized area should include at least the upper part of the vaginal wall and the pelvic viscera (uterus and ovaries) [30]. The atraumatic needles presently in use (e.g., Whitacre or Sprotte) decrease the incidence of postdural puncture headache (PDPH) to 1% [31–33] (see Fig. 7.23). Furthermore, use of low dose of local anesthetic in combination with narcotics as fentanyl or sufetanil can produce neuraxial blockade that decrease pain with preserved leg mobility [34–36].

Epidural anesthesia has the advantage of limited absorption of the anesthetic agents into the systemic circulation and has, therefore, been associated with minimal accumulation

---

[3] Rescue of a patient from a deeper level of sedation than intended is an intervention by a practitioner proficient in airway management and advanced life support. The qualified practitioner corrects adverse physiologic consequences of the deeper-than-intended level of sedation (such as hypoventilation, hypoxia, and hypotension) and returns the patient to the originally intended level of sedation. It is not appropriate to continue the procedure at an unintended level of sedation.

into the follicular fluid [37]. In addition, properly administered epidural anesthesia is associated with minimal respiratory depression.

7.7.1 Complication During Regional Anesthesia

Regional anesthesia is a safe technique, but like in all surgical procedures, however; rarely complications may occur (e.g., the cardiovascular, neurological, infectious, hematological, or total spinal anesthesia [38]).

– Hypotension is one of the cardiovascular complications of neuraxial technique. The most frequently applied definition is systolic arterial blood pressure less than 100 mmHg from baseline or if patient becomes symptomatic. Dense neuraxial blockade at the high sensory level, for example, fourth thoracic dermatome, includes sympathetic block and vasodilation that often results in hypotension. The hypotension can be prevented with low doses of local anesthetics in combination with intravenous fluid pre- or co-loading with crystalloids and ephedrine prophylaxis. Continuous hemodynamic monitoring should be applied [27, 39].
– Bradycardia and cardiac arrest are the most feared complications and have higher incidence in neuraxial than in general anesthesia. The blockade of the preganglionic cardioaccelerator fibers originating between vertebra T1 and T4 may progress in heart block or asystole. First-line therapy in this case is atropine, ephedrine is used when hypotension is associated with bradycardia or in unresponsive case to atropine.
– Postdural puncture headache (PDPH) is a common complication after inadvertent puncture of the dura mater. The risk factors included sex, young age, pregnancy, vaginal delivery, low body mass index, and being non-smoker. The PDPH is a postural headache that worsens with sitting or standing and improves with lying down. Conservative therapies, bed rest, hydration, and caffeine, are commonly used treatment and the blood epidural patch in the patients with unsuccessful conservative therapy [31, 32].
– Infective complications can occur if the meticulous aseptic technique during neuraxial block procedures in operating room has not been followed. The infection concerns the central nervous system such as arachnoiditis, meningitis, and abscess following spinal anesthesia. The source of infection is contamination by the hands or nasopharynx of the anesthesiologist that perform the neuraxial block. Using of sterile overalls, gloves, surgical cup, and face mask should be of procedural routine.
– Hematoma is a rare and well-recognized complication in patients who have received regional anesthesia. The

literature suggest that routine platelet count can predict anesthesia-related complications in patient with disorders associated with coagulopathy, or in patient in therapy with low molecular weight heparin, other factor Xa inhibitors, direct thrombin inhibitor, warfarin, aspirin, and GPIIb/IIIa antagonists [40, 41]. The American College of Obstetricians and Gynecologists (ACOG) Thrombocytopenia in Pregnancy Practice Bulletin recently concluded that neuraxial techniques are acceptable in parturients with platelet counts greater than 80,000 mm-3. Recently, it was suggested a safe neuraxial technique in patients whose platelet count was more than 56,000 mm-3 with normal thromboelastography value [42–46].
– Nausea and vomiting—Nausea is a common complaint during neuroaxial blocks. It is often related to hypotension from the sympathetic block, in which case restoring the blood pressure (with phenylephrine or ephedrine) should alleviate the nausea. Nausea and vomiting is common after spinal morphine (see Fig. 7.3) administration, but unlikely following neuraxial administration of lipophilic opioids (e.g., fentanyl, sufentanil) (see Fig. 7.26).
– Pruritus—Neuraxial opioids lead to pruritus in 60–100% of patient women. This may be resolved with small doses of intravenous opioid agonist-antagonist (e.g. nalbuphine 2.5–5 mg, butorphanol 1 mg), which may be followed by 2.2 mg/h infusion or antagonists (e.g. naloxone 40–100 mcg IV boluses), which may be followed by 0.25–1 mcg/kg/h infusion [47, 48].
– Total spinal anesthesia can happen when local anesthetic interferes with the normal neuronal function in the cervical spinal cord and brain stem. The onset is usually rapid and severe hypotension bradycardia, and respiratory arrest can occur. Management of total spinal anesthesia is mainly supportive: fluid administration, inotropic drugs

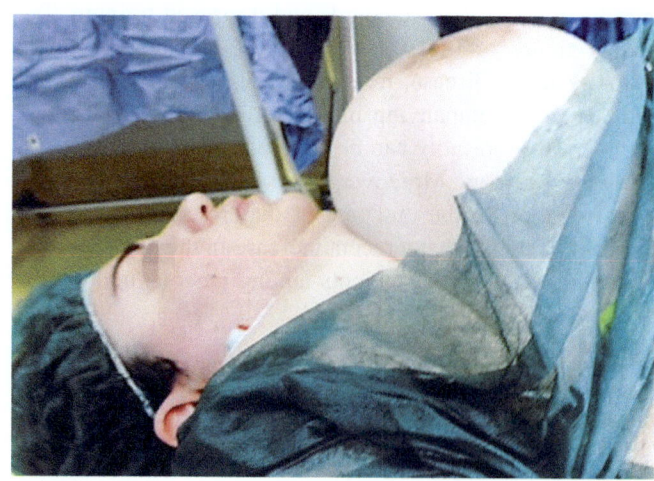

Fig. 7.27 Large breast in obesity patient and presupposed difficult airway management

or vasopressors to rise blood pressure, and atropine to treat bradycardia. Respiratory insufficiency may need tracheal intubation and mechanical ventilation [38].

About the problem of Regional Anesthesia, we can ask ourselves if we can talk about "complications or side-effects," because problems may be directly related to the performance of the technique (see Figs. 7.15, 7.24, and 7.25) or may result from poor management of the block. Pain at the moment of injection or paraesthesia while performing this technique are danger signals of potential injury and must not be ignored. Most complications of regional anesthesia are relatively minor, easily managed, and temporary (two third of paraplegias were transient) but in rare instances serious and permanent damage occurs. In literature, we found that permanent neurological injury is rare (0.02–0.07%); however, transient injuries do occur and were more common (0.01–0.8%) [49, 50].

Neuraxial anesthesia can be time consuming to perform and requires highly specialized anesthesia personnel, thus limiting its application outside a hospital environment.

7.8 Anesthesia and Analgesia for Oocyte Retrieval: What Is New and Important in the Literature?

Management of pain and anxiety in women undergoing oocyte retrieval procedures makes anesthesia and analgesia an important part of the in vitro fertilization (IVF) programs.

Multiple methods of conscious sedation and analgesia (CSA) have been used during oocyte retrieval in human in vitro fertilization (IVF). The choice of agent has been primarily influenced by the quality of CSA and by the concerns about possible detrimental effects of anesthesia on reproductive outcomes [51].

Kwan et al. assessed the effectiveness and safety of different methods of CSA for pain relief and pregnancy outcomes in women undergoing transvaginal oocyte retrieval [51]. The analysis (standard methodological procedures expected by Cochrane) included 24 randomized-controlled trials (RCTs) of 3160 women (N = 3160) in five comparisons. The authors concluded that the evidence in the literature does not support one particular method or technique over another in providing effective CSA for pain relief during, and what is equally important after oocyte retrieval. Simultaneous use of sedatives combined with analgesia such as the opiates, further enhanced by paracervical block or acupuncture techniques, resulted in better pain relief than occurred with one modality alone. Evidence was insufficient to show conclusively whether any of the interventions influenced pregnancy rates. All

techniques reviewed by the authors were associated with a high degree of patient intraoperative and postoperative satisfaction [51].

Morue et al. in a double-blinded RCT compared placebo vs low-dose ketamine infusion in addition to remifentanil target-controlled infusion (TCI) titrated to maintain a visual analogue pain score less than 30 mm for conscious sedation during oocyte retrieval in their institution [52]. After randomization, patients received either a ketamine infusion (40 µg kg min over 5 min followed by 2.5 µg kg min) or a 0.9% saline infusion in addition to the variable remifentanil TCI. No significant difference in the incidence of respiratory events was reported. In the ketamine group, visual analogue pain score and remifentanil concentrations were significantly reduced, but the latter remained above 2 ng mL. Postoperative nausea was less frequent in the ketamine group, 4 versus 15% (P = 0.038). The addition of ketamine did not influence the length of stay nor patient satisfaction. The authors concluded that the addition of low plasma levels of ketamine to a TCI remifentanil conscious sedation technique did not decrease the incidence nor the severity of respiratory depression. The authors also emphasized that continuous monitoring of capnography and oxygen saturation is always required during these procedures [52].

Özaltın et al. evaluated complications developing during and after transvaginal ultrasound-guided oocyte retrieval in 1031 patients (N = 1031) who underwent oocyte retrieval in the IVF unit of their hospital [53]. No anesthesia complications were reported. Vaginal bleeding was observed in 3.1% of the patients. There was no intra-abdominal bleeding or pelvic organ injuries requiring surgical intervention. Two patients developed pelvic abscesses. Ovarian hyperstimulation syndrome (OHSS) occurred in 1.45% of the patients. All of the patients tolerated the oocyte retrieval procedure well. After the procedure, only 2% of the patients described their postoperative pain as severe, and 0.4% described the postoperative pain as the worst pain they had ever experienced [53]. The authors concluded that the oocyte retrieval procedure can be considered a safe procedure. However; they emphasized that vaginal bleeding, which was easily controlled with pressure application still remained the most common complication during oocyte retrieval in their practice [53].

Rolland et al. [54] conducted a non-randomized prospective cohort study of the impact of the type of anesthesia on live birth rate, pain, and patient satisfaction in women undergoing IVF oocyte retrieval. Two groups of patients were prospectively included: the paracervical block (PCB) group (n = 234) and the general anesthesia (GA) group (n = 247). The type of anesthesia was selected by the patients. The primary endpoint was cumulative live birth rate by OR. Secondary endpoints were self-assessment of the patients' perioperative abdominal and vaginal pain vs. the doctors' evaluations during PCB, postoperative abdominal and vaginal pain level, and patient satisfaction in both groups. Pain levels were assessed with a numerical rating scale (NRS). The live birth rate was similar in both groups (19.8% in the GA group vs. 20.9% in the PCB group, $P = 0.764$). During oocyte retrieval in the PCB group, the physicians significantly under-estimated the vaginal pain experienced by the patients (3.04 ± 0.173 for patients vs. 2.59 ± 0.113 for surgeons, $P = 0.014$). Postoperative vaginal and abdominal pain were significantly greater in the PCB group compared to the GA group (2.26 ± 0.159 vs. 1.66 ± 0.123, respectively, $P = 0.005$, and 3.80 ± 0.165 vs. 3.00 ± 0.148, respectively, $P < 0.001$). Patients were more satisfied with GA than with PBC ($P < 0.001$). The authors concluded that given their results, the choice of anesthesia should be decided by the patients [54].

Zhao et al. [55] in a prospective double-blind randomized study evaluated the analgesic effect and potential effect on pregnancy rate of the nonsteroidal anti-inflammatory drug flurbiprofen axetil in 200 patients ($N = 200$) undergoing ultrasound-guided transvaginal oocyte retrieval under propofol-remifentanil anesthesia. The patients were randomly allocated to receive 1.5 mg/kg of flurbiprofen axetil (FA group) or placebo (control group) 30 min before the procedure. Postoperative pain scores, embryo implantation rate, and pregnancy rate were recorded. Neuroendocrine biomarkers and prostaglandin E2 levels in follicular fluid were tested after oocyte retrieval [54]. The authors concluded that flurbiprofen axetil given before ultrasound-guided transvaginal oocyte retrieval for patients under propofol-remifentanil general anesthesia relieves pain without any detrimental effect on clinical pregnancy rate [55].

After recent adverse effect of a paracervical block (cardiac arrest), which occurred during an oocyte retrieval (OR), Guillaume et al. [56] conducted an observational study with use of topical intravaginal lidocaine gel for pain management in 200 patients ($N = 200$). Pain was measured using a numeric pain scale during and after oocyte retrieval. The tolerance of the procedure was evaluated through a patient questionnaire. Median maximal pain was 5 ± 2.3 (0–10) pre-retrieval and 3 ± 2.2 (0–10) post-retrieval. The procedure was considered bearable by 85.5% of the patients and 81.5% of the patients indicated that they would choose this method in case of any future oocyte retrieval. No adverse effect occurred during the study. The authors concluded that the use of intravaginal lidocaine gel is an acceptable analgesic technique for oocyte retrieval [56].

Goutziomitrou et al. [57] studied propofol vs. thiopental sodium as anesthetic agents for oocyte retrieval in a randomized-controlled trial. One hundred and eighty patients undergoing ovarian stimulation with gonadotropins and gonadotropin-releasing hormone antagonists for IVF were randomized to receive either propofol ($n = 90$) or thiopental sodium ($n = 90$). No significant differences in baseline characteristics were present between the two groups. Time under anesthesia was significantly increased in the thiopental sodium group: median (IQR): 12 (5) versus 10 (4.5) min, $P = 0.019$ compared with the propofol group. Overall fertilization rates were similar between propofol and thiopental sodium groups. The authors concluded that use of propofol compared with thiopental sodium for general anesthesia during oocyte retrieval results in similar fertilization rates and IVF outcomes [57].

Lier et al. [58] in a randomized-controlled trial studied the use of patient-controlled remifentanil analgesia as alternative for pethidine with midazolam during oocyte retrieval in IVF procedures. Seventy-six women were randomized to receive pethidine (2 mg/kg i.m.) and midazolam (7.5 mg) induced conscious sedation ($n = 40$) or PCA with remifentanil and diclofenac (50 mg; $n = 36$). The Numeric Rating Scale, McGill Pain Questionnaire (MPQ), Ramsey Sedation Scale, and a 5-day pain-and-discomfort diary were used to evaluate pain and sedation levels [58]. There were no differences in baseline characteristics and reproductive outcomes between both groups. Periprocedural pain scores were comparable for remifentanil and pethidine groups (4 [3–7] vs. 6 [4–8]; $P = 0.13$). Pain scores in the pethidine group were significantly lower at 30 min after the procedure (1 [0–3] vs. 2 [1–5]; $P = 0.016$), but at cost of higher sedation levels when compared to remifentanil (4 [2–4] vs. 2 [2–2]; $P < 0.001$). Patient satisfaction was higher, and MPQ scores were lower in the remifentanil group. There were no differences in safety profiles between both analgesics. The authors concluded that patient-controlled analgesia with remifentanil showed a similar reduction in pain scores than pethidine with midazolam during oocyte retrieval, while pethidine induced the highest pain relief after the procedure. However, PCA remifentanil was associated with less sedation and a better patient satisfaction profile than pethidine.

Piroli et al. [59] compared the effects on patient physiology and oocyte competence of different anesthetic methodologies for sedation during in vitro fertilization procedures. Four analgesic techniques: EMLA cream, propofol, thiopental sodium, and sevoflurane were compared for effectiveness in in vitro fertilization (IVF) oocyte retrieval procedures [59]. The authors reported that most anesthetic parameters were not significantly different among the four treatments modalities. However; they noted that the highest rate of anomalous fertilization was observed in the propofol study group [59].

Circeo et al. [60] conducted a prospective, observational study of the depth of anesthesia during oocyte retrieval using a total intravenous anesthetic technique and the bispectral index monitor. Fifty patients ($N = 50$) scheduled to undergo IVF received a standard anesthetic of fentanyl and propofol for induction, followed by propofol infusion, with bispectral index values and modified Ramsey sedation scores recorded at 5-min intervals for the duration of anesthesia care. Moderate sedation was found only transiently during the first 5–10 min of the oocyte retrieval, but thereafter the level of sedation increased, with deep sedation and general anesthesia measured in all patients as determined by both the bispectral index scores and lack of response to painful stimulation [60].

In a prospective, randomized, double-blinded study Hong et al. [61] investigated the comparison of conscious sedation for oocyte retrieval between low-anxiety and high-anxiety patients. One hundred fifty consecutive women ($N = 150$) scheduled for oocyte retrieval under conscious sedation were included in the study. Anxiety scores were measured by an anesthesiologist who was not involved in sedation. The patients were divided into two groups, high-anxiety and low-anxiety, as determined by using the median of anxiety VAS scoring for assessment of preoperative anxiety (4.0 cm). The subjects were collected, 76 in high-anxiety group and 74 in low-anxiety group. An infusion of propofol with a preset target concentration of 2.5 μg/mL (−1) was started until the patient had reached and maintained a sedation level of 3 on a 5-point sedation scale. Hemodynamic variables were recorded by using standard monitors. The scorings of sedation, operability, and satisfaction were assessed by one of the anesthesiologists. The high-anxiety group required more for the induction of sedation and a larger amount of total dosage of propofol for sedation, as compared with the low-anxiety group. The concentrations of propofol on the Target-Controlled Infusion at sedation level 3 of the high-anxiety group were significantly higher than those of the low-anxiety group. Context-sensitive half time of high-anxiety group was also longer than that of the low-anxiety group. The postoperative pain score of the high-anxiety group was higher than that of the low-anxiety group. Increased preoperative anxiety was significantly correlated with postoperative wound pain ($r = 0.240$, $P = 0.009$) and previously experienced pain on same procedure ($r = 0.252$, $P = 0.031$), but not with pain on propofol injection ($r = −0.05$, $P = 0.58$) [47]. The authors concluded that the high-anxiety group of patients needs more sedative requirement of propofol for conscious sedation than the low-anxiety group of patients [61].

The role of routine anxiolytic premedication in anesthesia remains unclear and significant postoperative side-effects may result from its routine use. Ng et al. [62] in a randomized double-blinded placebo-controlled trial investigated the impact of anxiolytic premedication on preoperative anxiety and pain during oocyte retrieval. One hundred ($N = 100$) patients were randomized on the day of ultrasound-guided oocyte retrieval (TUGOR) by a computer-generated randomization list in sealed envelopes to receive either (1) 50 mg pethidine and 25 mg promethazine (premedication group) or (2) normal saline (placebo group) i.m. 30 min prior to TUGOR. Anxiety levels, pain levels, and severity of postoperative side-effects were recorded [62]. Preoperative anxiety level was significantly higher than the basal anxiety level in the placebo group only. The vaginal and abdominal pain levels during TUGOR and 4 h after TUGOR were significantly higher in the placebo group than the premedication group. Significantly, more patients complained of drowsiness after TUGOR in the premedication group than the placebo group and other side-effects were comparable in both groups [62]. The authors concluded that routine use of anxiolytic premedication prevented an increase of preoperative anxiety level, reduced pain levels during oocyte retrieval but was associated with a higher percentage of moderate/severe drowsiness in the postoperative period [62].

Singhal et al. [63] studied the patient experience with conscious sedation as a method of pain relief for transvaginal oocyte retrieval. Prospective cross-sectional study was conducted from October 2015 to January 2016 at a university-level hospital and 100 women ($N = 100$) were recruited. There was a moderate positive correlation between age and pain score on day 1 post-procedure. When the duration of procedure was >12 min, immediate post-procedure pain score was significantly higher compared to those whose procedure was for <12 min. There was no correlation between pain score and the number of oocytes retrieved (≤5, 6–15, and ≥16) and transmyometrial passage of needle. The VAS 10-point score immediately post-procedure, after 6 and 24 h post-procedure, and on day of embryo transfer was 2.83 (±1.67), 0.78 (±1.04), 0.39 (±1.09), and 0.14 (±0.58), respectively. Majority of the women (86%) preferred the same pain relief method for future analgesia. There were no major complications. The authors concluded that conscious sedation was associated with high satisfaction level and acceptance rate among patients undergoing transvaginal oocyte retrieval [63].

7.9 Summary

Oocyte retrieval is a procedure where sedation and analgesia is recommended and/or required. Provision of anesthesia, management of pain, and treatment of anxiety during oocyte retrieval makes an anesthesia provider an important member of the in vitro fertilization (IVF) team. From our literature analysis, evidence of serious toxicity of anesthetics used for in vitro fertilization in humans is not well established. Continuous monitoring of capnography and oxygen saturation (per institutional protocol) is always required. Currently, there is no gold standard for anesthesia care during oocyte retrieval. The evidence does not support one particular method or technique over another in providing effective conscious sedation and analgesia for pain relief during and after oocyte retrieval.

References

1. Ramsay MAE. John Snow, MD: anaesthetist to the Queen of England and pioneer epidemiologist. Proc (Bayl Univ Med Cent). 2006;19(1):24–8.
2. Steptoe PC, Edwards RG. Birth after the reimplantation of human embryo. Lancet. 1978;12:2–366.
3. Yentis S, May A, Malhotra S. Analgesia, anaesthesia and pregnancy. A practical guide. Cambridge: Cambridge University Press; 2001.
4. Baldini D, Savoia MV, Sciancalepore AG, Malvasi A, Vizziello D, Beck R, Vizziello G. High progesterone levels on the day of HCG administration do not affect the embryo quality and the reproductive outcomes of frozen embryo transfers. Clin Ter. 2018;169(3):e91–5. https://doi.org/10.7417/CT.2018.2060.
5. Gejervall AL, Lundin K, Stener-Victorin E, Bergh C. Effect of alfentanil dosage during oocyte retrieval on fertilization and embryo quality. Eur J Obstet Gynecol Reprod Biol. 2010;150(1):66–71. https://doi.org/10.1016/j.ejogrb.2010.01.007. Epub 2010 Mar 11.
6. Kuczkowski KM, Reisner LS, Benumof JL. Airway problems and new solutions for the obstetric patient. J Clin Anesth. 2003;15(7):552–63.
7. Malvasi A, Tinelli A, Di Renzo GC. Management and therapy of late pregnancy complications. Champaign: Springer; 2017.
8. Practice Guidelines for Obstetric Anesthesia: an updated report by the American Society of Anesthesiologists Task Force on Obstetric Anesthesia and the Society for Obstetric Anesthesia and Perinatology. Anesthesiology. 2016;124(2):270–300. https://doi.org/10.1097/ALN.0000000000000935.
9. Davies JM, Posner KL, Lee LA, Cheney FW, Domino KB. Liability associated with obstetric anesthesia: a closed claims analysis. Anesthesiology. 2009;110(1):131–9. https://doi.org/10.1097/ALN.0b013e318190e16a.
10. Cantwell R, Clutton-Brock T, Cooper G, Dawson A, Drife J, Garrod D, Harper A, Hulbert D, Lucas S, McClure J, Millward-Sadler H, Neilson J, Nelson-Piercy C, Norman J, O'Herlihy C, Oates M, Shakespeare J, de Swiet M, Williamson C, Beale V, Knight M, Lennox C, Miller A, Parmar D, Rogers J, Springett A. Saving Mothers' Lives: reviewing maternal deaths to make motherhood safer: 2006–2008. The eighth report of the confidential enquiries into maternal deaths in the United Kingdom. BJOG. 2011;118(Suppl 1):1–203. https://doi.org/10.1111/j.1471-0528.2010.02847.x.
11. D'Angelo R, Smiley RM, Riley ET, Segal S. Serious complications related to obstetric anesthesia: the serious complication repository project of the Society for Obstetric Anesthesia and Perinatology. Anesthesiology. 2014;120(6):1505–12. https://doi.org/10.1097/ALN.0000000000000253.
12. Irlbeck T, Zwißler B, Bauer A. ASA classification: transition in the course of time and depiction in the literature. [Article in German]. Anaesthesist. 2017;66(1):5–10. https://doi.org/10.1007/s00101-016-0246-4.
13. Soussis I, Boyd O, Paraschos T, Duffy S, Bower S, Troughton P, et al. Follicular fluid levels of midazolam, fentanyl, and alfentanil during transvaginal oocyte retrieval. Fertil Steril. 1995;64(5):1003–7.
14. Guasch E, Ardoy M, Cuadrado C, González Gancedo P, González A, Gilsanz F. Comparison of 4 anesthetic techniques for in vitro fertilization. [Article in Spanish]. Rev Esp Anestesiol Reanim. 2005;52(1):9–18.
15. Christiaens F, Janssenswillen C, Van Steirteghem AC, Devroey P, Verborgh C, Camu F. Comparison of assisted reproductive technology performance after oocyte retrieval under general anaesthesia (propofol) versus paracervical local anaesthetic block: a case-controlled study. Hum Reprod. 1998;13(9):2456–60.
16. Janssenswillen C, Christiaens F, Camu F, Van Steirtegem A. The effect of propofol on parthenogenetic activation, in vitro fertil- ization and early development of mouse oocytes. Fertil Steril. 1997;67(4):769–74.
17. Hammadeh ME, Wilhelm W, Huppert A, Rosenbaum P, Schmidt W. Effects of general anaesthesia vs. sedation on fertilization, cleavage and pregnancy rates in an IVF program. Arch Gynecol Obstet. 1999;263(1–2):56–9.
18. Sterzik K, Nitsch CD, Korda P, Sasse V, Rosenbusch B, Marx T, Traub E. The effect of different anesthetic procedures on hormone levels in women. Studies during an in vitro fertilization-embryo transfer (IVF-ET) program. [Article in German]. Anaesthesist. 1994;43(11):738–42.
19. Vricella LK, Louis JM, Mercer BM, Bolden N. Anesthesia complications during scheduled cesarean delivery for morbidly obese women. Am J Obstet Gynecol. 2010;203:276.e1–5. https://doi.org/10.1016/j.ajog.2010.06.022. Epub 2010 Jul 31.
20. American Society of Anesthesiologists. Continuum of depth of sedation: definition of general anesthesia and levels of sedation/analgesia. Developed by Committee on Quality Management and Departmental Administration. Approved by the ASA House of Delegates on October 13, 1999, and last amended on October 15, 2014.
21. Somerson SJ, Husted CW, Sicilia MR. Insights into conscious sedation. Am J Nurs. 1995;95(6):26–32.
22. Ditkoff EC, Plumb J, Selick A, Sauer MV. Anesthesia practices in the United States Common to in vitro fertilization (IVF) centers. J Assist Reprod Genet. 1997;14(3):145–7.
23. Yamakura T, Sakimura K, Shimoji K, Mishina M. Effects of propofol on various AMPA-, kainate- and NMDA-selective glutamate receptor channels expressed in Xenopus oocytes. Neurosci Lett. 1995;188(3):187–90.
24. Cotoia A, Mirabella L, Beck R, Matrella P, Assenzo V, Chazot T, Cinnella G, Liu N, Dambrosio M. Effects of closed-loop intravenous anesthesia guided by Bispectral Index in adult patients on emergence delirium: a randomized controlled study. Minerva Anestesiol. 2018;84(4):437–46. https://doi.org/10.23736/S0375-9393.17.11915-2. Epub 2017 Dec 13.
25. Dershwitz M. Intravenous and inhalation anesthetics. In: William HE, editor. Clinical anesthesia procedures of the Massachusetts General Hospital. 6th ed. Philadelphia: Lippincott Williams and Wilkins; 2002. p. 156–8.
26. Becker DE, Haas DA. Management of complications during moderate and deep sedation: respiratory and cardiovascular considerations. Anesth Prog. 2007;54(2):59–68.
27. Lehtinen AM, Laatikainen T, Koskimies AI, Hovorka J. Modifying effects of epidural analgesia or general anesthesia on the stress hormone response to laparoscopy for in vitro fertilization. J In Vitro Fert Embryo Transf. 1987;4(1):23–9.
28. Gottschalk A, Van Aken H, Zenz M, Standl T. Is anesthesia dangerous? Dtsch Arztebl Int. 2011;108(27):469–74. https://doi.org/10.3238/arztebl.2011.0469. Epub 2011 Jul 8.
29. Torpy JM, Lynm C, Golub RM. JAMA patient page. Regional anesthesia. JAMA. 2011;306(7):781. https://doi.org/10.1001/jama.306.7.781.
30. Covino BG. Comparative clinical pharmacology of local anesthetic agents. Anesthesiology. 1971;35(2):158–67.
31. Tubben RE, Jain S. Epidural blood patch. StatPearls [Internet]. Treasure Island: StatPearls Publishing; 2018.
32. Kwak KH. Postdural puncture headache. Korean J Anesthesiol. 2017;70(2):136–43. https://doi.org/10.4097/kjae.2017.70.2.136. Epub 2017 Feb 3.
33. Kuczkowski KM, Beck R. Anesthesia in labor and delivery. In: Di Renzo GC, Berghella V, Malvasi A, editors. Good practice and malpractice in labor and delivery: Edra Publisher; 2019. p. 379–92.
34. de Santiago J, Santos-Yglesias J, Giron J, Montes de Oca F, Jimenez A, Diaz P. Low-dose 3 mg levobupivacaine plus 10 microg fentanyl selective spinal anesthesia for gynecological outpatient

laparoscopy. Anesth Analg. 2009;109(5):1456–61. https://doi.org/10.1213/ANE.0b013e3181ba792e.

35. Coppejans HC, Vercauteren MP. Low-dose combined spinal-epidural anesthesia for cesarean delivery: a comparison of three plain local anesthetics. Acta Anaesthesiol Belg. 2006;57(1):39–43.

36. Gebhardt V, Kiefer K, Bussen D, Weiss C, Schmittner MD. Retrospective analysis of mepivacaine, prilocaine and chloroprocaine for low-dose spinal anaesthesia in outpatient perianal procedures. Int J Colorectal Dis. 2018;33(10):1469–77. https://doi.org/10.1007/s00384-018-3085-8.

37. Kogosowski A, Lessing JB, Amit A, Rudick V, Peyser MR, David MP. Epidural block: a preferred method of anesthesia for ultrasonically guided oocyte retrieval. Fertil Steril. 1987;47(1):166–8.

38. Palkar NV, Boudreaux RC, Mankad AV. Accidental total spinal block: a complication of an epidural test dose. Can J Anaesth. 1992;39(10):1058–60.

39. D'Ambrosio A, Cotoia A, Beck R, Salatto P, Zibar L, Cinnella G. Impedance cardiography as tool for continuous hemodynamic monitoring during cesarean section: randomized, prospective double blind study. BMC Anesthesiol. 2018;18(1):32. https://doi.org/10.1186/s12871-018-0498-4.

40. Vlahos NF, Giannakikou I, Vlachos A, Vitoratos N. Analgesia and anesthesia for assisted reproductive technologies. Int J Gynaecol Obstet. 2009;105(3):201–5. https://doi.org/10.1016/j.ijgo.2009.01.017. Epub 2009 Feb 26.

41. Vela Vásquez RS, Peláez Romero R. Aspirin and spinal haematoma after neuraxial anaesthesia: myth or reality? Br J Anaesth. 2015;115(5):688–98. https://doi.org/10.1093/bja/aev348.

42. Gogarten W. The influence of new antithrombotic drugs on regional anesthesia. Curr Opin Anaesthesiol. 2006;19(5):545–50.

43. Huang J, McKenna N, Babins N. Utility of thromboelastography during neuraxial blockade in the parturient with thrombocytopenia. AANA J. 2014;82(2):127–30.

44. Lee LO, Bateman BT, Kheterpal S, Klumpner TT, Housey M, Aziz MF, Hand KW, MacEachern M, Goodier CG, Bernstein J, Bauer ME, Multicenter Perioperative Outcomes Group Investigators. Risk of epidural hematoma after neuraxial techniques in thrombocytopenic parturients: a report from the multicenter perioperative outcomes group. Anesthesiology. 2017;126(6):1053–63. https://doi.org/10.1097/ALN.0000000000001630.

45. Pugliese PL, Cinnella G, Raimondo P, De Capraris A, Salatto P, Sforza D, Menga R, D'Ambrosio A, Fede RN, D'Onofrio C, Consoletti L, Malvasi A, Brizzi A, Dambrosio M. Implementation of epidural analgesia for labor: is the standard of effective analgesia reachable in all women? An audit of two years. Eur Rev Med Pharmacol Sci. 2013;17(9):1262–8.

46. Kuczkowski KM, Beck R. Labor analgesia. In: Di Renzo GC, Berghella V, Malvasi A, editors. Good practice and malpractice in labor and delivery: Edra Publisher; 2019. p. 361–77.

47. Kumar K, Singh SI. Neuraxial opioid-induced pruritus: an update. J Anaesthesiol Clin Pharmacol. 2013;29(3):303–7. https://doi.org/10.4103/0970-9185.117045.

48. Wu Z, Kong M, Wang N, Finlayson RJ, Tran QH. Intravenous butorphanol administration reduces intrathecal morphine-induced pruritus after cesarean delivery: a randomized, double-blind, placebo-controlled study. J Anesth. 2012;26(5):752–7. https://doi.org/10.1007/s00540-012-1421-7. Epub 2012 Jun 7.

49. Farag E, Mounir-Soliman L. Brown's regional anesthesia review. 1st ed. Elsevier—Health Sciences Division; Published Date: 28th May 2016.

50. Faccenda KA, Finucane BT. Complications of regional anaesthesia. Incidence and prevention. Drug Saf. 2001;24(6):413–42.

51. Kwan I, Wang R, Pearce E, Bhattacharya S. Pain relief for women undergoing oocyte retrieval for assisted reproduction. Cochrane Database Syst Rev. 2018;5:CD004829. https://doi.org/10.1002/14651858.CD004829.pub4.

52. Morue HI, Raj-Lawrence S, Saxena S, Delbaere A, Engelman E, Barvais LA. Placebo versus low-dose ketamine infusion in addition to remifentanil target-controlled infusion for conscious sedation during oocyte retrieval: a double-blinded, randomised controlled trial. Eur J Anaesthesiol. 2018;35(9):667–74. https://doi.org/10.1097/EJA.0000000000000826.

53. Özaltın S, Kumbasar S, Savan K. Evaluation of complications developing during and after transvaginal ultrasound—guided oocyte retrieval. Ginekol Pol. 2018;89(1):1–6. https://doi.org/10.5603/GP.a2018.0001.

54. Rolland L, Perrin J, Villes V, Pellegrin V, Boubli L, Courbiere B. IVF oocyte retrieval: prospective evaluation of the type of anesthesia on live birth rate, pain, and patient satisfaction. J Assist Reprod Genet. 2017;34(11):1523–8. https://doi.org/10.1007/s10815-017-1002-7. Epub 2017 Jul 28.

55. Zhao H, Feng Y, Jiang Y, Lu Q. Flurbiprofen axetil provides effective analgesia without changing the pregnancy rate in ultrasound-guided transvaginal oocyte retrieval: a double-blind randomized controlled trial. Anesth Analg. 2017;125(4):1269–74. https://doi.org/10.1213/ANE.0000000000002025.

56. Guillaume A, Schuller-Dufour E, Faitot V, Pirrello O, Rongières C, Ohl J, Nisand I, Bettahar K. Patient's experience of topical anesthesia by lidocaine vaginal gel for oocyte retrieval. [Article in French]. J Gynecol Obstet Biol Reprod (Paris). 2016;45(8):942–7. https://doi.org/10.1016/j.jgyn.2016.05.006. Epub 2016 Jun 16.

57. Goutziomitrou E, Venetis CA, Kolibianakis EM, Bosdou JK, Parlapani A, Grimbizis G, Tarlatzis BC. Propofol versus thiopental sodium as anaesthetic agents for oocyte retrieval: a randomized controlled trial. Reprod Biomed Online. 2015;31(6):752–9. https://doi.org/10.1016/j.rbmo.2015.08.013. Epub 2015 Sep 4.

58. Lier MC, Douwenga WM, Yilmaz F, Schats R, Hompes PG, Boer C, Mijatovic V. Patient-controlled remifentanil analgesia as alternative for pethidine with midazolam during oocyte retrieval in IVF/ICSI procedures: a randomized controlled trial. Pain Pract. 2015;15(5):487–95. https://doi.org/10.1111/papr.12189. Epub 2014 Apr 12.

59. Piroli A, Marci R, Marinangeli F, Paladini A, Di Emidio G, Giovanni Artini P, Caserta D, Tatone C. Comparison of different anaesthetic methodologies for sedation during in vitro fertilization procedures: effects on patient physiology and oocyte competence. Gynecol Endocrinol. 2012;28(10):796–9. https://doi.org/10.3109/09513590.2012.664193. Epub 2012 Mar 16.

60. Circeo L, Grow D, Kashikar A, Gibson C. Prospective, observational study of the depth of anesthesia during oocyte retrieval using a total intravenous anesthetic technique and the Bispectral index monitor. Fertil Steril. 2011;96(3):635–7. https://doi.org/10.1016/j.fertnstert.2011.06.010. Epub 2011 Jul 5.

61. Hong JY, Jee YS, Luthardt FW. Comparison of conscious sedation for oocyte retrieval between low-anxiety and high-anxiety patients. J Clin Anesth. 2005;17(7):549–53.

62. Ng EH, Miao B, Ho PC. Anxiolytic premedication reduces preoperative anxiety and pain during oocyte retrieval. A randomized double-blinded placebo-controlled trial. Hum Reprod. 2002;17(5):1233–8.

63. Singhal H, Premkumar PS, Chandy A, Kunjummen AT, Kamath MS. Patient experience with conscious sedation as a method of pain relief for transvaginal oocyte retrieval: a cross sectional study. J Hum Reprod Sci. 2017;10(2):119–23. https://doi.org/10.4103/jhrs.JHRS_113_16.

Monitoring Follicular Growth

8

Maria Elisabetta Coccia, Francesca Rizzello,
and Eleonora Ralli

Contents

M. E. Coccia
Department of Obstetrics and Gynecology, University of Firenze, Florence, Italy

F. Rizzello (✉)
Assisted Reproduction Center, Careggi University Hospital, University of Florence, Florence, Italy

E. Ralli
Department of Clinical and Experimental Biomedical Sciences, University of Florence, Florence, Italy
e-mail: Eleonora.ralli@unifi.it

Monitoring follicular growth usually involves a combination of hormonal assays and ultrasonic measurements of follicle size (Fig. 8.1). Nowadays, Transvaginal Ultrasound (TVUS) is the "gold standard" for monitoring ovarian ovulation in both spontaneous and stimulated cycles.

Accurate follicular monitoring is particularly important in In Vitro fertilization (IVF) plus Intracytoplasmic Sperm Injection (ICSI) program in order to:

© Springer Nature Switzerland AG 2020
A. Malvasi, D. Baldini (eds.), *Pick Up and Oocyte Management*, https://doi.org/10.1007/978-3-030-28741-2_8

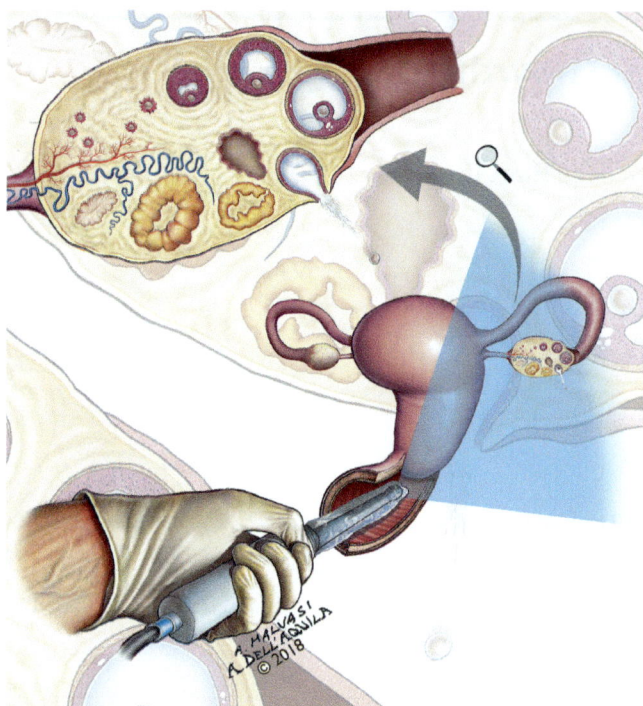

Fig. 8.1 Monitoring follicular growth usually involves a combination of hormonal assays and ultrasonic measurements of follicle size

- **predict ovarian responsiveness** to exogenous gonadotropins (it allows to individualize treatment protocols optimizing results and reducing complications)
- **evaluate the number, size** of developing follicles and their growth pattern before oocyte retrieval (predictive of oocytes competence)
- **estimate the appropriate time to trigger** the final oocyte maturation before ovum pickup
- **assess the risk of ovarian hyperstimulation syndrome (OHSS)**
- **make decisions on early cancellation of cycles** without proper ovarian response, thus avoiding unnecessary waste of resources

During a cycle of IVF/ICSI, women receive daily doses of gonadotropins (FSH, LH, hMG) to induce multifollicular development in the ovaries. Controlled ovarian hyperstimulation (COH) induces the growth of heterogeneous cohorts of follicles containing oocytes at different stages of maturity and competence and only few oocytes will be able to undergo meiosis, fertilization, and embryo development.

The proportion of competent oocytes is directly related to follicular size. Developmental competence refers to the oocyte's ability to mature, fertilize, and finally yield viable offspring [1].

In order to predict ovarian response, clinicians individualize the most suitable starting dose of gonadotropins on the basis of patient characteristics predictive of ovarian response such as age, clinical history, and other ovarian reserve tests (ORTs).

Nowadays, antral follicular count (AFC) and Anti-Müllerian hormone (AMH) appear to be the most useful markers of ovarian reserve in addition to chronological age. The retrieval of 5–15 oocytes is often considered a normal response to stimulation [2]. Poor and hyper-response to COH are significantly correlated with risk of cycle cancellation. Moreover, hyper-response is associated with increased risk of OHSS.

In this chapter, monitoring follicular growth during IVF/ICSI cycle will be presented.

8.1 Controlled Ovarian Stimulation: The Rational Basis

According to the model proposed by Baird (1987), during the menstrual phase the concentration of FSH rises to a level high enough to activate a single small antral follicle (2–4 mm) that secretes higher quantities of Estradiol (E32). The production of E2 and inhibin by the developing follicle is able to suppress the concentration of FSH below this threshold level (negative feedback). For a critical period, the dominant follicle becomes increasingly sensitive to FSH and consequently is less dependent on the level of plasma FSH. These conditions led to the growing of the dominant follicles and the inhibition of other follicles [3].

During COH, treatments with Clomiphene or gonadotropins maintain the period during which the level of FSH remains above this threshold allowing multiple follicular development. Under this condition, the follicles continue to grow at approximately the same rate, thus they are never completely synchronous (Fig. 8.2).

It has been demonstrated that FSH stimulates granulosa cells of early antral follicles and induces LH receptor forma-

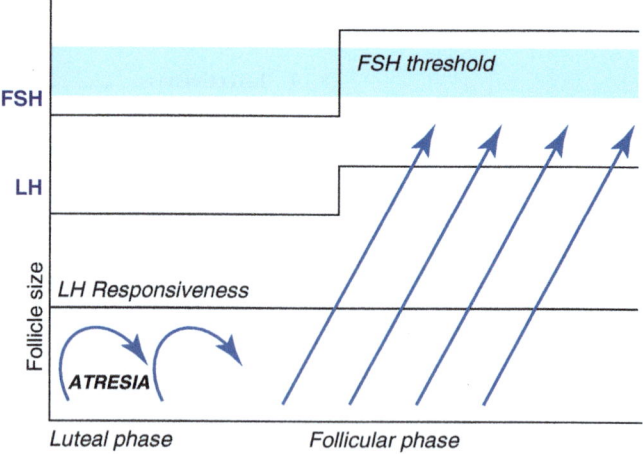

Fig. 8.2 FSH threshold concept in a stimulated cycle. During COH, levels of circulating FSH are elevated above threshold. The number of preovulatory follicles increases in an asynchronous manner

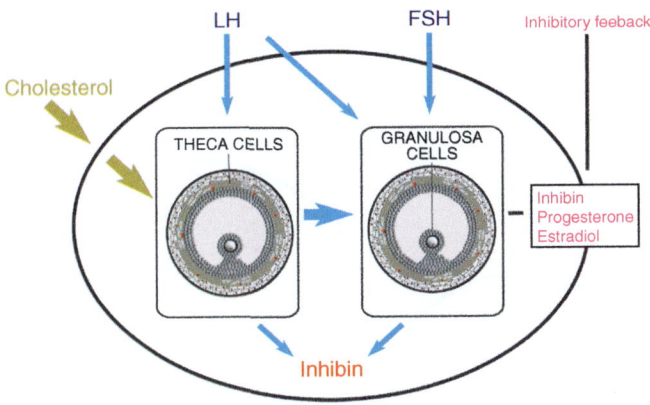

Fig. 8.3 The two-cells–two gonadotropins theory

tion on preovulatory follicle [4]. LH activates adenyl cyclase with the resulting production of cAMP that represents an amplified response to FSH [5]. Therefore, the maturing follicle reduces its dependency on FSH by acquiring LH receptors. The granulosa cells from early antral follicles are only responsive to FSH; granulosa cells from FSH-stimulated follicles are responsive to both FSH and LH [6].

The revised two-cells—two gonadotropins theory suggests a key role for LH not only in theca cells steroidogenesis stimulation, but also in follicle growth and maturation in the mid-luteal phase [7] (Fig. 8.3).

Ovarian stimulation protocols combine the use of human menopausal gonadotropin (hMG), urinary or recombinant FSH, recombinant LH with GnRH agonists or antagonists in order to increase oocyte number and to avoid premature LH surge. Given the physiological role of FSH and LH, the rational basis of controlled ovarian stimulation is to increase the duration that serum FSH concentrations are maintained above the threshold by direct administration of FSH.

8.2 Prediction of Ovarian Response

During an IVF/ICSI cycle, daily doses of gonadotropins (FSH, LH, hMG, Corifollitropin alfa, Follitropin delta) are used to induce multifollicular response in the ovaries. Although the number of eggs retrieved seems to depend on the starting/total doses of gonadotropins, individual woman's response differs [8, 9].

A low or poor ovarian response has been defined as the retrieval of three or fewer oocytes [10]. A hyper-response (or high response) is often described as the retrieval of 15–20 or more oocytes and is associated with an increase in the risk of OHSS [11, 12].

During fresh IVF cycles, some authors observed that the best chance of live birth was associated with the number of 5–15 eggs retrieved during oocyte pickup. Whereas a decline was observed after the retrieval of 20 or more oocytes [9].

In an effort to predict the response and outcome in couples prior to IVF/ICSI and counsel them, the estimation of ovarian reserve is routinely performed through various ovarian reserve tests or multifactorial algorithms [13].

Basal FSH (b-FSH), measured in serum in the early follicular phase of a menstrual cycle, is a simple and reliable test. It is less expensive than the other tests, easily applicable and is, therefore, the most widely used screening test in infertility programs. Previous studies demonstrated that a combination of early follicular FSH and age seems to be better than age alone in predicting outcome in women undergoing IVF [14]. B-FSH was later integrated with the AFC. AFC is measured by ultrasound and is a count of the number of antral follicles measuring about 2–10 mm (according to standard criteria) that are available in both ovaries [15].

More recently, AMH has emerged as a robust marker of ovarian function. It is a dimeric glycoprotein produced by granulosa cells of preantral (primary and secondary) and small antral follicles in the ovary.

The production of AMH starts following follicular transition from the primordial to the primary stage, and it continues until the follicles reach the antral stages, with diameters of 2–6 mm [16] (Fig. 8.4).

AMH represents a more direct and independent measure of the growing preantral and antral follicular pool and is not influenced by the menstrual cycle or pregnancy [17, 18]. The current evidence shows that AFC and AMH appear the most useful markers of ovarian reserve in addition to chronological age [19, 20].

According to the above-mentioned criteria, patients might be classified as predicted hyper-, normal, or hyporesponders:

8.3 Predicted Low Responders

According to Bologna criteria, two of these three criteria are required to define a patient as poor ovarian responder:

1. **advanced maternal age** (≥40 years) or any other poor ovarian response risk factor (genetic or acquired conditions, pelvic infection, ovarian endometriomas, and patients who have undergone ovarian surgery for ovarian cyst, chemotherapy, shortening of the menstrual cycle)
2. **a previous cycle with poor ovarian response** (≤3 oocytes with a conventional stimulation protocol)
3. **a low ovarian reserve test** in terms of AMH (<0.5–1.1 ng/mL) (<3.6–7.8 pmol/L) and AFC (<5–7 follicles)

Moreover, two cycles with poor ovarian response after maximal stimulation might classify a patient as a poor responder even in the absence of the other criteria [10]. More recently, the Poseidon Group (2016) suggested a more specific definition of "low prognosis" patients that introduces two new categories

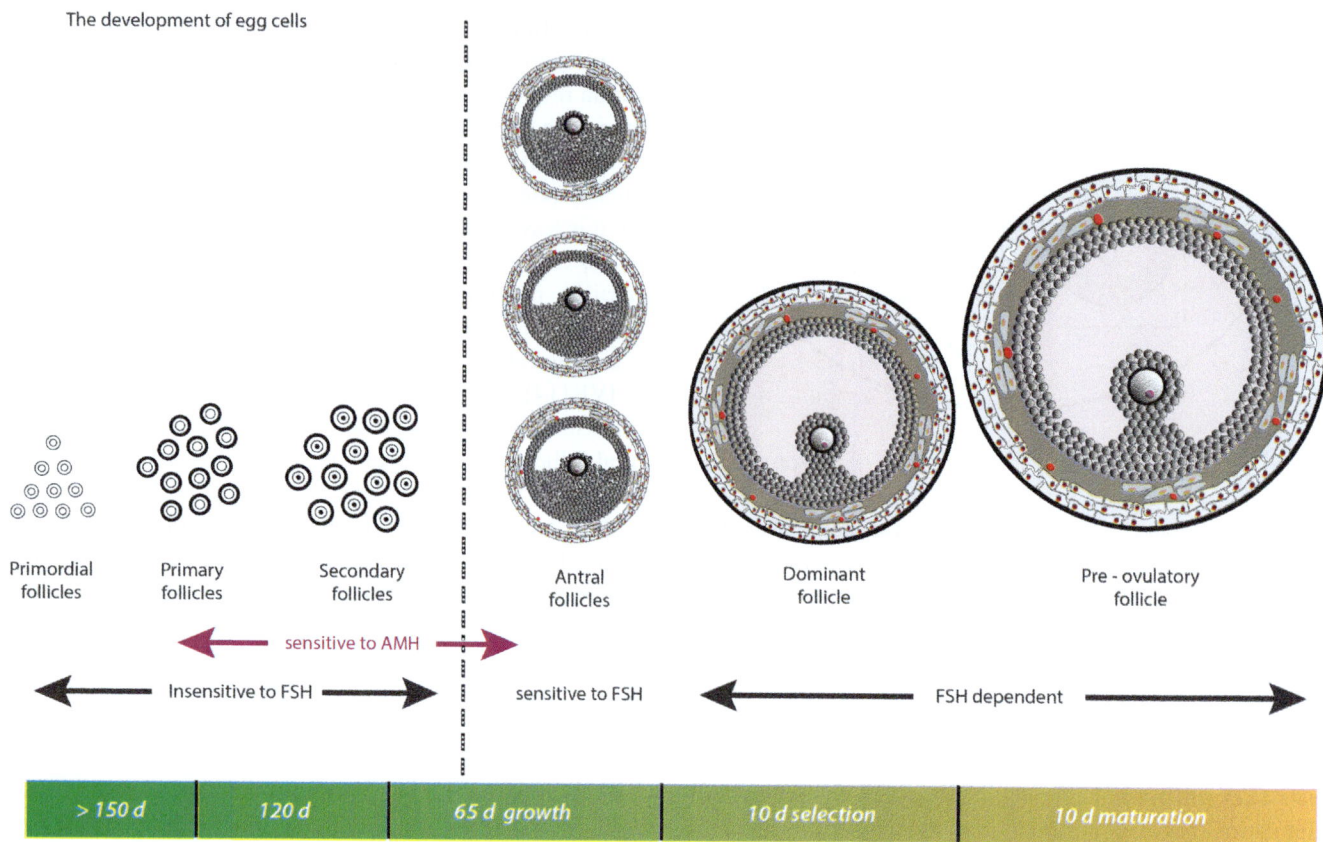

The development of egg cells

Primordial follicles | Primary follicles | Secondary follicles | Antral follicles | Dominant follicle | Pre - ovulatory follicle

sensitive to AMH

Insensitive to FSH   sensitive to FSH   FSH dependent

> 150 d | 120 d | 65 d growth | 10 d selection | 10 d maturation

Fig. 8.4 Follicular growth sensitive to FSH and AMH

Fig. 8.5 Differentiation into groups of low responders according to Poseidon criteria

The POSEIDON criteria: 4 groups of "Low Prognosis"

Poseidon group 1
Young patients <35 years with adequate ovarian reserve parameters (AFC≥5; AMH≥ 1.2 ng/ml) and with an unexpected poor or suboptimal ovarian response.
Subgroup 1a: <4 oocytes*
Subgroup 1b: 4-9 oocytes retrieved*

*after standard ovarian stimulation

Poseidon group 2
Older patients ≥35 years with adequate ovarian reserve parameters (AFC≥S; AMH≥ 1.2 ng/ml) and with an unexpected poor or suboptimal ovarian response.
Subgroup 2a: <4 oocytes*
Subgroup 2b: 4-9 oocytes retrieved*

*after standard ovarian stimulation

Poseidon group 3
Young patients <35 years with poor ovarian reserve pre-stimulation parameters (AFC<5; AMH< 1.2 ng/ml)

Poseidon group 4
Older patients ≥35 years with poor ovarian reserve pre-stimulation paramters (AFC≥5; AMH≥ 1.2 ng/ml)

of compromised response: "suboptimal response" and "hypo-response." "Suboptimal responders" include women with retrieval of 4–9 oocytes which is associated to a significantly lower live birth if compared to patients normoresponders (10–15 oocytes), regardless of age. On the other hand, when higher dose of gonadotropins and more prolonged stimulation are required to obtain more than three oocytes, patients are defined "hyporesponders" [21, 22] (Fig. 8.5). Lensen et al. (2018) in the last Cochrane reviews on individualized gonadotropin dose selection used the following cutoffs to categorize women as predicted low responders: AMH < 7 pmoL/L (0.98 ng/mL), AFC < 7, bFSH > 10 IU/L [2].

8.4 Predicted Hyper-Responders

1. age < 35 years old
2. low Body Mass Index (BMI) (<18.5 Kg/m²)
3. higher AMH levels (cutoff value 3.4 ng/mL)
4. AFC ≥ 24
5. polycystic ovarian syndrome (PCOS) (Fig. 8.6a, b)
6. history of OHSS

Lensen et al. (2018) adopted only AMH > 21 pmol/L (2.9 ng/mL) and AFC > 15 as predictors for high responders [2].

8.5 Predicted Normal Responders

Categorization of normal responders is frequently based on the exclusion of a poor or a hyper-response to ovarian stimulation, rather than by using specific inclusion criteria. Unfortunately, these criteria will include also patients with different prognosis (optimal and suboptimal) [21].

1. AFC 8–15
2. age 35–39 years
3. AMH >1.2 and <3.75 ng/mL

Lensens (2018) adopted the following inclusion criteria: AMH 7–21 pmol/L, AFC 7–15 categorized as predicted normal responders (bFSH was not included as it is not a reliable predictor for normal response) (Lensens 2018) (Table 8.1).

8.6 Protocols of Ovarian Stimulation

The main objective of a correct prediction of ovarian response is the personalization of ovarian stimulation to induce multifollicular development in the ovaries. Personalized treatment offers every single patient the best treatment tailored to her own unique characteristics, thus maximizing the chances of pregnancy, eliminating the iatrogenic and avoidable risks, such as OHSS, minimizing the risk of cycle cancellation and enabling clinicians to give women more accurate information on their prognosis [20].

Finally, and not least importantly, personalized therapy showed an important reduction of costs probably due to a reduced incidence of OHSS, drug consumption, and cancellation of cycles [23].

Dose increases during ovarian stimulation do not seem to affect the number of retrieved oocytes [24, 25]; therefore, the choice of an appropriate starting dose appears crucial for the final ovarian response.

Diverse therapeutic protocols have been suggested for the each category of patients. Usually, the gonadotropin starting dose is 150 IU for expected high responders, 200–225 for normal responders, and 300–450 IU for expected poor responders [2].

In recent times, clinical practice of infertility treatment is moving from standardized to individualized FSH dosing. Actually, new FSH preparations, as follitropin delta, integrate individualized dosing as part of the clinical managing. The dosing algorithm for follitropin delta aims to individualize the starting dose to each woman based on serum level of AMH and body weight, staying on the same dose throughout the whole stimulation cycle [26].

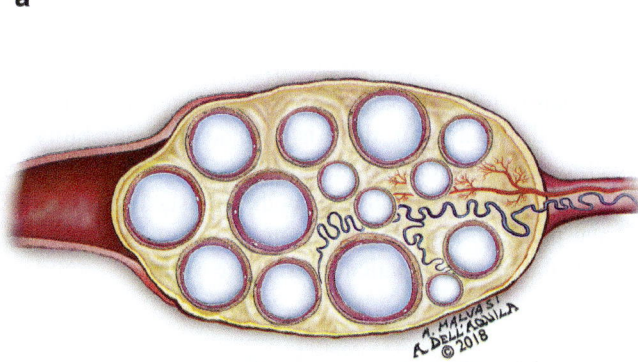
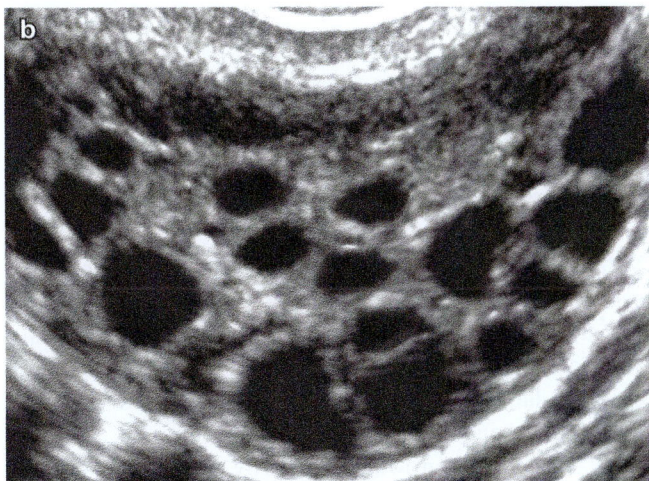

Fig. 8.6 (**a, b**) Schematic representation of micropolycystic ovary and its echographic appearance

Table 8.1 Criteria to categorize women into poor, hyper-, and normoresponders

Predicted response	Authors	Criteria

Poor responders	Bologna Criteria (Ferraretti 2014)	1. Advanced maternal age (≥40 years)
		Or any other poor ovarian response risk factor
		  – Genetic or acquired conditions
		  – Pelvic infection
		  – Ovarian endometriomas
		  – Ovarian surgery for ovarian cyst
		  – Chemotherapy
		  – Shortening of the menstrual cycle
		2. A previous cycle with poor ovarian response
		  – ≤3 oocytes with a conventional stimulation protocol
		3. A low ovarian reserve test
		  – AMH (<0.5–1.1 ng/mL) (<3.6–7.8 pmol/L)
		  – AFC (<5–7 follicles)
		  – Two previous cycles with poor ovarian response after a maximal stimulation (even in the absence of the other criteria)

	Poseidon Group (2016)	– AMH (<1.2 ng/mL) (<8.6 pmol/L) – AFC (<5 follicles) Or unexpected poor or suboptimal ovarian response Poor response: retrieval of <4 oocytes Suboptimal response: retrieval of 4–9 oocytes Hyporesponse: higher dose of gonadotropins and more prolonged stimulation to obtain more than 3 oocytes
	Lensen et al. (2018)	AMH < 7 pmol/L, AFC < 7, bFSH > 10 IU/L, it would be better numbering the list...)
Hyper-responders	ASRM (2016); Kwee J (2007)	1. Age < 35 years old 2. Low Body Mass Index (BMI) (BMI < 18.5 kg/m^2) 3. Higher AMH levels (cutoff value 3.36 ng/mL, 24 pmol/L) 4. AFC ≥ 24 5. Polycystic ovarian syndrome (PCOS) 6. History of OHSS
	Lensen et al. (2018)	1. AMH > 2.9 ng/ml (>21 pmol/L) 2. AFC > 15
Normal responders	Based on the exclusion of a poor or an hyper-response to ovarian stimulation	1. AFC 8–15 2. Age 35–39 years 3. AMH > 1.2 ng/mL (8.6 pmol/L) and <3.75 ng/mL (26.8 pmol/L)
	Lensens (2018)	1. AMH 0.98–2.9 ng/mL, (7–21 pmol/L) 2. AFC 7–15

8.7 Prediction of Oocyte Competence Through Monitoring Follicular Growth

TVUS follow-up of follicular growth is crucial for ART treatment. Counting and measuring growing follicles allows optimal dosage of hormones and correct timing of administration of the ovulation trigger. Early detection of ovarian hyperstimulation allows to freeze embryos and transfer frozen-thawed embryos later.

The evaluation of growing follicles by ultrasound includes (Fig. 8.7): follicle diameter, follicle growth pattern, follicular wall thickness, perifollicular vascularity, and perifollicular blood flow. A follicle that is >10 mm in diameter at the first scan, grows at a rate of 2–3 mm per day, has no internal echogenicity and has thin (pencil line) wall, is more likely to become a leading follicles [27].

Whether the follicles that are visualized represent potentially healthy follicles with competent oocytes has not been established. In addition, there is considerable variability in the clinical definition and technical methodology used to count and measure follicles in both published studies and clinical practice. As a further complication, more than one individual may scan a patient during one cycle.

8.8 Monitoring Follicular Growth

COH is monitored by serial TVUS plus serum E2 measurements performed every second day from stimulation day 5–6. The frequency of monitoring will depend on the biophysical parameters of follicular growth and hormonal parameters, principally E2 levels. The wall of mature ovarian follicles is a complex structure with endocrine function. It is constituted by two cell layers. The outer layer is comprised

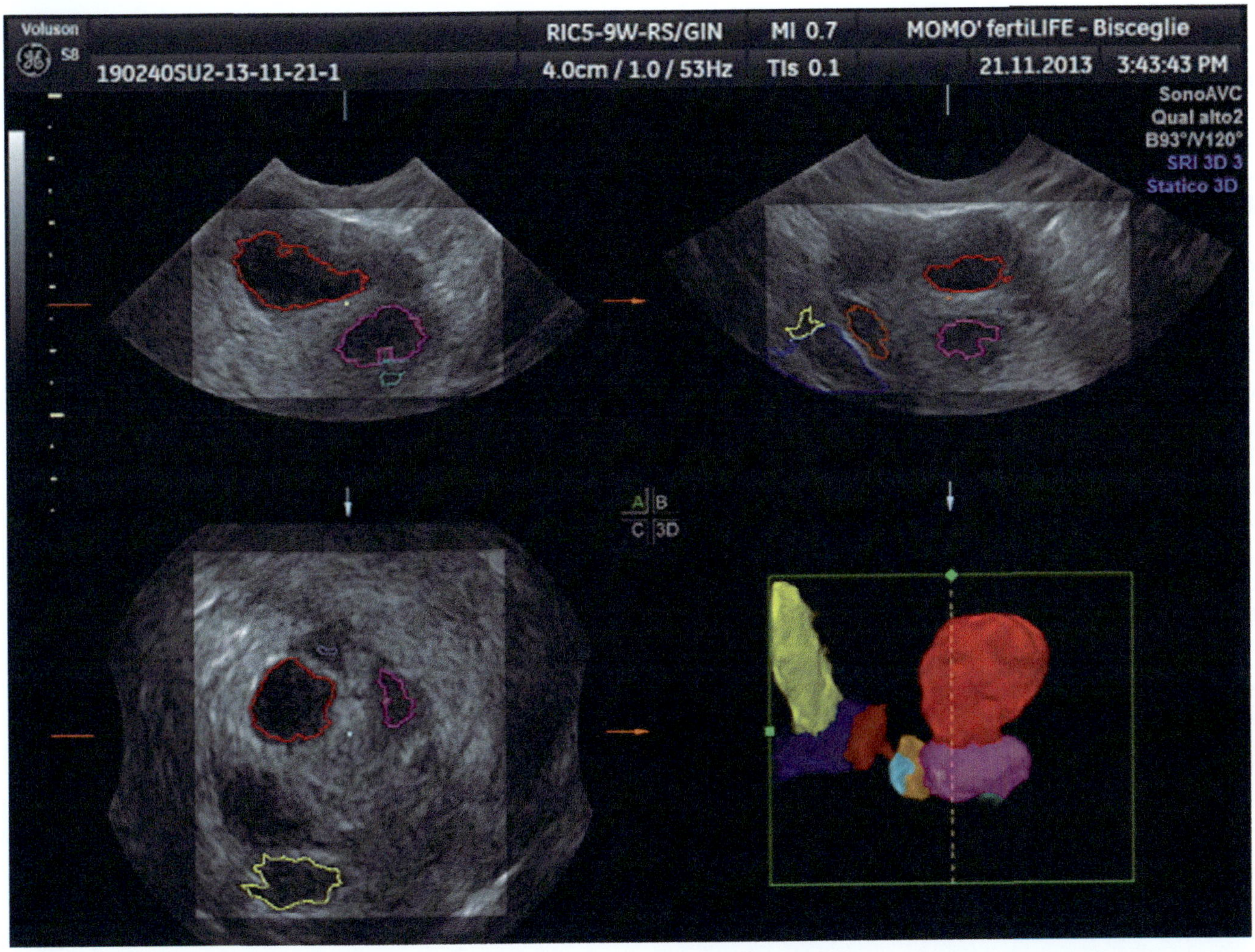

Fig. 8.7 The evaluation of growing follicles by ultrasound includes: follicle diameter, follicle growth pattern, follicular wall thickness, perifollicular vascularity, and perifollicular blood flow

of two types of cells and forms the theca: the theca interna contains cuboidal cells, synthesizing the androstenedione and is well vascularized; the theca externa mainly consists of connective tissue. The inner layer of the follicular wall is termed the granulosa and is composed of stratified cells which convert androstenedione into E2 through the action of the aromatase. The limit between the thecal layers and the granulosa is well defined histologically by a thick basal lamina [28]. The follicle wall is defined as the combined thicknesses of the stratum granulosa and theca. In order to measure the follicle size by the 2D-transvaginal scanning, the vaginal probe is placed as close as possible to the follicle to make follicle borders visualize clearly. The mean follicular diameter is calculated based on the mean of the two longest diameters. The two orthogonal diameters (d1 and d2) should be determined at the scanning plane corresponding to the largest follicle diameter, by placing the calipers on the fluid–follicle interface [29] (Fig. 8.8). Data on preferable placement of calipers on follicle borders (inner, outer, interface) are

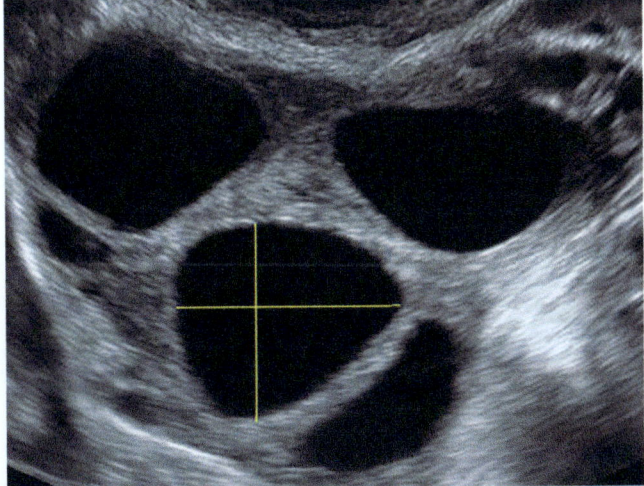

Fig. 8.8 Follicle size by the 2D-TVUS. The two orthogonal diameters (d1 and d2) should be measured at the scanning plane of the largest follicle diameter

scarce. Some authors measure follicular size using the internal diameters of the area [30]. The more accurate way of measurement will be probably clarified through studies on 3D ultrasound [31].

8.9 First Scan Under COH

Ovarian response can be identified early in the cycle. The first scan under COH for IVF-ICSI is performed on stimulation day 6–7.

Hodgen et al. classified ovarian response in the following way: "non-responders" as patients whose E2 levels did not reach 300 pg/mL by day 8 of stimulation; "slow responders" E2 levels were <300 pg/mL by day 5, but >300 pg/mL by day 8 of stimulation; "fast responders" with E2 levels >300 pg/mL by day 5 of stimulation [32] (Fig. 8.9).

Although debated, the practice of adjusting the dose on day 6–7 of stimulation, when cycle monitoring indicates that the ovarian response has been unsatisfactory, still represents a common practice. On the basis of both TVUS findings and E2 levels, gonadotropin dosages are adjusted up or down with 450 IU as the maximum daily dose allowed. How effective such dose increase or reduction is, is not well established [33]. Both very slow and very rapid estrogen growth rates, as calculated from the 4 days preceding oocyte retrieval were associated with a reduced pregnancy rate [34].

According to some authors, the dose of gonadotropin should not be altered as long as serial E2 levels increase between 50 and 100% every other day [35]. Suggested steps of dose adjustments ranges from 25–50 IU/day [36] to 75–100 IU/day. The dosage should be reduced by 75 IU if two consecutive E2 levels rise by >100% (Silverberg et al., 1991). From stimulation day 6–7 onward, COH continues until at least one dominant follicle reaches 18 mm diameter, with appropriate E2 levels (Fig. 8.10a, b).

8.10 Follicle Diameter and Anatomopathological Considerations

During follicular monitoring, clinicians should keep in mind that the size of follicles is related to the stage of oocytes. Prior to the widespread use of transvaginal sonography, morphometric data derived from studies of the entire follicular population of normal human ovaries (ovariectomy for carcinoma of the breasts or cervix, hysterectomy for fibroids) obtained at various stages of the menstrual period, allowed the development of a theoretical model of progression of follicles from the preantral to the ovulatory stage [37]. Follicular dimensions were measured with an ocular micrometer.

Histological examination of the human ovary revealed a great variety in the size of follicles from the preantral (0.1 mm) to the ovulatory stage (20 mm). Based on the number of granulosa cells, the entire follicular population was

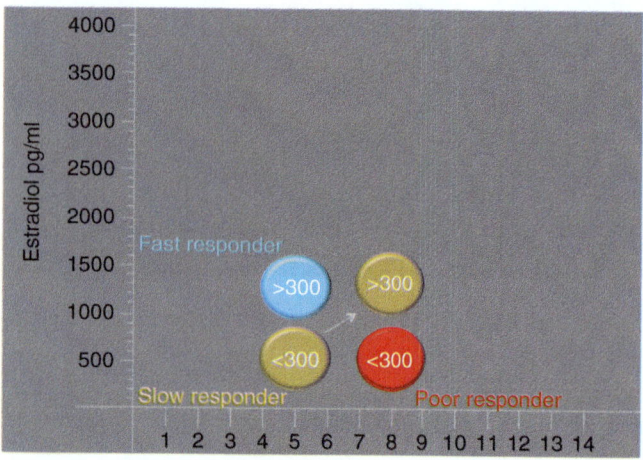

Fig. 8.9 Patients classification on day 8 of stimulation

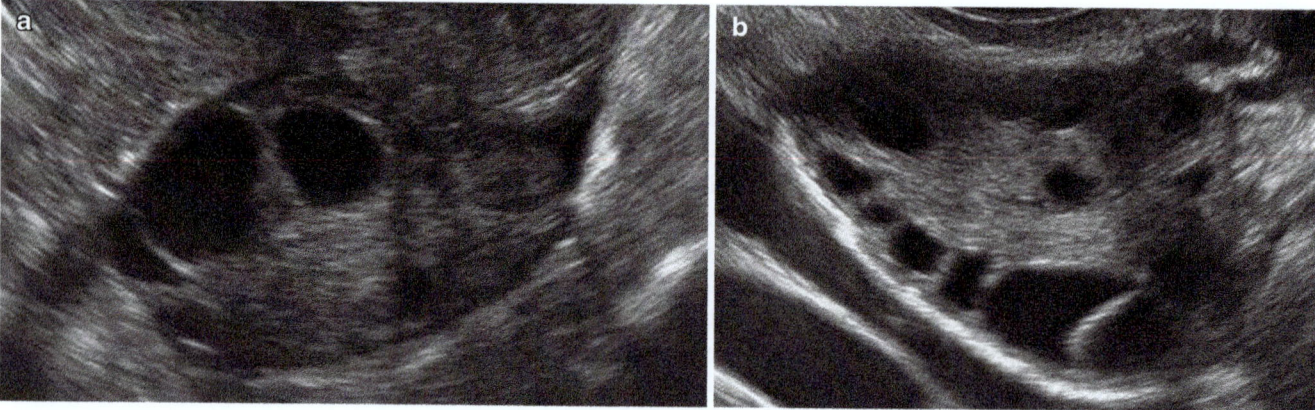

Fig. 8.10 Stimulation day 6, follicles measuring less than 14 mm: (**a**) POR patient; (**b**) woman with PCO

divided into classes representing the stages of follicular development. At each follicle diameter corresponded a number of granulosa cells (GC) (Figs. 8.11 and 8.12).

The numbers of preantral follicles throughout the cycle is more or less constant. Thus, the entry of follicles into this class is continuous during the cycle on the basis of a succession of waves, or cohorts, of growing follicles. Therefore, if an ovary is observed at any given point during the cycle, a large number of follicles of different diameter would be predictable, especially in young women (Table 8.2). In the early luteal phase (days 15–19), immediately after high levels of 17β-estradiol, the gonadotropins start the growth of follicles by the differentiation of the epitheloid cells in the theca interna (preantral follicles, 0.1–0.2 mm diameter).

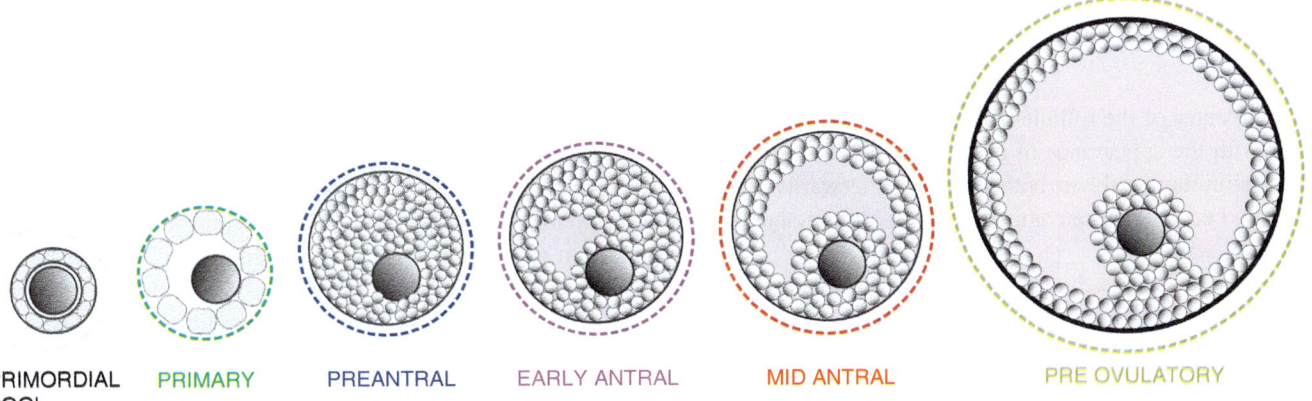

PRIMORDIAL POOL   PRIMARY   PREANTRAL   EARLY ANTRAL   MID ANTRAL   PRE OVULATORY

Fig. 8.11 Stages of folliculogenesis in the adult human ovary

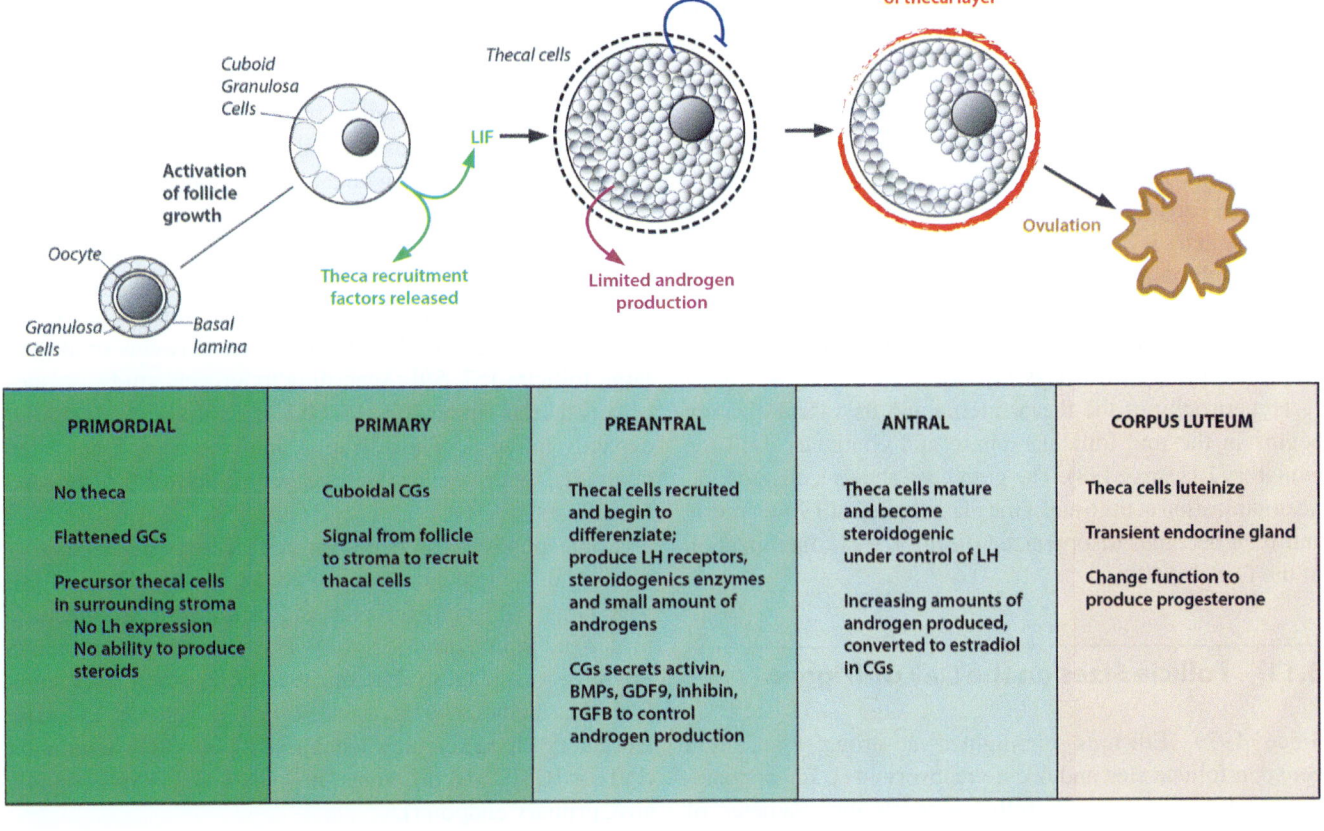

PRIMORDIAL	PRIMARY	PREANTRAL	ANTRAL	CORPUS LUTEUM
No theca Flattened GCs Precursor thecal cells in surrounding stroma No Lh expression No ability to produce steroids	Cuboidal CGs Signal from follicle to stroma to recruit thacal cells	Thecal cells recruited and begin to differenziate; produce LH receptors, steroidogenics enzymes and small amount of androgens CGs secrets activin, BMPs, GDF9, inhibin, TGFB to control androgen production	Theca cells mature and become steroidogenic under control of LH Increasing amounts of androgen produced, converted to estradiol in CGs	Theca cells luteinize Transient endocrine gland Change function to produce progesterone

Fig. 8.12 Stage of follicles maturation

Table 8.2 Follicular size and visualization by ultrasound

Stage	Follicular size
Primordial	0.03–0.04
Primary	0.05–0.06
Secondary	0.07–0.11
Preantral	0.12–0.20
Early antral	0.21–0.40
Antral	0.41–16.00
Preovulatory	16.1–20.00

Ovarian follicles larger than 2 mm in diameter can be observed by TVUS

The entry of the follicles into class 2 (0.2–0.4 mm diameter with the appearance of an antrum) is observed 25 days later simultaneously in both ovaries. Afterwards follicular growth becomes more complex with an asymmetry between the two ovaries.

Ovarian follicles larger than 2 mm in diameter can be observed by TVUS and are highly sensitive to gonadotropins. Follicles of 2–10 mm are related to the amount of the primordial follicle pool. Unfortunately, the same range 2–10 mm include also follicles at early stages of atresia and thus poorly responsive to gonadotropin.

As a consequence, the AFC tends to overestimate the number of gonadotropins responsive follicles. Healthy antral follicles tend to be 4–6 mm in diameter and might best represent the age-dependent proportion of the antral follicle pool. However, measuring the diameter of every follicle would require very long time.

The largest healthy follicles measure 2 and 5 mm in diameter at the end of the luteal phase and show a higher mitotic activity than the mid-luteal phase. The follicle destined to ovulate in the next cycle will be recruited among these follicles in the early follicular phase (days 1–5).

Its diameter is between 5.5 and 8.2 mm and increases significantly through cellular proliferation and accumulation of fluid in the antrum [38, 39]. During 2 weeks, it grows from 6.9 ± 0.5 mm (days 1–5) to 13.3 ± 1.2 mm (days 6–10) and then to 18.8 ± 0.5 mm (days 11–14).

Hypertrophy of the theca interna and its vascularization begins in the mid-follicular phase and continues until the ovulatory LH surge [38]. The granulosa shows a characteristic organization at the time of the plasma peak of 17β-estradiol and then becomes disorganized during the pre-luteinization of the follicle [40].

8.11 Follicle Sizes on the Day of Trigger

Since 1973, Edwards highlighted a strong association between follicle size and oocyte recovery [41]. In spontaneous cycles, preovulatory follicles reach the diameter of 17–25 mm in diameter [42]. During COH, the relationship between follicle size and oocyte maturity might be different.

It is more likely that a large follicle contains a free-floating cumulus-oocyte complex, compared to a small one [43–46]. In literature, data about ideal follicle size at the time of hCG are controversial and demonstrate the difficulty in defining a universally accepted threshold of follicle dimension to predict the presence of good competent oocytes. Generally, the incidence of mature oocytes increases with follicular size [47]; however, both too small and too large follicles are associated with low oocyte recovery, fertilization, and cleavage rates.

Table 8.2 summarizes data on oocyte competence and follicular size (Table 8.2). Oocytes are frequently found in the metaphase II (MII) when retrieved from follicles larger than 16 mm (approximately corresponding to a 2 mL volume). Some authors consider 18 mm as a better cutoff to discriminate follicles with higher chances of mature oocytes [48, 49].

In follicles below 12 mm a higher proportion of immature, germinal vesicle (GV) or metaphase I (MI) oocytes is found and some authors recommend not aspirate this pool of follicles [48, 50, 51].

Another study, reported that follicles from 11 to 15 mm sometimes can harbor mature oocytes [52]. Both in normal and PCO ovaries, follicles smaller than 14 mm diameter occasionally might contain MII oocytes [49–51, 53–56].

Discordant findings on the relationship between follicular size and embryo cleavage rates were reported [48, 51, 57, 58] (Table 8.3).

In case of oocytes obtained from smaller follicles, the rate of polyspermy with conventional IVF and the fragmentation rate were shown higher with a lower pregnancy rate [51].

These effects might be due to a reduced oocyte competence, to either safeguards from more than one sperm getting in and developing during the following cleavage stages. Other authors did not confirm any differences in oocyte recovery rate [58] or fertilization rate, between small and large follicles [57, 59]. According to a recent study, oocytes obtained from small follicles (0.3–0.9 mL) showed similar capacity in terms of fertilization and blastocyst rates when compared with oocytes from larger follicles (1–6 mL and >6 mL) [60].

Some publications demonstrated decreased fertilization rate and developmental competence in oocytes derived from very large (>23 mm) follicles, indicating adverse effects of prolonged stimulation [55, 61]. These controversial results might be attributed to differences in COH protocols, patient features, methods to measure follicular volume and size, laboratory characteristics, technique of oocyte insemination (IVF or ICSI), and difference in statistical analysis (sample size, primary endpoint).

Table 8.3 Human studies on follicle size and IVF outcomes

Author/year	Study design	Age (years)	COH protocol	IVF/ICSI	Number of oocytes	Mean diameter at HCG	Mean diameter at oocyte retrieval	% MII	Fertilization rate	Cleavage rate	% good quality embryos
Wittmaack, 1994	R	23–49	Long	Only IVF	6879	From 16 to 18 mm	21 mm	Worst <12 mm and >24 mm	Increasing from 12 mm onwards	Increasing from 12 mm onwards	None
Inaudi, 1995	R	28–37	Short	Only IVF	179	At least 3 foll > 16 mm	n.e.	None in the recovery rate	n.e.	n.e.	n.e.
Dubey, 1995	R	n.e.	Long	Only IVF	2429	At least 2 foll > 20 mm	n.e.	n.e.	Increasing from 16 mm onwards	n.e.	n.e.
Ectors, 1997	P	n.e.	Short	IVF/ICSI	2324	n.e.	n.e.	IVF: n.e.	IVF: increasing from 16 to 23, later decreasing	IVF: increasing from 16 to 23, later decreasing	IVF: increasing from 16 to 23, later decreasing
Bergh, 1998	P	33 mean	Long	IVF/ICSI	4159	n.e.	n.e.	n.e.	IVF: increasing	IVF: none	n.e. but increasing pregnancy rate only in IVF
Teissier, 2000	P	28 mean	Long	Only IVF	150	n.e.	n.e.	Increasing	n.e.	Increasing	n.e.
Triwitayakorn, 2003	P	31.4–40.5	Long-short	Only ICSI	991	At least 2 foll of 18 mm	n.e.	Always increasing together with oocyte recovery rate	None	n.e.	None
Rosen, 2008	P	28.2–40.0	Long-short	IVF/ICSI	2934	At least 2 foll of 18 mm	n.e.	IVF: n.e./ICSI: always increasing	IVF and ICSI: always increasing	n.e.	IVF and ICSI: always increasing
Lee, 2010	P	29.0–37.9	Long	Only ICSI	819	When 2–3 foll >18 mm	n.e.	Increasing from 18 mm onwards	None	None	None
Mehri, 2013	P	n.e.	Long	IVF/ICSI	360	At least 2 foll of 20 mm	n.e.	Increasing from 18 mm onwards	Increasing from 18 mm onwards	None	None
Wirleitner, 2018	P	<43	Long	Only IVF	1236	At least 2 foll of 18 mm	13–23 mm	Increasing	Similar results	Similar results	Similar results

Modified from Revelli (2014)

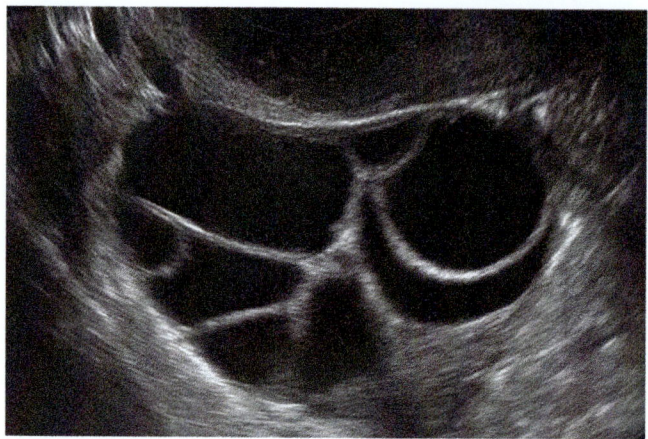

Fig. 8.13 Stimulation day 11, three follicles measuring 17–18 mm (day of HCG)

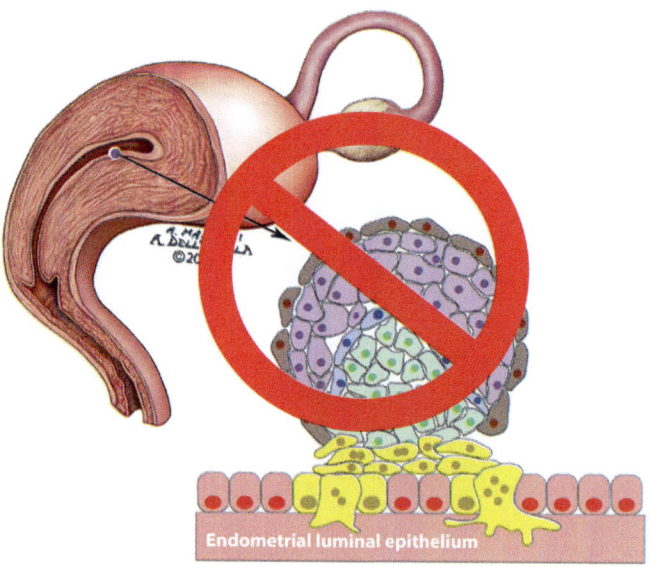

Fig. 8.14 The rise of progesteron during the final stage of IVF cycle can make the endometrium asynchronous

Moreover, few studies have analyzed the relationship between oocyte competence and follicular size following one-by-one follicle measurement.

Overall there is evidence that follicles having a mean diameter between 16 and 22 mm are those with the highest likelihood of containing MII oocytes, small follicles can seldom generate MII oocytes.

The most widely applied protocol is administering the trigger when at least two-three follicles have reached a diameter of ≥18 mm [62] or at least three leading follicles measure 17 mm (Wertheimer et al., 2018) (Fig. 8.13).

Furthermore, the number of adequate size follicles appears to be more important than the size of the leading follicle(s) for timing of hCG administration (Wittmaack et al., 1994).

8.12 Serum Progesterone Elevation During Follicular Growth

For over two decades, the potential adverse effect of serum progesterone elevation on the day of hCG administration on IVF/ICSI outcomes has been a matter of intense debate in the literature.

In early studies, no association between serum progesterone and pregnancy outcomes was observed [35, 63–68], whereas more recent studies reported a significant negative effect [69–76].

A large meta-analysis conducted on more than 60,000 cycles observed that adopting a threshold of 0.8 ng/mL, a decreased probability of pregnancy was associated with progesterone elevation on the day of hCG administration in fresh IVF cycles.

In contrast, no adverse effect was detected in the frozen–thawed and the donor/recipient cycles [77]. This data supported the hypothesis that progesterone rise does not influence the oocyte quality but somewhat endometrial receptivity [77].

The endometrial advancement of more than 3 days versus the actual day after ovulation leads to an asynchrony (Fig. 8.14) between the endometrium and the embryo [78]. Supraphysiological hormonal levels during ovarian stimulation for IVF might jeopardize the endometrial receptivity.

Previous studies performed on genomics evaluation of endometrial receptivity reported that progesterone rise on HCG day affects endometrial gene expression [79–81]. Nevertheless, recently published data highlight also a negative correlation between elevated progesterone and the rate of "top embryo quality." Huang et al. (2016) found that when serum progesterone levels were higher than 2.0 ng/mL, the number of top embryo quality was significantly reduced [82]. Another study observed that progesterone elevation on the day of hCG administration was more frequent in patients with recurrent IVF failure [83]. Furthermore, experimental research with animals revealed a crucial role of progesterone in oocyte acquisition of developmental competence [84, 85]. Thus, another possibility is that the elevated progesterone has negative effects on the quality of the oocyte or resulting embryo. However, the pathophysiology through which elevated progesterone levels might produce adverse effects on oocyte-embryo quality requires further studies. Similarly, the exact cause of progesterone elevation during the follicular phase of ovarian stimulation for IVF/ICSI remains still unclear. It does not seem to reflect a true luteinization event. It has been observed that progesterone elevation is associated with an increase in the total amount of gonadotropins used for ovarian stimulation, an increase in E2 levels on the day of hCG, GnRH agonist protocols, and the number of retrieved oocytes [77]. FSH has a direct stimulatory effect on the expression and the enzymatic activity of 3β-hydroxysteroid dehydrogenase (3β-HSD). Therefore, FSH stimulation increases the conversion of pregnenolone to progesterone in human mitotic granulosa cell line (in vitro study on human ovarian cortical samples). Pregnenolone and progesterone produced by granulosa cells should be converted into androgens by the theca cells. However, in the absence of LH support, 17-alpha-hydroxylase does not respond to FSH stimulation in human granulosa cell; thus, the amount of generated precursor steroids may exceed the ability of the ovary to effectively convert them into estrogen pathway producing their accumulation and leak into systemic circulation [86]. Some authors observed that ovarian stimulation with corifollitropin alpha (CFA) only might lead to a significantly reduced incidence of premature progesterone elevation on the day of final oocyte maturation. Pharmacokinetics and follicular dynamics of CFA might explain this result. Although maintaining the FSH activity above the threshold for 1 week, CFA reaches a peak concentration 2 days after the injection and then decreases progressively. Thus, a step-down protocol can be adopted in order to prevent the progesterone elevation. However, further studies are needed to support this approach [87, 88].

8.13 Threshold Level of Progesterone Elevation

There is no consensus about the exact threshold level of progesterone elevation affecting fresh IVF/ICSI cycles and a nonlinear effect has been suggested (Bosch et al., 2010). In the normal and in the poor responders, the negative effect of progesterone elevation appears already from progesterone concentrations of 0.8–1.1 ng/mL (OR: 0.79) and seems to be increased when progesterone concentration reaches value ≥1.2 ng/mL [77].

However, in the high responders, a detrimental effect of progesterone elevation is present only when the level of serum progesterone on the day of hCG reaches 1.9–3.0 ng/mL (Fig. 8.12). Thus, an increase in E2 levels or in the number of collected oocytes might compensate for the negative effect of progesterone elevation. As the E2 levels and the increase in mature follicles may be important factors affecting the progesterone threshold level, it has been proposed that the progesterone/E2 ratio might be a more efficient prognostic indicator [72, 89]. There are few studies investigating the value of progesterone/E2 ratio on predicting IVF/ICSI outcomes. In a recent retrospective cohort study, Golbasi et al. (2018) concluded that the progesterone/E2 ratio is not an efficient parameter for predicting the live birth rate in women with a progesterone value higher than 1.5 ng/mL. The same authors highlighted the limitations of

their study as the low number of included patients and suggested further research on this issue [90]. As the increase in total blood progesterone level was detrimental only if it resulted from an increase in the average progesterone secreted from each follicle and not from the recruitment of additional follicles, other more representative parameters have been proposed: Progesterone-to-follicle index (PFI) [91] and progesterone to a number of aspirated oocytes ratio (POI) [92].

The PFI was calculated by dividing the total blood progesterone level (nmol/L) by the number of follicles ≥14 mm in diameter on the hCG day [91]; POI was calculated by dividing the serum progesterone level on the day of hCG by the number of aspirated mature oocytes [92]. Both parameters need to be validated by further studies in order to be adopted in clinical practice.

8.14 Implications for Clinical Practice

The most frequently used method for managing progesterone elevation is freezing embryos and transferring them in a subsequent frozen–thawed cycle (the "freeze-all" strategy). Up to now no randomized controlled trial has evaluated the effectiveness of this intervention in women who exhibit progesterone raise on the day of hCG administration. Moreover, the "freeze-all" strategy has significant implications on the cost and the number of patients that require further testing and interventions. In order to make the decision to freeze-only as cost-effective, the threshold value should have strong positive predictive value.

Hill et al. (2018), through a threshold and cost analyses, observed a clinical benefit to a freeze-only approach above progesterone thresholds ranging from 1.5 to 2.0 ng/dL. At these thresholds, elevated progesterone has a demonstrable and clinically significant negative effect and makes the "freeze-only" a cost-effective option [93].

8.15 OHSS Risk Assessment During Monitoring Follicular Growth

OHSS is an uncommon but serious complication associated with COH. Moderate-to-severe OHSS occurs in approximately 1–5% of cycles [94].

The syndrome description includes a spectrum of findings, such as ovarian enlargement, ascites, hemoconcentration, hypercoagulability, and electrolyte imbalances (Figs. 8.15 and 8.16a, b). As recommended by the ASRM (2016) [94], every effort should be made to identify patients who are at the highest risk. The assessment of the risk of OHSS during monitoring of follicular growth is particularly important in the light of the prevention strategies that can be adopted as the use of GnRH agonist (with or without low-dose hCG) to trigger the final oocyte maturation of oocytes, the use of cabergoline, and cryopreservation of all embryos rather than transfer.

Ovarian stimulation parameters during monitoring follicular growth may aid in the prediction of patients who will develop OHSS.

A number of prospective studies observed that a high number of growing follicles is an independent predictor of OHSS. Development of ≥25 follicles and >19 large-/medium-sized follicles before hCG, E2 values >3500 pg/mL or ≥24 oocytes retrieved are related with an increased risk of OHSS [94].

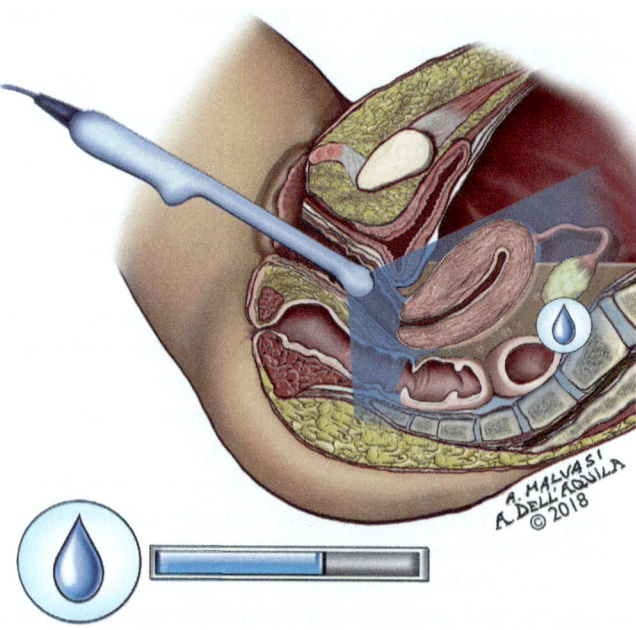

Fig. 8.15 Schematic representation the peritoneal fluid in OHSS

8.16 Three-Dimensional (3D) Ultrasonography

In late 1980s, the progress of 3D ultrasound allowed acquisition and analysis of volume data. A recent rendering technique, known as the inversion mode, allows the automatic identification and quantification of hypoechogenic ovarian follicles within the relatively hyperechoic ovarian tissue.

8.17 SonoAVC: The Technology

Sonography-based Automated Volume Calculation (SonoAVC, GE Medical Systems) was developed for follicle monitoring during COH. It is also used for AFC and other obstetric application.

The use of 3D TVUS allows to capture the entire volume of the ovary in a single sweep and allows to store the volume for re-evaluation of the follicles.

SonoAVC provides three flexible workflows of methods:

1. SonoAVC follicle
2. SonoAVC follicle semi-automated method
3. SonoAVC follicle manual method

In all cases, technology is based on the voxel count within the identified hypoechoic structure and calculates the following measurements:

1. the largest diameters in three orthogonal planes
2. the mean follicular diameter (MFD) (the arithmetic mean of the longest three orthogonal diameters)
3. the volume of the follicle
4. the volume-based diameter (d(V)) of the follicle (the diameter of a perfect sphere with the same volume of the follicle)

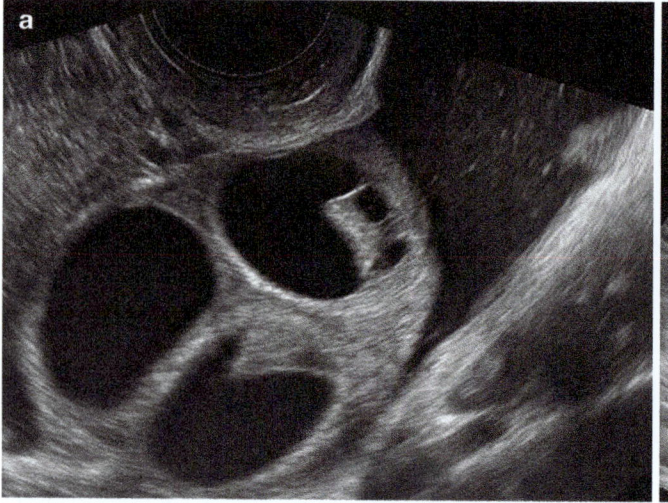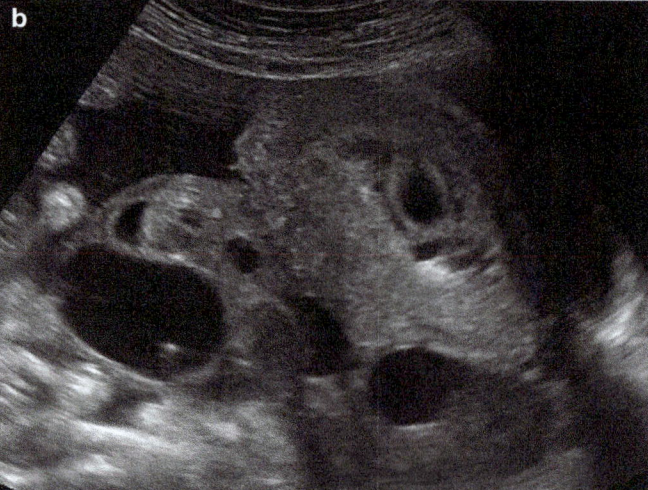

Fig. 8.16 (**a, b**) Pregnant woman with OHSS, ovarian enlargement, and ascites

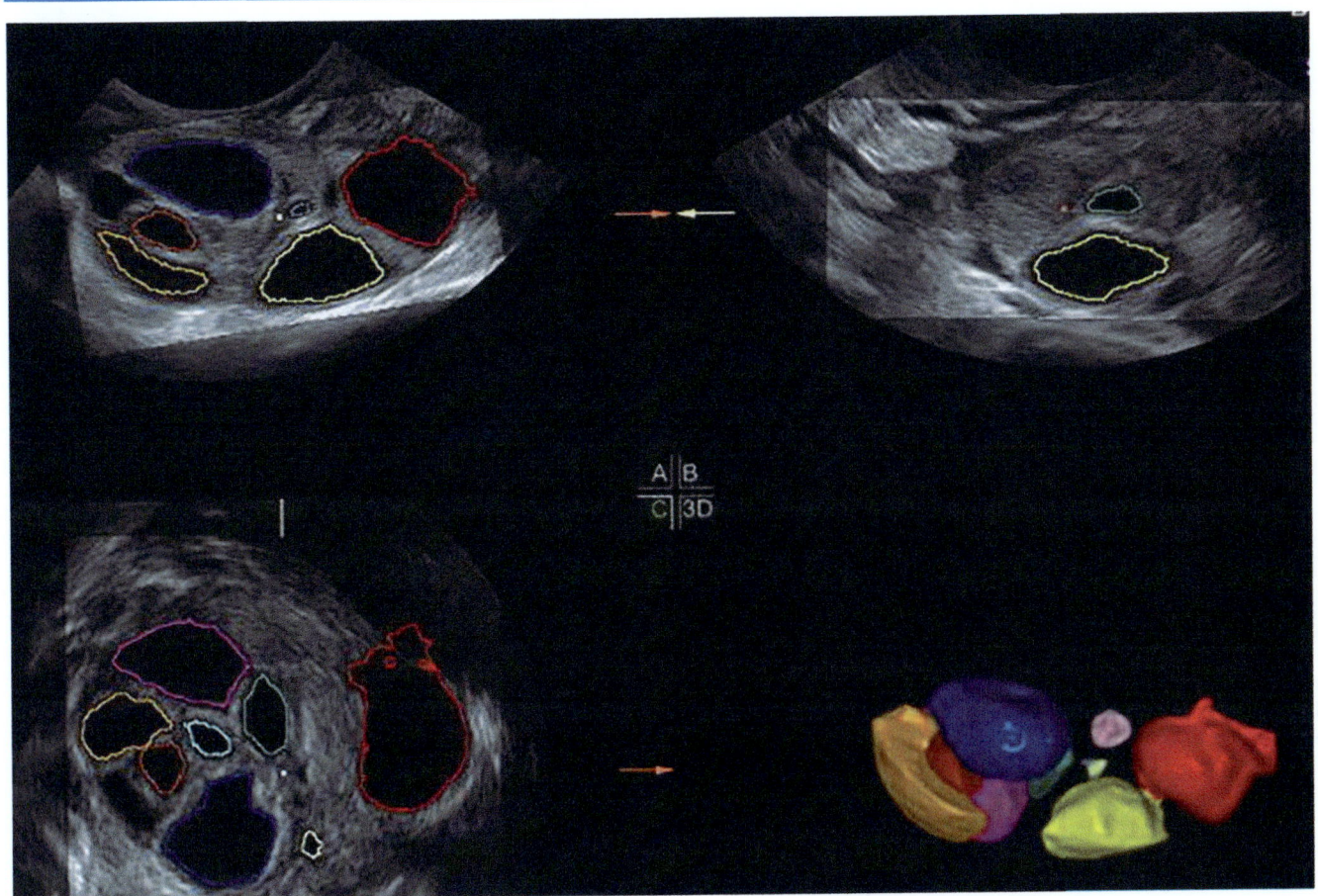

Fig. 8.17 SonoAVC analysis of a stimulated ovary. Automatically identified color-coded follicles in a stimulated ovary

After the capturing of a 3D image of an ovary, the user defines a region of interest (ROI) on the entire ovary, excluding extraovarian region. Once the volume of the ovary has been obtained, the operator selects the Volume Analysis and then the SonoAVC follicle with the preferred measurements methods (Fig. 8.17).

For SonoAVC follicle manual method, the operator firstly decides which ovary has to be calculated. Once this choice has been made, the volume will be shown in a single plane.

Through the use of the "Parallel Shift control," parallel sections of the ovary can be observed. Measurements can be performed through the calipers or the ellipse function. After completing all measurements of the follicles in a plane, we can shift to the following plane.

The SonoAVC follicle semi-automated method allows to control which follicle to measure by clicking on each follicle. The Shift control allows the access to other plane within the ovarian volume. At any time further measurement can be performed by selecting "follicle add manual."

For SonoAVC follicle, the "auto" option should be selected then the software will automatically measure the follicles within the ROI. It's up to the users to ensure that all the follicles have been included in the volume and if

they want to make correction, the "Add/remove" button can be used.

In the final report, individual follicles and their corresponding measurements are color coded and presented in descending order. The largest follicle is always shown in red, the second largest in blue, and the third in yellow (Fig. 8.18).

8.18 Accuracy of SonoAVC for Monitoring Follicular Growth and Clinical Advantageous

SonoAVC for Monitoring Follicular Growth has shown good agreement with conventional 2D TVUS. Data obtained from in Vitro Studies (ultrasound phantom that contained anechoic spheres, water-filled balloons in an ultrasound test reservoir) lead to conflicting results probably due to the use of different phantoms, equipment, and settings. Some authors highlighted a systematic underestimation by SonoAVC [95]. On the contrary, in vivo studies have demonstrated an excellent correlation between SonoAVC-calculated follicular volume and true follicular volume (with the volume of the follicular aspirate). When the follicles were categorized according to

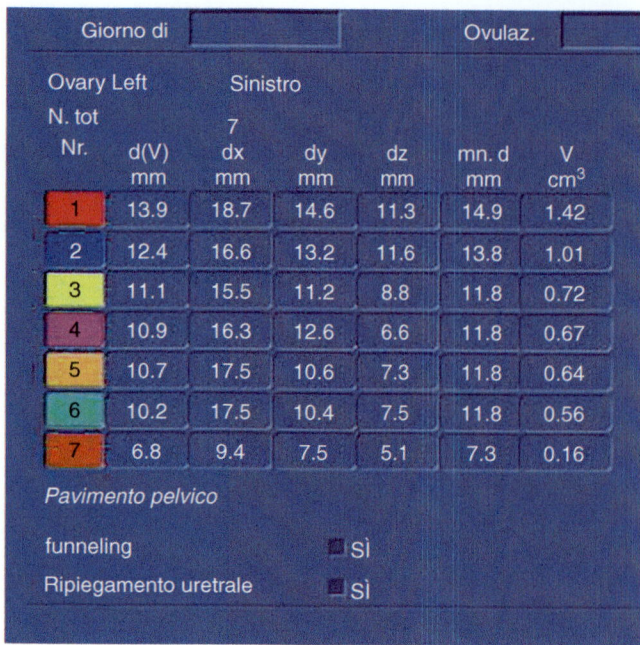

Giorno di				Ovulaz.			

Ovary Left   Sinistro

N. tot   7

Nr.	d(V) mm	dx mm	dy mm	dz mm	mn. d mm	V cm³
1	13.9	18.7	14.6	11.3	14.9	1.42
2	12.4	16.6	13.2	11.6	13.8	1.01
3	11.1	15.5	11.2	8.8	11.8	0.72
4	10.9	16.3	12.6	6.6	11.8	0.67
5	10.7	17.5	10.6	7.3	11.8	0.64
6	10.2	17.5	10.4	7.5	11.8	0.56
7	6.8	9.4	7.5	5.1	7.3	0.16

Pavimento pelvico

funneling   ☑Sì

Ripiegamento uretrale   ☑Sì

Fig. 8.18 Structured SonoAVC report. Each line corresponds to a follicle, from the largest to the smallest one. The lines are coded with the same colors as the corresponding follicles

their sizes, SonoAVC maintained its accuracy across subgroups. It appears that SonoAVC can accurately determine follicular size in stimulated ovaries [96, 97].

3D ultrasound imaging has potential advantages:

- *highly reproducible* with reduced observer and interobserver variability
- *less time* for ultrasound procedures
- the opportunity for post hoc *image analysis*
- *reduced variability* of measurements in non-spherical follicles
- *reduced chance of missing or double-counting* follicles
- *opportunity of quality control* [97]

Rodriguez-Fuentes et al. observed that with automated monitoring, women with >10 follicles would save an average of 7.6 min, and the sonographer would save 4 min per patient [98].

The advantage of decreasing examination time and facilitating workflow could be beneficial, especially in busy IVF units. Faster ultrasound examinations would decrease discomfort for patients, particularly when there are several follicles.

Unfortunately, a large number of patients require postprocessing and some follicles need manual measurement. Moreover this method, involves high quality image, is less accurate in identifying antral follicles smaller than 5–6 mm, and 3D imaging equipments have still high costs.

Follicle tracking with 3D sonographic follicular volume measurements does not achieve better fertility outcomes than standard 2D sonography [43, 99].

Therefore, the use of a fully automated 3D technology is limited in the field of reproductive medicine.

8.19 Effectiveness

Counting ovarian follicles and measurement by ultrasonography, and/or hormonal assessment, particularly serum E2 concentration, are used for monitoring COH. Monitoring COH by both TVUS and hormonal evaluation is associated with higher costs and discomfort for the patients. Whether hormonal assessment adds to efficacy and safety of COH is still matter of debate [100, 101].

For some authors, monitoring COH by ultrasonography alone is not likely to reduce the number of oocytes retrieved or to alter substantially the chances of achieving a clinical pregnancy. However, high E2 concentrations the day of ovulation induction are associated with increased probabilities for OHSS, irrespective of ultrasound findings [101–103].

Actually, there is no evidence from RCT to suggest that combined monitoring by TVUS and serum E2 is more efficacious than monitoring by TVUS alone, with regard to clinical pregnancy rates and the incidence of OHSS. Thus, a combined monitoring practice including both TVUS and serum E2 is still considered as good clinical practice [104].

References

1. Gilchrist RB, Thompson JG. Oocyte maturation: emerging concepts and technologies to improve developmental potential in vitro. Theriogenology. 2007;67(1):6–15.
2. Lensen SF, Wilkinson J, Leijdekkers JA, La Marca A, Mol BWJ, Marjoribanks J, Torrance H, Broekmans FJ. Individualised gonadotropin dose selection using markers of ovarian reserve for women undergoing in vitro fertilisation plus intracytoplasmic sperm injection (IVF/ICSI). Cochrane Database Syst Rev. 2018;2:CD012693.
3. Baird DT. A model for follicular selection and ovulation: lessons from superovulation. J Steroid Biochem. 1987;27(1–3):15–23.
4. Zeleznik AJ, Schuler HM, Reichert LE Jr. Gonadotropin-binding sites in the rhesus monkey ovary: role of the vasculature in the selective distribution of human chorionic gonadotropin to the preovulatory follicle. Endocrinology. 1981;109(2):356–62.
5. Goff AK, Armstrong DT. Stimulatory action of gonadotropins and prostaglandins on adenosine-3',5'-monophosphate production by isolated rat granulosa cells. Endocrinology. 1977;101(5):1461–7.
6. Zeleznik AJ, Hillier SG. The role of gonadotropins in the selection of the preovulatory follicle. Clin Obstet Gynecol. 1984;27(4):927–40.
7. Vegetti W, Alagna F. FSH and folliculogenesis: from physiology to ovarian stimulation. Reprod BioMed Online. 2006;12(6):684–94.
8. Andersen CY, Humaidan P, Ejdrup HB, Bungum L, Grøndahl ML, Westergaard LG. Hormonal characteristics of follicular fluid from women receiving either GnRH agonist or hCG for ovulation induction. Hum Reprod. 2006;21(8):2126–30.
9. Sunkara SK, Rittenberg V, Raine-Fenning N, Bhattacharya S, Zamora J, Coomarasamy A. Association between the number of

eggs and live birth in IVF treatment: an analysis of 400 135 treatment cycles. Hum Reprod. 2011;26(7):1768–74.

10. Ferraretti AP, Gianaroli L. The Bologna criteria for the definition of poor ovarian responders: is there a need for revision? Hum Reprod. 2014;29(9):1842–5.

11. Steward RG, Lan L, Shah AA, Yeh JS, Price TM, Goldfarb JM, Muasher SJ. Oocyte number as a predictor for ovarian hyperstimulation syndrome and live birth: an analysis of 256,381 in vitro fertilization cycles. Fertil Steril. 2014;101(4):967–73.

12. Youssef MA, Mourad S. Volume expanders for the prevention of ovarian hyperstimulation syndrome. Cochrane Database Syst Rev. 2016;(8):CD001302.

13. La Marca A, Papaleo E, Grisendi V, Argento C, Giulini S, Volpe A. Development of a nomogram based on markers of ovarian reserve for the individualisation of the follicle-stimulating hormone starting dose in in vitro fertilisation cycles. BJOG. 2012;119(10):1171–9.

14. Coccia ME, Rizzello F. Ovarian reserve. Ann N Y Acad Sci. 2008;1127:27–30.

15. Broekmans FJ, de Ziegler D, Howles CM, Gougeon A, Trew G, Olivennes F. The antral follicle count: practical recommendations for better standardization. Fertil Steril. 2010;94(3):1044–51.

16. Visser JA, de Jong FH, Laven JS, Themmen AP. Anti-Müllerian hormone: a new marker for ovarian function. Reproduction. 2006;131(1):1–9.

17. Seifer DB, MacLaughlin DT, Christian BP, Feng B, Shelden RM. Early follicular serum Müllerian-inhibiting substance levels are associated with ovarian response during assisted reproductive technology cycles. Fertil Steril. 2002;77(3):468–71.

18. van Rooij IA, Broekmans FJ, te Velde ER, Fauser BC, Bancsi LF, de Jong FH, Themmen AP. Serum anti-Müllerian hormone levels: a novel measure of ovarian reserve. Hum Reprod. 2002;17(12):3065–71.

19. Broer SL, Broekmans FJ, Laven JS, Fauser BC. Anti-Müllerian hormone: ovarian reserve testing and its potential clinical implications. Hum Reprod Update. 2014;20(5):688–701.

20. La Marca A, Sunkara SK. Individualization of controlled ovarian stimulation in IVF using ovarian reserve markers: from theory to practice. Hum Reprod Update. 2014;20(1):124–40.

21. Poseidon Group (Patient-Oriented Strategies Encompassing IndividualizeD Oocyte Number), Alviggi C, Andersen CY, Buehler K, Conforti A, De Placido G, Esteves SC, Fischer R, Galliano D, Polyzos NP, Sunkara SK, Ubaldi FM, Humaidan P. A new more detailed stratification of low responders to ovarian stimulation: from a poor ovarian response to a low prognosis concept. Fertil Steril. 2016;105(6):1452–3.

22. Esteves SC, Roque M, Bedoschi GM, Conforti A, Humaidan P, Alviggi C. Defining low prognosis patients undergoing assisted reproductive technology: POSEIDON criteria-the why. Front Endocrinol (Lausanne). 2018;9:461.

23. Yates AP, Rustamov O, Roberts SA, Lim HY, Pemberton PW, Smith A, Nardo LG. Anti-Mullerian hormone-tailored stimulation protocols improve outcomes whilst reducing adverse effects and costs of IVF. Hum Reprod. 2011;26(9):2353–62.

24. Khalaf Y, El-Toukhy T, Taylor A, Braude P. Increasing the gonadotrophin dose in the course of an in vitro fertilization cycle does not rectify an initial poor response. Eur J Obstet Gynecol Reprod Biol. 2002;103:146–9.

25. van Hooff MHA, Alberda AT, Huisman GJ, Zeilmaker GH, Leerentveld RA. Doubling the human menopausal gonadotrophin dose in the course of an in-vitro fertilization treatment cycle in low responders: a randomized study. Hum Reprod. 1993;8:369–73.

26. Bosch E, Havelock J, Martin FS, Rasmussen BB, Klein BM, Mannaerts B, Arce JC, ESTHER-2 Study Group. Follitropin delta in repeated ovarian stimulation for IVF: a controlled, assessor-blind Phase 3 safety trial. Reprod BioMed Online. 2019;38(2):195–205.

27. Panchal S, Nagori C. Comparison of anti-Mullerian hormone and antral follicle count for assessment of ovarian reserve. Hum Reprod Sci. 2012;5(3):274–8.

28. Blankstein J, Shalev J, Saadon T, Kukia EE, Rabinovici J, Pariente C, Lunenfeld B, Serr DM, Mashiach S. Ovarian hyperstimulation syndrome: prediction by number and size of preovulatory ovarian follicles. Fertil Steril. 1987;47(4):597–602.

29. Martinuk SD, Chizen DR, Pierson RA. Ultrasonographic morphology of the human preovulatory follicle wall prior to ovulation. Clin Anat. 1992;5:339–52.

30. La Marca A, Grisendi V, Giulini S, Argento C, Tirelli A, Dondi G, Papaleo E, Volpe A. Individualization of the FSH starting dose in IVF/ICSI cycles using the antral follicle count. J Ovarian Res. 2013;6(1):11.

31. Pan P, Chen X, Li Y, Zhang Q, Zhao X, Bodombossou-Djobo MM, Yang D. Comparison of manual and automated measurements of monodominant follicle diameter with different follicle size in infertile patients. PLoS One. 2013;8(10):e77095.

32. Hodgen GD. Biological basis of follicle growth. Hum Reprod. 1989;4(8 Suppl):37–46.

33. van Tilborg TC, Torrance HL, Oudshoorn SC, Eijkemans MJC, Koks CAM, Verhoeve HR, Nap AW, Scheffer GJ, Manger AP, Schoot BC, Sluijmer AV, Verhoeff A, Groen H, Laven JSE, Mol BWJ, Broekmans FJM. OPTIMIST study group. Individualized versus standard FSH dosing in women starting IVF/ICSI: an RCT. Part 1: the predicted poor responder. Hum Reprod. 2017;32(12):2496–505.

34. Dirnfeld M, Lejeune B, Camus M, Vekemans M, Leroy F. Growth rate of follicular estrogen secretion in relation to the outcome of in vitro fertilization and embryo replacement. Fertil Steril. 1985;43(3):379–8.

35. Silverberg KM, Burns WN, Olive DL, et al. Serum progesterone levels predict success of in vitro fertilization/embryo transfer in patients stimulated with leuprolide acetate and human menopausal gonadotropins. J Clin Endocrinol Metab. 1991;73:797–803.

36. van Tilborg TC, Eijkemans MJ, Laven JS, Koks CA, de Bruin JP, Scheffer GJ, van Golde RJ, Fleischer K, Hoek A, Nap AW, Kuchenbecker WK, Manger PA, Brinkhuis EA, van Heusden AM, Sluijmer AV, Verhoeff A, van Hooff MH, Friederich J, Smeenk JM, Kwee J, Verhoeve HR, Lambalk CB, Helmerhorst FM, van der Veen F, Mol BW, Torrance HL, Broekmans FJ. The OPTIMIST study: optimisation of cost effectiveness through individualised FSH stimulation dosages for IVF treatment. A randomised controlled trial. BMC Womens Health. 2012;12:29.

37. Dubey AK, Wang HA, Duffy P, Penzias AS. The correlation between follicular measurements, oocyte morphology, and fertilization rates in an in vitro fertilization program. Fertil Steril. 1995;64:787–90.

38. Inaudi P, Germond M, Senn A, De Grandi P. Timing of hCG administration in cycles stimulated for in vitro fertilization: specific impact of heterogeneous follicle sizes and steroid concentrations in plasma and follicle fluid on decision procedures. Gynecol Endocrinol. 1995;9:201–8.

39. Gougeon A. Dynamics of follicular growth in the human: a model from preliminary results. Hum Reprod. 1986;1(2):81–7.

40. Gougeon A, Lefèvre B. Evolution of the diameters of the largest healthy and atretic follicles during the human menstrual cycle. J Reprod Fertil. 1983;69(2):497–502.

41. Edwards RG. Studies on human conception. Am J Obstet Gynecol. 1973;117(5):587–601.

42. Hackelöer BJ, Fleming R, Robinson HP, Adam AH, Coutts JR. Correlation of ultrasonic and endocrinologic assessment of human follicular development. Am J Obstet Gynecol. 1979;135(1):122–8.

43. Revelli A, Martiny G, Delle Piane L, Benedetto C, Rinaudo P, Tur-Kaspa I. A critical review of bi-dimensional and three-dimensional ultrasound techniques to monitor follicle growth: do they help improving IVF outcome? Reprod Biol Endocrinol. 2014;12:107.

44. Scott RT, Hofmann GE, Muasher SJ, Acosta AA, Kreiner DK, Rosenwaks Z. Correlation of follicular diameter with oocyte recovery and maturity at the time of transvaginal follicular aspiration. J In Vitro Fert Embryo Transf. 1989;6(2):73–5.

45. Wittmaack FM, Kreger DO, Blasco L, Tureck RW, Mastroianni L Jr, Lessey BA. Effect of follicular size on oocyte retrieval, fertilization, cleavage, and embryo quality in in vitro fertilization cycles: a 6-year data collection. Fertil Steril. 1994;62(6):1205–10.

46. Triwitayakorn A, Suwajanakorn S, Pruksananonda K, Sereepapong W, Ahnonkitpanit V. Correlation between human follicular diameter and oocyte outcomes in an ICSI program. J Assist Reprod Genet. 2003;20(4):143–7.

47. Simonetti S, Veeck LL, Jones HW Jr. Correlation of follicular fluid volume with oocyte morphology from follicles stimulated by human menopausal gonadotropin. Fertil Steril. 1985;44(2):177–80.

48. Rosen MP, Shen S, Dobson AT, Rinaudo PF, McCulloch CE, Cedars MI. A quantitative assessment of follicle size on oocyte developmental competence. Fertil Steril. 2008;90(3):684–90.

49. Mehri S, Levi Setti PE, Greco K, Sakkas D, Martinez G, Patrizio P. Correlation between follicular diameters and flushing versus no flushing on oocyte maturity, fertilization rate and embryo quality. J Assist Reprod Genet. 2014;31(1):73–7.

50. Scott RT, Toner JP, Muasher SJ, Oehninger S, Robinson S, Rosenwaks Z. Follicle-stimulating hormone levels on cycle day 3 are predictive of in vitro fertilization outcome. Fertil Steril. 1989;51(4):651–4.

51. Bergh C, Broden H, Lundin K, Hamberger L. Comparison of fertilization, cleavage and pregnancy rates of oocytes from large and small follicles. Hum Reprod. 1998;13(7):1912–5.

52. Shmorgun D, Hughes E, Mohide P, Roberts R. Prospective cohort study of three- versus two-dimensional ultrasound for prediction of oocyte maturity. Fertil Steril. 2010;93(4):1333–7.

53. Teissier MP, Chable H, Paulhac S, Aubard Y. Comparison of follicle steroidogenesis from normal and polycystic ovaries in women undergoing IVF: relationship between steroid concentrations, follicle size, oocyte quality and fecundability. Hum Reprod. 2000;15(12):2471–7.

54. Lee TF, Lee RK, Hwu YM, Chih YF, Tsai YC, Su JT. Relationship of follicular size to the development of intracytoplasmic sperm injection-derived human embryos. Taiwan J Obstet Gynecol. 2010;49(3):302–5. https://doi.org/10.1016/S1028-4559(10)60065-4.

55. Ectors FJ, Vanderzwalmen P, Van Hoeck J, Nijs M, Verhaegen G, Delvigne A, Schoysman R, Leroy F. Relationship of human follicular diameter with oocyte fertilization and development after in-vitro fertilization or intracytoplasmic sperm injection. Hum Reprod. 1997;12:2002–5.

56. Akbariasbagh F, Lorzadeh N, Azmoodeh A, Ghaseminejad A, Mohamadpoor J, Kazemirad S. Association among diameter and volume of follicles, oocyte maturity, and competence in intracytoplasmic sperm injection cycles. Minerva Ginecol. 2015;67:397–403.

57. Nogueira D, Friedler S, Schachter M, Raziel A, Ron-El R, Smitz J. Oocyte maturity and preimplantation development in relation to follicle diameter in gonadotropin-releasing hormone agonist or antagonist treatments. Fertil Steril. 2006;85:578–83.

58. Salha O, Nugent D, Dada T, Kaufmann S, Levett S, Jenner L, Lui S, Sharma V. The relationship between follicular fluid aspirate volume and oocyte maturity in in-vitro fertilization cycles. Hum Reprod. 1998;13:1901–16.

59. Haines CJ, Emes AL. The relationship between follicle diameter, fertilization rate, and microscopic embryo quality. Fertil Steril. 1991;55:205–7.

60. Raine-Fenning N, Deb S, Jayaprakasan K, Clewes J, Hopkisson J, Campbell B. Timing of oocyte maturation and egg collection during controlled ovarian stimulation: a randomized controlled trial evaluating manual and automated measurements of follicle diameter. Fertil Steril. 2010;94:184–8.

61. Wertheimer A, Nagar R, Oron G, Meizner I, Fisch B, Ben-Haroush A. Fertility treatment outcomes after follicle tracking with standard 2-dimensional sonography versus 3-dimensional sonography-based automated volume count: prospective study. J Ultrasound Med. 2018;37(4):859–66.

62. Wirleitner B, Okhowat J, Vištejnová L, Králíčková M, Karlíková M, Vanderzwalmen P, Ectors F, Hradecký L, Schuff M, Murtinger M. Relationship between follicular volume and oocyte competence, blastocyst development and live-birth rate: optimal follicle size for oocyte retrieval. Ultrasound Obstet Gynecol. 2018;51(1):118–25.

63. Clark L, Stanger J, Brinsmead M. Prolonged follicle stimulation decreases pregnancy rates after in vitro fertilization. Fertil Steril. 1991;55:1192–4.

64. Edelstein MC, Seltman HJ, Cox BJ, et al. Progesterone levels on the day of human chorionic gonadotropin administration in cycles with gonadotropin-releasing hormone agonist suppression are not predictive of pregnancy outcome. Fertil Steril. 1990;54:853–7.

65. Check JH. Predictive value of serum progesterone levels for pregnancy outcome? Fertil Steril. 1994;62:1090–1.

66. Shechter A, Lunenfeld E, Potashnik G, Glezerman M. The significance of serum progesterone levels on the day of hCG administration on IVF pregnancy rates. Gynecol Endocrinol. 1994;8:89–94.

67. Ubaldi F, Smitz J, Wisanto A, et al. Oocyte and embryo quality as well as pregnancy rate in intracytoplasmic sperm injection are not affected by high follicular phase serum progesterone. Hum Reprod. 1995;10:3091–6.

68. Miller KF, Behnke EJ, Arciaga RL, et al. The significance of elevated progesterone at the time of administration of human chorionic gonadotropin may be related to luteal support. J Assist Reprod Genet. 1996;13:698–701.

69. Moffitt DV, Queenan JT Jr, Shaw R, Muasher SJ. Progesterone levels on the day of human chorionic gonadotropin do not predict pregnancy outcome from the transfer of fresh or cryopreserved embryos from the same cohort. Fertil Steril. 1997;67:296–301.

70. Fanchin R, de Ziegler D, Taieb J, et al. Premature elevation of plasma progesterone alters pregnancy rates of in vitro fertilization and embryo transfer. Fertil Steril. 1993;59:1090–4.

71. Papanikolaou EG, Kolibianakis EM, Pozzobon C, et al. Progesterone rise on the day of human chorionic gonadotropin administration impairs pregnancy outcome in day 3 single-embryo transfer, while has no effect on day 5 single blastocyst transfer. Fertil Steril. 2009;91:949–52.

72. Bosch E, Labarta E, Crespo J, et al. Circulating progesterone levels and ongoing pregnancy rates in controlled ovarian stimulation cycles for in vitro fertilization: analysis of over 4000 cycles. Hum Reprod. 2010;25:2092–100.

73. Kilicdag EB, Haydardedeoglu B, Cok T, et al. Premature progesterone elevation impairs implantation and live birth rates in GnRH-agonist IVF/ICSI cycles. Arch Gynecol Obstet. 2010;281:747–52.

74. Elgindy EA. Progesterone level and progesterone/E2 ratio on the day of hCG administration: detrimental cutoff levels and new treatment strategy. Fertil Steril. 2011;95:1639–44.

75. Xu B, Li Z, Zhang H, et al. Serum progesterone level effects on the outcome of in vitro fertilization in patients with different ovarian response: an analysis of more than 10,000 cycles. Fertil Steril. 2012;97:1321–7.

76. Ochsenkuhn R, Arzberger A, von Schonfeldt V, et al. Subtle progesterone rise on the day of human chorionic gonadotropin administration is associated with lower live birth rates in women undergoing assisted reproductive technology: a retrospective study with 2,555 fresh embryo transfers. Fertil Steril. 2012;98:347–54.

77. Nayak S, Ochalski ME, Fu B, et al. Progesterone level at oocyte retrieval predicts in vitro fertilization success in a short-antagonist protocol: a prospective cohort study. Fertil Steril. 2014;101:676–82.

78. Venetis CA, Kolibianakis EM, Bosdou JK, Tarlatzis BC. Progesterone elevation and probability of pregnancy after IVF:

a systematic review and meta-analysis of over 60 000 cycles. Hum Reprod Update. 2013;19(5):433–57.

79. Ubaldi F, Bourgain C, Tournaye H, Smitz J, Van Steirteghem A, Devroey P. Endometrial evaluation by aspiration biopsy on the day of oocyte retrieval in the embryo transfer cycles in patients with serum progesterone rise during the follicular phase. Fertil Steril. 1997;67(3):521–6.

80. Labarta E, Martinez-Conejero JA, Alama P, Horcajadas JA, Pellicer A, Simon C, Bosch E. Endometrial receptivity is affected in women with high circulating progesterone levels at the end of the follicular phase: a functional genomics analysis. Hum Reprod. 2011;26:1813–25.

81. Li R, Qiao J, Wang L, Li L, Zhen X, Liu P, Zheng X. MicroRNA array and microarray evaluation of endometrial receptivity in patients with high serum progesterone levels on the day of hCG administration. Reprod Biol Endocrinol. 2011;9:29.

82. Van Vaerenbergh I, Fatemi HM, Blockeel C, Van Lommel L, In't Veld P, Schuit F, Kolibianakis EM, Devroey P, Bourgain C. Progesterone rise on HCG day in GnRH antagonist/rFSH stimulated cycles affects endometrial gene expression. Reprod BioMed Online. 2011;22:263–71.

83. Huang B, Ren X, Wu L, Zhu L, Xu B, Li Y, et al. Elevated progesterone levels on the day of oocyte maturation may affect top quality embryo IVF cycles. PLoS One. 2016;11(1):e0145895. https://doi.org/10.1371/journal.pone.0145895.

84. Liu L, Zhou F, Lin XN, Li TC, Tong XM, Zhu HY, et al. Recurrent IVF failure is associated with elevated progesterone on the day of hCG administration. Eur J Obstet Gynecol Reprod Biol. 2013;171(1):78–83.

85. O'Shea LC, Mehta J, Lonergan P, Hensey C, Fair T. Developmental competence in oocytes and cumulus cells: candidate genes and networks. Syst Biol Reprod Med. 2012;58(2):88–101. https://doi.org/10.3109/19396368.2012.656217. Epub 2012/02/09. PMID: 22313243.

86. Fair T, Lonergan P. The role of progesterone in oocyte acquisition of developmental competence. Reprod Domest Anim. 2012;47(Suppl 4):142–7.

87. Oktem O, Akin N, Bildik G, Yakin K, Alper E, Balaban B, et al. FSH Stimulation promotes progesterone synthesis and output from human granulosa cells without luteinization. Hum Reprod. 2017;32(3):643–52.

88. Lawrenz B, Beligotti F, Engelmann N, Gates D, Fatemi HM. Impact of gonadotropin type on progesterone elevation during ovarian stimulation in GnRH antagonist cycles. Hum Reprod. 2016;31(11):2554–60.

89. Younis JS, Haddad S, Matilsky M, Ben-Ami M. Premature luteinization: could it be an early manifestation of low ovarian reserve? Fertil Steril. 1998;69:461–5.

90. Griesinger G, Mannaerts B, Andersen CY, Witjes H, Kolibianakis EM, Gordon K. Progesterone elevation does not compromise pregnancy rates in high responders: a pooled analysis of in vitro fertilization patients treated with recombinant follicle-stimulating hormone/ gonadotropin-releasing hormone antagonist in six trials. Fertil Steril. 2013;100:e1–3.

91. Golbasi H, Ince O, Golbasi C, Ozer M, Demir M, Yilmaz B. Effect of progesterone/E2 ratio on pregnancy outcome of patients with high trigger-day progesterone levels undergoing gonadotropin-releasing hormone antagonist intracytoplasmic sperm injection cycles: a retrospective cohort study. J Obstet Gynaecol. 2018;3:1–7.

92. Shufaro Y, Sapir O, Oron G, Ben Haroush A, Garor R, Pinkas H, Shochat T, Fisch B. Progesterone-to-follicle index is better correlated with in vitro fertilization cycle outcome than blood progesterone level. Fertil Steril. 2015;103(3):669–74.

93. Grin L, Mizrachi Y, Cohen O, Lazer T, Liberty G, Meltcer S, Friedler S. Does progesterone to oocyte index have a predictive value for IVF outcome? A retrospective cohort and review of the literature. Gynecol Endocrinol. 2018;34(8):638–43.

94. Hill MJ, Healy MW, Richter KS, Parikh T, Devine K, DeCherney AH, Levy M, Widra E, Patounakis G. Defining thresholds for abnormal premature progesterone levels during ovarian stimulation for assisted reproduction technologies. Fertil Steril. 2018;110(4): 671–679.e2.

95. Practice Committee of the American Society for Reproductive Medicine. Electronic address: ASRM@asrm.org; Practice Committee of the American Society for Reproductive Medicine. Prevention and treatment of moderate and severe ovarian hyperstimulation syndrome: a guideline. Fertil Steril. 2016;106(7):1634–47.

96. Ata B, Seyhan A, Reinblatt SL, Shalom-Paz E, Krishnamurthy S, Tan SL. Comparison of automated and manual follicle monitoring in an unrestricted population of 100 women undergoing controlled ovarian stimulation for IVF. Hum Reprod. 2011;26(1): 127–33.

97. Hernández J, Rodríguez-Fuentes A, Puopolo M, Palumbo A. Follicular volume predicts oocyte maturity: a prospective cohort study using three-dimensional ultrasound and SonoAVC. Reprod Sci. 2016;23(12):1639–43.

98. Vandekerckhove F, Vansteelandt S, Gerris J, De Sutter P. Follicle measurements using sonography-based automated volume count accurately predict the yield of mature oocytes in in vitro fertilization/intracytoplasmic sperm injection cycles. Gynecol Obstet Investig. 2013;76(2):107–12.

99. Rodriguez A, Guillén JJ, López MJ, Vassena R, Coll O, Vernaeve V. Learning curves in 3-dimensional sonographic follicle monitoring during controlled ovarian stimulation. J Ultrasound Med. 2014;33:649–55.

100. Wikland M, Borg J, Hamberger L, Svalander P. Simplification of IVF: minimal monitoring and the use of subcutaneous highly purified FSH administration for ovulation induction. Hum Reprod. 1994;9(8):1430–6.

101. Ellenbogen A, Rosenberg R, Shulman A, Libal Y, Anderman S, Jaschevatzky O, Ballas S. A follicular scoring system for monitoring ovulation induction in polycystic ovary syndrome patients based solely on ultrasonographic estimation of follicular development. Fertil Steril. 1996;65(6):1175–7.

102. Schoot DC, Hop WC, de Jong FH, van Dessel TJ, Fauser BC. Initial E2 response predicts outcome of exogenous gonadotropins using a step-down dose regimen for induction of ovulation in polycystic ovary syndrome. Fertil Steril. 1995;64(6): 1081–7.

103. Baldini D, Savoia MV, Sciancalepore AG, Malvasi A, Vizziello D, Beck R, Vizziello G. High progesterone levels on the day of HCG administration do not affect the embryo quality and the reproductive outcomes of frozen embryo transfers. Clin Ter. 2018;169(3):e91–5.

104. Kwan I, Bhattacharya S, McNeil A, van Rumste MM. Monitoring of stimulated cycles in assisted reproduction (IVF and ICSI). Cochrane Database Syst Rev. 2008;(2):CD005289.

Triggering Final Follicular Maturation for IVF Cycles

Raoul Orvieto

Contents

9.1 Introduction

In the course of the ovulatory cycle, sufficient production of estradiol by the preovulatory follicle induces the mid-cycle LH surge, which is followed by a loss of gap junctions between the oocyte and cumulus cells, cumulus expansion, germinal vesicle breakdown, resumption of meiosis, and luteinization of the granulosa cells (Figs. 9.1, 9.2, 9.3, 9.4, and 9.5). Moreover, the consequent increase in progesterone synthesis facilitates the positive feedback action of estradiol to induce the concomitant mid-cycle FSH peak [1]. This peak FSH has several roles, including the assurance of an adequate complement of LH receptors on the granulosa layer and the synthesis of hyaluronic acid matrix that facilitates the expansion and dispersion of the cumulus cells, allowing the oocyte-cumulus cell mass to become free-floating in the antral fluid [1].

9.2 Human Chorionic Gonadotropin, a Surrogate to the Naturally Occurring LH Surge

As part of a standard/conventional controlled ovarian hyperstimulation (COH) regimen, final follicular maturation is usually triggered by one bolus of human chorionic gonadotropin (hCG) (5000–10,000 units), that is administered as close as possible to the time of ovulation (i.e., 36 h before oocyte recovery) [2]. Human chorionic gonadotropin, a surrogate to the naturally occurring LH surge, induces luteinization of the granulosa cells, final oocyte maturation, and resumption of meiosis (Fig. 9.6).

Ovarian hyperstimulation syndrome (OHSS) almost always presents either 3–7 days after hCG administration

R. Orvieto (✉)
Infertility and IVF Unit, Department of Obstetrics and Gynecology, Sheba Medical Center, Ramat Gan, Israel
e-mail: raoul.orvieto@sheba.health.gov.il

© Springer Nature Switzerland AG 2020
A. Malvasi, D. Baldini (eds.), *Pick Up and Oocyte Management*, https://doi.org/10.1007/978-3-030-28741-2_9

Fig. 9.1 Ovulation

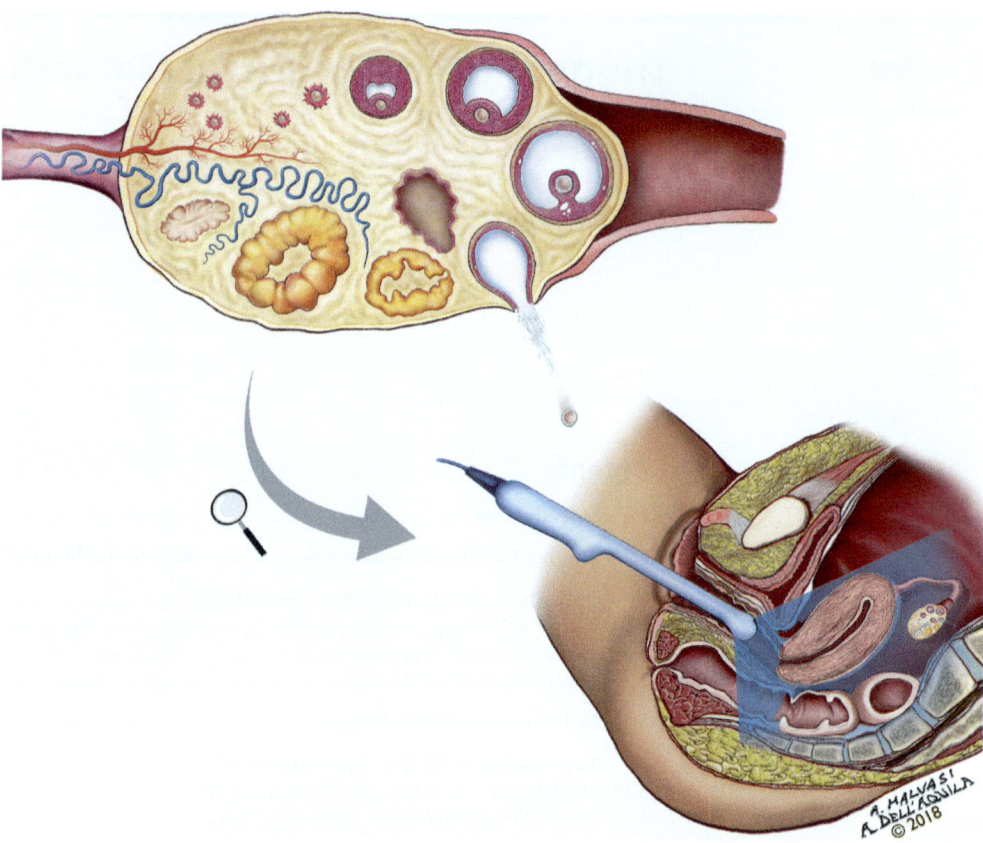

Fig. 9.2 FSH curve

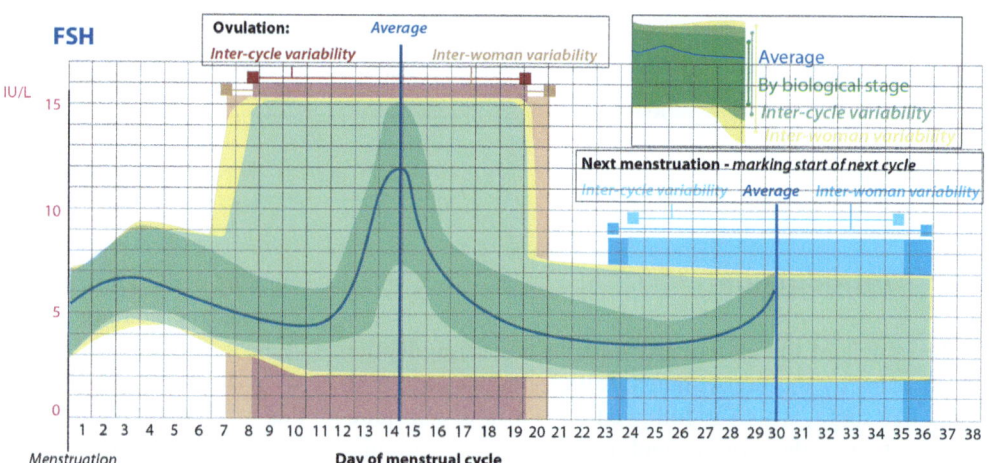

Fig. 9.3 LH curve

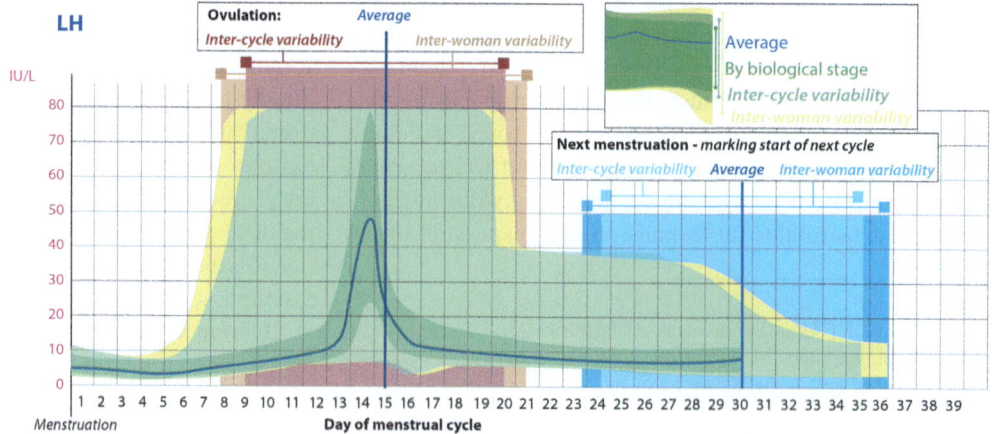

Fig. 9.4 Estradiol curve

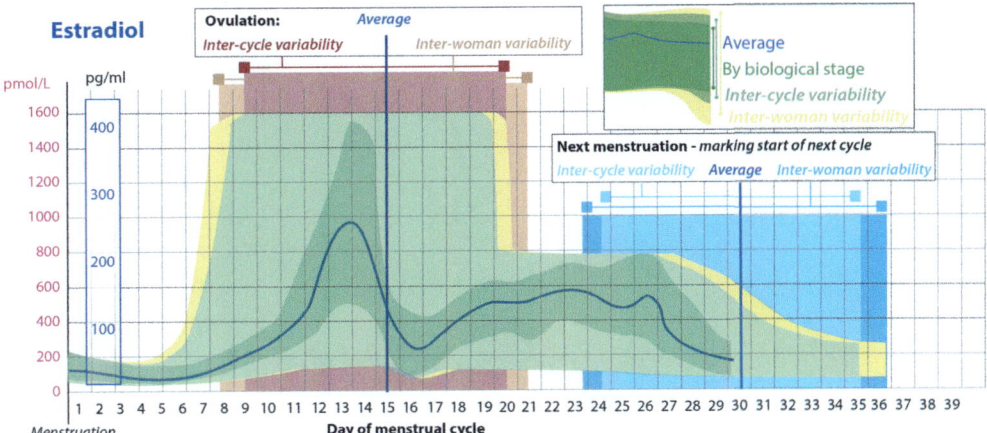

Fig. 9.5 Progesterone curve

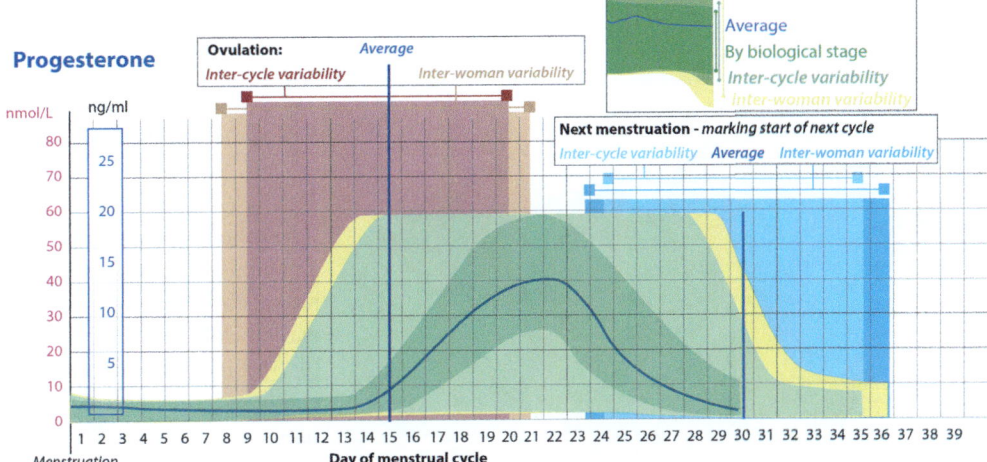

Fig. 9.6 LH/hCG receptor

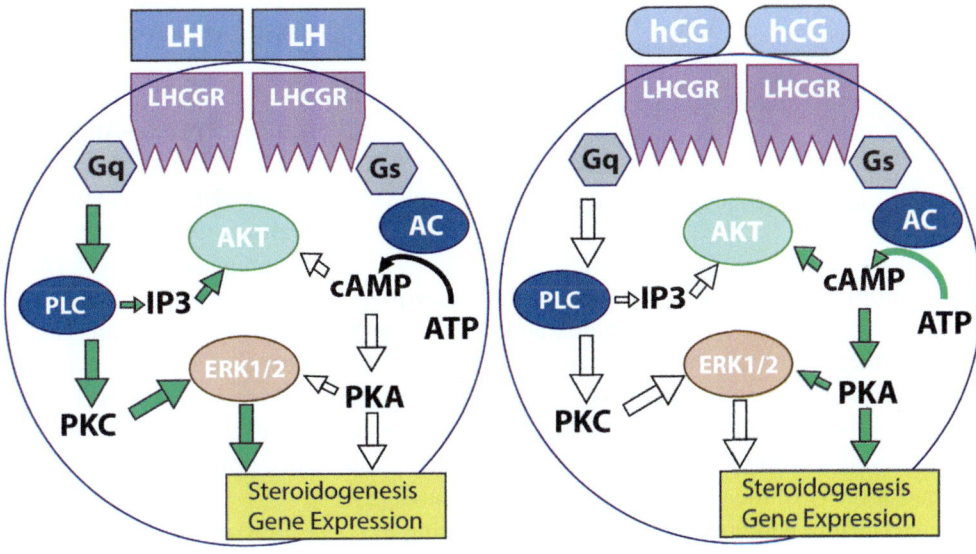

Fig. 9.7 Evaluation of OHSS with abdominal transducer

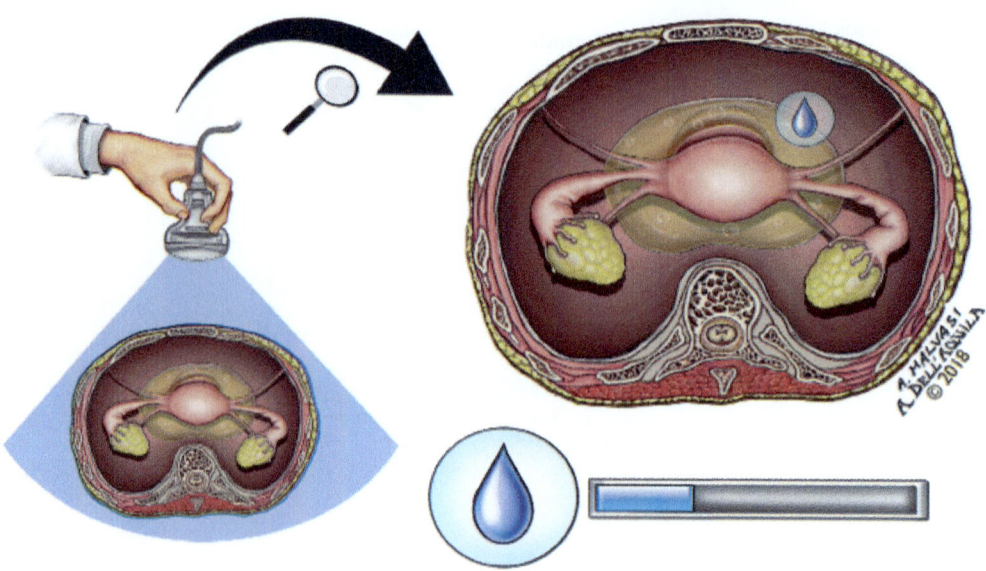

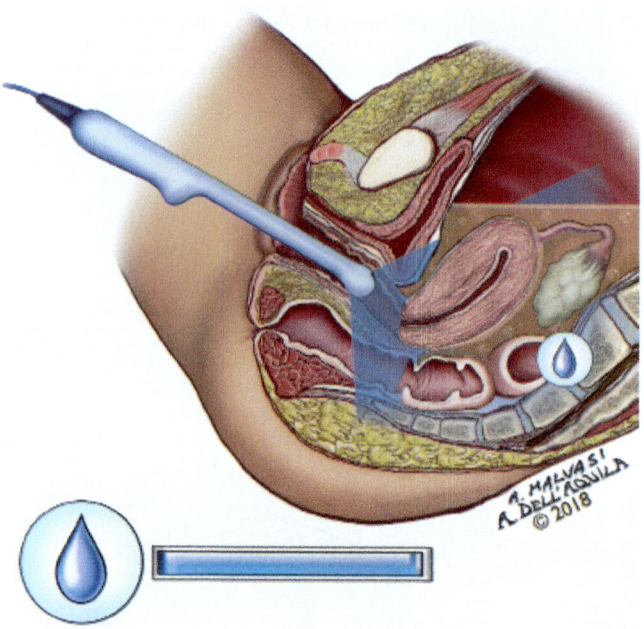

Fig. 9.8 Evaluation of OHSS with vaginal transducer

in susceptible patients (early onset) or during early pregnancy, 12–17 days after hCG administration (late onset). Individualization of treatment according to the specific risk factor and the specific response in the current cycle with the option of freezing of all embryos, or replacement of only a single embryo, has the potential of reducing the risk and severity of the syndrome in susceptible cases [3]. Moreover, while withholding the ovulation-inducing trigger of hCG may eliminate severe early OHSS, it denotes patients' frustration and is associated with time and money consuming.

9.3 Patients at Risk to Develop Severe OHSS

Controlled ovarian hyperstimulation which combines GnRH antagonist co-treatment and GnRH agonist (GnRHa) trigger has recently become a common tool aiming to eliminate severe early OHSS and to support the concept of an OHSS-free clinic [4, 5] (Figs. 9.7 and 9.8). However, due to the reported significantly reduced clinical pregnancy and increased first trimester pregnancy loss [6, 7], efforts have been made to improve reproductive outcome. While discussing the recent developments in GnRHa trigger, Kol and Humaidan [8] presented three optional strategies aiming to improve outcome: freeze-all policy; fresh transfer and intensive luteal support; and fresh transfer and low-dose HCG supplementation.

9.3.1 Freeze-All Policy

Freeze-all policy is offered in extreme cases [5] in an attempt to ensure OHSS risk-free and maintain a reasonable cumulative pregnancy rate [9]. However, despite the recent improvement in live birth rates after replacement of frozen-thawed vitrified oocytes/embryos, it should be emphasized that in most centers, there is still a gap in live birth rates between fresh and frozen/thawed cycles (in favor of fresh cycle).

Following the FIGO REI Committee (2015–2018), the good practice for freeze-all policy is:

- ≥20 oocytes are collected
- E2 above 15,000 pmol/L
- Patient unwell
- Ascites

Fig. 9.9 GnRH agonist vs. hCG:
11 RCT—1055 women

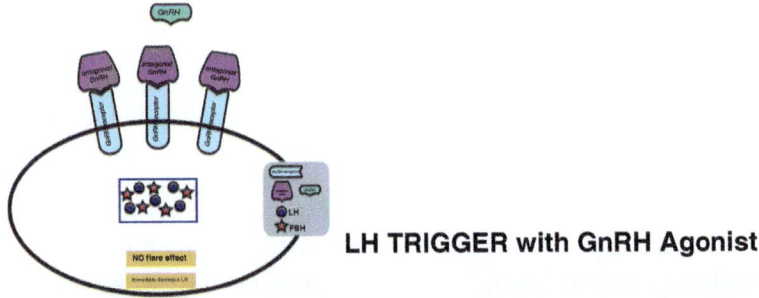

GnRH Agonist vs hCG : 1.055 women			
	Live birth	**Pregnancy**	**Moderate/ severe OHSS**
Fresh autologous cycles (8 RCT)	OR 0,44 (0,29-0,68)	OR 0,45 (0,31-0,65)	OR 0,10 (0,01-0,82)

Fig. 9.10 Intensive luteal support

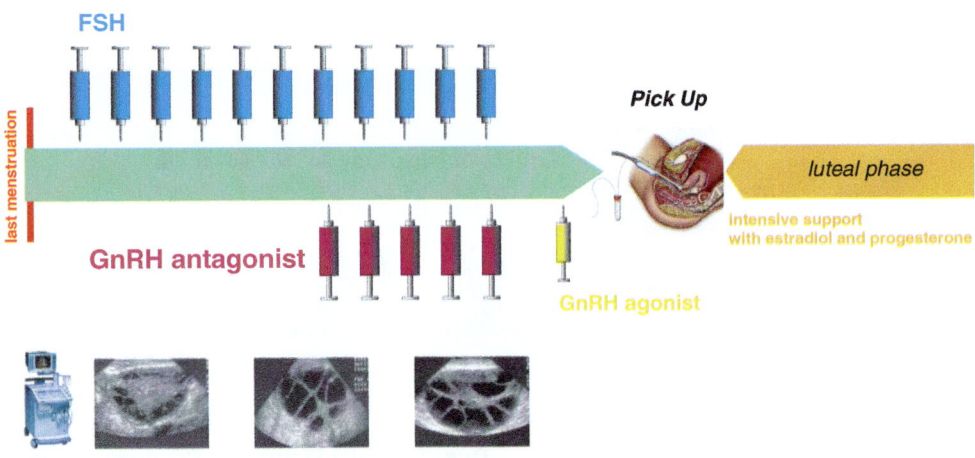

9.3.2 Intensive Luteal Support

Intense luteal support with estradiol and progesterone (E2) and progesterone, as described by Engmann et al. [10]. The data regarding the efficacy of luteal phase rescue after GnRHa trigger followed by intensive luteal phase support are intriguingly conflicting. We compared our experience with GnRHa trigger before [7] and after modifying our luteal-phase support to the intensive support with E2 and progesterone similar to the one reported by Engmann et al. [10]. We could not demonstrate any differences in peak E2 levels, fertilization rate, number of embryos transferred, or implantation and pregnancy rates, between the two luteal support regimens [11]. Of notice, that in both groups of luteal support following GnRH-a trigger, implantation and pregnancy rates were lower compared to HCG trigger [7] (Fig. 9.9).

9.3.3 One Bolus of 1500 IU hCG

One bolus of 1500 IU hCG 35 h after the triggering bolus of GnRHa, i.e., 1 h after oocyte retrieval [12, 13], was demonstrated to rescue the luteal phase, resulting in a reproductive outcome comparable with that of HCG triggering, and with no increased risk of OHSS [14]. However, when applied to patients at high risk to develop severe OHSS, 26% developed severe early OHSS requiring ascites drainage and hospitalization [15]. A figure that is comparable to the acceptable 20% prevalence of severe OHSS in ostensibly high-risk patients [16] (Fig. 9.10).

One bolus of 1500 IU hCG concomitant with GnRHa (dual trigger), 34–36 h before oocyte retrieval, was suggested as a method which improves oocyte maturation, while providing more sustained support for the corpus luteum than can be realized by the GnRHa-induced LH surge alone [17, 18] (Fig. 9.11). While acceptable rates of fertilization, implantation, clinical pregnancy, ongoing pregnancy rates, and early pregnancy loss were achieved in high responders after dual trigger [17, 18], the incidence of clinically significant OHSS was not eliminated, but rather reduced to 0.5% [18].

One bolus of hCG 1500 IU, 5 days following the GnRHa triggering of final follicular maturation [3, 19].

While the freeze-all policy was applied to all patients yielding more than 20 oocytes, those triggered with GnRHa, who achieved less than 20 oocytes, were instructed to start an intensive luteal support with estradiol and progesterone, the day following OPU, and were re-evaluated 3 days after oocyte retrieval (on the day of embryo transfer) for signs of early moderate OHSS (ultrasonographic signs of ascites as reflected by the appearance of fluid surrounding the uterus/ovaries, and/or Hct levels >40% for the degree of hemoconcentration). If no early signs of OHSS developed, one embryo was transferred, and the patients were instructed to inject 1500 IU of HCG. By deferring the hCG bolus by 3 days (5 days following GnRHa trigger), the corpus luteum was rescued, with an observed extremely high midluteal progesterone levels [19], reasonable pregnancy rate, with no patient developing severe OHSS.

However, while these preliminary results are promising, the small sample size mandates further large prospective randomized studies [19].

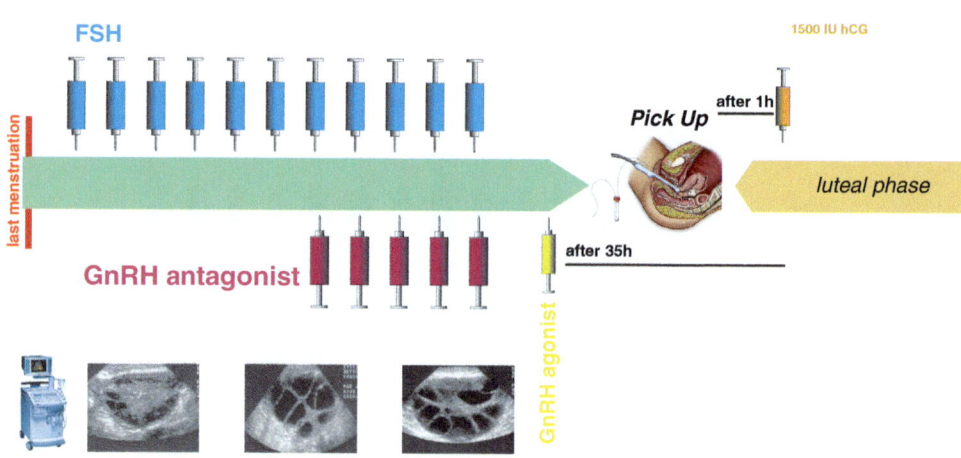

Fig. 9.11 One bolus of 1500 hCG

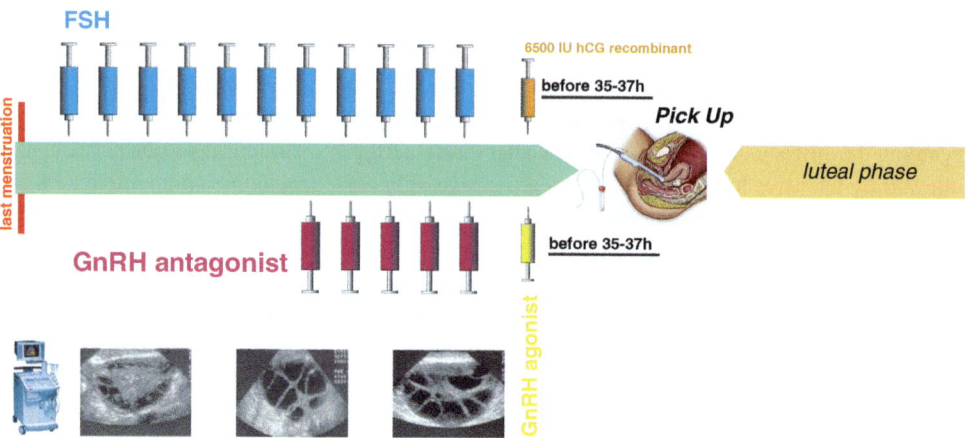

Fig. 9.12 Dual trigger: hCG and GnRHa 35–37 h before

9.4 hCG Versus GnRHa Trigger

While comparing the effect of hCG versus GnRHa trigger on the different follicular maturation variables following an IVF treatment cycle, studies have revealed that the number of oocytes retrieved, percentage of mature oocytes, and the number of top-quality embryos were either comparable or in favor of the GnRHa trigger.

Moreover, while studying the downstream effects of LH receptor activation by LH or hCG, it was demonstrated that LH has a greater impact on AKT and extracellular signal-regulated protein kinase (ERK1/2) phosphorylation, responsible for granulosa cell proliferation, differentiation, and survival, while hCG generates higher intracellular cAMP accumulation, which stimulates steroidogenesis (progesterone production) [20, 21].

Following the aforementioned observations, GnRHa combined with hCG trigger, for final follicular maturation has been implemented to clinical practice, and the different modes and timing of administration should be appropriately tailored to various subgroup of IVF patients.

9.5 Patients Not at Risk to Develop Severe OHSS

The aforementioned observations demonstrating a comparable or even better oocyte\embryos maturity and quality following GnRHa trigger, as compared to hCG trigger, and the different effects of LH and hCG on the downstream signaling of the LH receptor have led to a new strategy for final follicular maturation, the concomitant administration of both GnRHa and a standard bolus of hCG (5000–10,000 units) prior to oocyte retrieval, aiming to improve oocyte and embryo quality and the consequent IVF cycle outcome (Fig. 9.12).

9.5.1 Dual Trigger: Standard hCG Dose Concomitant with GnRHa, 35–37 h Before Oocyte Retrieval

Standard hCG dose concomitant with GnRHa (dual trigger), 35–37 h before oocyte retrieval. Lin et al. [22], in their retrospective cohort study, have compared IVF outcome in normal responders patients undergoing COH using the GnRH antagonist with either a standard dosage of hCG trigger (6500 IU of recombinant hCG) or the dual trigger (0.2 mg of triptorelin and 6500 IU of recombinant hCG) 35–36 h prior to oocyte retrieval.

The dual trigger group demonstrated statistically significantly higher number of oocytes retrieved, matured oocytes, and number of embryos cryopreserved, with the consequent significant increase in implantation, clinical pregnancy, and live-birth rates, as compared with the hCG-only trigger group.

In a subsequent prospective randomized controlled trial of normal responder patients, Decleer et al. [23] compared IVF outcome following either 5000 IU of hCG trigger or a combination of GnRHa plus 5000 IU of hCG concomitantly, 36 h prior to oocyte retrieval. While no in between group differences were observed in the mean number of oocytes retrieved, mature oocytes, or pregnancy rates, the number of patients who received at least one embryo of excellent quality and the number of cryopreserved embryos were significantly higher following the dual trigger.

Griffin et al. [24] evaluated the effect of the dual trigger (GnRHa and hCG 5000 IU or 10,000 IU, 35–37 h) prior to oocyte retrieval in patients with a previous history of >25% immature oocytes retrieved.

Despite a significantly higher proportion of mature oocytes retrieved with the dual trigger, the observed IVF outcome remained poor, probably due to patients' underlying oocyte dysfunction.

Fig. 9.13 Double trigger: GnRHa and hCG added 40 h and 34 h prior to OPU, respectively

Double trigger- GnRHa 40h and standard hCG added 34h prior to OPU

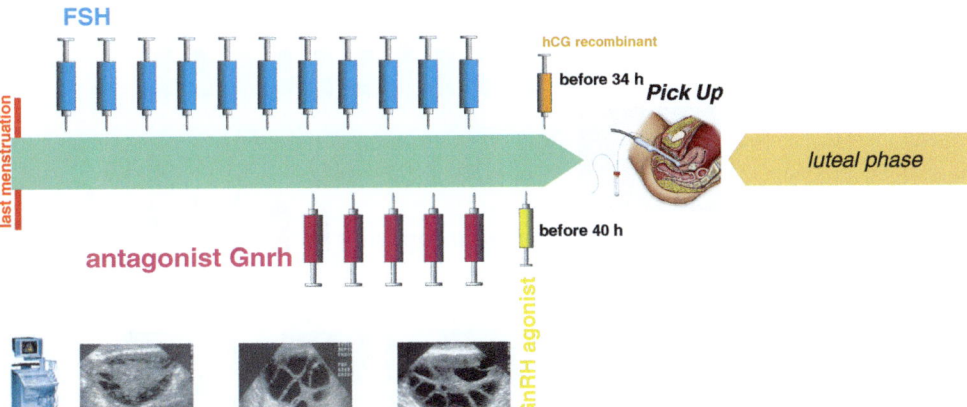

9.5.2 Double Trigger: GnRHa and Standard hCG Added 40 h and 34 h Prior to OPU, Respectively

GnRHa and standard hCG are added 40 h and 34 h prior to OPU (double trigger), respectively. Recently, Beck-Fruchter et al. [25] have described a case of recurrent empty follicle syndrome, successfully treated by ovulation trigger with GnRHa and hCG added 40 h and 34 h prior to oocyte retrieval, respectively.

They assumed that by prolonging the time between ovulation triggering and OPU [26] and the GnRHa trigger with the consequent simultaneous induction of an FSH surge, the "double trigger" could overcome any existing impairments in granulosa cell function, oocyte meiotic maturation, or cumulus expansion, resulting in successful aspiration of mature oocytes, pregnancy, and delivery.

Prompted by the aforementioned observations, we offered the double trigger to two group of patients demonstrating abnormal final follicular maturation despite normal response to COH, those with low (<50%) number of oocytes retrieved per number of dominant follicles >14 mm in diameter on the day of hCG administration [27], and those with low proportion of mature/metaphase-II (MII) oocytes (<66%) per number oocytes retrieved [28].

In the group of patients with low (<50%) number of oocytes retrieved per number of dominant follicles, following the double trigger, patients had significantly higher number of oocytes retrieved, number of 2PN, number of embryos transferred, and significantly higher proportions of the number of oocytes retrieved to the number of follicles >10 mm and >14 mm in diameter on the day of hCG administration, with a tendency toward a higher number of top-quality embryos, as compared to the hCG-only trigger cycles [27].

Moreover, in those with low proportion of MII oocytes (<66%) per number of oocytes retrieved, following the double trigger, patients yielded significantly higher number of MII oocytes and proportion of MII oocytes per number of oocytes retrieved, with the consequent significantly increased number of top-quality embryos, as compared to the hCG-only trigger cycles [28] (Figs. 9.13 and 9.14).

9.5.3 Standard hCG Dose Concomitant with GnRHa (Dual Trigger), 34 h Before OPU

According to the Bologna criteria, the minimal criteria needed to define poor ovarian response (POR) are the presence of at least two of the following three features: (1) Advanced maternal age (≥40 years) or any other risk factor for POR; (2) a previous POR (≤3 oocytes with a conventional stimulation protocol); and (3) an abnormal ovarian reserve test [29]. One of the major unnoticed concern in this group of poor responders is the observed high prevalence of premature luteinization\ovulation [30, 31], which may be overcome by early triggering of final follicular maturation, while approaching a follicular size of 15–16 mm, and by shortening the duration between the trigger and OPU.

However, since shortening the interval between hCG priming and oocyte retrieval may decrease the percentage of mature oocytes [26], an additional measure to improve the number of oocytes retrieved to the number of follicles >10 mm, and the proportion of mature oocytes should be implemented [27, 28]. One of the suggested measures that should be further studied is whether dual trigger (hCG and GnRHa) administered 34 h prior to OPU will provide the desired improved results (Fig. 9.15).

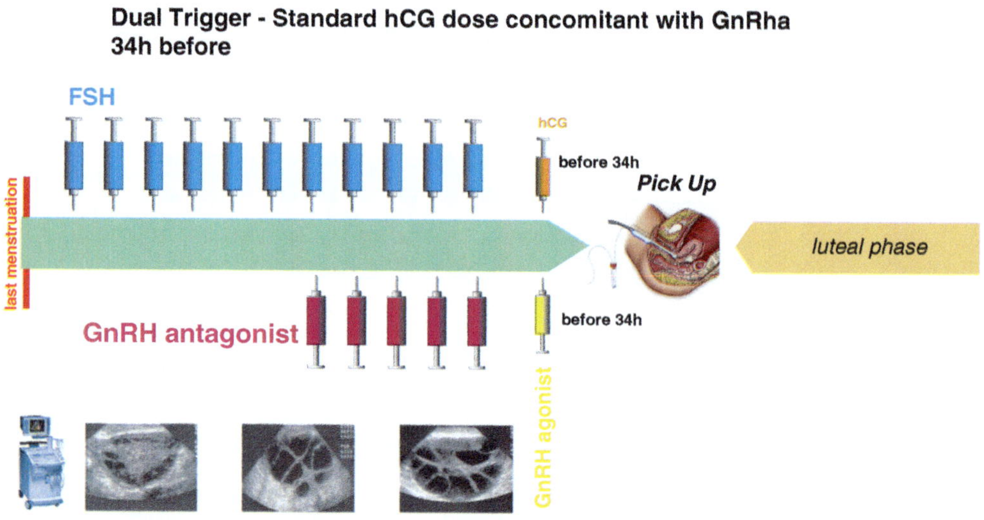

Fig. 9.14 Dual trigger: hCG and GnRHa added 34 h before OPU

Dual Trigger - Standard hCG dose concomitant with GnRha 34h before

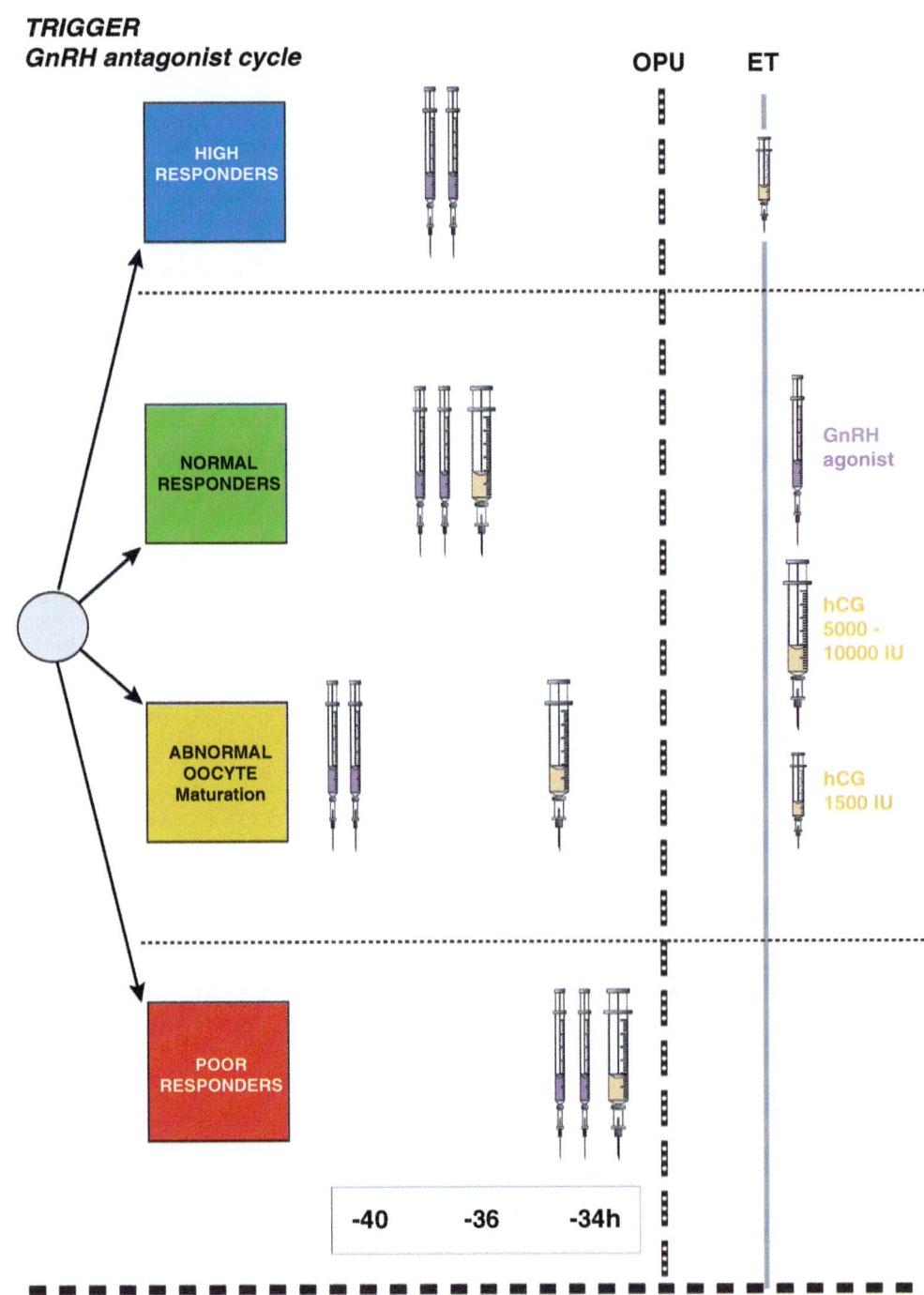

Fig. 9.15 Different modes of triggering ovulation with antagonist cycles

9.6   Conclusions

In the present chapter we analyzed and discussed the hitherto published studies relating to the different mode of GnRHa combined with hCG trigger—for final follicular maturation, aiming to elucidate how to tailor each mode to its appropriate subgroup of patients (Fig. 9.15, adapted from [32]).

One bolus of 1500 IU hCG, concomitant, and 35 h or 5 days after the triggering bolus of GnRHa were all demonstrated to rescue the luteal phase, resulting in improved reproductive outcome in patients at risk to develop severe OHSS, as compared to GnRHa trigger alone, with the questionable ability to eliminate severe OHSS.

Moreover, following the observations demonstrating a comparable or even better oocyte\embryo quality following GnRHa trigger as compared to hCG trigger, and the different effects of LH and hCG on the downstream signaling of the LH receptor, GnRHa is now offered concomitant to the standard hCG trigger dose, to improve oocyte/embryo yield and quality. GnRHa and hCG may be offered concomitantly,

34–37 h prior to oocyte retrieval (dual trigger) or 40 h and 34 h prior to oocyte retrieval, respectively (double trigger) in patients with abnormal final follicular maturation.

References

1. Regulation of the menstrual cycle. In: Fritz MA, Speroff L, editors. Clinical gynecologic endocrinology and infertility. 8th ed. Philadelphia: Lippincott Williams & Wilkins; 2011.
2. Ludwig M, Doody KJ, Doody KM. Use of recombinant human chorionic gonadotropin in ovulation induction. Fertil Steril. 2003;79:1051–9.
3. Orvieto R. Ovarian hyperstimulation syndrome—an optimal solution for an unresolved enigma. J Ovarian Res. 2013;6:77.
4. Orvieto R. Can we eliminate severe ovarian hyperstimulation syndrome? Hum Reprod. 2005;20:320–2.
5. Devroey P, Polyzos NP, Blockeel C. An OHSS-free clinic by segmentation of IVF treatment. Hum Reprod. 2011;6:2593–7.
6. Youssef MA, Van der Veen F, Al-Inany HG, Mochtar MH, Griesinger G, Nagi Mohesen M, Aboulfoutouh I, van Wely M. Gonadotropin-releasing hormone agonist versus HCG for oocyte triggering in antagonist-assisted reproductive technology. Cochrane Database Syst Rev. 2014;(10):CD008046.
7. Orvieto R, Rabinson J, Meltzer S, Zohav E, Anteby E, Homburg R. Substituting HCG with GnRH agonist to trigger final follicular maturation—a retrospective comparison of three different ovarian stimulation protocols. Reprod Biomed Online. 2006;13:198–201.
8. Kol S, Humaidan P. GnRH agonist triggering: recent developments. Reprod Biomed Online. 2013;26:226–30.
9. Griesinger G, Schultz L, Bauer T, Broessner A, Frambach T, Kissler S. Ovarian hyperstimulation syndrome prevention by gonadotropin-releasing hormone agonist triggering of final oocyte maturation in a gonadotropin-releasing hormone antagonist protocol in combination with a 'freeze-all' strategy: a prospective multicentric study. Fertil Steril. 2011;95:2029–33.
10. Engmann L, DiLuigi A, Schmidt D, Nulsen J, Maier D, Benadiva C. The use of gonadotropin-releasing hormone (GnRH) agonist to induce oocyte maturation after cotreatment with GnRH antagonist in high-risk patients undergoing in vitro fertilization prevents the risk of ovarian hyperstimulation syndrome: a prospective randomised controlled study. Fertil Steril. 2008;89:84–91.
11. Orvieto R. Intensive luteal-phase support with oestradiol and progesterone after GnRH-agonist triggering: does it help? Reprod Biomed Online. 2012;24:680–1.
12. Humaidan P, Bungum L, Bungum M, Yding Andersen C. Rescue of corpus luteum function with peri-ovulatory HCG supplementation in IVF/ICSI GnRH antagonist cycles in which ovulation was triggered with a GnRH agonist: a pilot study. Reprod Biomed Online. 2006;13:173–8.
13. Humaidan P, Bredkjaer HE, Westergaard LG, Andersen CY. 1,500 IU human chorionic gonadotropin administered at oocyte retrieval rescues the luteal phase when gonadotropin-releasing hormone agonist is used for ovulation induction: a prospective, randomized, controlled study. Fertil Steril. 2010;93:847–54.
14. Humaidan P, Papanikolaou EG, Kyrou D, Alsbjerg B, Polyzos NP, Devroey P, Fatemi HM. The luteal phase after GnRH-agonist triggering of ovulation: present and future perspectives. Reprod Biomed Online. 2012;24:134–41.
15. Seyhan A, Ata B, Polat M, Son WY, Yarali H, Dahan MH. Severe early ovarian hyperstimulation syndrome following GnRH agonist trigger with the addition of 1500 IU hCG. Hum Reprod. 2013;28:2522–8.
16. Orvieto R, Ben-Rafael Z. Role of intravenous albumin in the prevention of severe ovarian hyperstimulation syndrome. Hum Reprod. 1998;13:3306–9.
17. Shapiro BS, Daneshmand ST, Garner FC, Aguirr M, Thomas S. Gonadotropin-releasing hormone agonist combined with a reduced dose of human chorionic gonadotropin for final oocyte maturation in fresh autologous cycles of in vitro fertilization. Fertil Steril. 2008;90:231–3.
18. Shapiro BS, Daneshmand ST, Garner FC, Aguirre M, Hudson C. Comparison of "triggers" using leuprolide acetate alone or in combination with low-dose human chorionic gonadotropin. Fertil Steril. 2011;95:2715–7.
19. Haas J, Kedem A, Machtinger R, Dar S, Hourovitz A, Yerushalmi G, Orvieto R. HCG (1500IU) administration on day 3 after oocytes retrieval, following GnRH-agonist trigger for final follicular maturation, results in high sufficient mid luteal progesterone levels—a proof of concept. J Ovarian Res. 2014;7:35.
20. Casarini L, Lispi M, Longobardi S, Milosa F, La Marca A, Tagliasacchi D, Pignatti E, Simoni M. LH and hCG action on the same receptor results in quantitatively and qualitatively different intracellular signalling. PLoS One. 2012;7:e46682.
21. Haas J, Ophir L, Barzilay E, Machtinger R, Yung Y, Orvieto R, Hourvitz A. Standard human chorionic gonadotropin versus double trigger for final oocyte maturation results in different granulosa cells gene expressions: a pilot study. Fertil Steril. 2016;106:653–9.
22. Lin MH, Wu FS, Lee RK, Li SH, Lin SY, Hwu YM. Dual trigger with combination of gonadotropin-releasing hormone agonist and human chorionic gonadotropin significantly improves the live-birth rate for normal responders in GnRH-antagonist cycles. Fertil Steril. 2013;100:1296–302.
23. Decleer W, Osmanagaoglu K, Seynhave B, Kolibianakis S, Tarlatzis B, Devroey P. Comparison of hCG triggering versus hCG in combination with a GnRH agonist: a prospective randomized controlled trial. Facts Views Vis Obgyn. 2014;6:203–9.
24. Griffin D, Feinn R, Engmann L, Nulsen J, Budinetz T, Benadiva C. Dual trigger with gonadotropin-releasing hormone agonist and standard dose human chorionic gonadotropin to improve oocyte maturity rates. Fertil Steril. 2014;102:405–9.
25. Beck-Fruchter R, Weiss A, Lavee M, Geslevich Y, Shalev E. Empty follicle syndrome: successful treatment in a recurrent case and review of the literature. Hum Reprod. 2012;27:1357–67.
26. Wang W, Zhang XH, Wang WH, Liu YL, Zhao LH, Xue SL, Yang KH. The time interval between hCG priming and oocyte retrieval in ART program: a meta-analysis. J Assist Reprod Genet. 2011;28:901–10.
27. Haas J, Zilberberg E, Dar S, Kedem A, Machtinger R, Orvieto R. Co-administration of GnRH-agonist and hCG for final oocyte maturation (double trigger) in patients with low number of oocytes retrieved per number of preovulatory follicles—a preliminary report. J Ovarian Res. 2014;7:77.
28. Zilberberg E, Haas J, Dar S, Kedem A, Machtinger R, Orvieto R. Co-administration of GnRH-agonist and hCG for final oocyte maturation in patients with low proportion of mature oocytes. Gynecol Endocrinol. 2015;31:145–7.
29. Ferraretti AP, La Marca A, Fauser BC, Tarlatzis B, Nargund G, Gianaroli L, et al. ESHRE consensus on the definition of 'poor response' to ovarian stimulation for in vitro fertilization: the Bologna criteria. Hum Reprod. 2011;26:1616–24.
30. Martinez F, Barri PN, Coroleu B, Tur R, Sorsa-Leslie T, Harris WJ, Groome NP, Knight PG, Fowler PA. Women with poor response to IVF have lowered circulating gonadotrophin surge-attenuating factor (GnSAF) bioactivity during spontaneous and stimulated cycles. Hum Reprod. 2002;17:634–40.
31. Ben-Rafael Z, Orvieto R, Feldberg D. The poor-responder patient in an in-vitro fertilization-embryo transfer (IVF-ET) program. Gynecol Endocrinol. 1994;8:277–86.
32. Orvieto R. A simplified universal approach to COH protocol for IVF: ultrashort flare GnRH-agonist/GnRH-antagonist protocol with tailored mode and timing of final follicular maturation. J Ovarian Res. 2015;8:69.

Oocyte Retrieval

10

Domenico Baldini, Cristina Lavopa, Maria Matteo,
and Antonio Malvasi

Contents

D. Baldini (✉) · C. Lavopa
Center of Medically Assisted Procreation, MOMO' fertiLIFE,
Bisceglie, Italy

M. Matteo
Department of Obstetrics and Gynaecology, University of Foggia,
Foggia, Italy
e-mail: maria.matteo@unifg.it

A. Malvasi
Department of Obstetrics and Gynecology, GVM Care
and Research Santa Maria Hospital, Bari, Italy

Laboratory of Human Physiology, Phystech BioMed School,
Faculty of Biological and Medical Physics, Moscow Institute
of Physics and Technology (State University), Dolgoprudny,
Russia

In the last 40 years since the first successful human birth, ART has been continuously improved. Significant advances have been made in oocyte fertilization and embryo culture, resulting in an increase of the success rate and safety of ART treatments. Oocyte recovery aims to maximize the number of oocytes recruited from the ovarian follicles, while minimizing the patient surgical risks. In the early history of IVF experimentation, abdominal laparotomy was performed to collect oocytes during tubal ligation procedures. Techniques described for follicle aspiration involved puncturing follicles with a

© Springer Nature Switzerland AG 2020
A. Malvasi, D. Baldini (eds.), *Pick Up and Oocyte Management*, https://doi.org/10.1007/978-3-030-28741-2_10

diameter higher than 5 mm with a 20-gauge needle. The aspiration needle was connected to the tube and emptied into a test tube. Aspiration was achieved by covering the free opening in the three-way connector to create suction to 200 mmHg. Each follicle was finally transferred into an individual tube [1]. Although the laparotomic approach could be an option to obtain oocytes in certain cases, it may cause several surgical risks, such as bleeding, infection, pain, potential injury to the surrounding pelvic and abdominal organs, and longer recovery time, which encouraged the pursuit of alternative surgical options. In the 1950s and 1960s, there was a great interest in developing less invasive gynecologic techniques.

Until a few years ago, laparoscopy represented the election technique for the collection of oocytes to be initiated into extracorporeal fertilization. The laparoscopic technique is not very different from the traditional one; however, it should be noted that no instrument can be placed during the examination in the uterine cavity for the mobilization of the bowel; therefore, the patient is placed on the bed with the legs outstretched as for any gynecological intervention.

The laparoscopic technique is carried out under general anesthesia with an umbilical laparoscopic port and a second laparoscopic port placed 7–10 cm to the right of the midline between the pubic bone and the umbilicus (Fig. 10.1).

Fig. 10.1 Schematic representation of laparoscopic oocytes retrieval

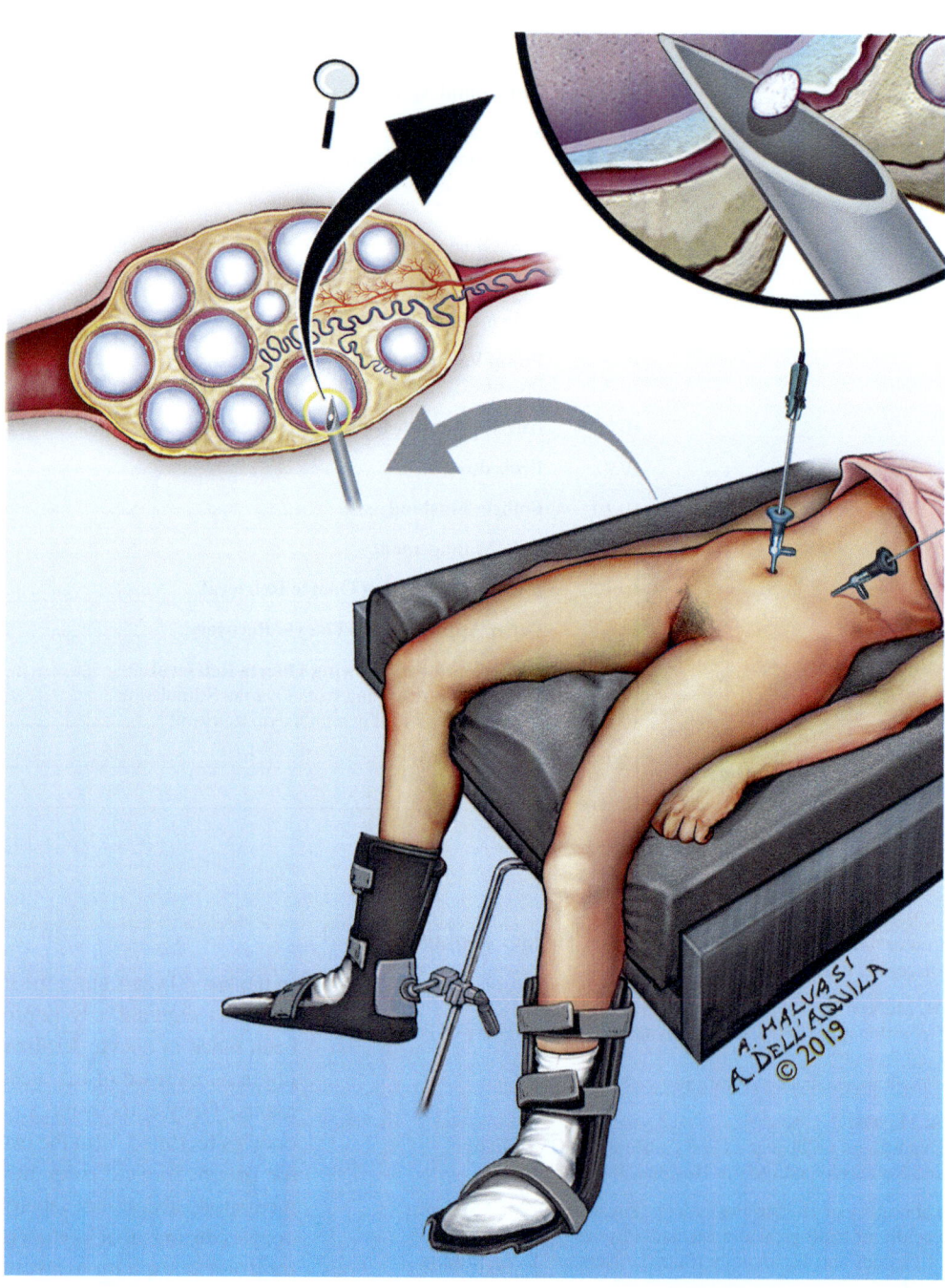

Using forceps to stabilize the ovary and by a rotation to obtain adequate visualization, the thin-walled follicles are aspirated using a 20-gauge needle and a syringe for suction.

A short bevel needle is placed directly through the skin into the abdominal cavity and then cleared of blood and tissue with a heparinized saline solution. By an outer guide to insert the aspiration needle, the follicles are punctured and the suction is obtained by placing a finger over a bypass valve on the aspiration needle. The needle and tube are cleaned after each follicle aspiration. The maximum pressure for the vacuum suction is 120 mmHg as higher pressures would damage the oocytes [2].

Laparoscopy has slowly gained a growing acceptance after studies demonstrating similar oocyte yields compared with the laparotomy approach. Lopata and colleagues [1] showed the absence of differences in the mean number of oocytes obtained per patient between laparoscopy and laparotomy.

When laparoscopy was performed with CO_2 pneumoperitoneum, there was no significant difference in oocyte fertilization rates. Advantages of laparoscopy include shorter recovery time, less bleeding, fewer infectious risks, and decreased pain. However, even with these improvements, the disadvantages of requiring general anesthesia and poor visualization of follicles within ovarian stroma led to improve the techniques of oocyte recovery [3].

10.1 Ultrasound Approach of Oocyte Retrieval

Advances in ultrasound-guided approach aimed to overcome the problem of a poor visualization of ovarian follicles. In 1972, Kratochwil's publication on the ultrasonic tomography of the ovaries opened a new window of opportunity [4]. The improved visualization of follicles offered a safer and more accurate method for oocyte retrieval, and in addition, ultrasound-guided approach is inexpensive and has minimal risks [5]. Using ultrasound guidance, various methods of oocyte retrieval including percutaneous [6], transvesical (Fig. 10.2) [6], per-urethral [7], and transvaginal follicle aspiration [8] have been developed (Table 10.1).

In 1982, Lenz and colleagues [6] reported the first ultrasound-guided transvesical route for oocyte recovery using local anesthesia.

The oocyte yield was comparable after transvesicular and laparoscopy aspiration, but because of the intentional route

Fig. 10.2 In the transvesical oocyte sampling, the needle passes through the urinary bladder

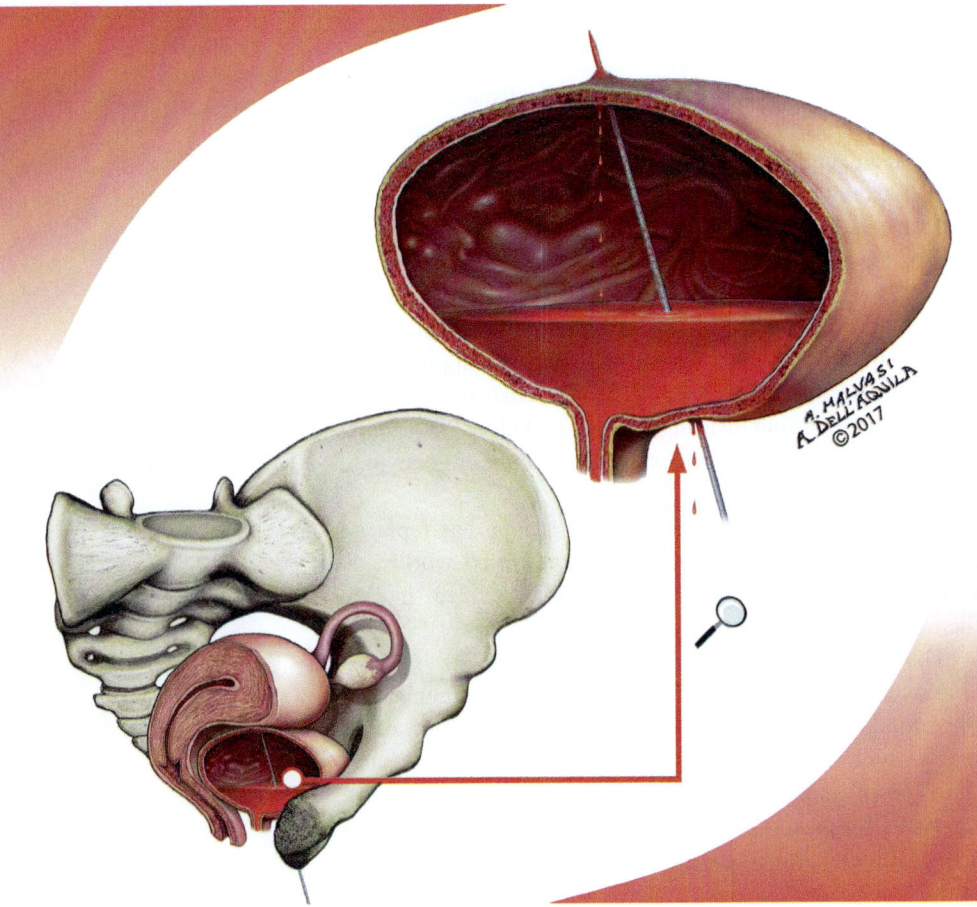

Table 10.1 Advantages of transvaginal ultrasound approach

Transvaginal oocyte retrieval offers the following advantages:
• *The distance to reach the ovary is **shorter***
• ***Higher-resolution pictures*** *that enable the identification of the ovaries and the aspiration follicles*
• *No risk of skin damage*
• *The procedure can be conveniently performed in the outpatient setting*
• ***Lower cost*** *than other techniques*
• ***Fewer staff*** *is required*
• ***Easy to learn*** *thanks to the use of ultrasound guidance*
• *All follicles can be visualized and punctured, even in case of severe pelvic adhesions*
• ***It gives more precision*** *than the abdominal approach*
• *Can be achieved by local anesthesia, under paracervical block, sedation or general anesthesia*
• ***It is well accepted by patients***

through the bladder, complications were reported, such as abdominal pain, exacerbation of preexisting pelvic inflammatory disease, mild hemoperitoneum, urinary tract infections, and transient macroscopic hematuria [9].

Despite these complications, this approach remained one of the preferred treatments among physicians and patients, as it allows to avoid the general anesthesia and is an outpatient procedure. In addition, this method is safer than laparoscopy in patients with extensive abdominal or pelvic adhesive disease, due to an increased accuracy and a closer proximity of the needle to the ovaries [10].

To overcome the inconvenience of the distance between the abdominal ultrasound probe and the ovaries, in 1985, Wikland and colleagues introduced for the first time the vaginal ultrasound probes [11].

Transvaginal oocyte retrieval is currently the most common method of oocyte collection in IVF cycles. In fact, this technique has been found to be the simple and fast (it takes about 20 min), while being less invasive and requiring minimal anesthesia, thus resulting the most effective approach for oocyte retrievals in ART clinics [12]. It consists in the aspiration of follicular fluid by using transvaginal ultrasonography; it is focused on obtaining the maximum number of oocyte to be fertilized.

As it is minimally invasive, this technique has replaced the laparoscopic approach and is currently used worldwide as the gold standard approach for oocyte retrieval in IVF therapy [13, 14].

The success of the technique depends on the inherent characteristics of the oocyte, which might be influenced by the actual process of oocyte collection, but also on other factors such as the length of the ovarian stimulation phase, the type of anesthesia used (local, sedation, or general), the type of aspiration needle (aspiration alone or aspiration with follicular flushing), and the experience of the clinician [15].

Finally, the number of embryos obtained relies on the number and inherent characteristics of the oocytes but also on other factors such as the length of the ovarian stimulation phase, the type of anesthesia used (local, sedation, or general), the type of aspiration needle magnitude, the needle used (wide or narrow bore or single or double channel), the aspiration mode (with or without follicular flushing), and the experience of the surgeon [16, 17].

10.2 Materials

10.2.1 Ultrasound Equipment and Probe

Ultrasound equipment (Fig. 10.3) with multifrequency, transvaginal (5–7.5 MHz) probe, which must be correctly configured. This frequency has the sufficient penetration

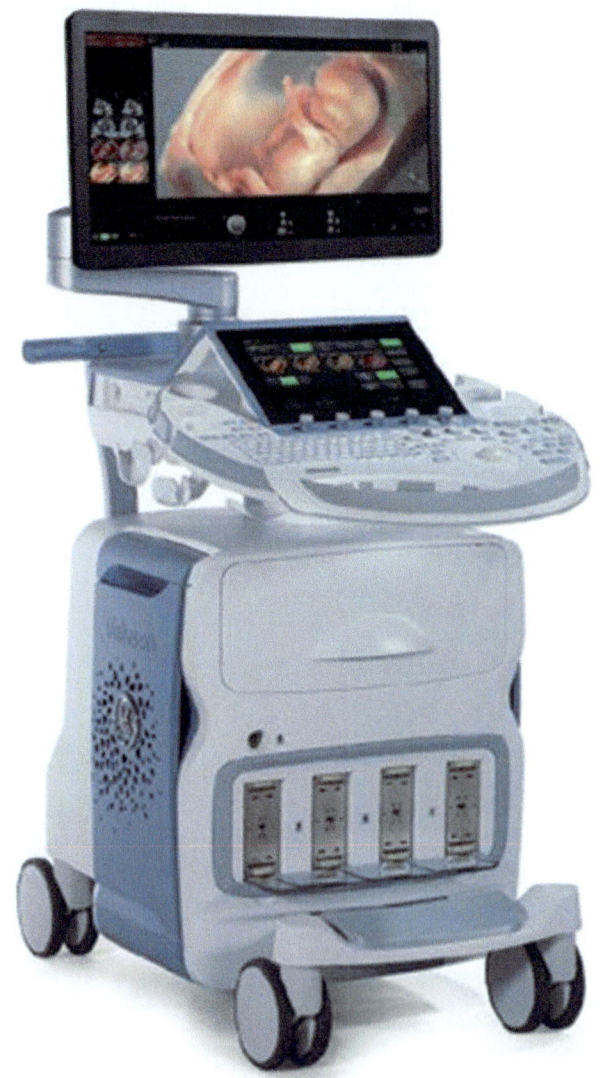

Fig. 10.3 New ultrasound machine

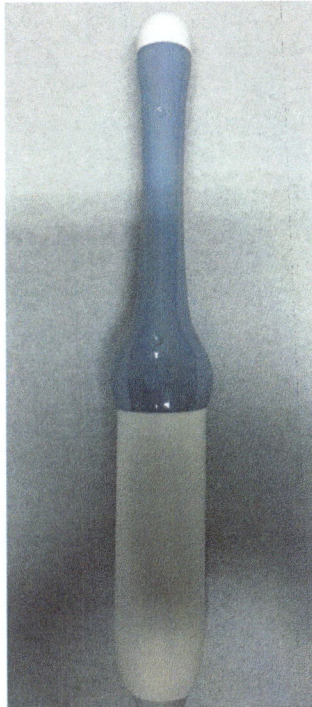

Fig. 10.4 Ultrasound vaginal probe

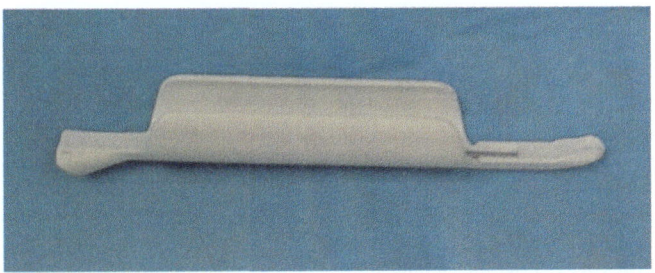

Fig. 10.5 Disposable endocavity needle guide

depth and enough resolution. The transducer (total length 40 cm) (Fig. 10.4) is easy to handle during the scanning and puncture procedure and has a shape easy to put into a slim sterile cover or a finger of a sterile surgical glove. It is equipped with a needle guide and crosshairs that is connected to the transducer and can be seen on the screen. The strict observation of rules for maintaining the sterility through the exclusive use of sterile supplies (namely needle guides (Fig. 10.5), vaginal probe covers, patient drapes) has become the standard practice during these procedures. Disinfection of the vaginal probe in between each patient has also been advocated to reduce bacterial contaminations.

Follicle aspiration set
1. Needle
2. Tubing

3. Sampling tubes
4. A thermoblock/heating block thermostat
5. Pump vacuum aspiration

10.3 Needle

The widespread diffusion of the ART techniques has recently driven the development of differently designed needles for oocyte retrieval (Fig. 10.6).

The main characteristics of commercially distributed needles are quite similar, while they can be differentiated on the basis of the length, gauge (thickness), and sharpness of the needle (Figs. 10.7 and 10.8); the presence of an echoreflective tip (Fig. 10.9); the presence of a single or double lumen (Fig. 10.10); and finally, the length of both the connector and the connector tubing (Figs. 10.11 and 10.12).

One of the most crucial factors of a pickup needle is the choice of an appropriate gauge, which should allow the passage of intact compact cumulus oocyte complexes without destroying them. The most frequently used gauge sizes range between 16 and 19, while lower values are chosen to aspirate smaller follicles for IVM (Fig. 10.13).

In theory, it should cause minimal tissue injury when passing through the vagina and ovary, by guarantying, at the same time, high visibility for the correct approach to the follicles of the clinician. The needle consists of a reduced part (tip) and unreduced part (body). The most used aspiration

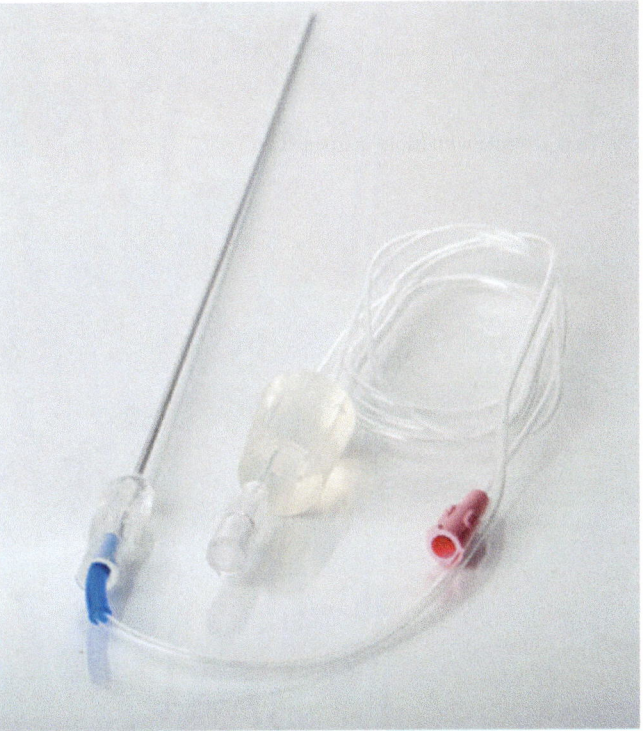

Fig. 10.6 Needle for transvaginal oocytes retrieval

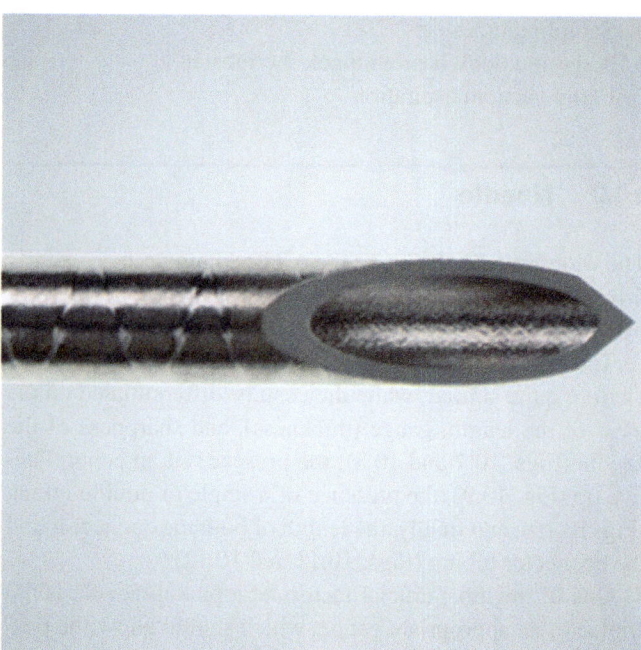

Fig. 10.7 Sharp tip of the needle

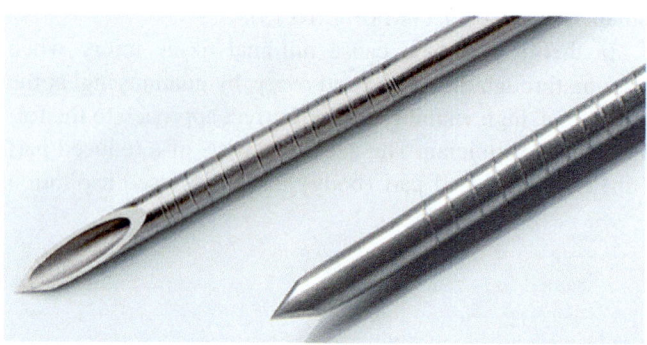

Fig. 10.8 Needle with triple sharpened tip

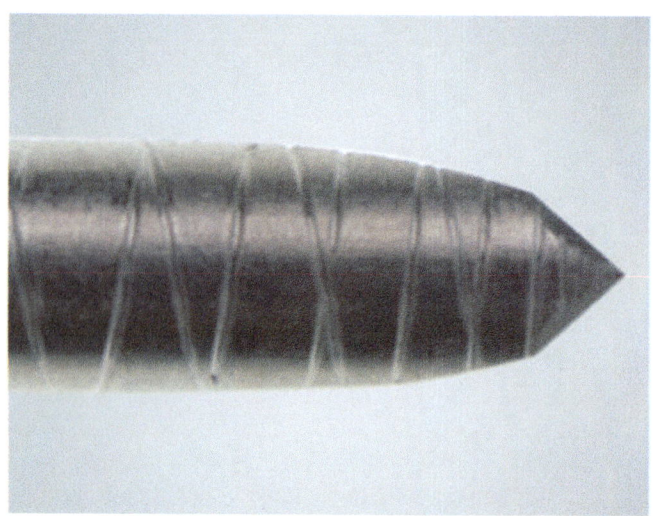

Fig. 10.9 Incision line on pickup needle to increase the echogenicity

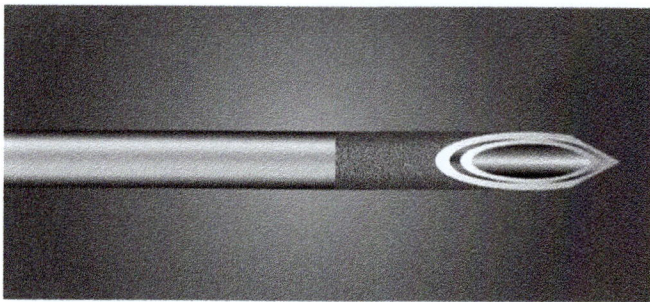

Fig. 10.10 Double lumen needle

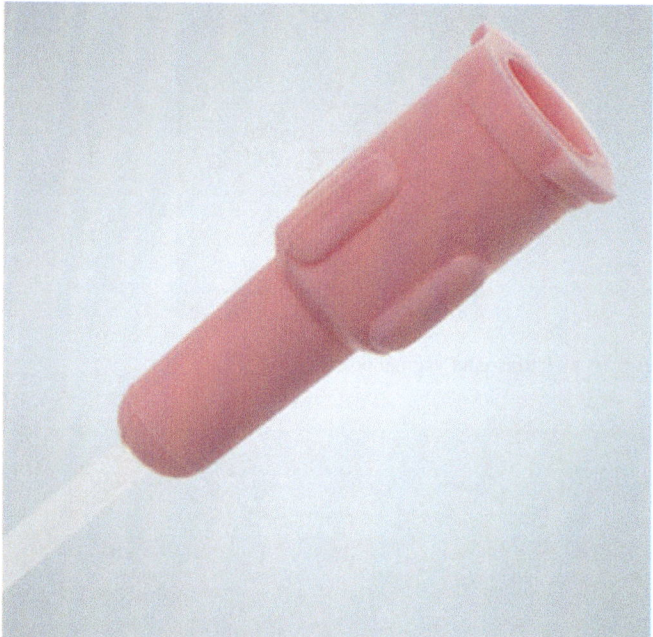

Fig. 10.11 Luer lock connector

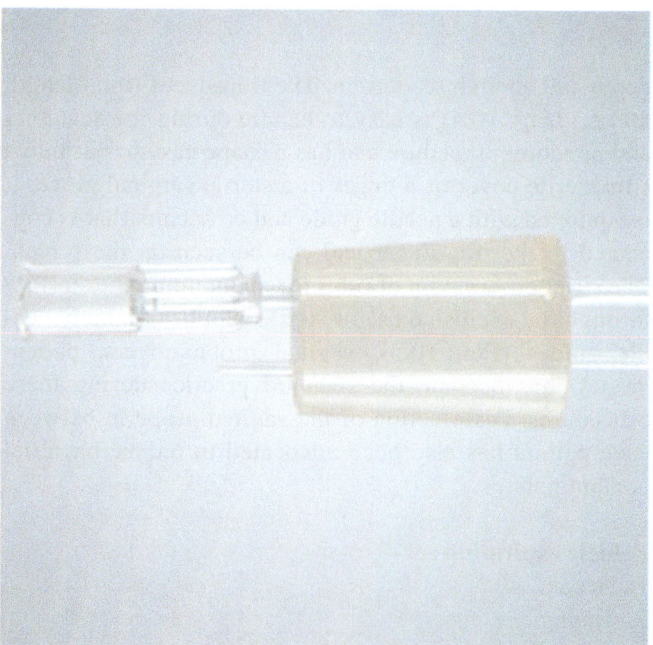

Fig. 10.12 Cap for sample tube

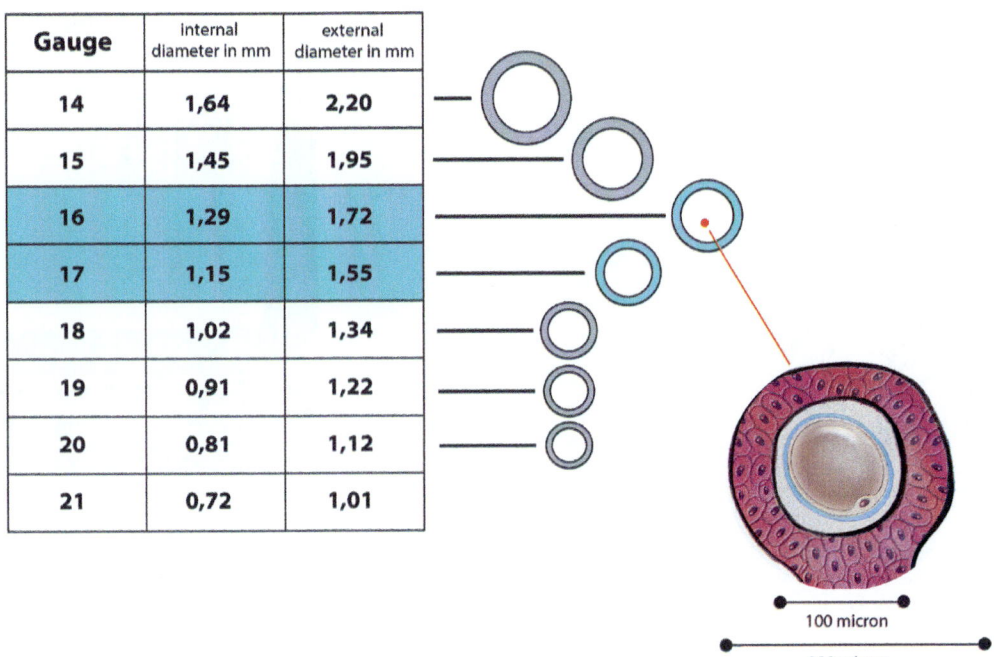

Fig. 10.13 Internal and external diameters of needles compared with the oocyte size

Gauge	internal diameter in mm	external diameter in mm
14	1,64	2,20
15	1,45	1,95
16	1,29	1,72
17	1,15	1,55
18	1,02	1,34
19	0,91	1,22
20	0,81	1,12
21	0,72	1,01

100 micron

200 micron

needles in IVF centers is with single lumen, which have a smaller diameter and causes less discomfort. The needles with double lumen allow a constant infusion of oocyte collection media into the follicles while the follicular fluid is being removed; increase the turbulence within the follicle; assist in dislodging the oocyte–cumulus complex from the follicle wall; and increase the chances of oocyte collection.

Few studies have evaluated the gauge of the needle used and the outcomes of the oocyte collection. One study compared transvaginal oocyte collections with 15-, 17-, or 18-gauge needles [18]. This prospective randomized study found that the number of oocytes collected was similar regardless of needle gauge, but more pain occurred with the 15-gauge than did with the 17- or 18- gauge needles [15]. A second study found a trend toward lower pain scores with transvaginal collections performed with a 19-gauge needle (used in in vitro maturation [IVM] retrievals) when compared with a 16- or 17-gauge needle (used in IVF retrievals), although not statistically significant [19]. The smaller needle may make for a more comfortable collection, despite more ovarian punctures and longer procedure time and the enlarged ovaries with multiple large follicles and higher aspiration pressure employed in IVF collection likely caused more pain. It is likely that within the range of conventional needles, smaller size results in less pain intra- and postoperatively, with a similar number of collected oocytes; however, more studies are needed to confirm this. There has been only a single randomized controlled trial comparing this needle to the traditional 19-gauge needle used for IVM. This study failed to find a difference in the number of oocytes aspirated [15]. Therefore, oocytes in the dead space do not seem to be lost by being returned to the follicle when flushing occurs. However, the single-lumen flushing needle resulted in statistically less ovarian punctures and less clot formation. Few studies have compared different needles for oocyte collection, and these studies should be added to the literature. It is difficult to select one needle over the other, and the current indications include cost and physician preference.

10.4 Tubing

The tubing, generally made of bend-resistant material, connects the follicle aspiration needle with the vacuum pump. In fact, all vacuum pump tubing has a male luer lock connection in one end for attaching the needle. The opposite end can be equipped with either an open end or female/male luer lock connection. The tubing should be sterile, and are intended for single use.

10.5 Sampling Tubes

After being aspirated, the follicular fluid is transferred through the tubing to the sampling tubes. A typical sampling tube used in oocyte retrieval is a disposable, sterile, and conical tube with a screw cap. It is generally made of transparent polystyrene and with a maximum volume of 15 mL (Fig. 10.14). As the oocytes contained in the collected samples are very sensitive to temperature changes, after filling the tubes, they are immediately transferred to a warmer device.

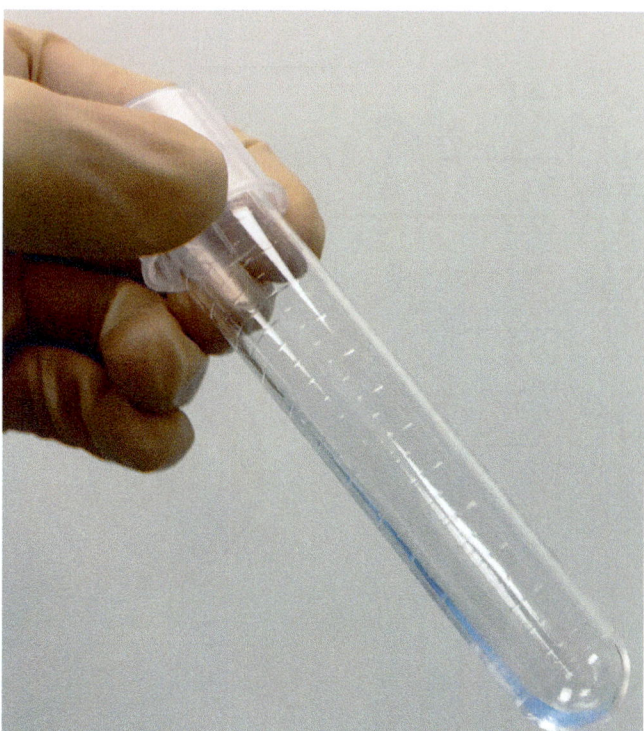

Fig. 10.14 Sampling tubes

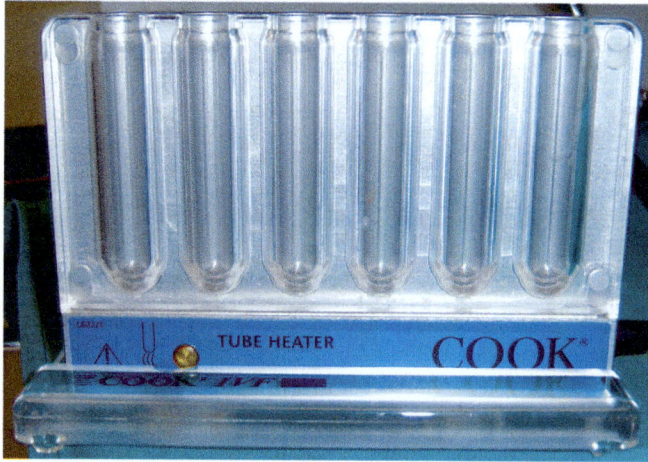

Fig. 10.16 Heating block thermostat (Cook)

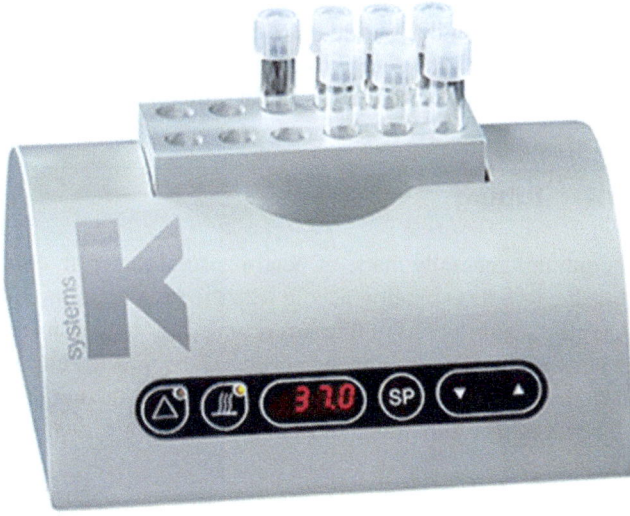

Fig. 10.15 Heating block thermostat (K Systems)

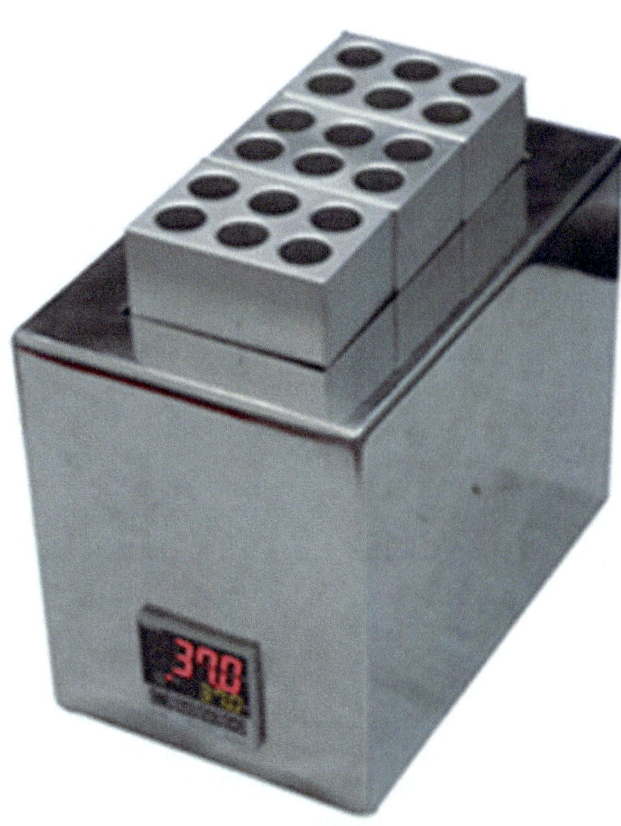

Fig. 10.17 Heating block thermostat

10.6 Thermoblock/Heating Block

After the retrieval, oocytes need to be kept at body temperature (36–37 °C) as much as possible. The mostly used heating devices consist of a sampling tube holder equipped with a heating unit (Figs. 10.15, 10.16, and 10.17), temperature sensor, and, in some cases, additional sensors to detect the fluid level (Fig. 10.18). The thermoblocks are used in the IVF laboratory to hold tubes containing the follicular fluid with the oocytes, to ensure them a constant temperature once the oocyte is aspirated out of its in vivo environment. Evidences from bovine studies [20] have demonstrated that heat shock can affect the ultrastructural morphology of early embryos and, consequently, the cleavage and blastocyst formation [21, 22]. Moreover, it has been shown that temperature fluctuations might cause changes in meiotic spin-

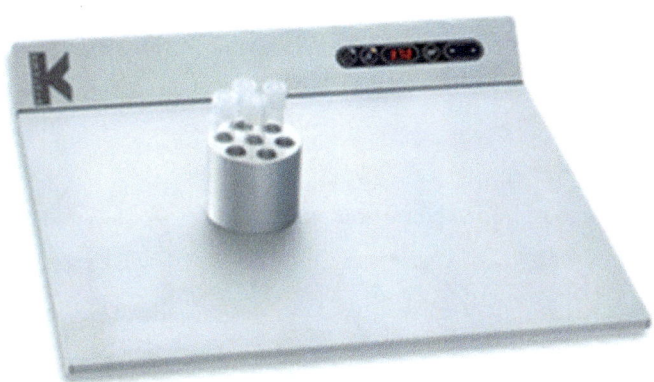

Fig. 10.18 Thermostated table

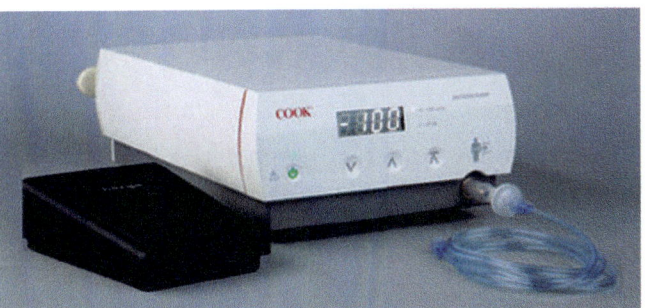

Fig. 10.19 Pump vacuum aspiration

dles which may in turn lead to abnormal fertilization and altered embryo development [23]. It is important to underline that the longer the follicular fluids remain in the thermoblock waiting for inspection, the more dependent the process is from the efficiency of the warming device. Therefore, as a general rule for obtaining oocytes in good conditions, aspirates should be divided into small samples and analyzed as soon as possible.

10.7 Pump Vacuum Aspiration

10.7.1 Pressure

As the quality of the retrieved oocytes depends on both their intrinsic characteristics and the methods used for oocyte retrieval, the aspiration of oocyte is a crucial step of ART. In particular, the aspiration pressure used for oocyte retrieval can affect the integrity of the oocyte cumulus complex.

The optimal follicle aspiration setup including the needle, pump vacuum aspiration, and media culture has not been definitively established. The pump vacuum aspiration ends with a black pedal used for turning on/off the aspiration function and a white pedal used to activate the suction pump in order to deliver the predefined negative pressure (Figs. 10.19, 10.20, and 10.21).

IVF and IVM researchers frequently indicate the aspiration pressures they used, but this information can be misleading or not easily reproducible. In fact, the pressure at the exit of the aspiration device is different from the pressure experienced by the oocyte at the needle tip [19]. Different factors such as needle gauge, length of needle, connecting tube gauge, length of connecting tube, size of the collection tube, and size of the vacuum reservoir in the pump play a role in determining the pressure experienced within the needle from the aspiration device.

Horne et al. [24] calculated the velocity of the fluid within a pickup needle, by using a model incorporating the Hagen–Poiseuille's law and taking into account the shear stress phenomenon.

Therefore, for a given pressure, the velocity of a fluid is described by the following equation:

$$av^2 + bv + c = 0$$

where v is the velocity of the fluid, and a is the loss due to changes of cross section, calculated as follows:

$$a = \rho / 2 \left[1 + K_2 + A_1^2 / A_1^2 * K_1 \right]$$

where ρ is the density of the fluid, K_1 the loss factor for the inlet to the needle, K_2 the loss factor for the interface between the needle and line, A_1 the cross-sectional area of the needle, and A^2 the cross-sectional area of the aspiration line.

b is the frictional resistance of the needle and line, calculated as follows:

$$b = 32 \mu L_2 / D_2^2 + A_2 / A_1 * 32 \mu L_1 / D_1^2$$

where L_1 is the length of the needle, L_2 the length of the aspiration line, D_1 the diameter of the needle, and D^2 the diameter of the aspiration line.

Finally, c is the pressure and gravitational driving force, calculated as follows:

$$c = (P_3 - P_5) + \rho g (z_3 - z_5)$$

where P_3 is the pressure at the collection tube, P_5 the pressure at the follicle, z_3 the vertical distance at the collection tube from a datum, and z_5 the vertical distance at the follicle from a datum.

They also calculated the flow rate, Q, as:

$$Q = vA$$

where v is the velocity of the fluid and A the internal cross-sectional area of the needle or line, finding that while the flow remained laminar, the flow rates predicted by the model were within ±5% of the observed flows.

Fig. 10.20 Pump vacuum aspiration

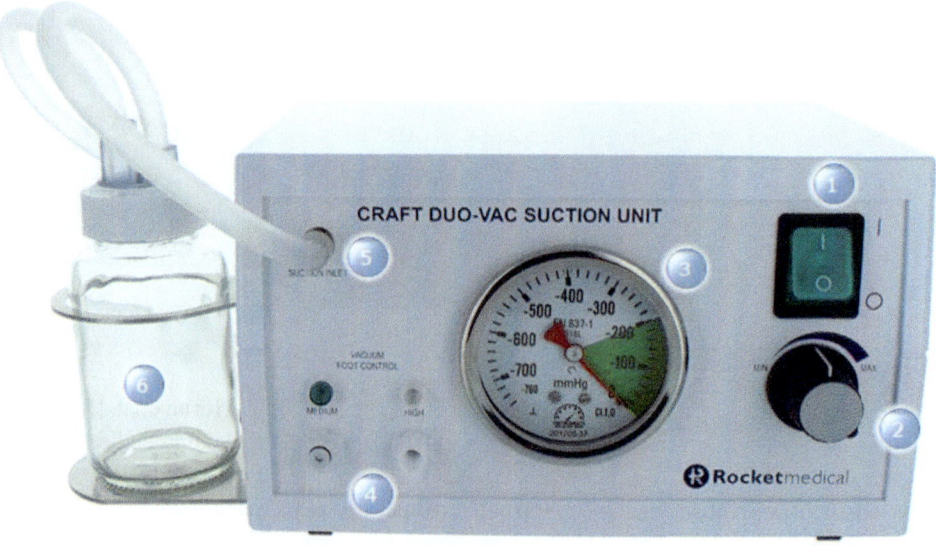

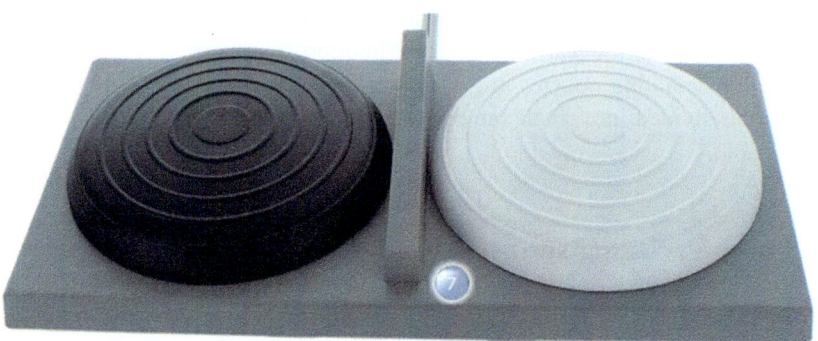

1. Illuminated O/I Mains Power On/Off
2. Vacuum Control Dial – clockwise to increase, anticlockwise to decrease the set value
3. Vacuum Display mmHg^{-1}
4. Footswitch connection ports
5. Water trap connection port for use with R57685 Rocket Craft Pump Water Trap Sets
6. R57685 Rocket Craft Pump Water Trap Set
7. Medium Vacuum (Standard) 50-250mmHg^{-1} & High Vacuum 440mmHg^{-1} foot-switch

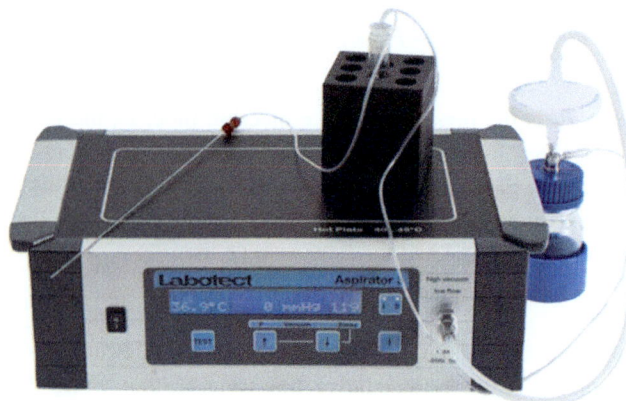

Fig. 10.21 Pump vacuum aspiration

In addition, with needles having an i.d. <1.4 mm, laminar flow occurred over the range of vacuums 5–40 kPa (37.5–300 mmHg). At vacuums >50 kPa (375 mmHg) the model predicted velocities (and hence flow rates) in excess of those observed.

They also evaluated the effect of increasing the length of the needle by using a 16-gauge needle with an internal diameter of 1.2 mm coupled with a 60 cm Teflon line on velocity and flow rates at different vacuums, finding that by increasing the length of the needle, both the velocity and flow rates decreased.

As regarding the evaluation of IVF outcomes using different collection pressures, the work of Fry and collaborators examined in bovine oocytes the use of various needle sizes

(17- and 20-g) and aspiration pressures (25, 50, 75, and 100 mmHg) to evaluate the impact on the quantity and quality of recovered immature oocytes [25].

In that study, the authors aspirated 5827 follicles from 720 ovaries with 17- and 20-gauge needles and found that the highest recovery occurred at the highest aspiration pressures with 46% at 25 mmHg and 59% at 100 mmHg. Another study by Bols et al. [26], which included 3000 aspirated follicles, reported a similar finding where higher pressures were associated with a higher recovery (55.5% at 50 mmHg vs. 67% at 130 mmHg).

It should be noted that in in vitro maturation (IVM) retrievals, a lower aspiration pressures with respect to the one used in IVF treatments improve the recovery as oocytes are denuded of the cumulus oophorus cells at higher pressures, and furthermore, the negative impact of increasing aspiration pressures is greater in larger-gauge needles [27].

Morphologically altered oocytes have been found at aspiration around 180 mmHg, which were usually used during laparoscopic oocyte retrieval [25]. Aspiration pressure higher than 180 mmHg was related with oocyte damage and poor embryogenesis [28]. On the contrary, lower aspiration pressures between 90 and 120 mmHg have been associated with good oocyte quality and minimal damage [29].

In particular, when the lower aspiration vacuum was used, the number of immature oocytes increased, as well as the numbers of intact cumulus cells, fertilized oocytes, and cleaved and transferable embryos increased (Table 10.2). On the contrary, when the aspiration vacuum exceeds a threshold, the number of retrieved oocytes decreased, probably due to local turbulence caused by inflow and coagulation of blood in the tube.

The presence of an intact cumulus resulted a crucial factor in the oocyte resistance to the damage. In fact, in a study carried out with bovine cumulus, Horne and collaborators showed that the morphology of bovine cumulus was unchanged after in vitro aspiration at vacuum and velocities comparable to those used in vivo, if the cumulus was regular and compact. Differently, the cumulus was less resistant if it was damaged or degenerated [24].

A special attention should be paid to the aspiration pressure and the oocyte retrieval method in patients with low antral follicle count (AFC) (≤10). Kumaran and colleagues [30] compared oocyte retrieval outcomes using three methods of aspiration:

1. Direct aspiration pressure of 120 mmHg in women with normal AFC
2. Direct aspiration pressure at 140 mmHg in women with low AFC
3. Aspiration pressure of 120 mmHg with flushing in women with low AFC

In this study, they showed that a slight increase of aspiration pressure to 140 mmHg did not affect the oocyte and embryo yield when compared with standard aspiration pressure (120 mmHg), thus concluding that it could be promising to improve the pregnancy outcomes in women with a low AFC, in which the alternative practice of flushing showed discouraging outcome [31].

Similarly, there is not a wide agreement over the most effective culture media for oocyte in vitro culture. Currently, most media are supplemented with pyruvic acid with essential and nonessential amino acids. However, further studies need to be performed to help the optimization of this setup [32].

10.8 Anesthesia with Oocyte Retrieval

The use of anesthesia is an integral part of performing oocyte retrievals. Anesthetic options include general anesthesia, neuraxial anesthesia, paracervical block, and conscious sedation. The choice of an anesthetic agent should be based on the ease of administration and monitoring with short-term reversible effects [33]. In addition, the agent of choice should not have any toxic effects on the oocytes and embryos. An adequate pain control is critical not only for the well-being of the patient but also for the safety of the procedure as the retrieval needle is inserted near adjacent vital organs and vessels [34].

With laparoscopic oocyte recovery, general anesthesia with endotracheal intubation and intermittent positive pressure ventilation are required to ensure airway protection, to assist with the maintenance of normocarbia and to provide muscle paralysis [35]. With less invasive techniques of oocyte recovery (transvesical and transvaginal routes), the need for general anesthesia has declined allowing for methods such as regional anesthesia. Advantages of regional anesthesia include limited absorption of anesthetic agents into the circulation and thus minimal effects on the oocytes [36]. However, adverse effects such as spinal headache, back pain, urinary retention, hypotension, high spinal, epidural hematoma, abscess, and significant nerve damage limit its potential use [37].

For transvaginal oocyte retrieval procedures, local anesthesia is commonly used. However, local anesthesia in the

Table 10.2 Recommended pressure values

	Single lumen		Double lumen	
	16 G	17 G	18 G	17 G
Tube set length, cm	Recommended vacuum, mmHg			
55	80	110	130	150
70	90	130	150	170
90	100	150	170	190

form of a paracervical block has been found to be inadequate for many women. Moreover, 28% of patients required additional analgesia to complete the procedure. Despite the decreased cost and ease of administration, a paracervical block is best used in conjunction with another form of anesthesia to provide adequate pain relief [37].

10.9   Procedure

Ovarian pickup (OPU) is scheduled when there are >3 follicles of sizes >17 mm or at least one follicle 20 mm, provided that the total number of follicles measuring >14 mm is ≥8 follicles [38].

Oocyte retrieval must be scheduled with great precision: oocyte maturation is completed at 25–30 h after the preovulatory LH surge (or HCG injection or GnRH agonist administration). Follicular rupture occurs on average within 37 h. Following HCG administration, the earliest follicular rupture is about 39 h, and the latest is about 41 h [39, 40].

After that patient has been transferred into the operating room and anesthetized, the pickup procedure can start. It is important that the clinician, knowing the patient to treat,

might select the proper aspiration kit, choosing the monolumen kit with or without flushing, the double lumen with flushing, the needle length, gauge, and connector.

Before starting the surgery, the team will check the surgical equipment and flush the aspiration system, and then the needle is rinsed with flushing media for removing potential debris or contaminations inside the needle (Figs. 10.22, 10.23, 10.24, and 10.25). The vacuum pressure is verified as higher pressure could affect oocyte integrity, thus decreasing their quality and increasing the proportion of oocytes without zona pellucida. At least one operator (gynecologist) and one assistant (nurse) are needed to perform this technique. While one is performing the follicle aspiration, the assistant will be changing the tubes for each of the follicles aspirated.

When a general intravenous or local anesthesia is administered, the patient is placed in a gynecological position, and the procedure begins (Fig. 10.26), once the patient is asleep; before the procedure starts, the patient is advised to empty her bladder, in order to reduce the risk of urinary bladder injury and facilitate the access to the ovaries during transvaginal oocyte retrieval (TVOR). Intraoperatively, if one or both ovaries are found to be inaccessible and the bladder is full, a disposable catheter

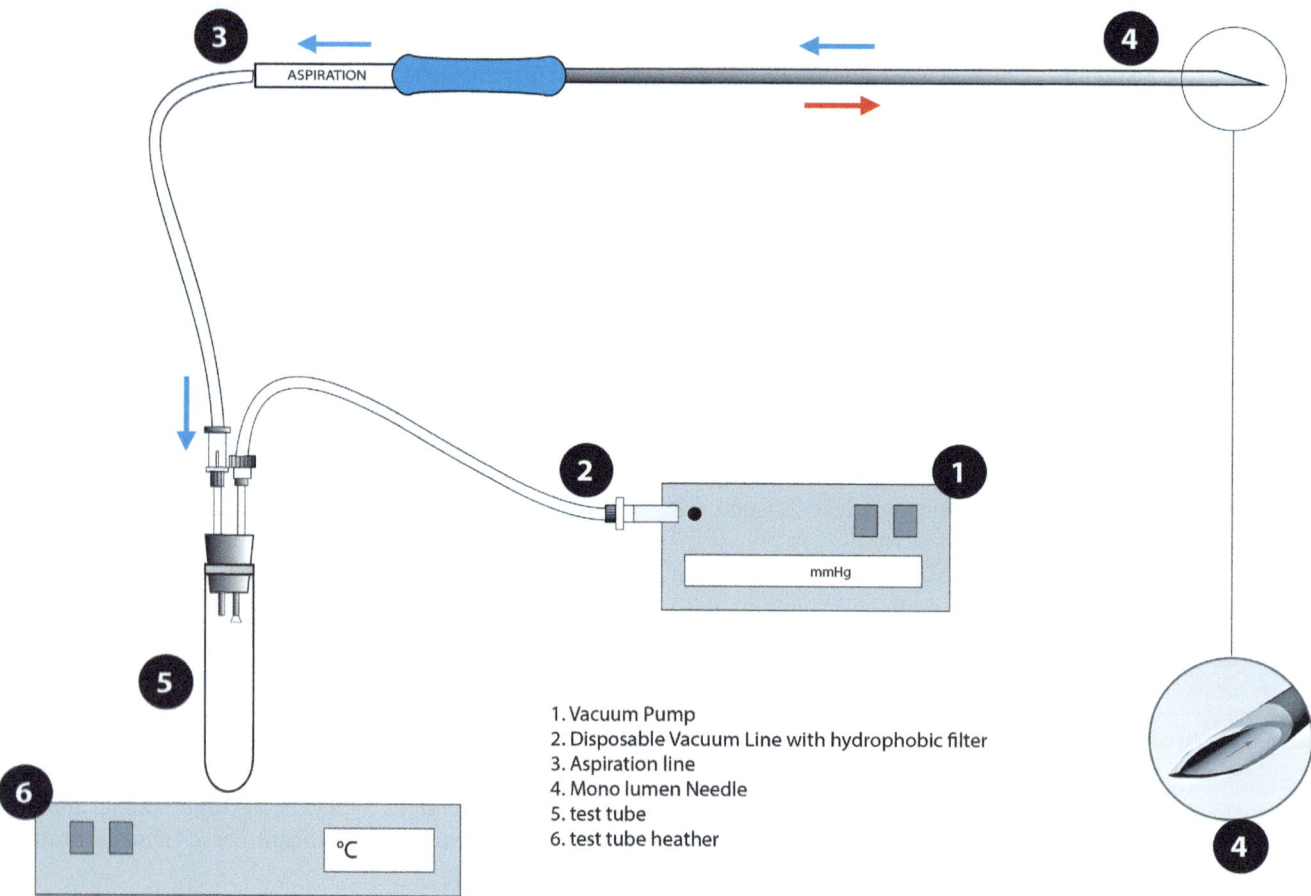

1. Vacuum Pump
2. Disposable Vacuum Line with hydrophobic filter
3. Aspiration line
4. Mono lumen Needle
5. test tube
6. test tube heather

Fig. 10.22 Kit mono-lumen needle without the follicular flushing system

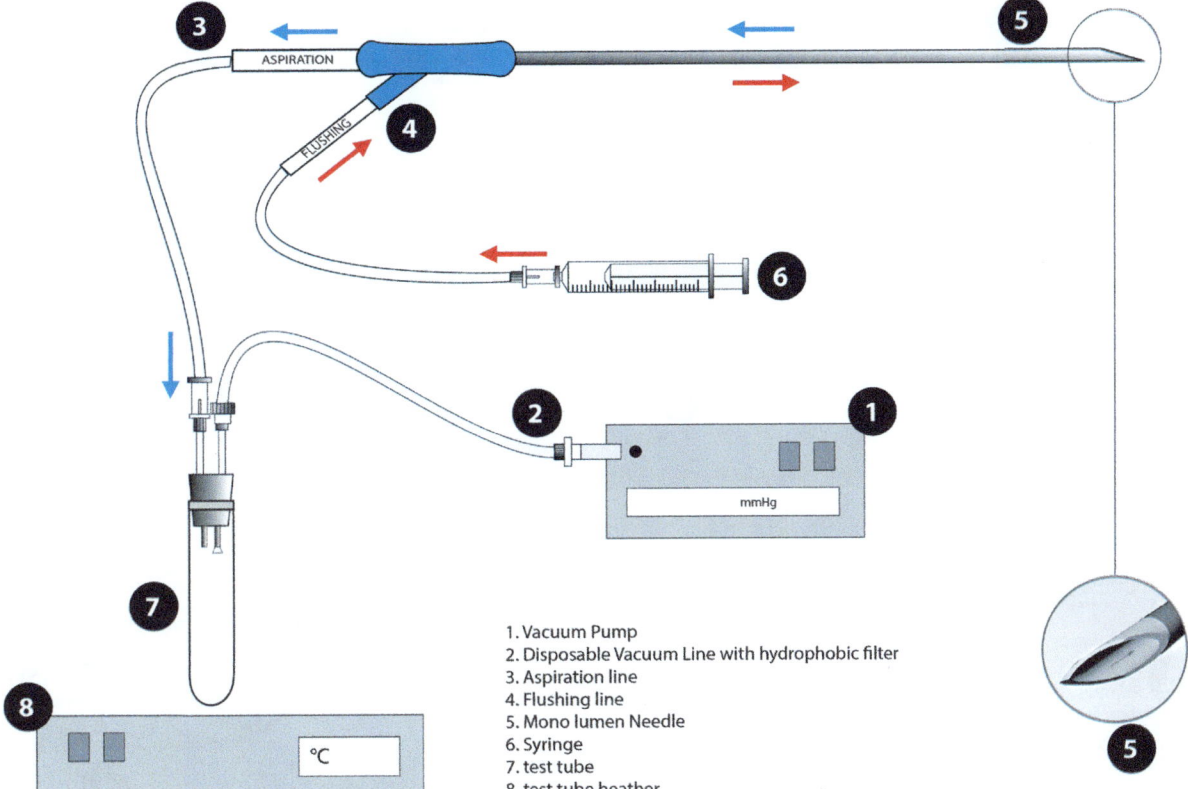

Fig. 10.23 Kit mono-lumen needle equipped with the follicular flushing system

1. Vacuum Pump
2. Disposable Vacuum Line with hydrophobic filter
3. Aspiration line
4. Flushing line
5. Mono lumen Needle
6. Syringe
7. test tube
8. test tube heather

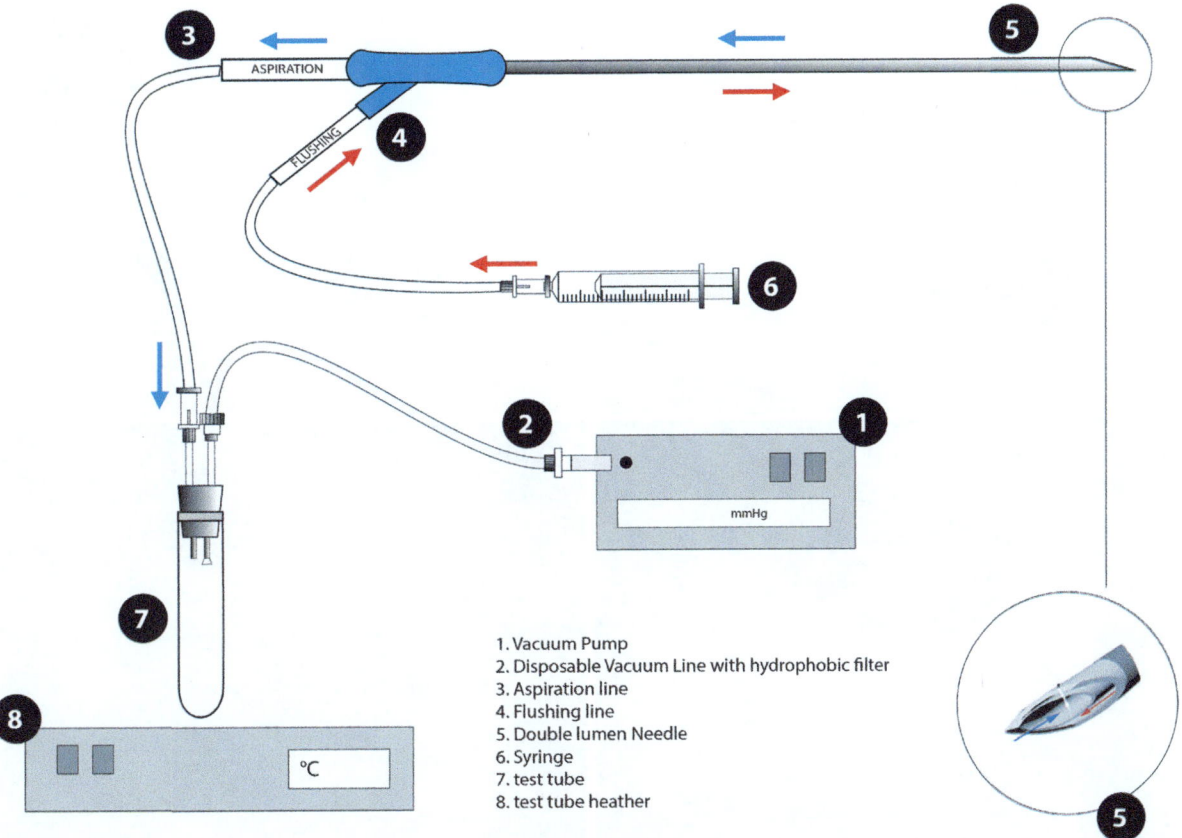

Fig. 10.24 Kit double lumen needle without the follicular flushing system

1. Vacuum Pump
2. Disposable Vacuum Line with hydrophobic filter
3. Aspiration line
4. Flushing line
5. Double lumen Needle
6. Syringe
7. test tube
8. test tube heather

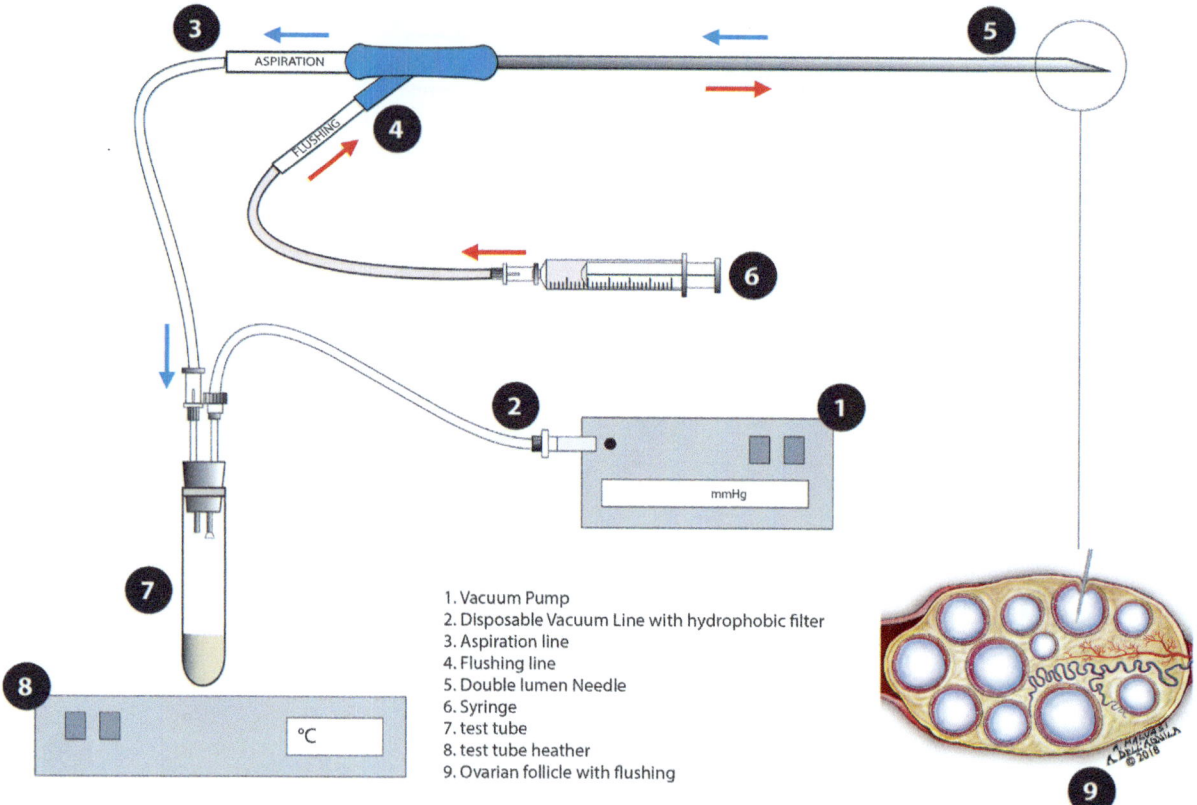

1. Vacuum Pump
2. Disposable Vacuum Line with hydrophobic filter
3. Aspiration line
4. Flushing line
5. Double lumen Needle
6. Syringe
7. test tube
8. test tube heather
9. Ovarian follicle with flushing

Fig. 10.25 Kit double lumen needle equipped with the follicular flushing using washing media

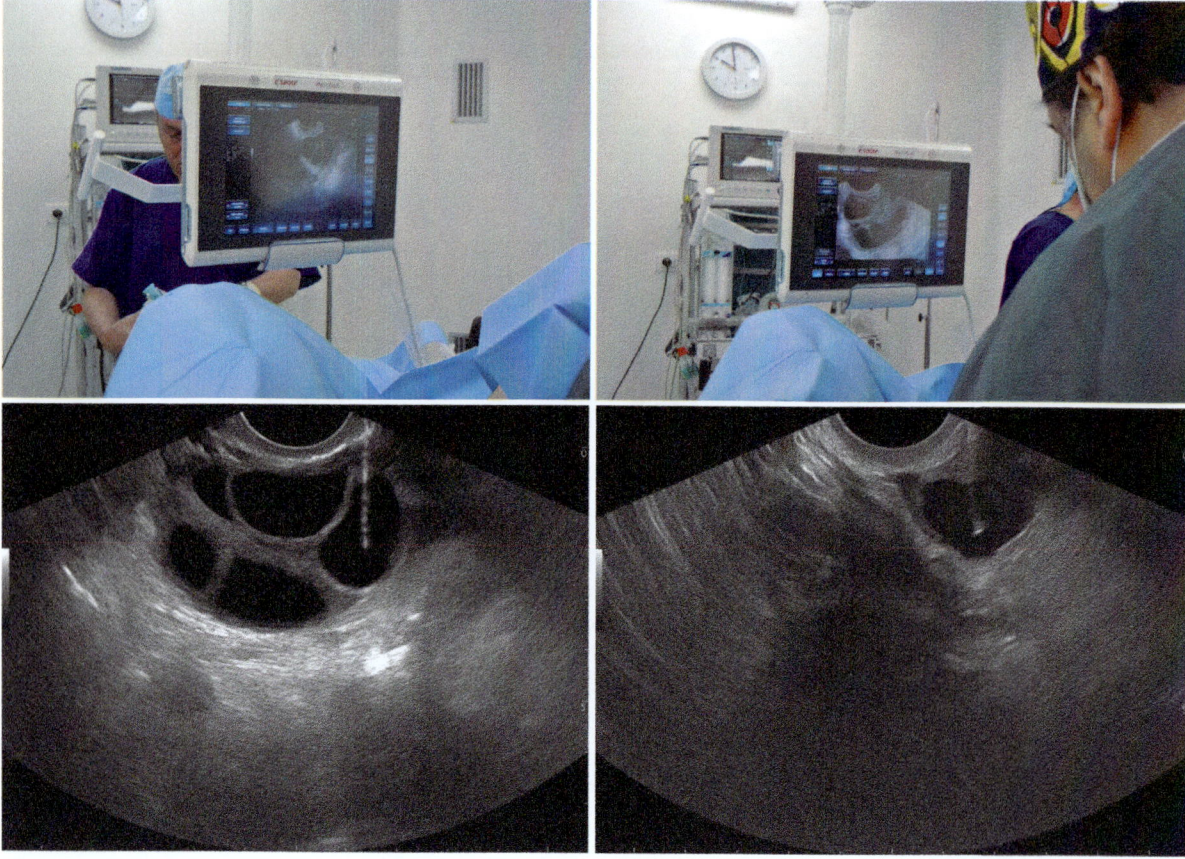

Fig. 10.26 Ultrasound images showing the puncture of two follicles in two different moments in the same patient

should be used to empty the bladder as this can bring the ovaries closer to the vagina and render them accessible.

A vaginal speculum is then placed, and saline solution (at 35–37 °C) (Fig. 10.27) [40] or non-cytotoxic antiseptic agents (such as chlorhexidine) are flushed to clean the area. It is not advisable to use iodide agents since they can be potentially cytotoxic, but to use gauze pads and Foerster ring forceps. In fact, vaginal preparation solutions used to reduce vaginal microbial concentrations prior to oocyte retrievals have been shown to impact pregnancy outcomes. The two most common disinfectants are 1% povidone-iodine and normal saline solution [41].

The question of prophylactic antibiotics arises for all gynecologic surgeries and procedures. Specifically for oocyte retrievals, studies have shown a potential benefit for antibiotics prior to this procedure. Currently, no data convincingly support the use of prophylactic antibiotics to improve pregnancy outcomes. Additional research is needed to evaluate live birth rates as the primary outcome and to assess microbial colonization as a secondary outcome to be able to fully offer recommendations [42].

The transvaginal probe must be carefully inserted, and an ultrasound scan is made in order to visualize the pelvic area to confirm the number and size of follicles according to previous follicle tracking scans (Figs. 10.28 and 10.29). It consists of the insertion of a small needle with an attached ultrasound probe covered with an ultrasound gel into the vagina which is slightly moved by means of the top wall of the vagina. The uterus is located and examined, together with the ovaries and pelvic vessels, in order to determine the best way to approach the ovaries and assess any potential risks (full bladder, retrouterine ovaries, cysts, endometrial fibroids, uterine fibroids, etc.) that could hinder oocyte recovery.

Then, the gloves must be changed, and if possible, power-free gloves should be used.

The ultrasound probe allows visualizing the follicles on the ultrasound screen, and then the needle is inserted into every follicle to extract the follicular fluid and collect it into a tube [43, 44]. The improved visualization of the ovaries due to the proximity of the ultrasound probe led to more precise oocyte aspiration. Once the most accessible ovary is selected, the needle is penetrated through the vaginal fornix into the follicle, by applying a steady inward pressure, with the vaginal probe, in order to directly access as closer as possible to the ovary (1–3 cm distance) and immobilize the ovaries and avoid movements, reduce the risk of intraoperative rupture of the ovarian capsule and keep bowel loops away. Before penetrating the tissue, the probe should be rotated to 90° from the midsagittal plane in order to reduce the risk of lesions of the vessels of the vaginal wall. Also Doppler ultrasound guidance (Fig. 10.30) can be used to avoid vascular injury. When the biggest follicle is visualized on the

Fig. 10.27 Surgical carriage for oocyte pickup

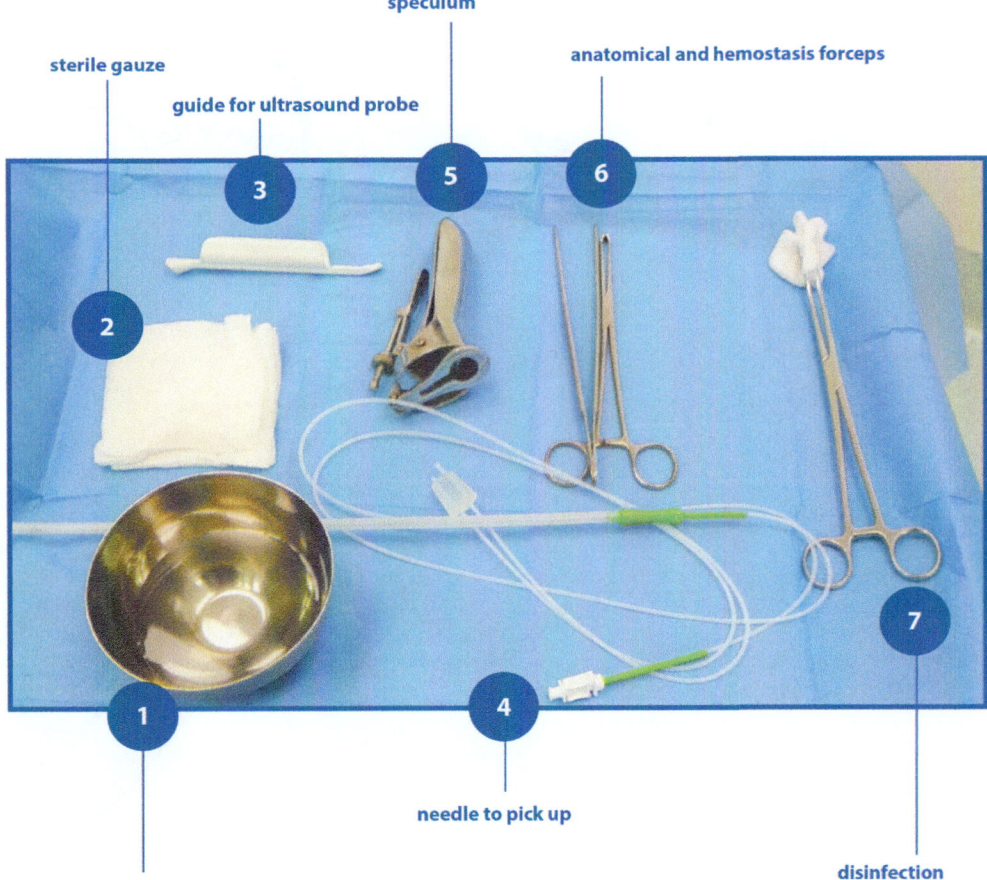

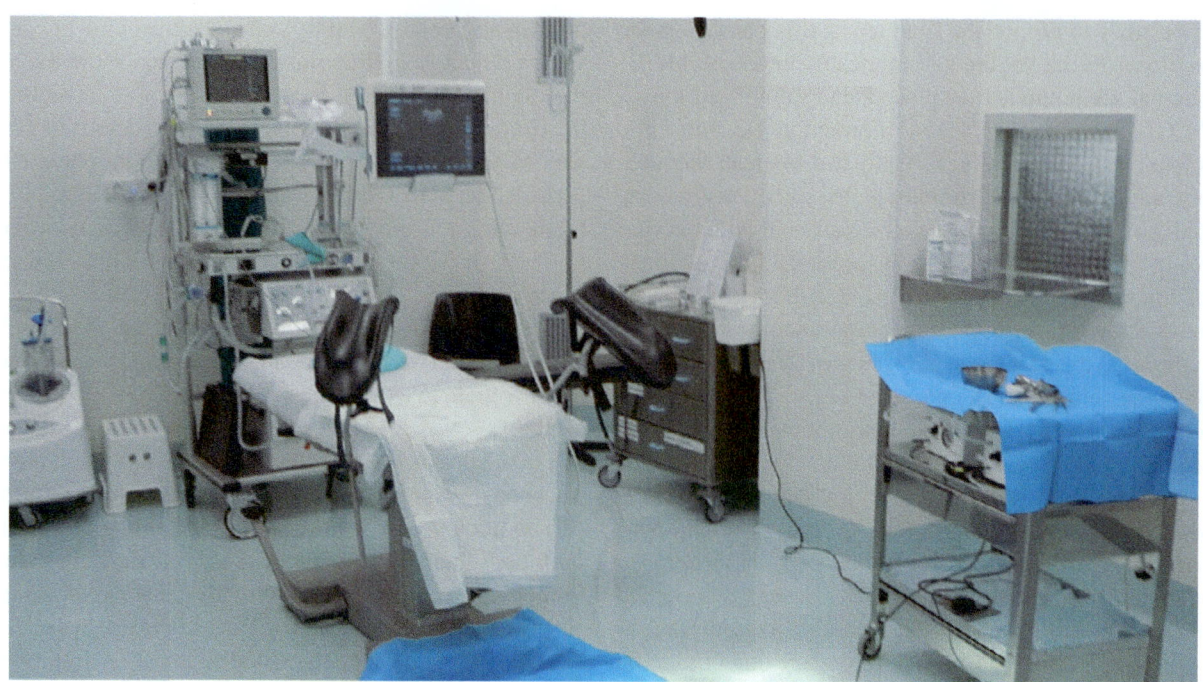

Fig. 10.28 Surgery room (theater pickup)

Fig. 10.29 Schematic representation of the oocyte retrieval under transvaginal ultrasound guidance

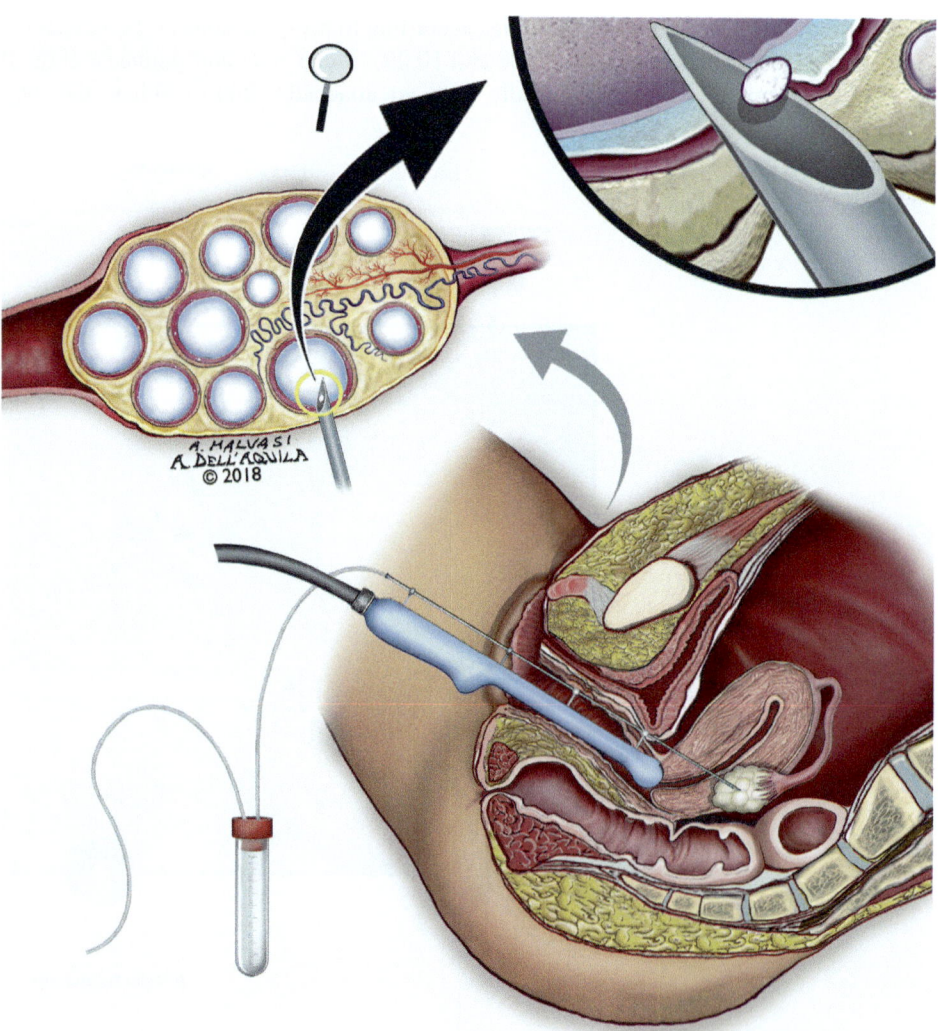

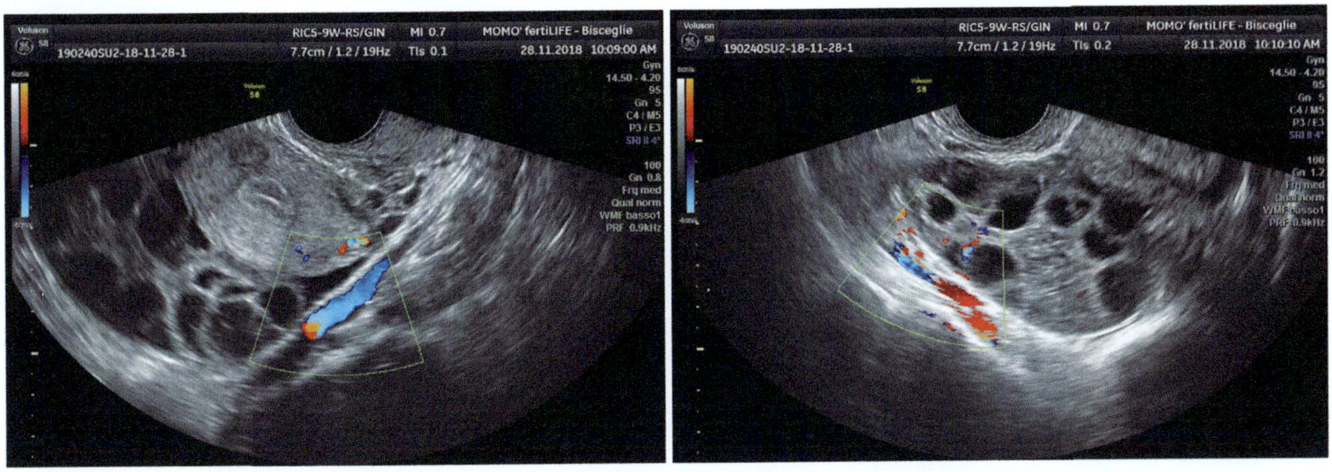

Fig. 10.30 The use of the Doppler during the oocyte retrieval can help avoid sting the vessels near the ovaries or the vessels of the ovaries

ultrasound screen, once the needle is inserted, a controlled vacuum is applied to the needle and the follicular fluid is aspirated from the ovary and aspiration of the other follicles is performed without removing the needle from the ovary, following the same approach.

Whenever possible (Fig. 10.26, 10.31, 10.32, and 10.33), a single puncture of each ovary should be performed also for the other follicles [45]. After puncture, bleeding in the ovarian capsule often occurs; therefore, the number of punctures should be limited to reduce the risk of post-retrieval bleeding. Oocyte aspiration is often completed at the end of the procedure, aspirating thick and viscous fluid (granulosa cells of the corona radiata and cumulus) (Fig. 10.34).

Another management option is the use of appropriate pressure, with or without concomitant abdominal pressure, in order to bring an inaccessible ovary closer to the vaginal wall. Sometimes, reverse Trendelenburg position and lateral table tilt can also help. Sometimes the ovary is firmly fixed behind the uterus and, despite various maneuvers, the only possible way would be through the uterus, by a transvaginal-transmyometrial approach in order to aspirate the follicles of a retroverted ovary [46] (Table 10.3).

The follicular fluid is collected in the sterile tubes placed in the thermal block set at 37 °C. Once three quarters of the tube is full, it is transferred to the IVF lab in a thermoblock in order to maintain the temperature. Follicular fluid obtained is analyzed by the biologists under the microscope, who will confirm the presence and the number of oocytes. After the puncture of both ovaries, the pelvic cavity is assessed with the transvaginal probe in order to confirm the absence of bleeding.

Accumulation of blood in the pouch of Douglas is frequently found after oocyte retrieval, up to 100 mL is normal [48, 49]. The liquid is removed before completing the surgical procedure; this routine would help to reduce postoperative pain caused by peritoneal irritation (Fig. 10.35).

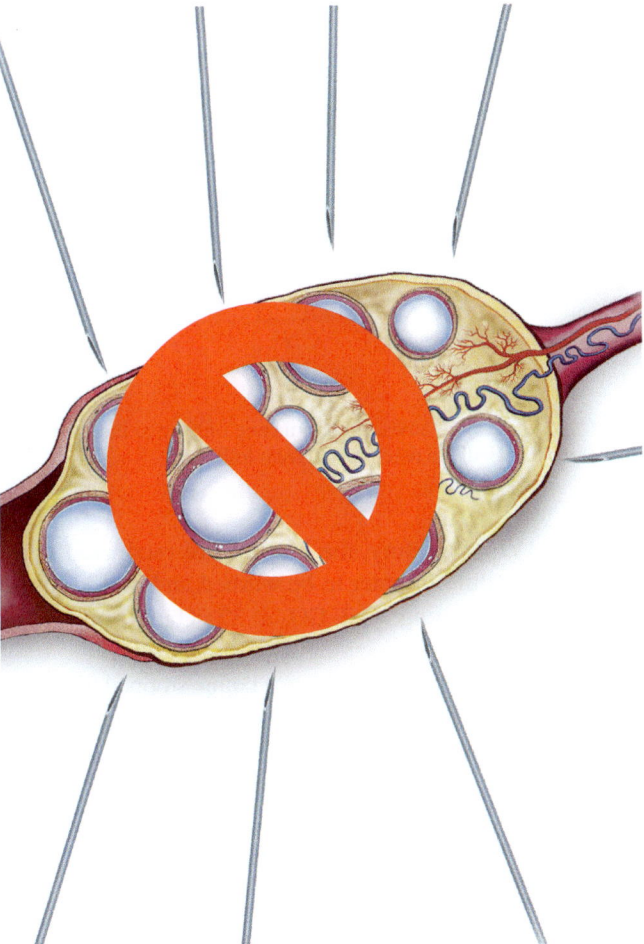

Fig. 10.31 Several ovarian punctures are not recommended

Visual examination of the posterior fornix and cervix for lesions and/or bleeding is performed. Flush the vagina with 0.9% saline solution. Press firmly for a few seconds with a swab to stop bleeding [50, 51]. Remove vaginal speculum.

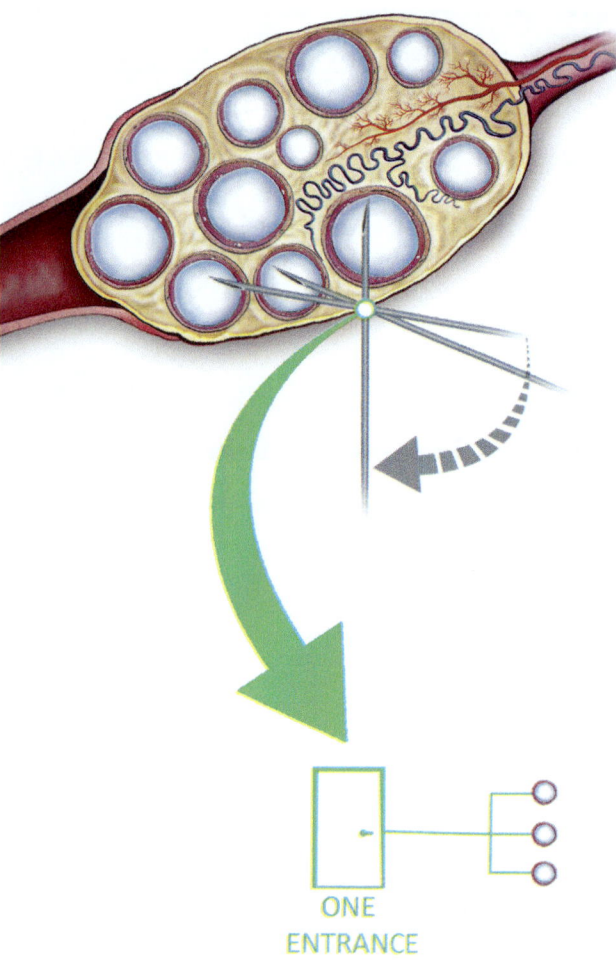

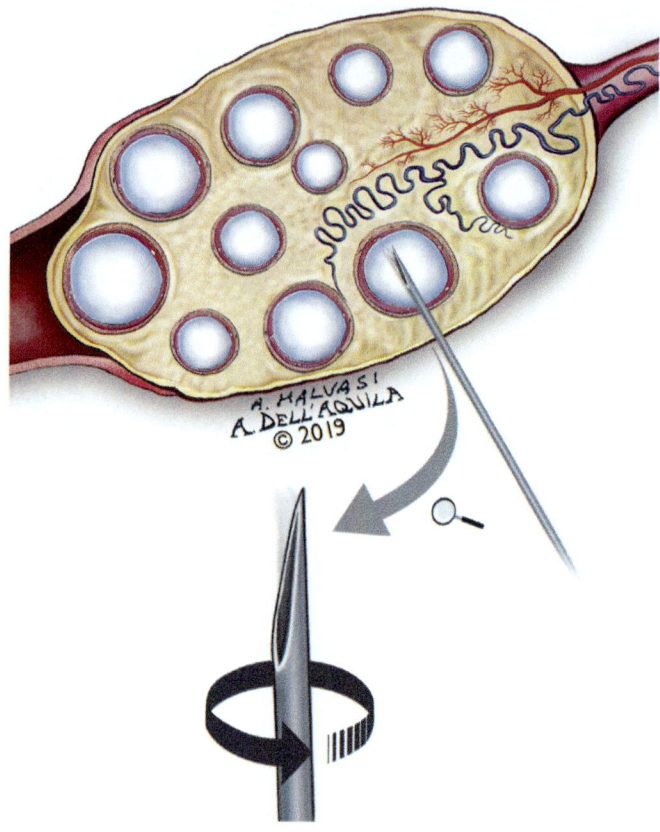

ONE
ENTRANCE

Fig. 10.32 It is more advisable to puncture only once the ovary and then move the needle to reach the adjacent follicles

Fig. 10.33 During aspiration a slow rotary movement can help to complete the oocyte recovery

In the IVF laboratory, the oocytes are recovered from the follicular fluid in order to be washed and placed in the incubator maintaining a 5% CO_2 at 37 °C until insemination or ICSI.

In case of vaginal bleeding not being stopped with the hemostatic gauze, the surgeon applies the hemostatic clamp by using ring forceps (Fig. 10.36). If the bleeding lasts longer than 5 min, it is necessary to make a suture.

10.10 Follicle Flushing

The purpose of oocyte retrieval is to maximize the number of oocytes recovered at the end of the procedure. In the past decade, there have been attempts to refine the equipment, thus increasing the number of oocytes retrieved. The double lumen retrieval needle was developed to reintroduce additional fluid into an aspirated follicle and increase the likelihood of recovering a retained oocyte (Fig. 10.37) [52].

To maximize the number of oocytes recovered, follicular aspiration followed by flushing, has been suggested [53]. Also, double lumen needles, which have one channel for flushing fluid into the follicle and another channel for aspiration of the oocyte, have also been developed [54].

The potential benefit of follicular flushing is the increased number of oocytes collected, which may possibly increase the pregnancy and live birth rates. However, potential disadvantages include longer procedure time with more anesthetics and more tissue handling. Flushing may also in theory remove some of the follicular cells that could potentially serve an important endocrine luteal support function. There have been several reviews on the effectiveness of follicular flushing in human IVF.

A comprehensive Cochrane review performed in 2010 [47] has found that follicle flushing does not appear to improve ART outcomes in normal-responding patients and that it increases the length of the procedure and time under anesthesia. Thus, follicle flushing is not recommended in this population [31, 55]. It is felt that this benefit may occur because cumulus oocyte complexes in poor responding women have less luteinizing hormone receptor responsiveness and may not be released from the follicle wall as easily compared to women who are normal responders.

Fig. 10.34 Schematic drawing of the oocyte with corona radiata and corresponding stereomicroscope picture

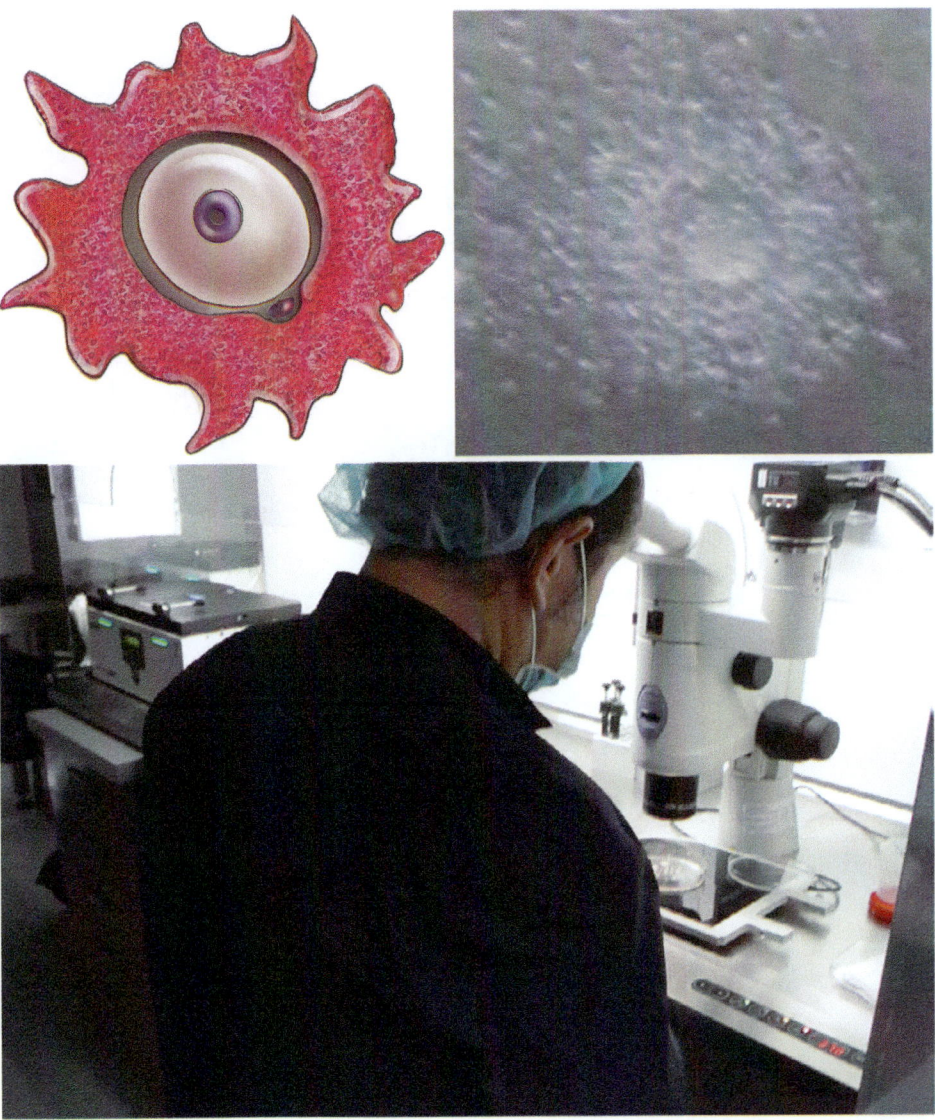

Table 10.3 Safety measures that should be taken during ovum pickup

*When inserting the needle, **color Doppler ultrasound guidance should be used***

***The tip of the needle should always be visualized** to prevent injury to the adjacent pelvic structures. The follicle should be completely aspirated before passing to another follicle*

***Do not make any sudden or lateral movements** once the ovary has been punctured*

*Once the needle has entered the ovarian cortex, follicles should be punctured in a fan-shaped manner starting from the entering point, by **starting with the follicle showing the biggest diameter***

Once the aspiration of follicles in one ovary is completed, the other ovary should be punctured

The aspiration needle must be removed and flushed with washing media

Regarding the proportion of oocytes recovered by this surgical approach, at least 80% of the oocytes are collected [47]

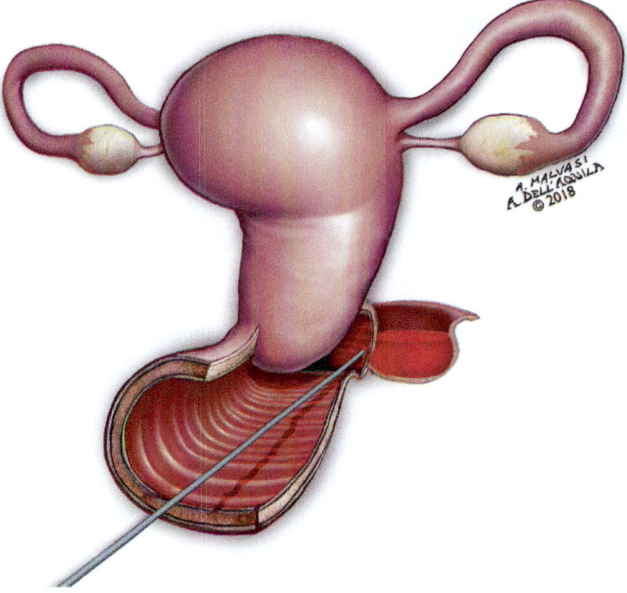

Fig. 10.35 Blood aspiration from the pouch of Douglas at the end of the procedure

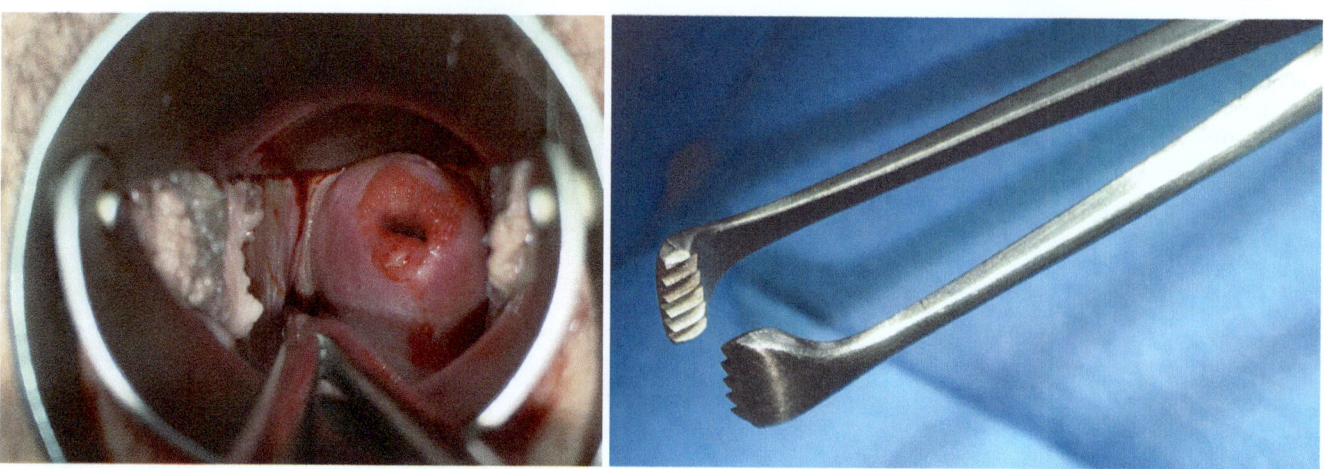

Fig. 10.36 In some cases when there is blood loss from the vaginal wall, it is possible to clamp the area of the loss for a few minutes

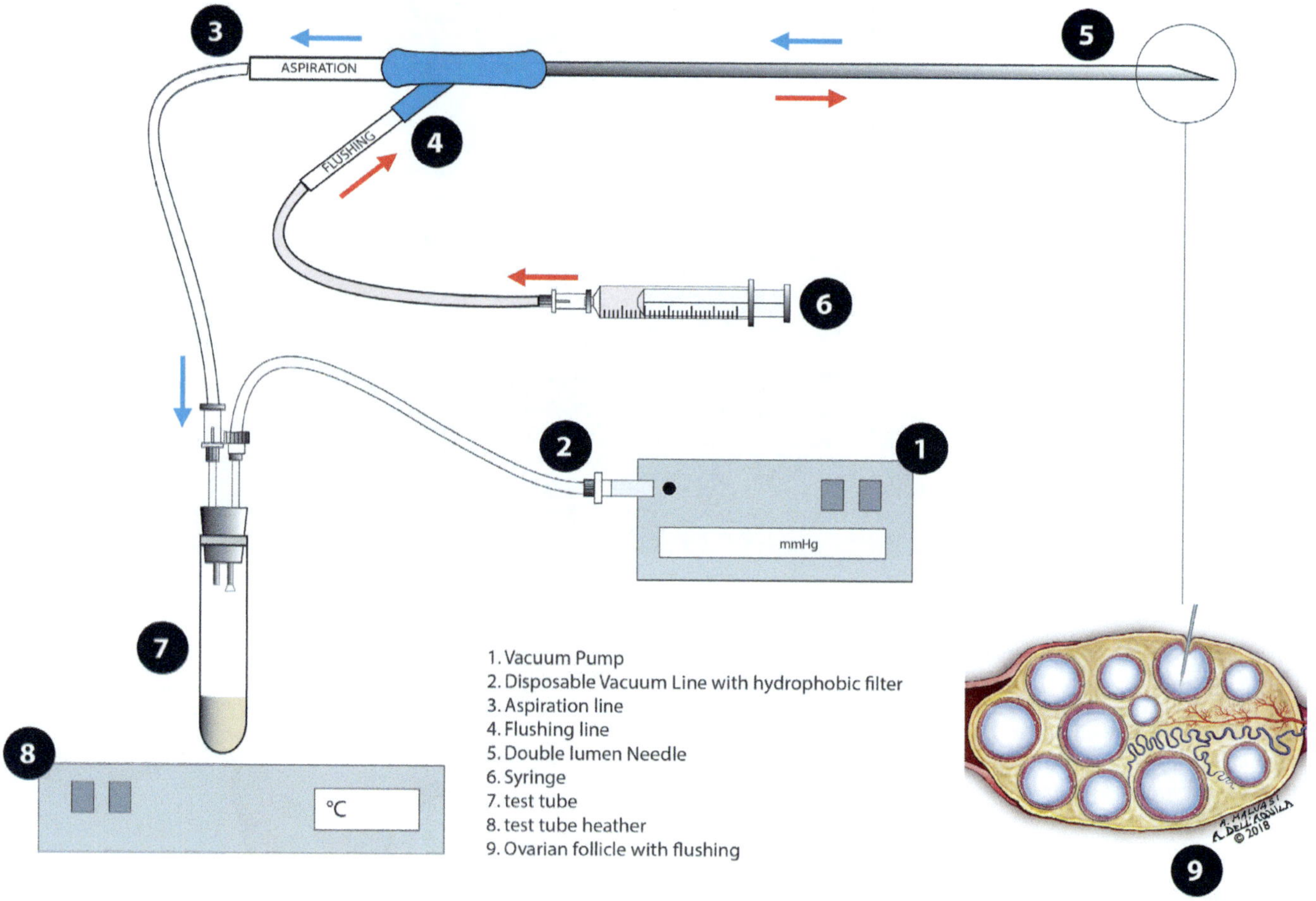

ASPIRATION
FLUSHING
mmHg
°C
1. Vacuum Pump
2. Disposable Vacuum Line with hydrophobic filter
3. Aspiration line
4. Flushing line
5. Double lumen Needle
6. Syringe
7. test tube
8. test tube heather
9. Ovarian follicle with flushing

Fig. 10.37 Follicle aspiration kit with double lumen needle for flushing

This procedure is reserved for cases of low oocyte recovery [56]. If flushing is interrupted, the needle must be rotated 45° to restore the flow of liquid (this can happen when the tip of the aspiration needle is attached to the follicular wall).

Alternatively, the increase of the aspiration pressure should help to restore the flow. The needle could also be removed from the ovary in order to flush the aspiration system if there is the suspect of a potential occlusion caused by blood clots and/or ovarian tissue before continuing with the procedure [57, 58].

10.11 Pain Management

One of the main aspects of post oocyte retrieval care is the management of pain, which is although difficult to evaluate, might be influenced by many factors, such as fear of pain, anxiety, surgical skills of the doctor, operation time, and other technical factors, such as needle diameter and the sharpness during ovum pickup (OPU) [59].

After OPU, 3% of patients experience from severe to very severe pain and 2% of patients still suffer severe pain 2 days after the procedure [14, 37, 51]. Intraoperative analgesia should be indicated and routine postoperative analgesic regime should be given in order to minimize postoperative pain.

Post-harvesting oocyte pain is often a constant related to repeated perforations of the ovarian cortex, but before thinking that pain in general is due to this, it is important to exclude pain related mainly to ongoing blood loss or injury to other organs.

So far, very little attention has been given to the technical aspects related to the pain relief, as for example the effect of the needle size [60].

Only a few studies have investigated the relationship between the needle size and pain experience in patients undergoing the oocyte pickup, finding that a significantly less pain was experienced when the needle size was reduced from 15 and 16 gauge to 17 and 18 gauge. On the other hand, an excessive reduction of the needle diameter (<0.8 mm) might cause damages to the oocyte or increase the technical difficulty of the retrieval.

In a recent study, to overcome these inconveniences a newly designed needle has been proposed, having only the last 50 mm with a reduced diameter.

Wikland (Fig. 10.38) and colleagues demonstrated a significant decrease of the overall pain as well as a reduction of vaginal bleeding with such a thinner needle respect to a standard needle. Based on this advantage, Vitrolife, an international medtech company focused on IVF field, has recently proposed the "Sense" needle, with an unreduced body (17 gauge) and a reduced tip (20 gauge). In this configuration, where only the tip is reduced, the rigidity of the needle is maintained, ensuring an accurate control of the oocyte retrieval, while reducing the patient pain and bleeding.

After ovum pickup, the patient rests for 2 h at the clinic under observation to discard circulatory complications and determine the need of further analgesia. The patient is then discharged if there are no complications.

For donors who yield >20 oocytes or present high serum estradiol levels (E2 > 3500 pg/mL) or in the event of difficult oocyte retrieval or patients who report any symptoms, a follow-up visit is scheduled.

Clear postoperative instructions are given to the patients, along with information on emergency contact telephone numbers (24 h) in case of bleeding, temperature, feeling of weakness, dizziness, or poor general condition [60].

10.12 Factors Influencing Oocyte Retrieval

Several physiological or pathological female factors might adversely affect the number and quality of the recovered oocytes, which, in turns, consequently influence the preimplantation embryo development and pregnancy outcomes.

If all transvaginal attempts fail, then other approaches to oocyte recovery could be used on one or both ovaries without sacrificing safety or efficacy and is useful in cases where vaginal access to the ovaries is denied [13]. Transvaginal inaccessibility of the ovaries is uncommon and ranges from 0.4% [12] to 1.7% of cases [61]. Nevertheless, the transvaginal approach becomes unfeasible if the ovaries of infertile patients are not easily accessible by transvaginal ultrasonography, due to changes in the anatomy of pelvic organs which may be caused, for example, by biological variations or pelvic disease [62].

Pathological conditions in patients with, for example, previous pelvic surgery, uterine adhesions, which may distort the pelvic anatomy and the normal ovarian location, including endometriosis, uterine fibroids (Fig. 10.39 and 10.40), or congenital anomalies of the genital tract, such as Müllerian anomaly can make the procedure almost impossible [63–65]. Those patients with previous history of inaccessible ovaries at transvaginal oocyte retrieval might be more prone to have this problem; however, it should not be relied upon to accurately predict their occurrence.

It is important to identify such factors, paying special attention to the position of ovaries and the vaginal accessibility during transvaginal follicular monitoring at the ovarian

Fig. 10.38 A needle of equal length but with a reduced caliber, however, allows a normal oocyte recovery and a reduced presence of post-pick pains

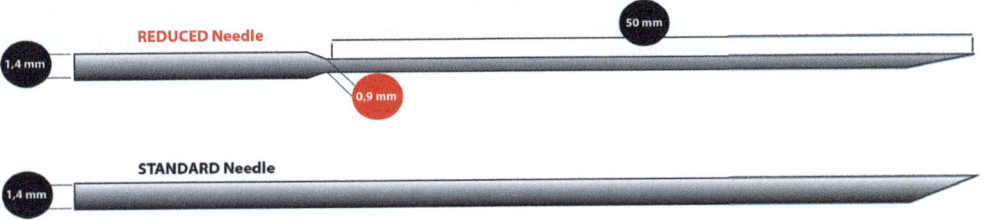

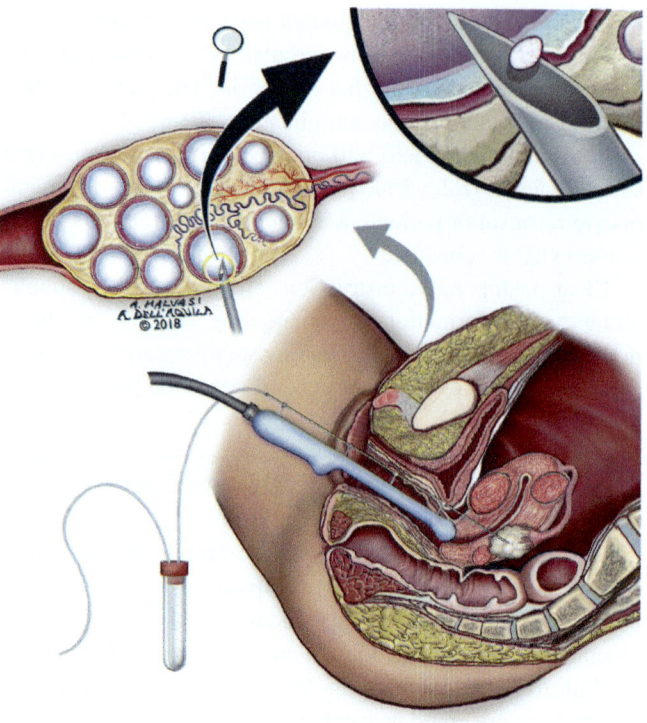

Fig. 10.39 In some cases, the patients to be submitted to the oocyte collection have uterine fibroids, in these cases the operator must be able to perform the oocyte retrieval avoiding the fibroids

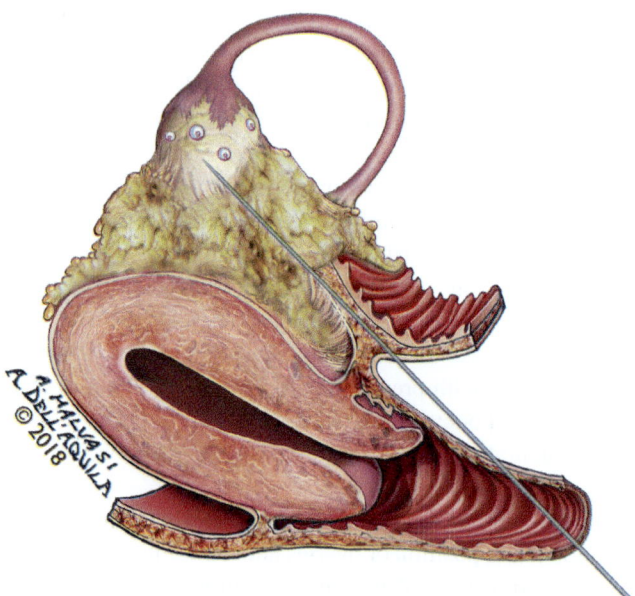

Fig. 10.40 Following the displacement of the ovaries due to physiological causes or contracted adhesions, the ovaries may sometimes be difficult to access with the transvaginal approach

stimulation stage in order to identify those patients at high risk of transvaginal inaccessible ovaries. This information should be documented in the patient's record; most of the times, the professional performing the scan might not be the same one carrying out the OPU.

10.13 Other Approaches to Oocyte Recovery

The decisive element for a good pickup is the surgical accessibility to the ovaries. As such, transvaginal ultrasound-guided aspiration has become the standard of care in women undergoing oocyte retrieval during IVF [12]. Problems arise when the ovaries are not transvaginal accessible (Fig. 10.41). Historically, in these cases laparoscopy has been performed for oocyte retrieval, or these women were not considered candidates for IVF.

An alternative retrieval method is the transabdominal ultrasound-guided retrieval in women whose ovaries are not accessible by transvaginal ultrasonography in either one or both ovaries, despite the usual technique of applying abdominal pressure to push the ovaries into the pelvis [64, 65]. Transabdominal follicular aspiration (Fig. 10.42) can be considered a safe and feasible route for the pickup also in patients undergoing a mixed oocyte retrieval procedure. In fact, when transvaginal aspiration was unfeasible for one ovary, it was attempted to reach the ovary transvaginally by standard procedures for example by applying an abdominal pressure to push ovaries into the pelvis. In the study of Baldini et al., it has been demonstrated that if such procedure fails, the same operator might carry out the transabdominal aspiration to the patient subjected to the same conscious sedation used for transvaginal aspiration. To this aim, patient abdomen is treated with a betadine solution, which is washed off with physiological solution and dried with sterile dressing. The operator moves the same transvaginal ultrasound probe (Fig. 10.43) over the abdomen in correspondence to the ovary and inserts the retrieval needle coupled with a needle guide through the abdomen skin [66]. It should be noted that for all transabdominal aspirations, a single ovarian puncture was requested to retrieve all oocytes. This is an important aspect of this study, since the low elasticity of the abdominal wall might require multiple ovarian punctures through different abdominal wall entries, which may cause pain and increase the risk of abdominal residual scar or injury to the viscera [61].

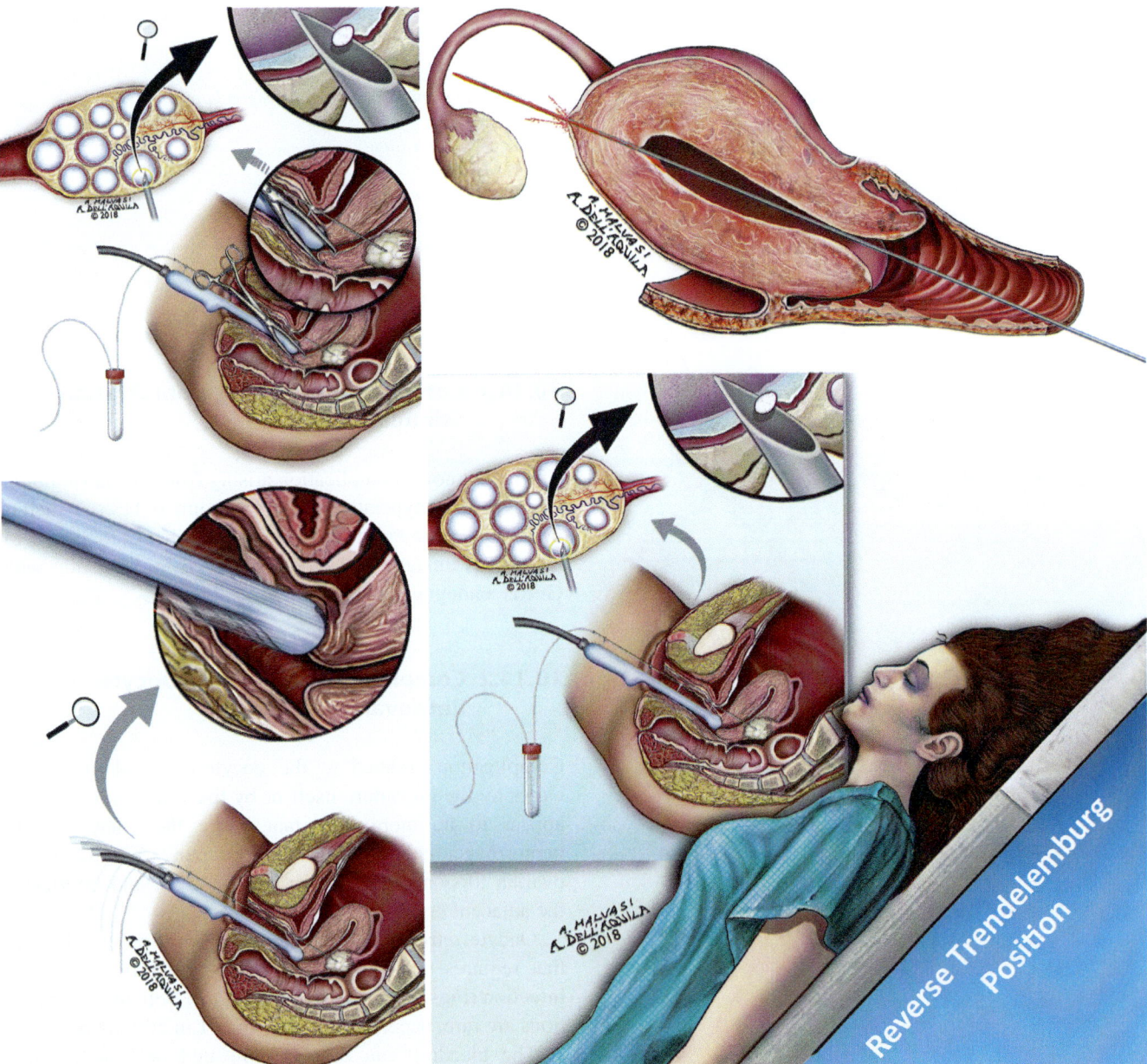

Fig. 10.41 Transmyometrial oocyte retrieval

Although a slight decrease in the total number of oocytes retrieved transabdominally has been reported, this did not translate into fewer mature oocytes or fewer embryos. Furthermore, no increase in oocyte damages was observed [67].

In some cases, when the ovaries are behind or fixed to the uterus, it might be necessary to carry out a transmyometrial oocyte retrieval (Fig. 10.43 and Table 10.4).

10.14 Complications Following Oocyte Retrieval

Short-term complications are usually divided into two categories.

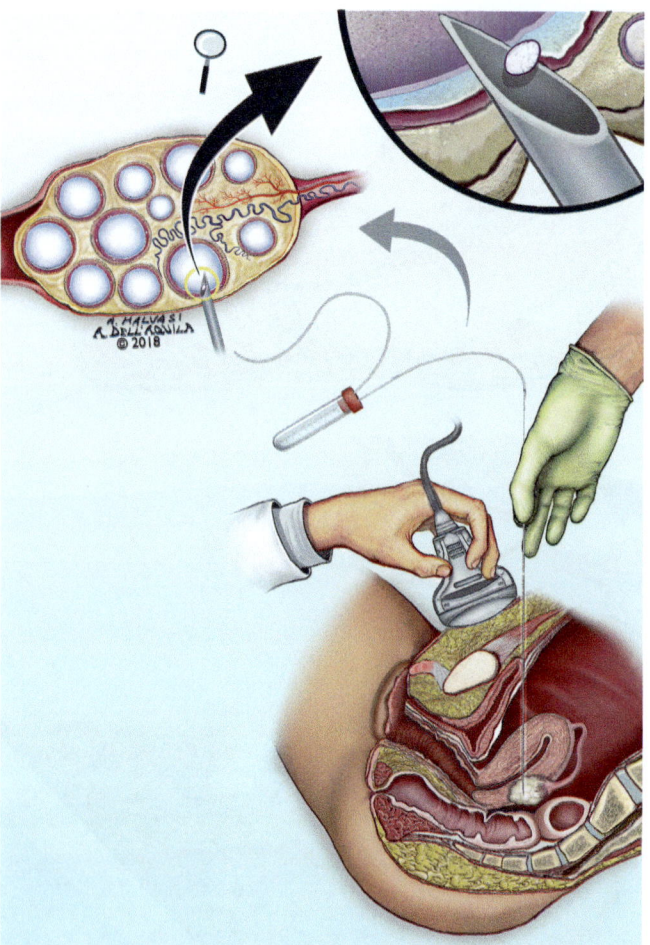

Fig. 10.42 Schematic representation of transmyometrial oocyte retrieval

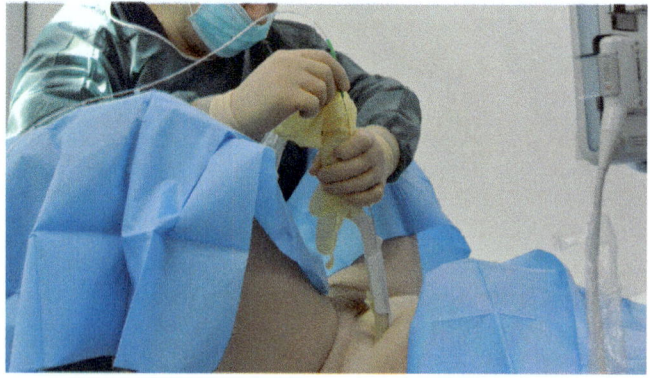

Fig. 10.43 In rare cases of transabdominal pickup in which the transabdominal probe is not available, it is possible to use the transvaginal probe, especially if the ovary is superficially located, since the high frequency of the probe allows a better vision at short distance

Table 10.4 Sequence of maneuver carried out for oocyte retrieval in patients with inaccessible ovaries

1th Maneuver
Bimanual abdominal pressure and vaginal probe pressure
2th Maneuver
Trendelenburg position
3th Maneuver
Cervical clamp traction
4th Maneuver
Transabdominal oocyte retrieval
5th Maneuver
Transmyometrial oocyte retrieval

10.14.1 Complications Arising from Ovarian Stimulation

The main known complication arising from ovarian stimulation is ovarian hyperstimulation syndrome (OHSS), which is nowadays a rare event in oocyte donors, thanks to the use of the GnRH antagonist protocol followed by induction with GnRH analogue [68–70].

10.14.2 Complications Following Oocyte Retrieval

Complications related to the oocyte retrieval procedure, either by the procedure itself or by the venous blood areas, appear to be more important, since they may lead to hemorrhage, pelvic infections (occurring in 0.01–0.6%), ovarian torsion (occurring in 0.08–0.13%), and injuries of the adjacent organs, mainly.

Oocyte retrieval can be associated with pelvic bleeding that requires transfusion or surgical exploration or pelvic infection (Figs. 10.44, 10.45, and 10.46). Both the complications are rare, occurring in fewer than 1 in 500 cases.

The bleeding can be uncomplicated or loss (median: 72 mL; maximum: ≤200 mL; Hgb reduction ≤2 g/day; pelvic free fluid ≤200 mL [48]). The vaginal bleeding requires compression >1 min (2.7%) or tamponade >2 h (0.1%) for vaginal discharge ≥100 mL. Laparoscopy or laparotomy approach is necessary for heavy bleeding.

The intra-abdominal hemorrhage is possible from ovarian vessels or capsule puncture sites or other pelvic vessels. A large prospective study of 2670 oocyte retrievals reported vaginal hemorrhage in 8.6% of cases, with a significant loss (estimated at greater than 100 mL) in 22 (0.8%).

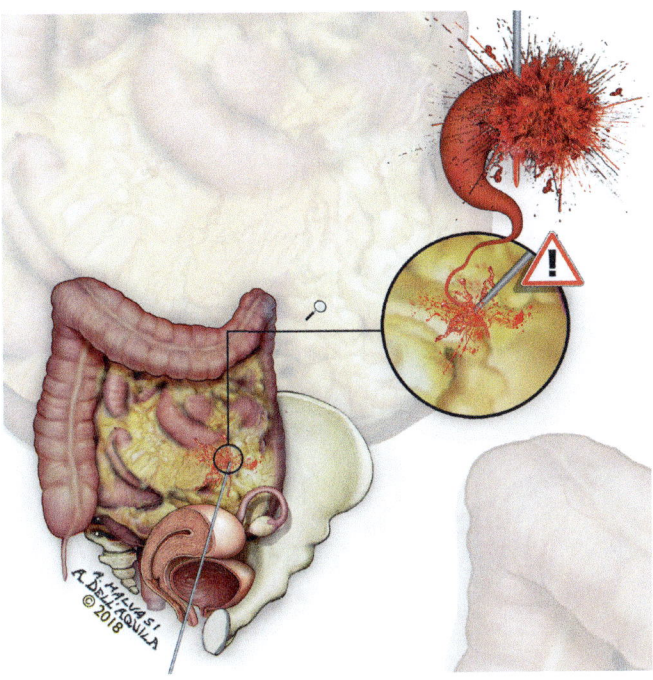

Fig. 10.44 Bleeding complication after oocyte pickup

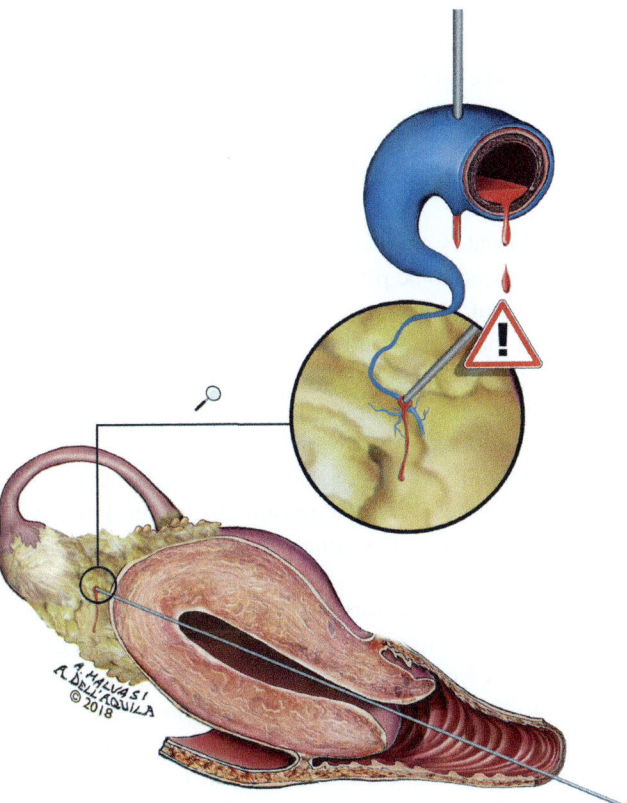

Fig. 10.45 Bleeding complication after oocyte pickup

There were two cases of post procedure bleeding from an ovary causing hemoperitoneum. One case required emergency laparotomy. There was one case of pelvic hematoma formation which did not require intervention [71].

The risk factors are:
- **Lean patients with PCOS: 4.5% (68)**
- **Lower BMI**
- **History of surgery**

In this contest is necessary multidisciplinary approach with early hemodynamic monitoring, transfusion, and surgical management with laparoscopy (blood is aspirated from the peritoneal cavity bleeding site is identified on the ovary follicle is aspirated) or laparotomy [72, 73].

For the prevention of bleeding, it is important to visualize a peripheral follicle in cross section by:

1. **Aspirating all follicles without withdrawing the needle tip from the ovary**
2. **Gently manipulating the needle**
3. **Properly visualizing the tip of the needle**

If color Doppler is available, puncture of blood vessels can be avoided. It is important to prevent the overdistension of follicles during flushing. A routine coagulation screening is however necessary to avoid bleeding before OR in cases with an abnormal coagulation test result. [13]. Pelvic infection following retrieval is also uncommon, occurring in fewer than 1 in 500 cases.

The most common types of pelvic infections are: pelvic abscesses, ovarian abscesses, or infected endometriotic cysts. These complications depend on the technique of vaginal puncture, the presence of pelvic infections or pelvic endometriosis, the puncture of hydrosalpinx or bowel during the procedure, the preoperative vaginal preparation by 10% povidone-iodine or normal saline, and the use of the prophylactic antibiotics. Also, the presence of pelvic adhesions could be associated with pelvic infections after TVOR.

Postoperative pelvic infections occurred in 18 (0.6%) cases and included nine patients with pelvic abscess formation. The examination of the pus from these cases suggested the inoculation of vaginal organisms into the peritoneal cavity through the oocyte retrieval needle.

The use of a proper antibiotic prophylaxis is important to prevent the infections, as well as the cryopreservation and the delayed embryo transfer in the presence of clinical infection signs. It is recommendable before starting an IVF treat-

Fig. 10.46 Oocyte retrieval can be associated with pelvic bleeding that requires transfusion or surgical exploration or pelvic infection

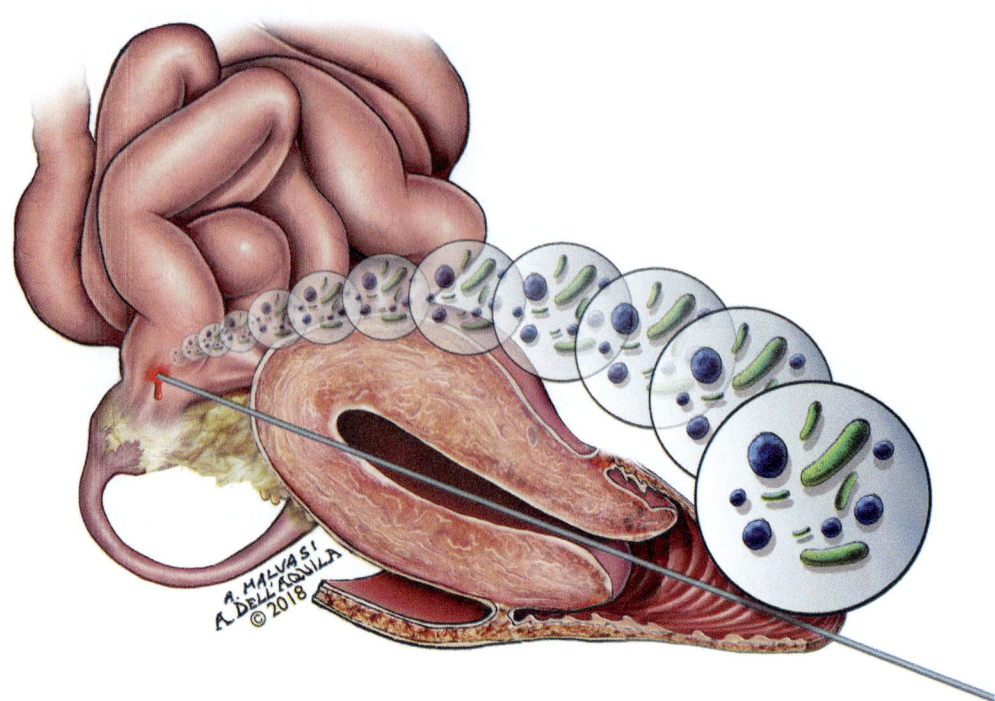

ment to perform a culture for vaginal infections and to proceed only after a negative result [74].

Only 0.7% of patients had severe postprocedural pain requiring hospital admission, and it is possible that these patients did have postoperative bleeding as hemoperitoneum after retrieval causes significant pain.

Rare complications

1. Ruptured endometriotic or dermoid cysts → acute abdominal symptoms → laparotomy.
2. Acute appendicitis due to puncture holes in the appendix.
3. Injury to the ureter: ureterovaginal fistula or ureteral obstruction. Bowel and urinary system injuries to the bladder or ureter have also been reported, but are exceptionally rare.
4. Rectus sheath hematoma.
5. Vaginal perforation in older patients with a history of repeated OR, particularly when the ovaries are difficult to visualize.
6. Vertebral Osteomyelitis: Severe Low Back Pain: Antibiotics.

Additional complications may result from the administration of intravenous sedation or general anesthesia. These include asphyxia caused by airway obstruction, apnea, hypotension, and pulmonary aspiration of stomach contents [75–77]. Another risk of oocyte retrieval is that no oocytes might be obtained. The incidence of this event likely depends on ovarian reserve and response to stimulation and trigger medica-

tions, but even among patients with ultralow AMH values, defined as less than 0.17 ng/mL, the rate of failed retrieval was found to be only 3.3%.

10.15 Conclusions

Oocyte retrieval is affected by the interaction of the several aspects that need to be planned for the execution of the procedure. Vaginal sonography allows the visualization of all follicles on the screen, and therefore, the procedure can be continued for all the remaining follicles.

Vaginal scanning is not influenced by obesity or unfavorable location of the ovaries. Laparoscopic puncture might be difficult in cases of adhesions or unfavorable position of the ovaries. Another reason for the high recovery rate of oocytes by transvaginal follicular aspiration is the small distance between the ovaries and the vaginal probe. As the vaginal probe is introduced into the posterior fornix of the vagina, it is located close to the ovaries. As a consequence, higher frequencies can be used, and the accuracy of imaging follicles is improved. The vaginal probe which was used for our investigations can be easily placed in the posterior fornix of the vagina and can be moved to any angle. In contrast with other sonographically guided aspiration methods or laparoscopy, with vaginal ultrasound no scars remain and the vaginal probe does not enter the urinary bladder. Since transvaginal puncture is a less-invasive procedure, it can be repeated as often as necessary. It is preferred by the patients because of the absence of the typical shoulder pain due to the pneumoperitoneum. Patients can leave the hospital 4–5 h after puncture. In summary, transvaginal follicular aspiration provided a remarkably simple and successful method for oocyte retrieval. The method is rapid, technically simple, and easy to learn.

References

1. Lopata A, Johnston IW, Leeton JF, Muchnicki D, Talbot JM, Wood C. Collection of human oocytes at laparoscopy and laparotomy. Fertil Steril. 1974;25(12):1030–8.
2. Steptoe PC, Edwards RG. Laparoscopic recovery of preovulatory human oocytes after priming of ovaries with gonadotrophins. Lancet. 1970;1(7649):683–9.
3. Khan I, Devroey P, Van den Bergh M, et al. The effect of pneumoperitoneum gases on fertilization, cleavage and pregnancy inhuman in-vitro fertilization and gamete intra-fallopian transfer. Hum Reprod. 1989;4(3):323–6.
4. Kratochwil A, Urban G, Friedrich F. Ultrasonic tomography of the ovaries. Ann Chir Gynaecol Fenn. 1972;61(4):211–4.
5. Wikland M, Hamberger L. Ultrasound as a diagnostic and operative tool for in vitro fertilization and embryo replacement (IVF/ER) programs. J In Vitro Fert Embryo Transf. 1984;1(4):213–6.
6. Lenz S, Lauritsen JG. Ultrasonically guided percutaneous aspiration of human follicles under local anesthesia: a new method of collecting oocytes for in vitro fertilization. Fertil Steril. 1982;38(6):673–7.
7. Parsons J, et al. Oocyte retrieval for in-vitro fertilisation by ultrasonically guided needle aspiration via the urethra. Lancet. 1985;1(8437):1076–7.
8. Dellenbach P, Nisand I, Moreau L, et al. Transvaginal, sonographically controlled ovarian follicle puncture for egg retrieval. Lancet. 1984;1(8392):1467.
9. Ashkenazi J, Ben David M, Feldberg D, Shelef M, Dicker D, Goldman JA. Abdominal complications following ultrasonically guided percutaneous transvesical collection of oocytes for in vitro fertilization. J In Vitro Fert Embryo Transf. 1987;4(6):316–8.
10. Lenz S. Percutaneous oocyte recovery using ultrasound. Clin Obstet Gynaecol. 1985;12(4):785–98.
11. Wikland M, Enk L, Hamberger L. Transvesical and transvaginal approaches for the aspiration of follicles by use of ultrasound. Ann N Y Acad Sci. 1985;442:182–94.
12. Barton SE, et al. Transabdominal follicular aspiration for oocyte retrieval in patients with ovaries inaccessible by transvaginal ultrasound. Fertil Steril. 2011;95(5):1773–6.
13. Roman-Rodriguez CF, et al. Comparing transabdominal and transvaginal ultrasound-guided follicular aspiration: a risk assessment formula. Taiwan J Obstet Gynecol. 2015;54(6):693–9.
14. Ozaltin S, Kumbasar S, Savan K. Evaluation of complications developing during and after transvaginal ultrasound-guided oocyte retrieval. Ginekol Pol. 2018;89(1):1–6.
15. Leung AS, Dahan MH, Tan SL. Techniques and technology for human oocyte collection. Expert Rev Med Devices. 2016;13(8):701–3. ISSN 1745-2422; 1743-4440.
16. Lenz S, Lauritsen JG, Kjellow M. Collection of human oocytes for in vitro fertilisation by ultrasonically guided follicular puncture. Lancet. 1981;1(8230):1163–4.
17. Wiseman DA, Short WB, Pattinson HA, et al. Oocyte retrieval in an in vitro fertilization-embryo transfer program: comparison of four methods. Radiology. 1989;173:99–102.
18. Awonuga A, Waterstone J, Oyesanya O, et al. A prospective randomized study comparing needles of different diameters for transvaginal ultrasound-directed follicle aspiration. Fertil Steril. 1996;65:109–13.
19. Rose BI. Approaches to oocyte retrieval for advanced reproductive technology cycles planning to utilize in vitro maturation: a review of the many choices to be made. J Assist Reprod Genet. 2014;31:1409–19.
20. Yeung QS, Briton-Jones CM, Tjer GC, Chiu TT, Haines C. The efficacy of test tube warming devices used during oocyte retrieval for IVF. J Assist Reprod Genet. 2004;21(10):355–60.
21. Rivera RM, Kelley KL, Erdos GW, Hansen PJ. Alterations in ultrastructural morphology of two-cell bovine embryos produced in vitro and in vivo following a physiologically relevant heat shock. Biol Reprod. 2003;69:2068–77.
22. Shi DS, Avery B, Greve T. Effects of temperature gradients on in vitro maturation of bovine oocytes. Theriogenology. 1998;50(4):667–74.
23. Rivera RM, Hansen PJ. Development of cultured bovine embryos after exposure to high temperatures in the physiological range. Reproduction. 2001;121(1):107–15.
24. Horne R, Bishop CJ, Reeves G, Wood C, Kovac GT. Aspiration of oocytes for in-vitro fertilization. Hum Reprod Update. 1996;2(1):77–85.
25. Fry RC, Niall EM, Simpson TL, et al. The collection of oocytes from bovine ovaries. Theriogenology. 1997;47:977–9879.
26. Bols PEJ, Ysebaert MT, Van Soom A, de Kruif A. Effects of needle tip bevel and aspiration procedure on the morphology and developmental capacity of bovine compact cumulus oocyte complexes. Theriogenology. 1997;47:1221–36.
27. Hashimoto S, Fukuda A, Murata Y, et al. Effect of aspiration vacuum on the developmental competence of immature human oocytes retrieved using a 20-gauge needle. Reprod Biomed Online. 2007;14(4):444–9.
28. Belaisch-Allart JC, Hazout A, Guillet-Rosso F, Glissant M, Testart J, Frydman R. Various techniques for oocyte recovery in an in vitro fertilization and embryo transfer program. J In Vitro Fert Embryo Transf. 1985;2:99–104.
29. Jeffcoat N. Infertility and assisted reproductive technologies. In: Kumar P, Malhotra N, editors. Jeffcoate's principles of gynaecology. 7th ed. New Delhi: Jaypee; 2008. p. 721–3.
30. Kumaran A, Narayan PK, Pai PJ, Ramachandran A, Mathews B, Adiga SK. Oocyte retrieval at 140-mmHg negative aspiration pressure: a promising alternative to flushing and aspiration in assisted reproduction in women with low ovarian reserve. J Hum Reprod Sci. 2015;8:98–102.
31. Wongtra-Ngan S, Vutyavanich T, Brown J. Follicular flushing during oocyte retrieval in assisted reproductive techniques. Cochrane Database Syst Rev. 2010;(9):CD004634.
32. Practice Committees of the American Society for Reproductive Medicine and the Society for Assisted Reproductive Technology. In vitro maturation: a committee opinion. Fertil Steril. 2013;99(3):663–6.
33. Vlahos NF, Giannakikou I, Vlachos A, Vitoratos N. Analgesia and anesthesia for assisted reproductive technologies. Int J Gynaecol Obstet. 2009;105(3):201–5.
34. Healy MW, Hill MJ, Levens ED. Optimal oocyte retrieval and embryo transfer techniques: where we are and how we got here. Semin Reprod Med. 2015;33(2):83–91.
35. Ohlgisser M, Sorokin Y, Heifetz M. Gynecologic laparoscopy. A review article. Obstet Gynecol Surv. 1985;40(7):385–96.
36. Marco AP, Yeo CJ, Rock P. Anesthesia for a patient undergoing laparoscopic cholecystectomy. Anesthesiology. 1990;73(6):1268–70.
37. Kogosowski A, Lessing JB, Amit A, Rudick V, Peyser MR, David MP. Epidural block: a preferred method of anesthesia for ultrasonically guided oocyte retrieval. Fertil Steril. 1987;47(1):166–8.

38. Hammarberg K, Wikland M, Nilsson L, Enk L. Patients' experience of transvaginal follicle aspiration under local anesthesia. Ann N Y Acad Sci. 1988;541:134–7.

39. Bodri D, et al. Comparison between a GnRH antagonist and a GnRH agonist flare-up protocol in oocyte donors: a randomized clinical trial. Hum Reprod. 2006;21(9):2246–51.

40. Andersen AG, et al. Time interval from human chorionic gonadotrophin (HCG) injection to follicular rupture. Hum Reprod. 1995;10(12):3202–5.

41. Taymor ML, et al. Ovulation timing by luteinizing hormone assay and follicle puncture. Obstet Gynecol. 1983;62(2):191–5.

42. Ludwig AK, et al. Perioperative and post-operative complications of transvaginal ultrasound-guided oocyte retrieval: prospective study of >1000 oocyte retrievals. Hum Reprod. 2006;21(12):3235–40.

43. Kroon B, Hart RJ, Wong BM, Ford E, Yazdani A. Antibiotics prior to embryo transfer in ART. Cochrane Database Syst Rev. 2012;(3):CD008995.

44. Cohen J, Debacte C, Pez JP, Junca AM, Cohen-Bacrie P. Transvaginal sonographically controlled ovarian puncture for oocyte retrieval for IVF. J In Vitro Fert Embryo Transfer. 1986;3:309–13.

45. Dellenbach P, Nisand I, Moreau L, Feger B, Plumere C, et al. Transvaginal sonographically controlled follicle puncture for oocyte retrieval. Fertil Steril. 1985;44:656–62.

46. Gembruch U, Diedrich K, Welker B, et al. Transvaginal sonographically guided oocyte retrieval for in-vitro fertilization. Hum Reprod. 1988;3(Suppl 2):59–63.

47. El Hussein E, Balen AH, Tan SL. A prospective study comparing the outcome of oocytes retrieved in the aspirate with those retrieved in the flush during transvaginal ultrasound directed oocyte recovery for in-vitro fertilization. Br J Obstet Gynaecol. 1992;99:841–4.

48. Davis LB, Ginsburg ES. Transmyometrial oocyte retrieval and pregnancy rates. Fertil Steril. 2004;81(2):320–2.

49. Aragona C, et al. Clinical complications after transvaginal oocyte retrieval in 7,098 IVF cycles. Fertil Steril. 2011;95(1):293–4.

50. Ragni G, et al. Blood loss during transvaginal oocyte retrieval. Gynecol Obstet Investig. 2009;67(1):32–5.

51. Siristatidis C, et al. Clinical complications after transvaginal oocyte retrieval: a retrospective analysis. J Obstet Gynaecol. 2013;33(1):64–6.

52. Nakagawa K, et al. The effect of a newly designed needle on the pain and bleeding of patients during oocyte retrieval of a single follicle. J Reprod Infertil. 2015;16(4):207–11.

53. Rose BI, Laky D. A comparison of the cook single lumen immature ovum IVM needle to the Steiner-Tan pseudo double lumen flushing needle for oocyte retrieval for IVM. J Assist Reprod Genet. 2013;30(6):855–60.

54. Miller KA, Elkind-Hirsch K, Benson M, Bergh P, Drews M, Scott RT. A new follicle aspiration needle set is equally effective and as well tolerated as the standard needle when used in a prospective randomized trial in a large in vitro fertilization program. Fertil Steril. 2004;81(1):191–3.

55. Haydardedeoglu B, Cok T, Kilicdag EB, et al. In vitro fertilization-intracytoplasmic sperm injection outcomes in single versus double-lumen oocyte retrieval needles in normally responding patients: a randomized trial. Fertil Steril. 2011;95:812–4.

56. Roque M, Sampaio M, Geber S. Follicular flushing during oocyte retrieval: a systematic review and meta-analysis. J Assist Reprod Genet. 2012;29(11):1249–54.

57. Levy G, Hill MJ, Ramirez CI, et al. The use of follicle flushing during oocyte retrieval in assisted reproductive technologies: a systematic review and meta-analysis. Hum Reprod. 2012;27(8):2373–9.

58. Levens ED, Whitcomb BW, Payson MD, Larsen FW. Ovarian follicular flushing among low-responding patients undergoing assisted reproductive technology. Fertil Steril. 2009;91(4 Suppl):1381–4.

59. Moklin E, et al. Follicular flushing and in vitro fertilization outcomes in the poorest responders: a randomized controlled trial. Hum Reprod. 2013;28(11):2990–5.

60. Seyhan A, et al. Comparison of complication rates and pain scores after transvaginal ultrasound-guided oocyte pickup procedures for in vitro maturation and in vitro fertilization cycles. Fertil Steril. 2014;101(3):705–9.

61. Wikland M, Blad S, Bungum L, Hillensjo T, Karlstrom PO, Nilsson S. A randomized controlled study comparing pain experience between a newly designed needle with a thin tip and a standard needle foe oocyte aspiration. Hum Reprod. 2011;26(6):1377–83.

62. Donoso P, Devroey P. Low tolerance for complications. Fertil Steril. 2013;100(2):299–301.

63. Centers for Disease Control and Prevention, American Society for Reproductive Medicine, Society for Assisted Reproductive Technology. Assisted reproductive technology success rates: national summary and fertility clinic reports. 2010 ed. Atlanta: Department of Health and Human Services; 2008.

64. Seifer D, Collins R, Paushter D, George C, Quigley M. Follicular aspiration: a comparison of an ultrasonic endovaginal transducer with fixed needle guide and other retrieval methods. Fertil Steril. 1988;49:462–7.

65. Damario MA. Transabdominal-transperitoneal ultrasound-guided oocyte retrieval in a patient with Mullerian agenesis. Fertil Steril. 2002;78:189–91.

66. Raziel A, Vaknin Z, Schachter M, Strassburger D, Herman A, et al. Ultrasonographic-guided percutaneous transabdominal puncture for oocyte retrieval in a rare patient with Rokitansky syndrome in an in vitro fertilization surrogacy program. Fertil Steril. 2006;86:1760–3.

67. Baldini D, Lavopa C, Vizziello G, Sciancalepore AG, Malvasi A. The safe use of the transvaginal ultrasound probe for transabdominal oocyte retrieval in patients with vaginally inaccessible ovaries. Front Women Health. 2018;3(2):1–3.

68. Los AG, et al. Single operator ultrasound guided transabdominal oocyte retrieval in patients with ovaries inaccessible transvaginally: a modified technique. Gynecol Obstet. 2014;4:1000214.

69. Baron KT, et al. Emergent complications of assisted reproduction: expecting the unexpected. Radiographics. 2013;33(1):229–44.

70. Pena JE, et al. Usefulness of Doppler sonography in the diagnosis of ovarian torsion. Fertil Steril. 2000;73(5):1047–50.

71. Castillo JC, Garcia-Velasco J, Humaidan P. Empty follicle syndrome after GnRHa triggering versus hCG triggering in COS. J Assist Reprod Genet. 2012;29(3):249–53.

72. Sismanoglu A, et al. Ovulation triggering with GnRH agonist vs. hCG in the same egg donor population undergoing donor oocyte cycles with GnRH antagonist: a prospective randomized cross-over trial. J Assist Reprod Genet. 2009;26(5):251–6.

73. Maxwell KN, Cholst IN, Rosenwaks Z. The incidence of both serious and minor complications in young women undergoing oocyte donation. Fertil Steril. 2008;90(6):2165–71.

74. Elizabeth S. Ginsburg, Catherine Racowsky, in Yen & Jaffe's reproductive endocrinology (7th ed.), 2014.

75. Liberty G, et al. Ovarian hemorrhage after transvaginal ultrasonographically guided oocyte aspiration: a potentially catastrophic and not so rare complication among lean patients with polycystic ovary syndrome. Fertil Steril. 2010;93(3):874–9.

76. Christiaens F, Janssenswillen C, Verborgh C, Moerman I, Devroey P, Van Steirteghem A, Camu F. Propofol concentrations in follicular fluid during general anaesthesia for transvaginal oocyte retrieval. Hum Reprod. 1999;14(2):345–8.

77. El-Shawarby S, et al. A review of complications following transvaginal oocyte retrieval for in-vitro fertilization. Hum Fertil (Camb). 2004;7(2):127–33.

78. Wikland M. Oocyte retrieval. In: Gardner DK, editor. In vitro fertilization a practical approach. New York: Informa Healthcare USA, Inc.; 2006. p. 120–8.

Oocyte Retrieval in Double Stimulation

11

Qiuju Chen and Yanping Kuang

Contents

11.1 Basic Physiology of Follicle Development

11.1.1 Endocrine Control of Follicular Development

Follicle growth from the resting primordial stage until the pre-ovulatory phase takes several months; only the last 2 weeks of this long trajectory are dependent on gonadotropin support (Fig. 11.1) [1]. If maturing antral follicles achieve a distinct stage of development, they are programmed to die, but if serum FSH levels surpass a threshold, these follicles are rescued from atresia, i.e., gain gonadotropin dependence and continue their development [2]. Under normal conditions, elevated FSH levels above the threshold occur during the luteo-follicular transition. The subsequently follicular estradiol secretion inhibits pituitary secretion of FSH, which in turn causes the FSH concentration in the developing cohort follicles to drop below the threshold, the decreased FSH concentrations during the follicular phase are crucial for single dominant follicle selection (Fig. 11.2) [2]. The number of follicles recruited can be increased if endogenous FSH levels are augmented by exogenous gonadotropins or can be reduced if FSH levels are sufficiently diminished [3].

Although of course FSH is the crucial hormone for follicular rescue, LH is necessary for fully functional follicles. The maturing dominant follicle may become less dependent on FSH because of the ability to respond to LH. Basic and clinical experimental evidences indicate that development of ovarian follicles requires a threshold of LH stimulation for adequate follicular development and maturation [4]. The amount of LH required seems to be very low (1–10 IU/L),

Q. Chen (✉) · Y. Kuang
Department of Assisted Reproduction, Shanghai Ninth People's Hospital, Shanghai Jiaotong University School of Medicine, Shanghai, China

© Springer Nature Switzerland AG 2020
A. Malvasi, D. Baldini (eds.), *Pick Up and Oocyte Management*, https://doi.org/10.1007/978-3-030-28741-2_11

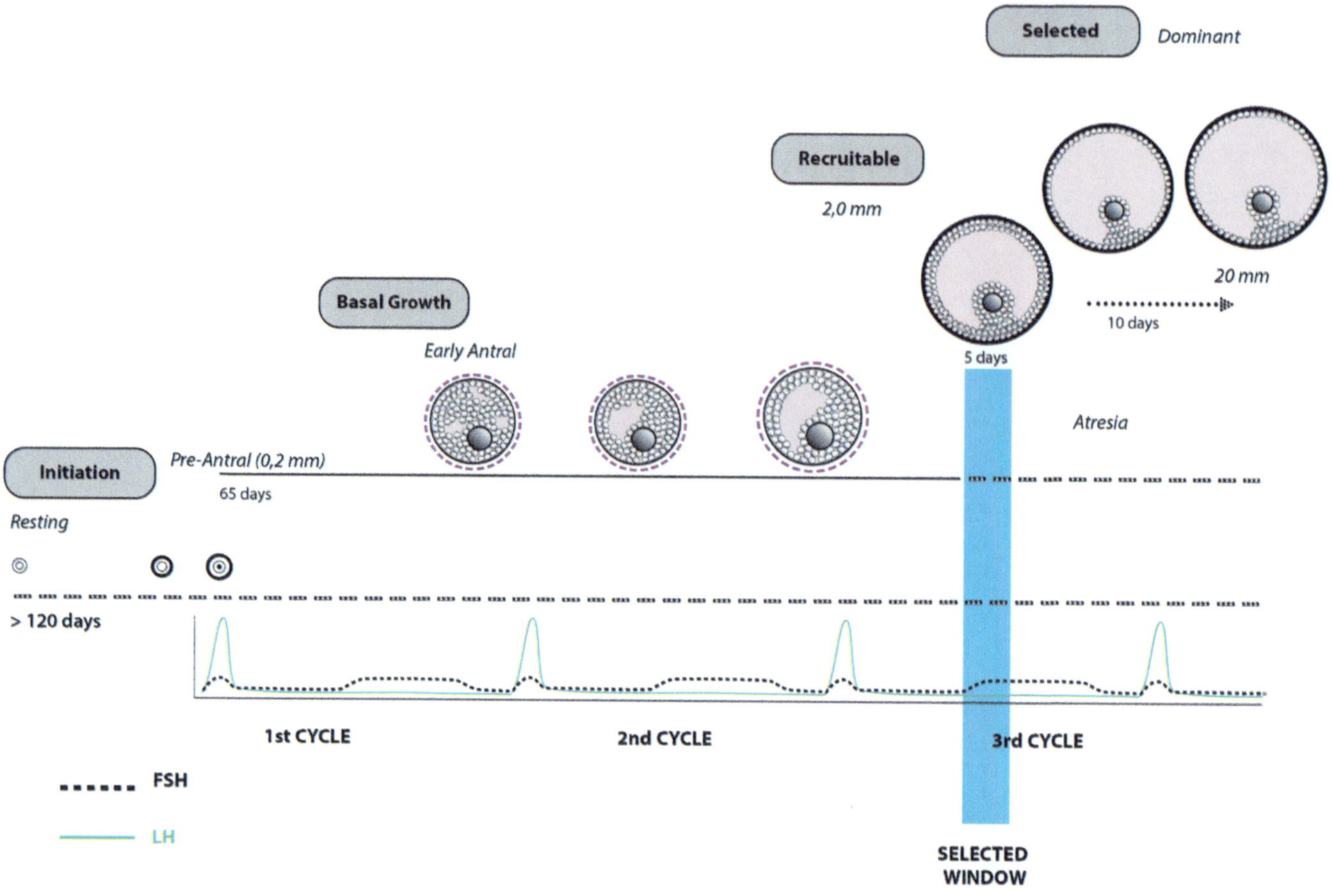

Selected *Dominant*

Recruitable

2,0 mm

20 mm

10 days

Basal Growth

Early Antral

5 days

Atresia

Initiation

Pre-Antral (0,2 mm)

65 days

Resting

> 120 days

1st CYCLE   2nd CYCLE   3rd CYCLE

- - - - - **FSH**

———— LH

SELECTED WINDOW

Fig. 11.1 The profile of follicular development

Fig. 11.2 The different stages of follicle in the ovary

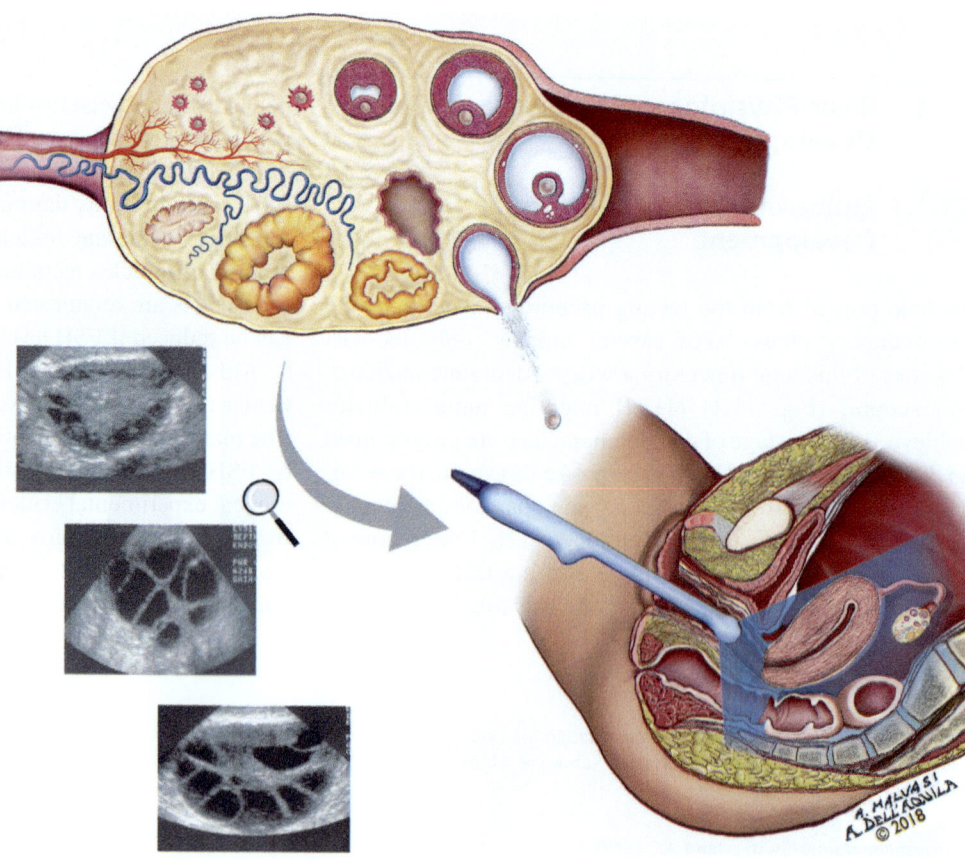

since only 1% of the LH receptors need to be occupied in order to induce the maximal steroidogenic response from theca cells [5]. LH rise then initiates ovulation, and it is necessary for oocyte mature and follicle rupture [6].

11.1.2 Ovarian Hormones Regulate Gonadotropin Secretion

11.1.2.1 Estradiol Regulates FSH and LH Secretion

Estradiol has a dual function in regulating gonadotropin secretion. At low circulating levels, it exerts rapidly expressed, negative feedback control over FSH and LH. At higher, maintained circulating levels, positive feedback becomes the dominant force and a relatively delayed LH and FSH surge is induced.

11.1.2.2 Progesterone Regulates FSH and LH Secretion

Progesterone has multiple effects for regulating gonadotropin secretion [7].

- **First**, the high plasma concentration of progesterone, such as is seen in the luteal phase (4–8 ng/mL in humans) enhances the negative feedback effects of estradiol, FSH, and LH secretion being held down to a very low level [8].
- **Second**, progesterone blocks the positive feedback effect of estradiol on gonadotropin release. The physiologic plasma levels of progesterone, whether achieved by normally functioning corpora lutein or the artificial imposture by progestin implant during the follicular phase of the cycle, prevent the estrogen-induced gonadotropin discharge in intact rhesus macaque [9, 10] (Fig. 11.3). The same blocking effect of progesterone is observed when progesterone is simultaneously administered with estradiol benzoate to castrated women of fertile age with uninterrupted estradiol replacement [11]. This anti-positive feedback of progesterone requires an intact hypothalamus, for the physiological levels of progesterone fail to block the positive feedback in monkeys with hypothalamic lesions on a replacement regimen of exogenous GnRH [12]. Moreover, progesterone does not interfere with the negative feedback inhibition of gonadotropin secretion by estrogen [9].

- **Third**, progesterone plays a facilitatory role in the initiation of the pre-ovulatory gonadotropin surge after a period of estrogen priming in female monkey, ewes, and human [9, 13–15]. Leyendecker et al. provide experimental evidences in women that progesterone—at low serum levels around 1–2 ng/mL, with a short latency phase of about 3 h, and with adequate estrogen priming—can induce a positive feedback effect in advance, since estradiol benzoate alone induces an LH surge at this stage of the cycle after a considerably longer latency phase (Fig. 11.4) [16, 17]. Also in the rhesus macaque, the positive feedback can, as in women, be augmented and advanced by additional and properly timed administration of progesterone [18].

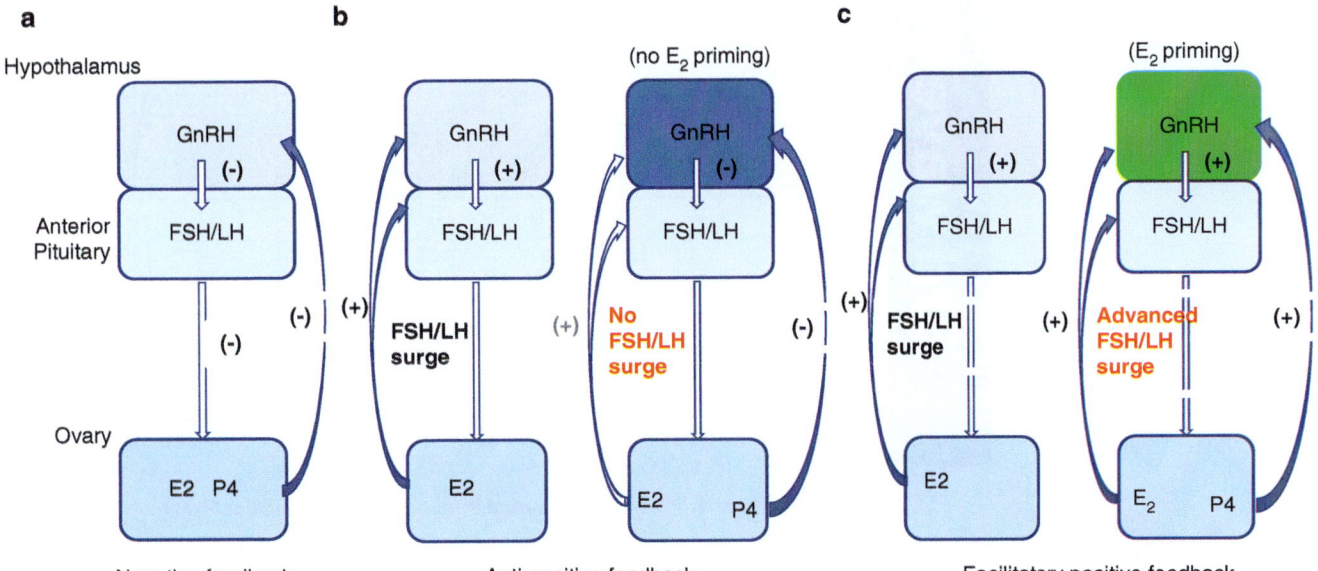

Fig. 11.3 Progesterone has multiple effects for regulating gonadotropin secretion. (**a**) Progesterone enhances the negative feedback effects of estrogen in the luteal phase (negative feedback). (**b**) Progesterone blocks the estrogen-induced LH surge in human or monkeys with intact gonad axis and no existing estrogen priming (anti-positive feedback); (**c**) Progesterone plays a facilitatory role in the initiation of LH surge after a period of estrogen priming in human (facilitatory positive feedback)

Fig. 11.4 The follicle morphologic changes occurring in association with the development of follicle waves during the human menstrual cycle. Sixty-eight percent of women with regular cycles have two waves of follicular growth during a single menstrual cycle, and 32% of women have three waves through daily ultrasound monitoring

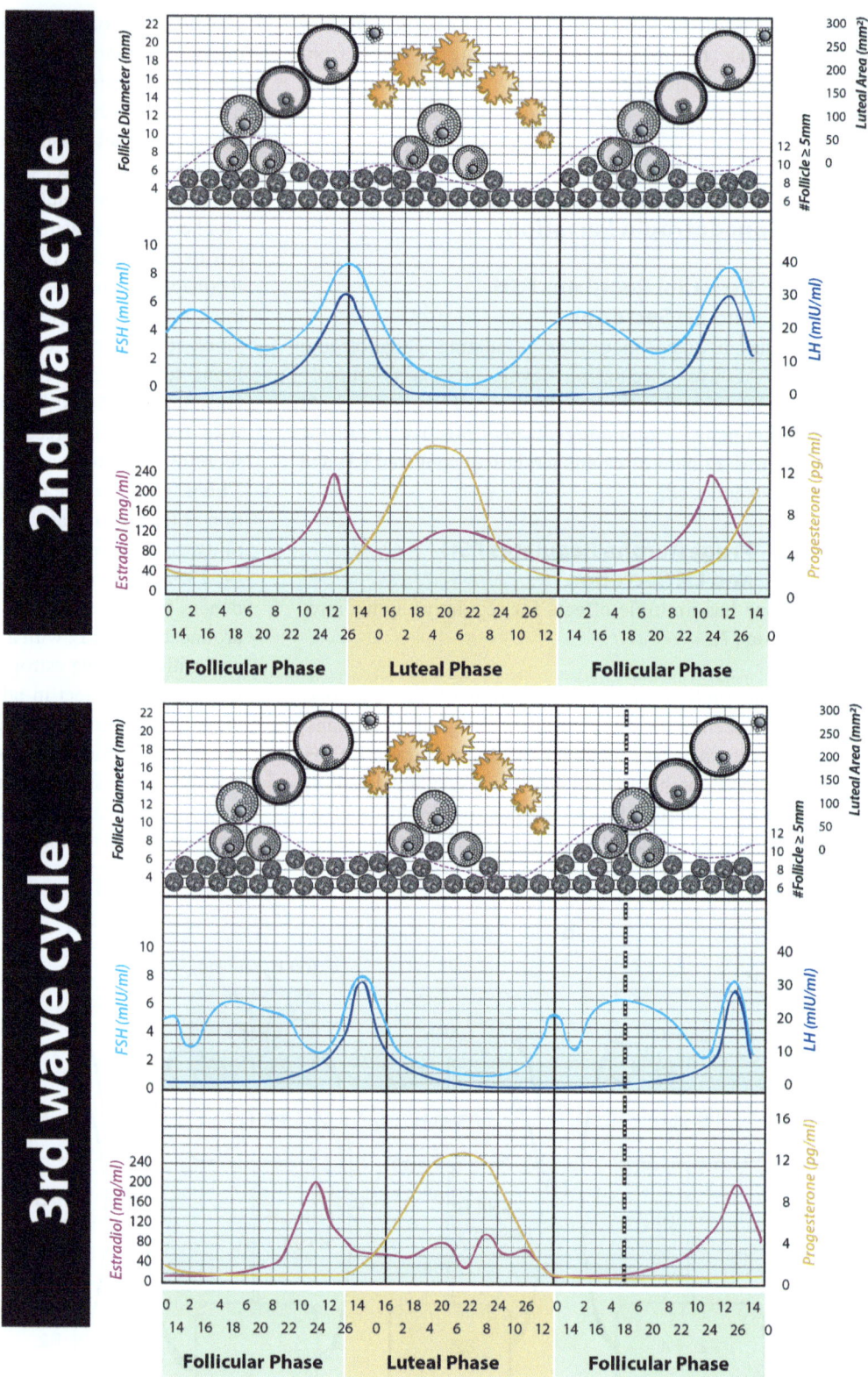

Thus, the actions of progesterone that could occur at the hypothalamus to enhance or inhibit the GnRH secretion depend on the relative time of the rise of progesterone and estrogen [9, 13–15]. Progesterone exerts its facilitatory effect at the level of the pituitary and its blocking effect at the level of the central nervous system from a series of experiments performed in acyclic, but gonad-intact, rhesus females given exogenous GnRH after hypothalamic lesioning [10, 19, 20].

11.1.3 The Antral Follicles in the Luteal Phase

During the luteal phase, LH and FSH levels are comparatively low and are insufficient to maintain antral follicle development, so follicular atresia occurs. After luteolysis, a new cycle then begins as tonic gonadotropin levels are elevated and progesterone is low. In humans, the follicular phase is about 10–14 days, while in many species such as cow, pig, sheep, and horse, the follicular phase is brief and the major part of follicular growth occurs during the luteal phase of the previous cycle, because FSH and LH levels in these species do not fall to such low levels during the luteal phase [21].

The competence of the antral follicles in normal human ovaries during the luteal phase is not distinguishable from atretic follicles in terms of the number, size range, and steroidogenic activities [22]. The mean number of antral follicles (AFC) was not different in the early-follicular, late-follicular, and luteal phase [23, 24]. Granulosa cells from the luteal phase follicles are responsive to FSH with respect to progesterone and estradiol biosynthetic activity, the aromatase system in the cells from the mid- to late-luteal phase follicles is significantly more responsive to FSH than that in cells from late follicular or early luteal phase follicles [22]. Another evidence about the competence of cumulous oocyte complexes (COCs) retrieved during the luteal phase is that the potential of COCs or in vitro mature (IVM) is comparable whatever the phase of the cycle at which immature eggs in breast cancer patients [25–27]. In addition, some studies show that immature oocytes retrieved during cesarean section (with exposure to high serum progesterone concentrations) are capable of IVM and could lead to live births after fertilization [28, 29]. These materials confirm that during the luteal phase, remaining small antral follicles may be in the early stages of follicular development, suggesting that the ovary could be continuously stimulated during the menstrual cycle.

11.1.4 Waves of Folliculogenesis During the Menstrual Cycle

Contrary to the traditional theory that a single cohort of antral follicles grows only at the early follicular phase, it has been demonstrated that there are two or three waves (namely cohorts) of follicular growth in a single menstrual cycle. Baerwald et al. have shown that 68% of women with regular cycles have two waves of follicular growth during a single menstrual cycle, and 32% of women have three waves through daily ultrasound monitoring (Fig. 11.4) [30, 31].

These waves can be differentiated between major and minor, depending on whether one follicle shows dominance over the others or not, most women having just one major wave with dominance [32]. The follicular wave that emerges in the early to middle follicular phase is ovulatory while the waves emerging in the luteal phase are anovulatory. An elevation in circulating FSH appears to precede the recruitment of each follicular wave during the interovulatory interval in women [30]. The development potential of anovulatory follicles in the luteal phase occurs as a result of progesterone-mediated inhibition of LH secretion to levels that allow follicular development to proceed to the antral or late antral stage, but do not allow the LH surge and ovulation to occur. Anovulatory follicles do not grow as large, on average, as ovulatory follicles. However, a notable number of women exhibited anovulatory follicles that grew to an ostensibly preovulatory diameter [31]. A preliminary trial showed that using pharmacological (recombinant hCG administration) and mechanical (aspiration of dominant follicle) interventions were efficient to induce follicular wave emergence in infertile women [33].

The role of the corpus luteum (CL) in regulating follicular wave dynamics has been studied in women and domestic farm animals (Fig. 11.5). No differences in the size or lifespan of the CL, progesterone, or estradiol secretion were detected in women with two versus three waves or in women with major versus minor waves preceding the ovulatory wave [34]. However, the presence of the CL appeared to influence dominant follicle selection in women with three waves. Luteal regression and progesterone withdrawal occur later in cows with three versus two follicular waves, at which time the viable dominant follicle present goes on to ovulate [35, 36].

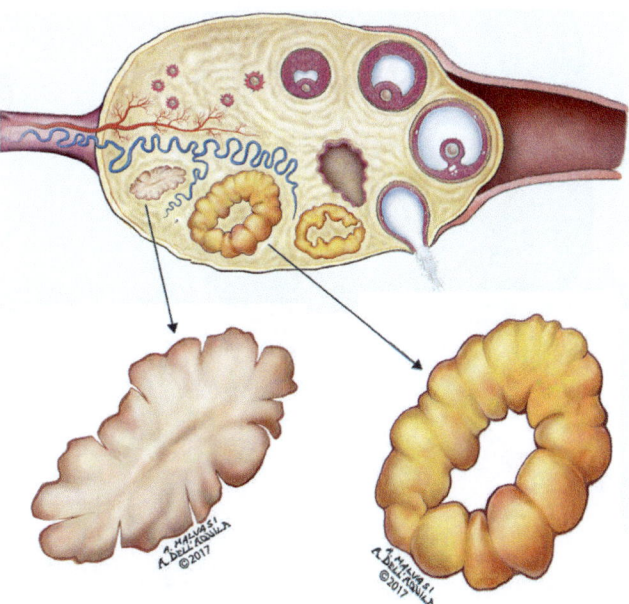

Fig. 11.5 Two stages of corpus luteus

It is important to recognize that folliculogenesis is a discontinuous process, independent from the rhythm of the menstrual cycle. The competence of antral follicle in the luteal phase is comparable with those in the follicular phase in previous reports of IVM or in vitro culture. So we presume that the antral follicles in the luteal phase are not atresic, but may be unawakened due to the suppressed FSH/LH, and they have the potential to response to gonadotropin. Follicles can be stimulated to ongoing and gonadotropin-dependent development when the appropriate endocrine signal (i.e., elevated serum FSH levels) is operative [37]. It could, therefore, be speculated that the developing follicles in the luteal phase have the potential to ovulate in the presence of an exogenous LH surge. This is the basic principle to introduce new strategies for ovarian stimulation.

11.2 Controlled Ovarian Stimulation

Based on the vitrification and freeze-all policy, new stimulation approaches together with advanced cryopreservation techniques allow for a total "disarticulation" between the time of the menstrual cycle, ovarian stimulation start, and embryo transfer [38, 39].

In addition to conventional protocols, new regimens are emerging with ovarian stimulation starting in the late follicular phase, luteal phase, random-start ovarian stimulation, and double stimulation.

11.2.1 Follicular Phase Ovarian Stimulation

Conventional ovarian stimulation regimens use gonadotropins to promote multifollicular development and GnRH analogue to prevent the LH surge and premature ovulation [40]. The analogue improves the success of IVF cycles by optimizing oocyte retrieval and synchronization of the endometrium. Ovarian stimulation in these protocols starts in the early follicular phase or equivalent. The mild stimulation is performed using a low dose of gonadotropin with or without clomiphene/letrozole; it also begins at the early follicular phase and results with less oocyte yields but with the advantages of patient-friendly and safety [41].

11.2.2 Luteal-Phase Ovarian Stimulation

The luteal-phase ovarian stimulation protocol is originally used for urgent fertility preservation in cancer patients (Fig. 11.6) [42, 43]. Recently they have been tested outside of this context, in normal and poor responders [44–46].

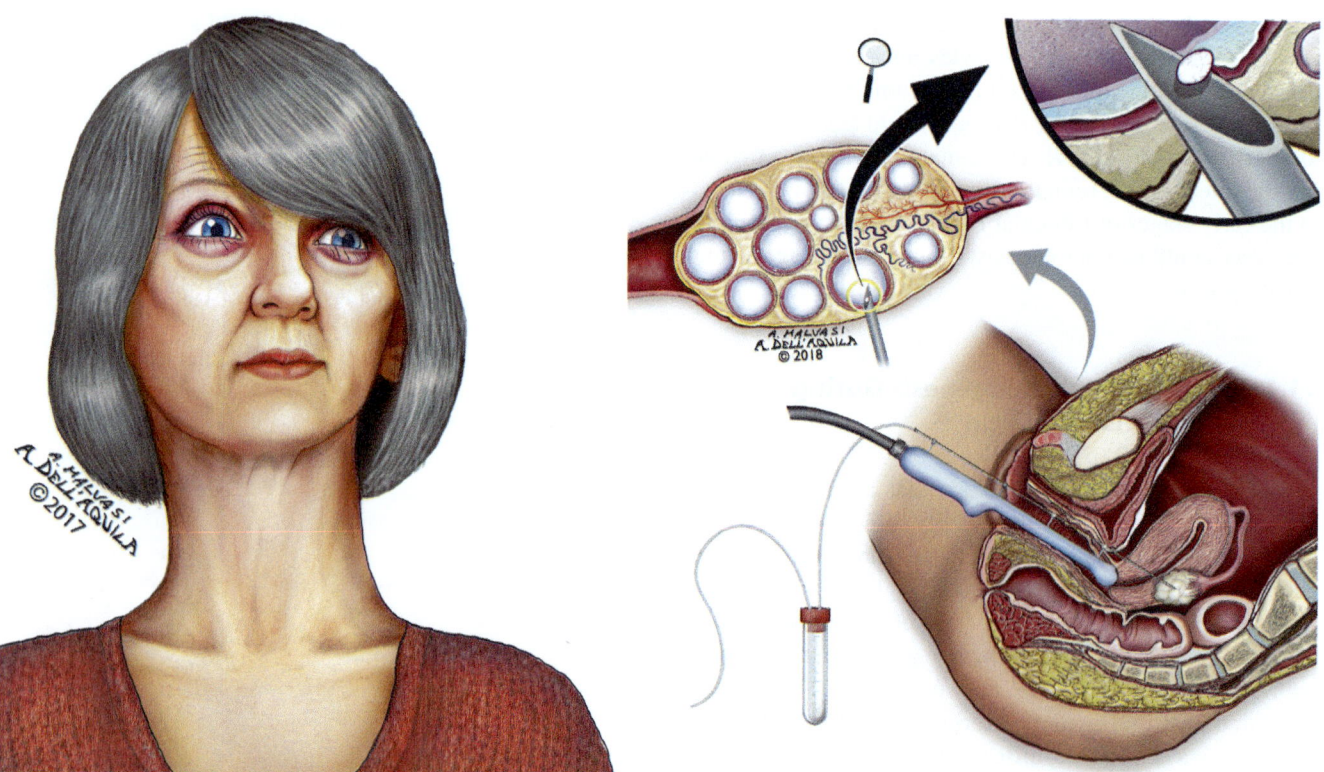

Fig. 11.6 The luteal-phase ovarian stimulation protocol is originally used for urgent fertility preservation in cancer patients

Table 11.1 The follicle growth and endocrinological changes in the case of luteal-phase ovarian stimulation

Cycle days	3	4	5	6	7	8	9	10	11	12	13	14	15	16	17	18	19	21
Letr. 2.5 mg/day		+	+	+	+	+	+	+	+	+							Trigger with GnRhA 0.1 mg	OPU
HMG 150 IU/day		+	+	+	+	+	+	+	+	+	+	+	+	+	+	+		
FSH (IU/L)	8.53							14.83						9.36			8.83	
LH (IU/L)	2.59							6.36						0.61			0.7	
E2 (pg/L)	87							56						208			507	
P (ng/L)	0.2							2.1						19.2			6	
Ultrasound																		
Follicles																		
Right	10.4							7									21.8	
	8							3.7						10.4			14.6	
								3.7						8.9*2			11.7	
														6.1*2			10.3	
Left	3.9													5.9			9	
														5.9			8.7	

The first live birth of embryos developed from oocytes retrieved following luteal phase stimulation was reported in 2009 [47]. A 40-year-old woman with a 10-year history of primary infertility was given hMG 150 IU and letrozole 2.5 mg from cycle day 3 onwards. Her cycle spontaneously transitioned into the luteal phase beginning on cycle day 10 but the follicles continued growth with hMG stimulation. GnRH agonist 0.1 mg was given for the final stage of oocyte maturation, resulting into four mature oocytes and two top-quality embryos for vitrified cryopreservation (Table 11.1). Two months later, the two embryos were transferred during a natural cycle, creating a twin pregnancy and a favorable delivery. Three-year follow-up showed that the physical and psychomotor development of the twin babies were in the normal range of children conceived naturally [47]. This case report documents favorable outcomes of oocyte development competence following luteal-phase stimulation and opens the door to generalize the successful outcome from luteal-phase stimulation into a routine setting.

After this, Prof. Yanping Kuang and his team attempted to stimulate the luteal-phase existing antral follicles in patients who did not respond well during the follicular phase stimulation or with diminished ovarian reserve. They faced the first problem that the luteal-phase antral follicles were not sensitive to the exogenous gonadotropin stimulation compared with conventional protocols, the duration of hMG in some cases was very long (20.6 days) with low efficiency, then they attempted to increase the ovarian response by adjuvant usage of letrozole in luteal-phase ovarian stimulation. The improved effects after letrozole administration were obvious. Then a prospective trial of 242 women with normal ovarian function and undergoing their first IVF/ICSI treatment was initiated using letrozole and HMG for luteal-phase stimulation after spontaneous ovulation, the protocol of luteal-phase ovarian stimulation is shown in (Fig. 11.7). All participants succeeded in producing oocytes, and 227 women had highest-quality embryos to cryopreserve (93.8%).

The average number of oocytes retrieved was 13.1, producing an average of 4.8 good embryos. The mean duration of hMG stimulation was 10.2 ± 1.6 days, with a mean dose of 2211.3 ± 422.7 IU, so adjuvant administration of letrozole in luteal-phase ovarian stimulation appeared to increase the sensitivity of follicles to gonadotropins and reduce the stimulation duration, but the specific mechanism should be further investigated.

For the outcome of frozen embryo transfers (FETs), the clinical pregnancy rate, ongoing pregnancy rate, and implantation rate were, respectively, 55.46% (127/229), 48.91% (112/229), and 40.37% (174/431) [48]. Clomiphene citrate also has the same effects as letrozole in luteal-phase ovarian stimulation, but the relevant data are rarely reported.

Unexpectedly, no cases experienced a premature LH surge during the luteal-phase ovarian stimulation cycles [48] (Fig. 11.8). The serum LH on the trigger day was only 1.9 mIU/mL (range 0.1–11.0 mIU/mL) in 242 women, the endogenous increased estrogen levels did not induce LH surge but a GnRH agonist-induced LH surge appeared, which provided a sound evidence of modest-extent pituitary suppression during the luteal-phase stimulation (Fig. 11.9). The phenomenon has far-reaching significance in removing the scruples of blocking an endogenous LH surge for IVF treatment. It primarily simplifies ovarian stimulation protocols and makes it easy to handle procedure monitoring.

The first European feasibility study [49] was a prospective case–control study of good prognosis patients with ten in each arm. Luteal phase stimulation was started between day 19 and 21 of a spontaneous menstrual cycle, with 300 IU FSH and a daily GnRH antagonist, while in the control group the starting dose was 150–225 IU. The rates of maturity, fertilization, and embryo development were identical in the two groups. It found a lack of significance for this strategy because of the higher dose of FSH required for luteal-phase stimulation. However, the comparison of the two groups was

Fig. 11.7 The protocol of luteal-phase ovarian stimulation is shown. Luteal-phase ovarian stimulation in combination with freeze-all was confirmed its efficacy and safety

Protocol of luteal-phase ovarian stimulation

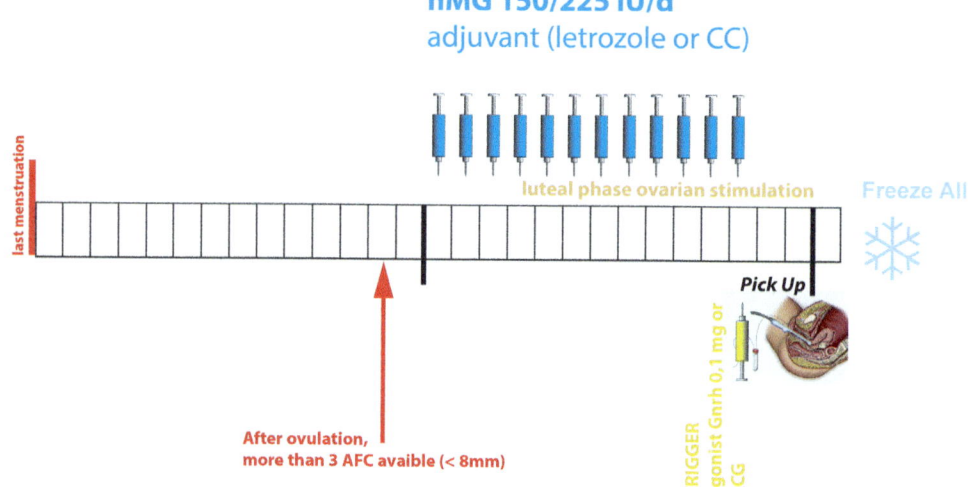

Fig. 11.8 The endogenous increased estrogen levels did not induce LH surge in luteal-phase ovarian stimulation but a GnRH agonist-induced LH surge appeared, which provided a sound evidence of modest-extent pituitary suppression during the luteal-phase stimulation

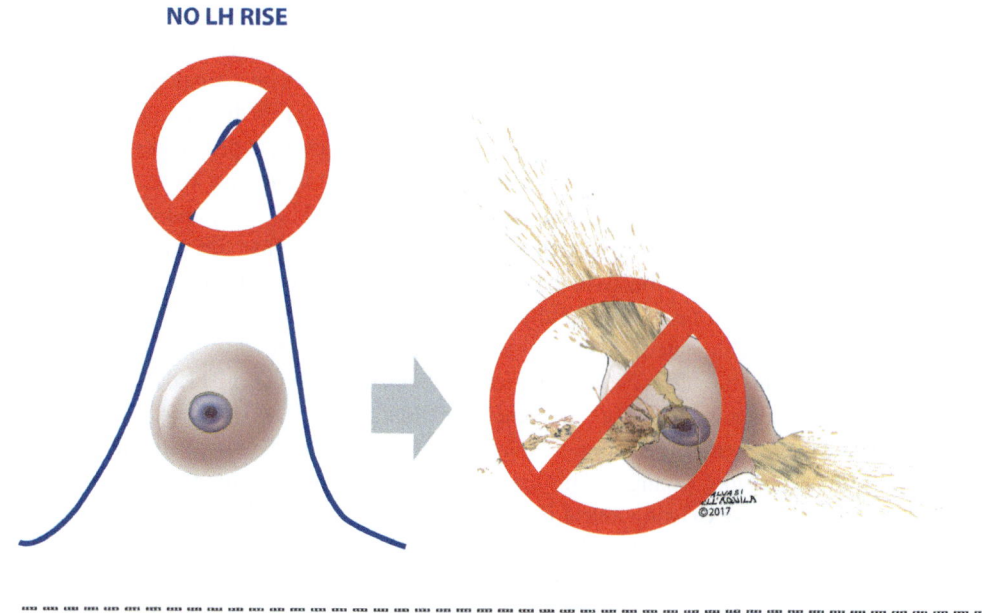

flawed because of a higher starting dose for luteal stimulation.

In a large retrospective study of luteal stimulation in normalovulatory patients [50], the comparison of three protocols (luteal stimulation versus mild stimulation versus the short agonist protocol) confirmed that the duration of stimulation and total dose were higher (Fig. 11.10) with luteal-phase stimulation but were accompanied by a higher number of mature oocytes and top-quality embryos.

Moreover, the study shows on a large scale that the use of an agonist or antagonist is not necessary in the luteal phase

and that endogenous progesterone alone is sufficient to block the LH surge. In this retrospective study with good-prognosis women, the implantation rates are identical with luteal-phase stimulation (35.5%) and mild stimulation (34.8%), but significantly lower with the standard short agonist protocol (31.8%). Birth rates were also lower with the short agonist protocol, and the levels of miscarriage were identical among the three groups. The health of children born following the luteal-phase stimulation was confirmed by the comparable gestational age, birth weight, neonatal anomalies, or number of malformations [51].

Fig. 11.9 The early protocol of double stimulation for oncological patients

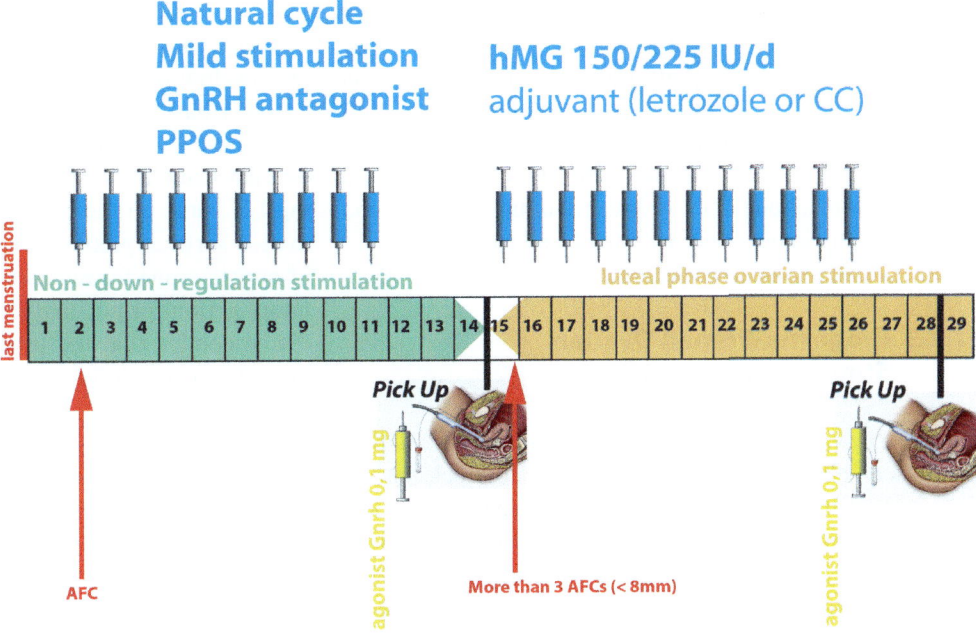

Fig. 11.10 Difference between the proliferative phase and the luteal phase

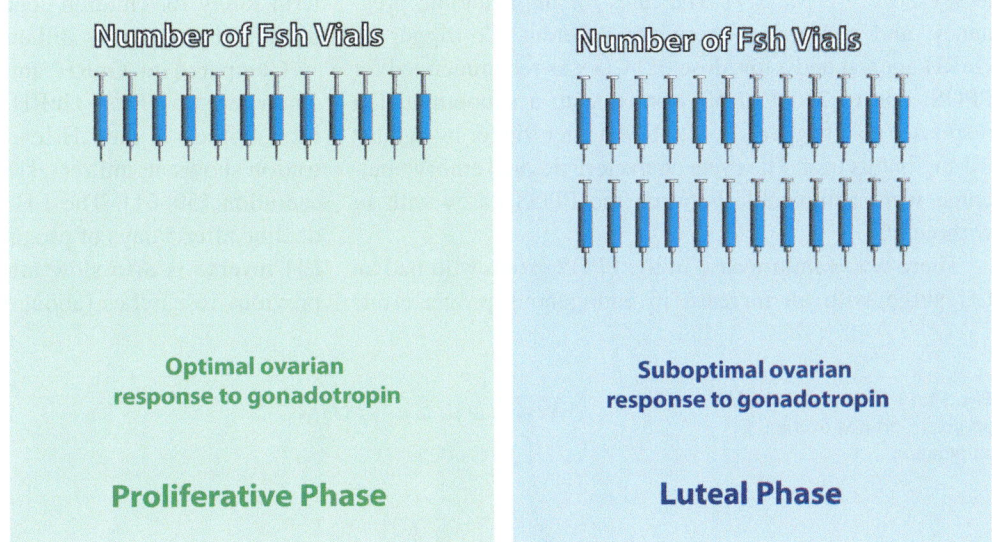

These studies demonstrate that the protocol of luteal-phase ovarian stimulation is able to produce competent oocytes/embryos, with optimal pregnancy outcome from the subsequent FET. These data also approve that no spontaneous LH surge in the luteal-phase ovarian stimulation occurs, and the use of a GnRH antagonist is not necessary in the luteal phase [48, 50, 52]. But there are also some disadvantages in performing luteal-phase stimulation.

First, the recognition of entering into early luteal phase is not as obvious and easily recognizable as menstruation, but dependent on urine LH kit, ultrasound examination, or serum hormone measurement.

Second, the luteal-phase stimulation is not suitable for the cases who show diverse-size follicles after spontaneous ovulation, and this status is not predictable at advance.

Third, the slightly higher gonadotropin consumption in luteal-phase stimulation than conventional stimulation reflects the suboptimal ovarian response to gonadotropin stimulation, and it is another adverse factor (Fig. 11.10).

The clinical experiences about luteal-phase ovarian stimulation make a privilege and chance to study the role of progesterone in preventing premature LH surge. After the transition stage of using luteal-phase ovarian stimulation, the improved protocol of progestin-primed ovarian stimulation (PPOS) is released to perform ovarian stimulation by simultaneously using exogenous progestin and gonadotropins from the early follicular phase, which rapidly becomes a dominant protocol due to its advantages of high efficacy and patient-friendly in our clinic with freeze-all strategy.

11.2.3 Progestin-Primed Ovarian Stimulation (PPOS)

PPOS is a new regimen of ovarian stimulation using oral progestin as an alternative of GnRH analogue to block the LH surge and premature ovulation [52–57]. The specific protocol is shown in Fig. 11.11. Kuang et al. reported a randomized clinical trial of PPOS versus short protocol in women with normal ovarian function. The results showed that the duration of stimulation was significantly longer by 1 day, and the total dose of HMG was higher (~+400 IU) with PPOS, but the numbers of mature oocytes and viable embryos were not significantly different in a population of normal responders (9.9 vs. 9.0; 4.3 vs. 3.7). The rates for implantation, pregnancy, and miscarriage were not different. Co-trigger by GnRH agonist and a low dose of hCG was recommended for PPOS, due to 3 out of 50 women with a suboptimal LH response (post-trigger LH < 20 IU/L) after trigger by agonist 0.1 mg in this trial. The cycle characteristics and embryo outcome were comparable between the PPOS cases with or without hCG.

There was a failure case in the PPOS group who had an LH surge with an increase in endogenous progesterone (1/150). In her case, stimulation was nevertheless continued, and oocyte retrieval enabled collection of a number of oocytes that was similar to the group average. This case had a higher basic estrogen level at the earlier follicular phase (85 pg/mL), so the action of exogenous progestin during ovarian stimulation spontaneously converted into facilitating LH surge on the basis of estrogen-priming, not blocking LH surge as predesigned. It is described as the third role of progesterone for regulating pituitary function (the facilitatory action for positive feedback) in Sect. 11.1.2. So it is recommended that the progestin has to be started before estradiol rises (<50–70 pg/mL) for controlled ovarian stimulation.

Multiple types of oral progestin can be used as gonadotropin adjuvant in PPOS. Medroxyprogesterone acetate (MPA) is replaced with utrogestan or dydrogesterone in large-sample clinical trials, resulting into the well-controlled LH levels and comparable pregnancy outcomes [52, 55–57]. A retrospective cohort study including 4596 newborns from PPOS, agonist short protocol, and mild stimulation suggested that compared with conventional ovarian stimulations, PPOS neither compromised neonatal outcomes of IVF newborns nor increased the prevalence of congenital malformations [58]. The long-term safety for children conceived with ovarian stimulation using oral progestin is still under investigation.

Compared to GnRH antagonist, PPOS has its unique characteristics. First, GnRH antagonist administration rapidly suppresses the LH level while progesterone administration shows an indirect, slow suppression on pituitary LH secretion [59–61]. The LH level in PPOS is recorded to decline after 5 days of progesterone administration, and the LH reverse is also slow after progesterone withdrawal in previous researches (about 5–7 days). Second, the role of

Fig. 11.11 The protocol of progestin-primed ovarian stimulation

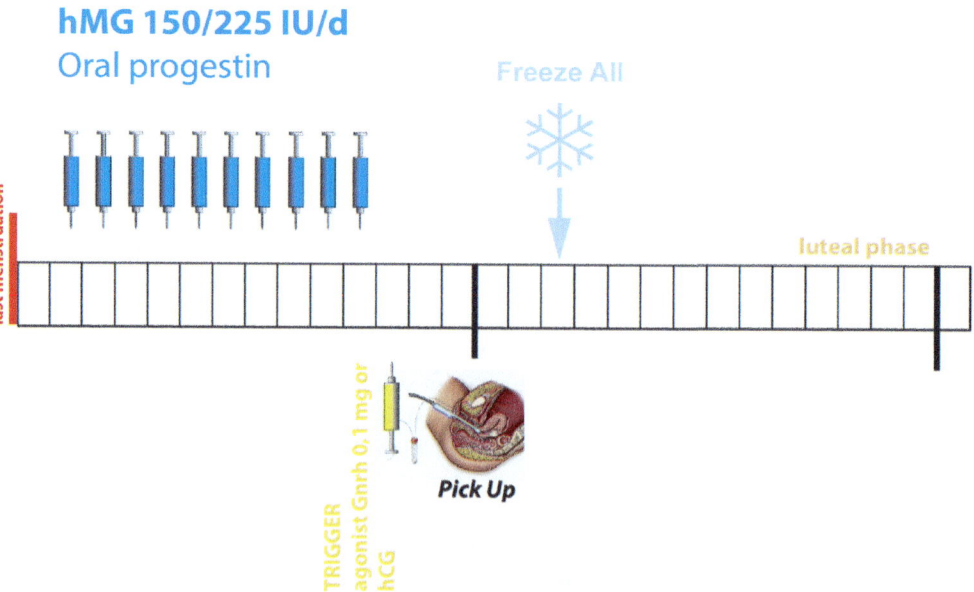

progesterone's inhibition of LH surge is highly dependent on the estrogen status and duration as detailed in the first section, so in controlled ovarian stimulation, progestin has to be administered from the early follicular phase (before estrogen priming). The indication of PPOS is not recommended for the cases with higher basal estradiol levels (>70 pg/mL) [52]. Third, the trigger by GnRH agonist alone is sufficient in mostly PPOS cases except that 2.71% of all cases show a sub-optimal LH response in a large-sample retrospective trial [62], which is in parallel with the reports of GnRH antagonist protocol [63, 64], so the co-trigger by GnRHa and low dose of hCG is recommended in PPOS.

11.2.3.1 Randomized-Start Ovarian Stimulation

The concept of "random-start" or "flexible-start" protocols means starting stimulation at any time in the menstrual cycle rather than precisely in the early follicular phase or after downregulation. The "random-start" stimulation has led to shorter ovarian stimulation protocols and may be beneficial for the cases whose time constraints are associated with emergency fertility preservation before starting oncology treatments [65–70].

Whether the random start of stimulation might alter the size of the oocyte crop, its competence, or both? The oocyte yields of the "random-start" protocols are found to equal as those of ovarian stimulation started in the early follicular phase in several reports [71, 72]. A case series study reported that using random-start GnRH antagonist cycles started in the late follicular or luteal phase, the duration of controlled ovarian hyperstimulation ranged between 8 and 13 days, and a total of 14–40 oocytes were retrieved and 5–20 embryos cryopreserved for each patient [73]. But the questions still need some high-qualified data to confirm although the current several literatures support its value.

Another retrospective trial compared three initiation times (the early follicular phase, late follicular phase, and after spontaneous ovulation) using a combination of HMG, clomiphene, and MPA in women with normal ovary reserve [74]. For those of "late follicular" group, a GnRH agonist injection was given to collapse the existing dominant follicle, then launch new stimulation with clomiphene, MPA, and HMG. Qin et al. showed that the duration of stimulation was two more days longer in the late follicular and luteal groups compared with conventional group but that the number of oocytes collected, metaphase II oocytes, and viable embryos were identical in the three groups. However, the cancelation rate was lower in the conventional group (10% vs. 22% vs. 16%), the reported ongoing pregnancy rate per transfer was not different among three groups but a large-sample prospective trial is needed to provide more sound evidence [74].

11.3 Double Ovarian Stimulation

Is it possible to combine the follicular-phase ovarian stimulation with luteal-phase stimulation in a single menstrual cycle? The answer is "Yes" based on the strategy of freeze-all policy [45, 48, 69, 75, 76].

To design the protocol for double stimulation, we not only take account of controlling serum FSH and LH for two retrievals, but also have to consider the natural connection of the first stimulation and second stimulation. All the down-regulation protocols are not ready for the second stimulation in a single cycle, in which GnRH agonist receptor inaction results into the over-suppression of ovary, and the recovery of the pituitary from downregulation during the luteal phase is slow [77]. So the non-downregulation protocols such as the natural cycle, minimal/mild stimulation, GnRH antagonist protocols, and progestin-primed ovarian stimulation have the potential to continue stimulation after first retrieval in a single menstrual cycle (Fig. 11.12).

We have to notice that the status of ovary should be examined again after first retrieval, if there are several small uniform antral follicles available (recommended as 3–8 mm follicle at least 3), it is ready to continue the second stimulation. But the size and number of antral follicles are not able to predict in advance, it have to examine on the trigger day or after the first oocyte retrieval, the synchronous small antral follicles are one of pre-requirements before deciding to perform the second stimulation, for the bigger developing follicle has a more chance to present sufficient LH receptor and may be luteinized by the increasing LH levels after first trigger. The asymmetrical antral follicles in the early luteal phase may produce suboptimal results if the second stimulation is conducted.

The protocols of double stimulation during the follicular and luteal phases in women with poor ovarian response (Shanghai protocol) are shown in Fig. 11.13. It combines a mild stimulation and a subsequent luteal-phase ovarian stimulation. A pilot study of 38 women began with mild ovarian stimulation; after the first oocyte retrieval, hMG and letrozole were administered to stimulate luteal-phase antral follicle development, and oocyte retrieval was carried out a second time when dominant follicles had matured. The first trigger preferred to use GnRH agonist rather than hCG, for hCG has a relative longer half-life and is possible to luteinize the subsequent dominant follicles. The primary outcome measured was the number of oocytes retrieved: stage 1, 1.7 ± 1.0; stage 2, 3.5 ± 3.2. The more oocytes retrieved in stage 2 were associated with more gonadotropin used in the second stimulation. From the double stimulation, 167 oocytes were collected and 26 out of 38 women (68.4%) succeeded in producing 1–6 viable embryos. Twenty-one women underwent 23 FETs, resulting in 13 clinical pregnan-

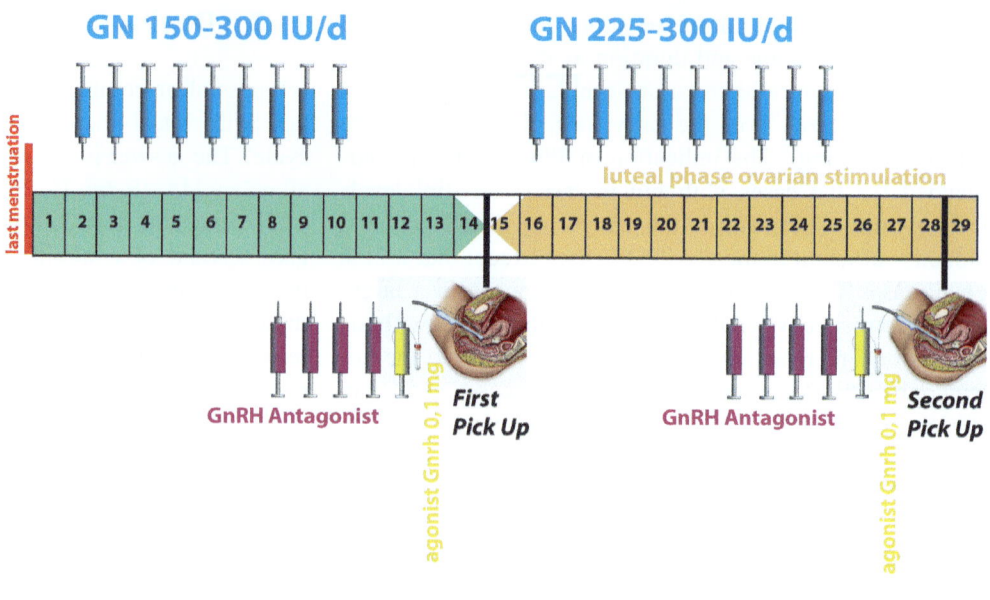

Fig. 11.12 The double stimulation represents two continuous ovarian stimulation in a single menstrual cycle, including a non-downregulation protocol in the first stimulation and luteal-phase ovarian stimulation in the second stimulation

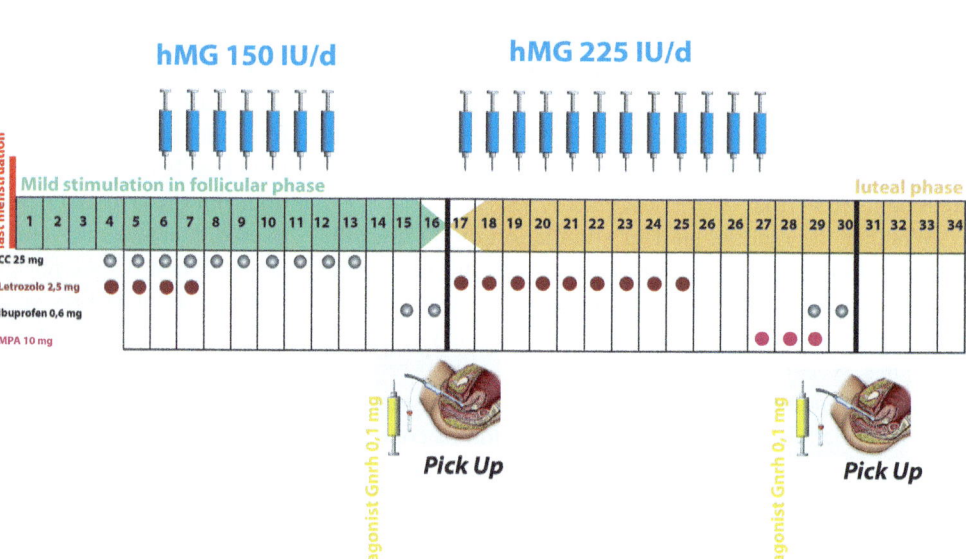

Fig. 11.13 The protocols of double stimulation during the follicular and luteal phases in women with poor ovarian response is shown (namely Shanghai protocol)

cies. The study shows that double ovarian stimulations in the same menstrual cycle provide more opportunities for retrieving oocytes in poor responders [48]. The stimulation can start in the luteal phase resulting in retrieval of more oocytes in a short period of time.

The hormone profiles during the double stimulation are shown in Fig. 11.14. The fluctuation of serum estrogen and progesterone levels showed that it naturally converted into luteal phase after first retrieval. The elevated progesterone level was preserved during the whole second stimulation. GnRH antagonist is not necessary for the luteal-phase ovarian stimulation for the endogenous progesterone from corpus lutein and has the capacity to inhibit the spontaneous LH surge. The FSH surge and LH surge induced by the same dose of GnRH agonist were much lower in the second trigger than the first trigger. This data presumed that the pituitary function and ovarian sensitivity to gonadotropin

stimulation was significantly reduced during the second stimulation [48].

Another retrospective study by Liu et al. collected 103 women aged 38 years or older whose first retrieval included GnRH agonist short protocol, GnRH antagonist protocol, mild stimulation, and progestin-primed ovarian stimulation. The subsequent luteal phase stimulation was performed with 225 hMG daily within 1–3 days of oocyte retrieval. Both triggering were made with 250 IU rhCG. The number of oocytes retrieved (5.8 ± 4.6), MII oocytes (4.7 ± 4.0), and cleaved embryos (4.0 ± 3.4) in double stimulation increased and the cancelation rate of no available embryos reduced (37.07% vs. 18.10%) significantly compared with standard follicular phase stimulation [78].

There are other published protocols of double stimulation with GnRH antagonist two times in a single menstrual cycle [69, 75, 79]. Martínez et al. [75] reported a pilot study of

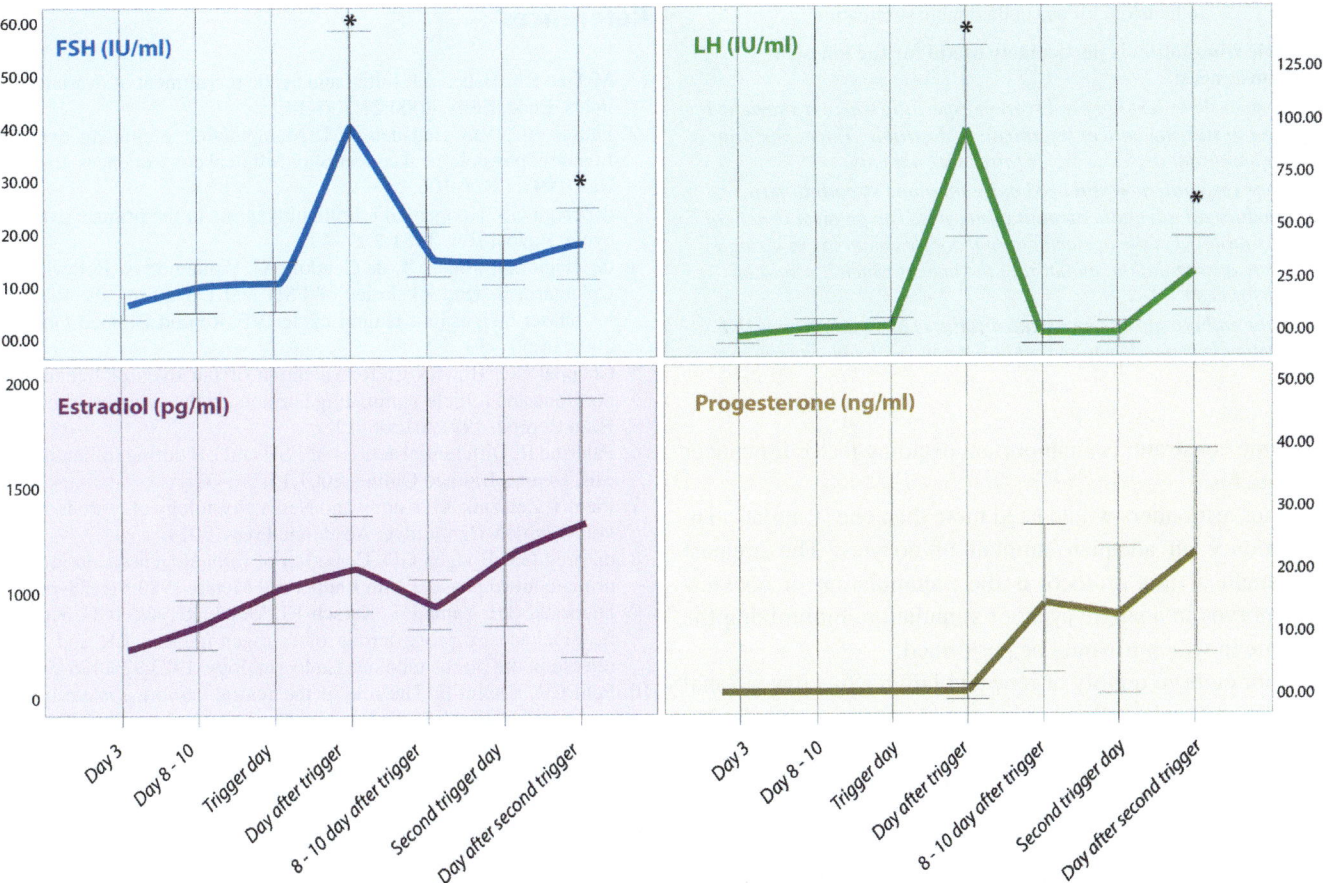

Fig. 11.14 The hormone profiles during the double stimulation are shown. The cycle naturally converted into luteal phase after first retrieval. The elevated progesterone level was preserved during the whole second stimulation. The FSH/LH surge induced by the same dose of GnRH agonist were much lower in the second trigger than the first trigger. This data presumed that the pituitary function was significantly reduced during the second stimulation. (From Kuang et al., 2014)

nine donors using GnRH antagonist two times in a single menstrual cycle, with the trigger by GnRH agonist and the oocytes being vitrified. The data for follicular and luteal phase stimulation did not show any difference regarding the number of mature oocytes (14.0 ± 7.0 vs. 16.9 ± 7.5) or the fertilization rate (77.3% vs. 76.5%). In this trial, the duration and consumption of FSH were not increased in the follicular vs. luteal phase (10.4 vs. 9.9 days; 2261 vs. 2147 IU), but the number of days for antagonist was doubled depending on the protocol applied (5.1 vs. 9.9). Ubaldi et al. used the same duplex protocols to compare the euploid blastocyst formation rates obtained after follicular phase versus luteal phase stimulation in patients with reduced ovarian reserve. One reassuring argument for the competence of oocytes obtained in the luteal phase is the absence of an increased risk of aneuploidy in 43 patients with a genetic diagnosis of aneuploidy by trophectoderm biopsy. The rate of euploid blastocysts biopsied was 46.9% in the follicular phase compared to 44.8% in the luteal phase [80].

Double stimulation was tested in oncologic patients [81]. Patients diagnosed with a malignancy commenced a random start antagonist stimulation protocol. The initial dose of gonadotropin was 150–450 IU of hMG depending on the basic status of ovary. The final maturation of oocytes was triggered by 5000 IU of hCG. On the day of oocyte collection, the patients were offered the option of a second stimulation starting the same day or after a few days. The dose of gonadotropin was the same or increased, depending on the ovarian response in the first stimulation cycle. The increased number of mature oocytes were retrieved with double stimulation for oncology patients, without delaying cancer treatment [81].

As a new approach to ovarian stimulation, double stimulation in combination with freeze-all is not recommended for women with normal ovarian reserve, for these good-prognosis women have higher chance of pregnancy by accomplishing a single ovary stimulation, and the existing multiple corpus lutea after first retrieval would add difficulties for the second stimulation. Double stimulation is particularly useful for the following circumstances:

1. Women seeks fertility preservation especially where a shortened time to starting cancer treatments is desirable.

Table 11.2 Indicazioni all'uso della double stimulation

Double stimulation is particularly useful for the following circumstances:
1. *Women seeks fertility preservation especially where a **shortened time to starting cancer treatments is desirable**. Time constraint is an important deciding factor for cancer patients*
2. ***Poor responders would need more than one stimulation to produce an adequate amount of oocytes**. The greatest benefit of this protocol is the accumulation of oocytes/embryos in a single cycle of stimulation, minimizing the time in which it would be performed*
3. ***Poor embryo quality or repeated failures by conventional IVF protocols** is another proposed indication for double stimulation*

Time constraint is an important deciding factor for cancer patients.

2. Poor responders would need more than one stimulation to produce an adequate amount of oocytes. The greatest benefit of this protocol is the accumulation of oocytes/embryos in a single cycle of stimulation, minimizing the time in which it would be performed.

3. Poor embryo quality or repeated failures by conventional IVF protocols is another proposed indication for double stimulation. For women with unsatisfactory egg factors in which repeated immature eggs, recurrent fertilization failure, or very poor-quality embryos are found using the conventional stimulation protocols, to change the stimulation strategy may be unexpectedly useful although there is no measurable indicator or sound rationale in routine clinic (Table 11.2).

11.4 Summary

Double ovarian stimulation makes it possible to complete two oocyte retrievals in a single menstrual cycle, the first retrieval may use non-down-regulation protocols, LH suppression is reached with or without GnRH antagonist, the second stimulation is accomplished in the luteal phase and endogenous progesterone has the capability to inhibit spontaneous LH surge. Double stimulation is originally applied in cancer patients with the requirement of emergency fertility preservation and is now indicated not only for fertility preservation in a limited time but also for women who has repeated IVF failures due to impaired oocyte or embryo qualities, or poor ovarian reserve. In conclusion, double ovarian stimulation provides another alternative to the conventional assisted reproductive techniques and increases the flexibility of ovarian stimulation. Well-designed randomized control trials are necessary to confirm these preliminary findings.

References

1. McGee EA, Hsueh AJ. Initial and cyclic recruitment of ovarian follicles. Endocr Rev. 2000;21:200–14.
2. Fauser BC, Van Heusden AM. Manipulation of human ovarian function: physiological concepts and clinical consequences. Endocr Rev. 1997;18:71–106.
3. diZerega GS, Hodgen GD. Folliculogenesis in the primate ovarian cycle. Endocr Rev. 1981;2:27–49.
4. de Ziegler D, Fraisse T, de Candolle G, Vulliemoz N, Bellavia M, Colamaria S. Outlook: roles of FSH and LH during the follicular phase: insight into natural cycle IVF. Reprod Biomed Online. 2007;15:507–13.
5. Chappel SC, Howles C. Reevaluation of the roles of luteinizing hormone and follicle-stimulating hormone in the ovulatory process. Hum Reprod. 1991;6:1206–12.
6. Palermo R. Differential actions of FSH and LH during folliculogenesis. Reprod Biomed Online. 2007;15:326–37.
7. Plant T, Zeleznik AJ. Knobil and Neil's physiology of reproduction, vol. 1. 4th ed. Cambridge: Academic Press; 2014.
8. diZereg GS, Hodgen GD. Cessation of folliculogenesis during the primate luteal phase. J Clin Endocrinol Metab. 1980;51:158–60.
9. Dierschke DJ, Yamaji T, Karsch FJ, Weick RF, Weiss G, Knobil E. Blockade by progesterone of estrogen-induced LH and FSH release in the rhesus monkey. Endocrinology. 1973;92:1496–501.
10. Pohl CR, Knobil E. The role of the central nervous system in the control of ovarian function in higher primates. Annu Rev Physiol. 1982;44:583–93.
11. March CM, Goebelsmann U, Nakamura RM, Mishell DR Jr. Roles of estradiol and progesterone in eiliciting the midcycle luteinizing hormone and follicle-stimulating hormone surges. J Clin Endocrinol Metab. 1979;49:507–13.
12. Gougeon A. Regulation of ovarian follicular development in primates: facts and hypotheses. Endocr Rev. 1996;17:121–55.
13. Richter TA, Robinson JE, Evans NP. Progesterone treatment that either blocks or augments the estradiol-induced gonadotropin-releasing hormone surge is associated with different patterns of hypothalamic neural activation. Neuroendocrinology. 2001;73:378–86.
14. Richter TA, Robinson JE, Lozano JM, Evans NP. Progesterone can block the preovulatory gonadotropin-releasing hormone/luteinising hormone surge in the ewe by a direct inhibitory action on oestradiol-responsive cells within the hypothalamus. J Neuroendocrinol. 2005;17(3):161–9.
15. Attardi B, Scott R, Pfaff D, Fink G. Facilitation or inhibition of the oestradiol-induced gonadotrophin surge in the immature female rat by progesterone: effects on pituitary responsiveness to gonadotrophin-releasing hormone (GnRH), GnRH self-priming and pituitary mRNAs for the progesterone receptor A and B isoforms. J Neuroendocrinol. 2007;19:988–1000.
16. Lasley BL, Wang CF, Yen SS. The effects of estrogen and progesterone on the functional capacity of the gonadotrophs. J Clin Endocrinol Metab. 1975;41:820–6.
17. Leyendecker G, Wildt L, Gips H, Nocke W, Plotz EJ. Experimental studies on the positive feedback effect of progesterone, 17 alpha-hydroxyprogesterone and 20 alpha-dihydroprogesterone on the pituitary release of LH and FSH in the human female. The estrogen priming of the progesterone feedback on pituitary gonadotropins in the eugonadal woman. Arch Gynakol. 1976;221:29–45.
18. Helmond FA, Simons PA, Hein PR. The effects of progesterone on estrogen-induced luteinizing hormone and follicle-stimulating hormone release in the female rhesus monkey. Endocrinology. 1980;107:478–85.

19. Knobil E. Regulation, by feedback, of gonadotropin hormone secretion in rhesus monkeys. Probl Actuels Endocrinol Nutr. 1974;18:37–8.

20. Wildt L, Hutchison JS, Marshall G, Pohl CR, Knobil E. On the site of action of progesterone in the blockade of the estradiol-induced gonadotropin discharge in the rhesus monkey. Endocrinology. 1981;109:1293–4.

21. Johnson MH. Essential reproduction. 6th ed. Blackwell Publishing; 2007. Chapter 5.

22. McNatty KP, Hillier SG, van den Boogaard AM, Trimbos-Kemper TC, Reichert LE Jr, van Hall EV. Follicular development during the luteal phase of the human menstrual cycle. J Clin Endocrinol Metab. 1983;56:1022–31.

23. Pache T, Wladimiroff J, Dejong F, Hop W, Fauser B. Growth patterns of nondominant ovarian follicles during the normal menstrual cycle. Fertil Steril. 1990;54:638–42.

24. Van Disseldorp J, Lambalk CB, Kwee J, Looman CW, Eijkemans MJ, Fauser BC, Broekmans FJ. Comparison of inter- and intra-cycle variability of anti-Mullerian hormone and antral follicle counts. Hum Reprod. 2010;25:221–7.

25. Rao GD, Chian RC, Son WS, Gilbert L, Tan SL. Fertility preservation in women undergoing cancer treatment. Lancet. 2004;363:1829–30.

26. Chian RC, Buckett WM, Tan SL. In vitro maturation of human oocytes. Reprod Biomed Online. 2004;8:148–66.

27. Grynberg M. The challenge of fertility preservation in cancer patients: a special focus issue from future oncology. Future Oncol. 2016;12:1667–9.

28. Chian RC, Chung JT, Downey BR, Tan SL. Maturational and developmental competence of immature oocytes retrieved from bovine ovaries at different phases of folliculogenesis. Reprod Biomed Online. 2002;4:127–32.

29. Chian RC, Huang JY, Gilbert L, Son WY, Holzer H, Cui SJ, Buckett WM, Tulandi T, Tan SL. Obstetric outcomes following vitrification of in vitro and in vivo matured oocytes. Fertil Steril. 2009;91:2391–8.

30. Baerwald A, Adams G, Pierson R. Characteristics of ovarian follicular wave dynamics in women. Biol Reprod. 2003;69:1023–31.

31. Baerwald AR, Adams GP, Pierson RA. Ovarian antral folliculogenesis during the human menstrual cycle: a review. Hum Reprod Update. 2012;18:73–91.

32. Baerwald A, Adams G, Pierson R. A new model for ovarian follicular development during the human menstrual cycle. Fertil Steril. 2003;80:116–22.

33. Bianchi PH, Viera LM, Gouveia GR, Rocha AM, Baruselli PS, Baracat EC, Serafini PC. Study of two strategies to induce follicular wave emergence for assisted reproductive treatments (ART)—a preliminary trial. J Assist Reprod Genet. 2015;32:543–9.

34. Baerwald AR, Adams GP, Pierson RA. Form and function of the corpus luteum during the human menstrual cycle. Ultrasound Obstet Gynecol. 2005;25:498–507.

35. Adamsa GP, Jaiswalb R, Singha P, Malhic J. Progress in understanding ovarian follicular dynamics in cattle. Theriogenology. 2008;69(1):72–80.

36. Viana JH, Dorea MD, Siqueira LG, Arashiro EK, Camargo LS, Fernandes CA, Palhão MP. Occurrence and characteristics of residual follicles formed after transvaginal ultrasound-guided follicle aspiration in cattle. Theriogenology. 2013;79:267–73.

37. de Mello Bianchi PH, Serafini P, Monteiro da Rocha A, Assad Hassun P, Alves da Motta EL, Sampaio Baruselli P, Chada Baracat E. Review: follicular waves in the human ovary: a new physiological paradigm for novel ovarian stimulation protocols. Reprod Sci. 2010;17:1067–76.

38. Edgar DH, Gook DA. A critical appraisal of cryopreservation (slow cooling versus vitrification) of human oocytes and embryos. Hum Reprod Update. 2012;18:536–54.

39. Massin N. New stimulation regimens: endogenous and exogenous progesterone use to block the LH surge during ovarian stimulation for IVF. Hum Reprod Update. 2017;23:211–20.

40. Macklon NS, Stouffer RL, Giudice LC, Fauser BC. The science behind 25 years of ovarian stimulation for in vitro fertilization. Endocr Rev. 2006;27:170–207.

41. Fauser BC, Devroey P, Yen SS, Gosden R, Crowley WF Jr, Baird DT, Bouchard P. Minimal ovarian stimulation for IVF: appraisal of potential benefits and drawbacks. Hum Reprod. 1999;14:2681–6.

42. Maman E, Meirow D, Brengauz M, Raanani H, Dor J, Hourvitz A. Luteal phase oocyte retrieval and in vitro maturation is an optional procedure for urgent fertility preservation. Fertil Steril. 2011;95:64–7.

43. Decanter C, Robin G. Fertility preservation strategies in young women in case of breast cancer or hematologic malignancy. Gynecol Obstet Fertil. 2013;41:597–600.

44. Kuang Y, Hong Q, Chen Q, Lyu Q, Ai A, Fu Y, Shoham Z. Luteal-phase ovarian stimulation is feasible for producing competent oocytes in women undergoing in vitro fertilization/intracytoplasmic sperm injection treatment, with optimal pregnancy outcomes in frozen-thawed embryo transfer cycles. Fertil Steril. 2014;101:105–11.

45. Zhang J. Luteal phase ovarian stimulation following oocyte retrieval: is it helpful for poor responders? Reprod Biol Endocrinol. 2015;13:76.

46. Li Y, Yang W, Chen X, Li L, Zhang Q, Yang D. Comparison between follicular stimulation and luteal stimulation protocols with clomiphene and HMG in women with poor ovarian response. Gynecol Endocrinol. 2016;32:74–7.

47. Kuang Y, Chen QJ, Hong QQ, Lyu QF, Fu YL, Ai A, Shoham Z. Luteal-phase ovarian stimulation case report: three-year follow-up of a twin birth. J IVF Reprod Med Genet. 2013;1:106.

48. Kuang Y, Chen Q, Hong Q, Lyu Q, Ai A, Fu Y, Shoham Z. Double stimulations during the follicular and luteal phases of poor responders in IVF/ICSI programmes (Shanghai protocol). Reprod Biomed Online. 2014;29:684–91.

49. Buendgen NK, Schultze-Mosgau A, Cordes T, Diedrich K, Griesinger G. Initiation of ovarian stimulation independent of the menstrual cycle: a case-control study. Arch Gynecol Obstet. 2013;288:901–4.

50. Wang N, Wang Y, Chen Q, Dong J, Tian H, Fu Y, Ai A, Lyu Q, Kuang Y. Luteal-phase ovarian stimulation vs conventional ovarian stimulation in patients with normal ovarian reserve treated for IVF: a large retrospective cohort study. Clin Endocrinol. 2016;84:720–8.

51. Chen H, Wang Y, Lyu Q, Ai A, Fu Y, Tian H, Cai R, Hong Q, Chen Q, Shoham Z, Kuang Y. Comparison of live-birth defects after luteal-phase ovarian stimulation vs. conventional ovarian stimulation for in vitro fertilization and vitrified embryo transfer cycles. Fertil Steril. 2015;103:1194–201.

52. Kuang Y, Chen Q, Fu Y, Wang Y, Hong Q, Lyu Q, Ai A, Shoham Z. Medroxyprogesterone acetate is an effective oral alternative for preventing premature luteinizing hormone surges in women undergoing controlled ovarian hyperstimulation for in vitro fertilization. Fertil Steril. 2015;104:62–70.

53. Dong J, Wang Y, Chai WR, Hong QQ, Wang NL, Sun LH, Long H, Wang L, Tian H, Lyu QF, Lu XF, Chen QJ, Kuang YP. The pregnancy outcome of progestin-primed ovarian stimulation using 4 versus 10 mg of medroxyprogesterone acetate per day in infertile women undergoing in vitro fertilisation: a randomised controlled trial. BJOG. 2017;124:1048–55.

54. Chen Q, Wang Y, Sun L, Zhang S, Chai W, Hong Q, Long H, Wang L, Lyu Q, Kuang Y. Controlled ovulation of the dominant follicle using progestin in minimal stimulation in poor responders. Reprod Biol Endocrinol. 2017;15:71.

55. Zhu X, Ye H, Fu Y. Use of utrogestan during controlled ovarian hyperstimulation in normally ovulating women undergoing in vitro fertilization or intracytoplasmic sperm injection treatments in combination with a "freeze all" strategy: a randomized controlled dose-finding study of 100 mg versus 200 mg. Fertil Steril. 2017;107:379–86.

56. Zhu X, Ye H, Fu Y. Duphaston and human menopausal gonadotropin protocol in normally ovulatory women undergoing controlled ovarian hyperstimulation during in vitro fertilization/intracytoplasmic sperm injection treatments in combination with embryo cryopreservation. Fertil Steril. 2017;108:505–12.

57. Yu S, Long H, Chang HY, Liu Y, Gao H, Zhu J, Quan X, Lyu Q, Kuang Y, Ai A. New application of dydrogesterone as a part of a progestin-primed ovarian stimulation protocol for IVF: a randomized controlled trial including 516 first IVF/ICSI cycles. Hum Reprod. 2018;33:229–37.

58. Zhang J, Mao X, Wang Y, Chen Q, Lu X, Hong Q, Kuang Y. Neonatal outcomes and congenital malformations in children born after human menopausal gonadotropin and medroxyprogesterone acetate treatment cycles. Arch Gynecol Obstet. 2017;296:1207–17.

59. Erb K, Klipping C, Duijkers I, Pechstein B, Schueler A, Hermann R. Pharmacodynamic effects and plasma pharmacokinetics of single doses of cetrorelix acetate in healthy premenopausal women. Fertil Steril. 2001;75:316–23.

60. Sitruk-Ware R. New progestogens for contraceptive use. Hum Reprod Update. 2006;12:169–78.

61. D'Arpe S, Di Feliciantonio M, Candelieri M, Franceschetti S, Piccioni MG, Bastianelli C. Ovarian function during hormonal contraception assessed by endocrine and sonographic markers: a systematic review. Reprod Biomed Online. 2016;33:436–48.

62. Lu X, Hong Q, Sun L, Chen QJ, Fu Y, Ai A, Lyu Q, Kuang Y. Dual trigger for final oocyte maturation improves the oocyte retrieval rate of suboptimal responders to gonadotropin-releasing hormone agonist. Fertil Steril. 2016;106:1356–62.

63. Kummer NE, Feinn RS, Griffin DW, Nulsen JC, Benadiva CA, Engmann LL. Predicting successful induction of oocyte maturation after gonadotropin-releasing hormone agonist (GnRHa) trigger. Hum Reprod. 2013;28:152–9.

64. Youssef MA, Van der Veen F, Al-Inany HG, Mochtar MH, Griesinger G, Nagi Mohesen M, et al. Gonadotropin-releasing hormone agonist versus HCG for oocyte triggering in antagonist assisted reproductive technology. Cochrane Database Syst Rev. 2014;(10):CD008046.

65. von Wolff M, Thaler CJ, Frambach T, Zeeb C, Lawrenz B, Popovici RM, et al. Ovarian stimulation to cryopreserve fertilized oocytes in cancer patients can be started in the luteal phase. Fertil Steril. 2009;92:1360–5.

66. Sönmezer M, Türkçüoğlu I, Coşkun U, Oktay K. Random-start controlled ovarian hyperstimulation for emergency fertility preservation in letrozole cycles. Fertil Steril. 2011;95:2125.

67. Ozkaya E, San Roman G, Oktay K. Luteal phase GnRHa trigger in random start fertility preservation cycles. J Assist Reprod Genet. 2012;29:503–5.

68. Ethics Committee of American Society for Reproductive Medicine. Fertility preservation and reproduction in patients facing gonadotoxic therapies: a committee opinion. Fertil Steril. 2013;100:1224–31.

69. Vaiarelli A, Venturella R, Vizziello D, Bulletti F, Ubaldi FM. Dual ovarian stimulation and random start in assisted reproductive technologies: from ovarian biology to clinical application. Curr Opin Obstet Gynecol. 2017;29(3):153–9.

70. Danis RB, Pereira N, Elias RT. Random start ovarian stimulation for oocyte or embryo cryopreservation in women desiring fertility preservation prior to gonadotoxic cancer therapy. Curr Pharm Biotechnol. 2017;18:609–13.

71. Cakmak H, Rosen MP. Ovarian stimulation in cancer patients. Fertil Steril. 2013;99:1476–84.

72. Pereira N, Voskuilen-Gonzalez A, Hancock K, Lekovich JP, Schattman GL, Rosenwaks Z. Random-start ovarian stimulation in women desiring elective cryopreservation of oocytes. Reprod Biomed Online. 2017;35:400–6.

73. Nayak SR, Wakim AN. Random-start gonadotropin-releasing hormone (GnRH) antagonist-treated cycles with GnRH agonist trigger for fertility preservation. Fertil Steril. 2011;96:e51–4.

74. Qin N, Chen Q, Hong Q, Cai R, Gao H, Wang Y, Sun L, Zhang S, Guo H, Fu Y, et al. Flexibility in starting ovarian stimulation at different phases of the menstrual cycle for treatment of infertile women with the use of in vitro fertilization or intracytoplasmic sperm injection. Fertil Steril. 2016;106:334–41.

75. Martínez F, Clua E, Devesa M, Rodríguez I, Arroyo G, González C, Solé M, Tur R, Coroleu B, Barri PN. Comparison of starting ovarian stimulation on day 2 versus day 15 of the menstrual cycle in the same oocyte donor and pregnancy rates among the corresponding recipients of vitrified oocytes. Fertil Steril. 2014;102:1307–11.

76. Cardoso MCA, Evangelista A, Sartório C, Vaz G, Werneck CLV, Guimarães FM, Sá PG, Erthal MC. Can ovarian double-stimulation in the same menstrual cycle improve IVF outcomes? JBRA Assist Reprod. 2017;21:217–21.

77. Smitz J, Van Den AE, Bollen N, Camus M, Devroey P, Tournaye H, Van Steirteghem AC. The effect of gonadotrophin-releasing hormone (GnRH) agonist in the follicular phase on in-vitro fertilization outcome in normo-ovulatory women. Hum Reprod. 1992;7:1098–102.

78. Liu C, Jiang H, Zhang W, Yin H. Double ovarian stimulation during the follicular and luteal phase in women ≥38 years: a retrospective case-control study. Reprod Biomed Online. 2017;35:678–84.

79. Moffat R, Pirtea P, Gayet V, Wolf JP, Chapron C, de Ziegler D. Dual ovarian stimulation is a new viable option for enhancing the oocyte yield when the time for assisted reproductive technology is limited. Reprod Biomed Online. 2014;29:659–61.

80. Ubaldi FM, Capalbo A, Vaiarelli A, Cimadomo D, Colamaria S, Alviggi C, Trabucco E, Venturella R, Vajta G, Rienzi L. Follicular versus luteal phase ovarian stimulation during the same menstrual cycle (DuoStim) in a reduced ovarian reserve population results in a similar euploid blastocyst formation rate: new insight in ovarian reserve exploitation. Fertil Steril. 2016;105:1488–95.

81. Tsampras N, Gould D, Fitzgerald CT. Double ovarian stimulation (DuoStim) protocol for fertility preservation in female oncology patients. Hum Fertil (Camb). 2017;20:248–53.

Oocyte Retrieval in IVM

12

Mario Mignini Renzini, Claudio Brigante, Mara Zanirato,
Maria Beatrice Dal Canto, Fausta Brambillasca,
and Rubens Fadini

Contents

Transvaginal oocyte retrieval during assisted reproductive technologies (ARTs) was first introduced in 1981, replacing both surgical egg collection and laparoscopic retrieval but also previous different approaches such as the transurethral ultrasound-guided route. It is well known that the number of oocytes retrieved depends on many factors: type of aspiration needle (wide or narrow bore or single or double channel), aspiration pressure, follicular flushing, timing of HCG triggering, and experience and skills of the surgeon.

In IVM critical factors are the aspiration pressure and the gynecological skills because the target is the collection of oocytes from sometimes primed but not properly stimulated ovaries with smaller follicular size; the follicle's volume varies by the cube of its radius: for instance, a 5 mm and a 10 mm follicle contain 1/8th and 1/64th the volume of a 20 mm diameter follicle, respectively (Table 12.1).

Thus antral follicles of 3 mm may contain a competent oocyte, but will have approximately 1/300th the amount of fluid of a normal dominant follicle, with practical consequences on the oocyte aspiration technique [1].

Trounson et al. suggested that compared to conventional IVF in IVM, there are many factors that affect quality and number of retrieved oocytes:

- **Needle length**
- **Bevel of the needle**
- **Rigidity of the needle**
- **Aspiration pressure**

Critical aspects to deal with are also the higher risk of bleeding and pain for the patient during and after the collection of immature eggs.

Conventional IVF oocyte retrieval is a bloody operation in which a patient's blood loss is not easily visualized; Dessole et al. analyzed the reduction of plasmatic hemoglobin on a sample of 220 IVF patients estimating an average

M. M. Renzini (✉) · C. Brigante · M. Zanirato · M. B. Dal Canto
F. Brambillasca · R. Fadini
CMR Biogenesi, Istituti Clinici Zucchi, Monza, Italy
e-mail: mariomigninirenzini@biogenesi.it; claudio.brigante@
fastwebnet.it; dalcanto@biogenesi.it

© Springer Nature Switzerland AG 2020
A. Malvasi, D. Baldini (eds.), *Pick Up and Oocyte Management*, https://doi.org/10.1007/978-3-030-28741-2_12

Table 12.1 Follicle diameter and fluid volume

Follicle diameter (mm)	Fluid volume (mL)	Hemisphere surface area (mm²)
4	0.034	25
6	0.113	56
8	0.263	101
10	0.524	157
12	0.955	226
14	1.437	306
20	4.189	625

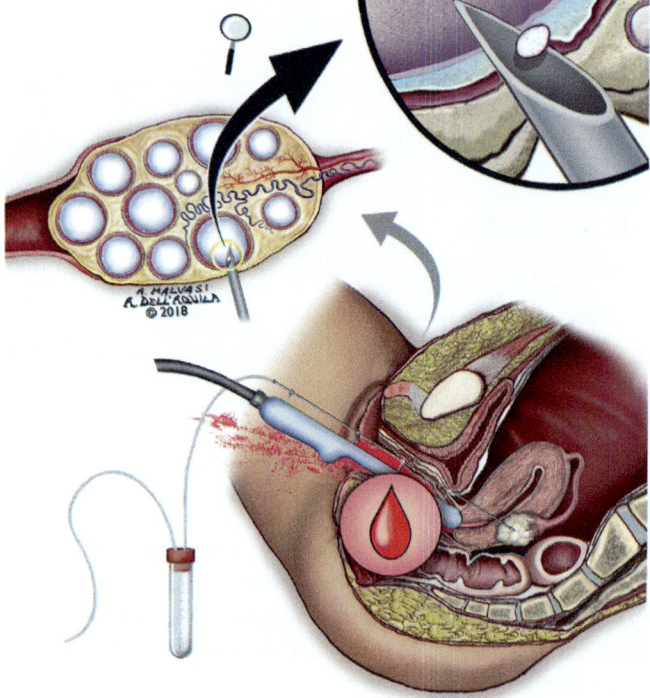

Fig. 12.1 Limiting blood loss may be especially important in IVM cases since PCO patients are at greater risk for ovarian hemorrhage after conventional IVF retrievals

blood loss of about 230 mL after 24 h of uncomplicated oocyte retrieval procedure [2]. Limiting blood loss may be especially important in IVM (Fig. 12.1) cases since PCO patients are at greater risk for ovarian hemorrhage after conventional IVF retrievals; a retrospective analysis performed by Liberty et al. in PCO patients showed higher risk of bleeding compared to all other patients (odds ratio 50, 95% confidence interval 11–250) [3].

12.1 Needle

Different parameters are to be taken in account looking at the characteristics of an optimal IVM needle:

- **Gauge**
- **Bevel length**

- **Angle**
- **Tip**
- **Stiffness**
- **Dead space**

The needle gauge could affect the outcome of the oocyte collection in terms of number of retrieved eggs, tissue trauma, and consequent bleeding (Fig. 12.2). Early studies reported that higher number of oocyte recovery corresponded to larger gauge needles used, but afterwards Awonuga et al. compared transvaginal oocyte retrievals with 15-, 17-, or 18-gauge needles founding similar results for number of collected oocytes, but less pain with smaller size needles [4].

Seyhan et al. analyzed pain scores with different gauge needles comparing a 19-gauge needle for IVM with a 16- or 17-gauge IVF needle: they found a trend of lower pain scores with 19-gauge needle, although not statistically significant; they suggested that smaller needles could give a more comfortable collection, even if in IVF enlarged ovaries with multiple large follicles and higher aspiration pressure could cause more pain. It is likely that within the range of conventional needles, smaller size results in less pain intra- and postoperatively, with a similar number of collected oocytes [5].

This may be particularly important in ART settings in which limited anesthesia is available for the patient. Seyhan et al. compared IVM patients in cases using a 19-gauge needle to IVF patients in cases using a 16- or 17-gauge needle. Records on 375 patients were reviewed retrospectively.

There were several approaches to anesthesia, but 233 patients received conscious sedation with midazolam and fentanyl together with a paracervical block.

12.2 Gauge

Patients ranked the amount of pain they experienced during the procedure on a scale of 1 to 10. There was no difference in the pain experience of the groups. Note that in addition to different gauge needles, this study compared different aspiration procedures since IVF required passage of the needle through the vagina and into each ovary only once, whereas IVM required a number of punctures in each ovary.

The authors viewed the results as showing that a smaller gauge needle was less traumatic since multiple insertions of the 19-gauge needle caused no more pain than two insertions of the larger needle. Several studies from the IVF literature also suggest that smaller needles cause less pain for women who are lightly sedated during retrieval; however, more studies are needed to confirm this.

Given the same needle **bevel length** (Fig. 12.3) (measured along the outer horizontal barrel edge), a smaller gauge needle will form a smaller angle and thus be sharper, passing easily through tissue; experimental data on tissue–needle interaction found that when a beveled needle has a smaller

Fig. 12.2 Internal and external dimensions of the needles in relation to the gauge

Gauge	internal diameter in mm	external diameter in mm
14	1,64	2,20
15	1,45	1,95
16	1,29	1,72
17	1,15	1,55
18	1,02	1,34
19	0,91	1,22
20	0,81	1,12
21	0,72	1,01

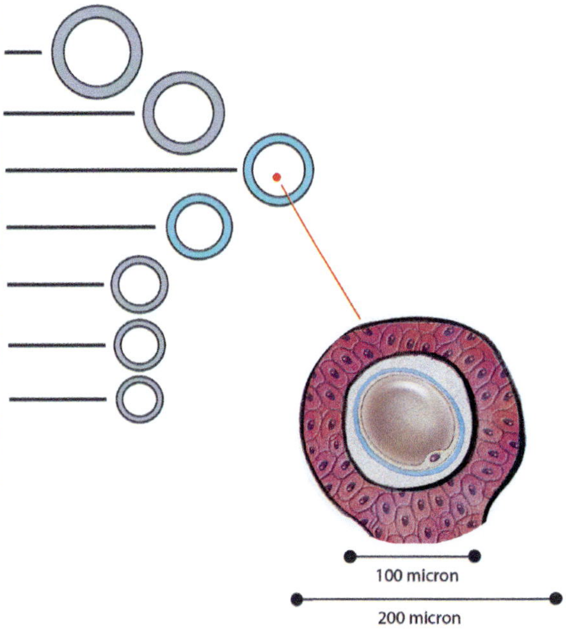

100 micron

200 micron

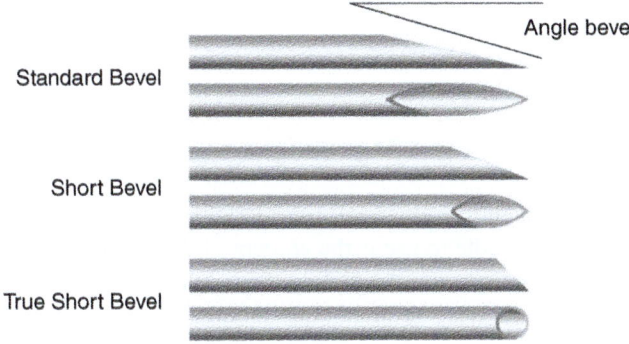

Fig. 12.3 The angle bevel and length of bevel

angle, there is less tissue deformation before the needle pierces that structure and less deformation of the follicle during entry, making placement of the end of the needle in the middle of the follicle easier [6].

The bevel length for many conventional IVF needles is about 3 mm (Table 12.2); the surface area of the scoring on the bevel is 50% of a segment of the needle barrel of that length, but can only be seen in the orientation where the back of the needle faces the probe.

The surgeon has to adjust his or her idea of where the end of the needle is, and if the needle is not axial, it could easily lie in the wall of the follicle.

For Cook's 19-gauge immature ovum aspiration needle set (K-OPS-7035-RWH-ET, Cook Medical, Spencer IN) (Fig. 12.4), the ultrasound scoring begins 2 mm above the top of the bevel. A smaller gauge needle is sharper for a given length bevel, since the **angle of the bevel** to the barrel of the needle is smaller. These special needles were with a

shorter length and stiffer that the ones used for traditional IVF (K-OPS-7035-RWH-ET, Cook Medical, Spencer IN). However, as can be seen in Table 12.2, different programs were successfully carried out with a range of different sized needles.

The fact that the target follicles in IVM are smaller than the target follicles in IVF could not represent an important reason to use a smaller gauge needle for IVM than for IVF, but the bevel angle and length are important because it defines the way the needle enters a follicle axially and it passes through the follicle's center, given it the opportunity to occupy a portion of the entire diameter of the follicle.

Finally **needle thickness** is the primary variable determining the pressure that an oocyte experiences at the needle tip (for a given pump aspiration pressure). Needle tip pressure should vary so significantly with needle diameter as predicted by the Hagen–Poiseuille law for steady flow through pipes, even though this physical law does not fully explain the more complicated systems used for oocyte aspiration [8].

Some beveled needles utilize a diamond cut to make them sharper without increasing the bevel length (Table 12.2). This is done by making two cuts at right angle to the barrel at the end of the needle, making it sharper by reducing its thickness at the end. A minor disadvantage of this is that it makes a scored tip of the needle slightly harder to see by ultrasound.

Another issue to consider is **needle stiffness**: the wall diameter of a 17-gauge needle is 0.203 mm, whereas a 19-gauge needle has a wall thickness 0.191 mm. An obvious problem with decreased needle thickness occurs for those surgeons who find it helpful in some patients to apply external pressure on the ovaries: there are commercial alternatives

Table 12.2 Needle characteristics

Manufacturer (identification number)	Gauge	Lumen	Needle length (cm)	Bevel length (mm)	Bevel angle (degrees)[a]	Needle dead space (mL)[a]	Total dead space (mL)	Length ultrasound scoring (mm)	Ultrasound scoring begins	Diamond tip?	Flow rate (mL/s)[b]
Cooper-Smith, Trumbull, CT(AR-N1695)	16	Single	35	5	18.3	0.392	1.57	22	Tip	Angled bevel	0.78
Cook Medical, Spencer, IN (K-OPSD-1635-A-S-US)	16	Double	41	5	18.3	0.291[c]	1.31	5	1 mm above bevel top	No	0.45
Smiths. Medical, Kent, UK (Wallace, 0NS1733LL-500)	17	Single	36	3	26.2	0.322	0.93	23	Tip	Yes	0.42
Smiths Medical, Kent, UK (Wallace, ONS18333LL-500)	18	Single	36	3	22.9	0.199	0.74	23	Tip	Yes	0.31
Cook Medical, Spencer, IN (K-OPS-7035-RWH-ET)	15	Single	41	3	19.6	0.152	0.58	5	2 mm above bevel top	Yes	0.21
IVFETFLEX.com, Ganz, Austria (Steiner-Tan 21 gauge)	21	Pseudo-double	8	3	15.3	0.017	0.012[d]	9	0.5 mm above bevel top	Yes	0.30

[a]Using data from [7] and length measurement
[b]Using a craft suition unit aspiration pump with pressure set at 1 CO mmHg
[c]Measured
[d]Tubing and larger sheathed needle were not counted as dead space since they can be flushed

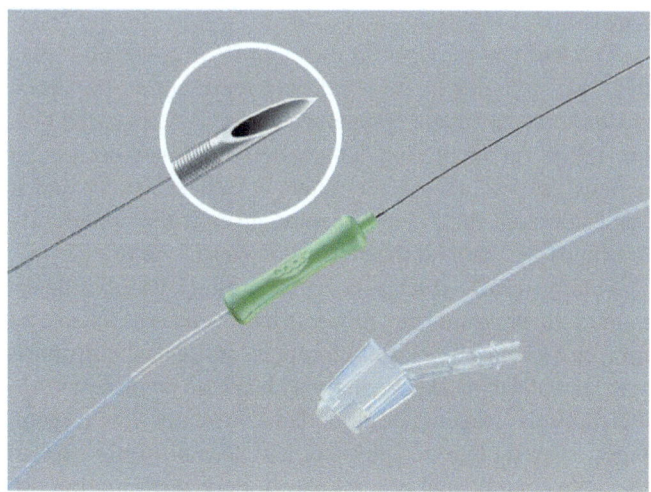

Fig. 12.4 Cook medical needle—K-OPS-7035-RWH-ET

that provide sharp thin needles within the ovary while providing a stiffer thicker needle for outside the ovary. Two of these are the Steiner-Tan pseudo-double lumen needles which provides a 21- or 19-gauge needle mounted on a larger needle that does not enter the ovary (Steiner-Tan Needle 21 gauge, IVFETFLEX.com, Graz, Austria) and Cook's Immature Ovum Aspiration Set (K-IOPS-2035-1730, Cook Medical, Spencer, IN) which uses a double needle. This aspiration set uses a 17-gauge needle to pass through the vagina and ovary and uses a 20-gauge inner needle to aspirate the follicles.

Likely a more important consideration in choosing the gauge of a needle to use is the amount of **dead space in the needle**. Dead space is defined by the volume of the cylinder created by the cross-sectional interior area of the needle and the length.

This is more significant for IVM than for IVF in terms of comparing the volume of the follicle aspirated with the amount of dead space in the needle (Table 12.2).

For larger gauge needles, several follicles may need to be aspirated before enough fluid is able to enter the collecting tube (attached to the bung).

For example, it would take the fluid from 14, 5 mm follicles to just fill a Wallace 17-gauge needle and the tubing proximal to the collecting tube; it would take five such follicles just to see the fluid in the tubing where it is attached to the needle. Depending on the speed of the surgeon, prolonged residence of the aspirate in the dead space of the needle and tubing may lead to clotting in the needle and loss of oocytes or to exposure of oocytes to nonoptimal environmental conditions.

A smaller dead space is obviously an advantage over a larger dead space. The IVM needle and collection device with the smallest dead space is the Steiner-Tan needle, which also allows for simultaneous emptying of the needle outside the vagina and the tubing attached to the needle without removing the needle from the ovary [7]. The genuine dead space is limited to an 8 cm segment of 21-gauge needle and has a volume of 0.017 mL. It also partly overcomes the stiffness issue and its bevel length is approximately 3 mm and bevel angle is 15.3° (based on declaimed characteristics) [9].

12.3 Aspiration Pressure (Fig. 12.5), Fluid Velocity, and Flow Rate

The majority of IVM programs used a reduced aspiration pressure for IVM oocyte retrieval compared to the pressure they use for IVF retrieval (Table 12.3).

Most commonly this is 7.5 kPa (approximately 56 mmHg), as suggested by Trounson et al., original studies: in their opinion "this [lower pressure] improved the recovery of immature oocytes in preliminary studies" [10].

These data are in conflict with the results suggested in different studies using a bovine model; Fry et al. aspirated 5827 follicles from 720 ovaries with 17- and 20-gauge needles [11]. More than 5000 of these follicles were 2–4 mm in diameter. The rest were 5–15 mm. With 17-gauge needles, 56% of the follicles yielded oocytes, but with 20-gauge needles recovery dropped to 45%. The highest recovery also

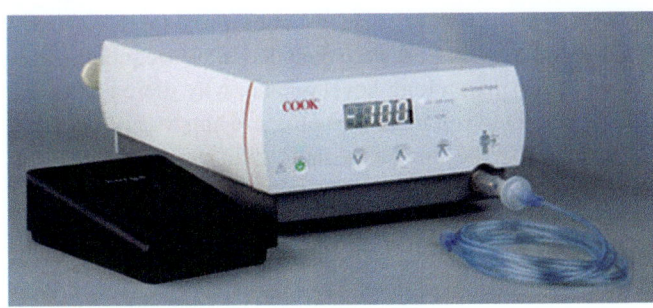

Fig. 12.5 Pump aspiration with digital display

Table 12.3 Aspiration pressure and needle type

Study	Needle type	Aspiration vacuum[a]
Trounson et al. (1984)	Not given	7.5 kPa
Wynn et al. (1998)	16-gauge double lumen	80 mmHg
Mikkelsen et al. (1999)	17-gauge single lumen	7.5 kPa
Chian et al. (1999)	17-gauge single lumen	7.5 kPa
Suikkari et al. (2000)	17-gauge single lumen	7.5 kPa
Cha et al. (2000)	Not given (specially designed needle)	7.5 kPa
Mikkelsen and Linden berger (2001)	17-gauge single lumen	Syringe pump
Child et al. (2001)	17-gauge single lumen	7.5 kPa
Lin et al. (2001)	17-gauge double lumen	7.5 kPa
Dal Canto et al. (2006)	17-gauge single lumen	80 mmHg
Hashimoto et al. (2007)	20-gauge single lumen	300 or 180 mmHg

[a]7.5 kPa, 56 mmHg

occurred with the highest aspiration pressures. The pressures evaluated ranged from 25 to 100 mmHg. Recovery was 46% at 25 mmHg and 59% at 100 mmHg.

Fry et al. concluded that the optimal pressure to maximize recovery of bovine CCOCs was 55 mmHg with a 17-gauge needle and 77 mmHg for a 20-gauge needle. Bols et al. aspirated 3000 follicles 3–8 mm in diameter with 18-, 19-, and 21-gauge needles using aspiration pressures of 50–130 mmHg. Oocyte recovery increased from 52.7% for 21-gauge needles to 74.4% for 18-gauge needles. Recovery was only 55.5% with a pressure of 50 mmHg, but increased to a maximum at the three highest pressure levels (67% at 90 mmHg, 69.5% at 110 mmHg, and 67% at 130 mmHg) [12].

In these bovine studies the increasing aspiration revealed an improvement in recovery rate, but as aspiration pressures increased, the recovered oocytes were increasingly denuded of cumulus cells. This loss of cumulus cells also occurred at lower aspiration machine pressures using larger diameter needles compared to smaller diameter needles, suggesting that needle gauge and pressure are independent variables that both contributed to the outcome.

Looking at the human IVM technique of aspiration, at the beginning of IVF, aspiration with hand-helding syringes was shown to cause detrimental fractures of the zona pellucida [13].

The type of damage caused by the low pressures used in these studies appears to be more unique to IVM in that oocytes tightly enclosed by granulosa cells; in human IVM, naked oocytes are less likely to mature, fertilize, or cleave as embryos [14].

An old study looked at oocyte retrieval by laparoscopy using a 24 cm 20-gauge needle with a 45° bevel: an aspiration pressure of 200 mmHg produced higher oocyte recovery than lower pressures (grouped together as pressures of 120–180 mmHg).

This study aspirated follicles of all sizes, but the majority came from follicles with diameters 7–9 mm, with an aspiration pressure estimated to be greater than 400 mmHg; the conclusion of the authors was that a pressure of 200 mmHg was better than higher pressures that damaged oocytes and removed surrounding cumulus cells [15].

A small study with human subjects (43 cycles) compared oocyte recovery for IVM using a 20-gauge needle with aspiration pressures of 180 or 300 mmHg [16]. These aspiration pressures are both higher than the pressures used in the bovine studies cited above and most published clinical human IVM studies (Table 12.2). More oocytes were retrieved with more cumulus cells with the lower pressure retrievals; a limit of the study is that half of the patients in the lower pressure aspiration group received FSH for priming. FSH priming increases growth of the granulosa cells in follicles, making the antral follicle easier to visualize and aspirate since it increases the number of granulosa cells in the follicle [17].

These studies suggested that in IVM retrievals lower aspiration pressures compared with IVF could improve recovery as oocytes become denuded of cumulus cells at higher pressures, and furthermore, the negative impact of increasing aspiration pressures is greater in larger-gauge needles: naked oocytes are uncommonly observed in current conventional IVF practice, but occur to some degree in IVM recovery with any needle size or pressure.

In human models, the system of aspiration have a lot of variables that determine the pressure experienced by the oocyte at the needle tip: needle gauge, length of needle, connecting tube gauge, length of connecting tube, size of the collection tube, and size of the vacuum reservoir in the pump; as demonstrated by Horne et al. using bovine ovaries, Hagen–Poiseullie law (for steady flow through pipes) does not adequately predict flow and pressure in the more complex system required for oocyte aspiration [8].

Poiseullie law says that increasing the length of the tube decreases pressure at the end in proportion to the percentage that the length was increased; decreasing the interior diameter of the needle or tube decreases the pressure by the fourth power of the decreased percentage of the diameter (i.e., decreasing the diameter of pipes by 10% results in decreasing the pressure to 65.6% of what it was). The best way to refer to a stable parameter comparable between different studies could be the use of the fluid flow rate; flow rate is an expression of the velocity of fluid at the tip of the needle, and it is easier to measure and adjust. The flow rate commonly used for IVF with a Wallace 17-gauge needle using a Craft suction unit (Rocket Medical plc., Watford. Herts, England) aspiration pump set at 100 mmHg is 0.42 mL/s (aspirates 10 mL of water in 24 s).

A common flow rate used for IVM with the pump at 50 mmHg is 0.12 mL/s: it takes about 0.5 s after pressure is applied before 75% of the maximal pressure is attained and about 5 s before the maximal pressure is reached [7]. Since the aspiration of a follicle usually takes less than 5 s, we measured flow by recording the time it takes to aspirate 10 mL from the onset of suction. The average velocity of the fluid moving in the needle does not completely explain the forces acting on the oocyte during aspiration: laminar flow within a needle has a parabolic distribution of velocities with fluid along the inner wall of the needle moving slowest (due to friction) and fluid in the center of the needle moving fastest.

In a 17-gauge needle, a typical COC (cumulus oocyte complex) will occupy more than 25% of the diameter of the needle. The shear stress force acting on the COC is the force component perpendicular to the flow, which varies related to how far the COC is from the center of the needle. The magnitude of the shear stress that a COC may experience depends on the velocity of the fluid and on the diameter of the needle: the theory of flow dynamics suggests that with sufficient velocity, fluid flow in the needle can change from laminar flow to turbulent flow, which exposes the COC to more severe randomly directed forces (since the Reynolds number is proportional to the velocity and the Reynolds number predicts when flow becomes turbulent).

However, most flow rates commonly used for IVF and IVM (Table 12.2) are likely to keep flow within the needle laminar. Otherwise an IVM program that used FSH to prime the oocytes leads to more oocytes with expended cumulus that is harder to strip [8].

The stripping of cumulus cells from the oocyte likely occurs either when the oocyte leaves the follicle wall or during passage through the needle.

The entry of the COC into the beveled tip of the needle generally involves a change of direction for the COC while it undergoes rapid changes in velocity. This will result in turbulent flow before entry into the needle and for the first few millimeters of flow inside the needle until laminar flow is established. This period of turbulent flow exerts stronger forces on the COC that are differently directed and at times causes the COC to hit the walls and bevel of the needle. The strength of these forces increases with increased velocity (increased flow rate) due to increased pressure. Rapid radial movement of the needle (twisting) or vigorous flushing, as some surgeons do, may also increase the magnitude of the force exerted on the COC. Consideration of the forces acting on COCs due to flow characteristics provides a unifying explanation of why COCs are denuded more frequently with a short rather than a long bevel needle, why there is a linear relationship between increased pressure and loss of cumulus cells, and why the impact of increasing pressure has more impact with thicker rather than thinner needles. Increasing pressure increases volume of flow and the velocity of the fluid much more rapidly in a larger than in a smaller gauge needle. Turbulent flow occurs over a longer distance in long bevel compared to short bevel needles. The turbulence to entry into the needle exerts randomly directed forces on the COC, which with increased velocity, may overcome the adherence of the cumulus cells to the oocyte.

12.4 Flushing

To maximize the number of oocytes recovered, follicular aspiration followed by flushing has been suggested in IVF, even if several meta-analysis studies show that there is no difference in oocyte recovery with and without flushing [18–21].

Also, double-lumen needles (Fig. 12.6), which have one channel for flushing fluid into the follicle and another channel for aspiration of the oocyte, have also been developed [22].

The potential benefit of follicular flushing is increased number of oocytes being collected, which may possibly increase pregnancy and live birth rates; however, potential

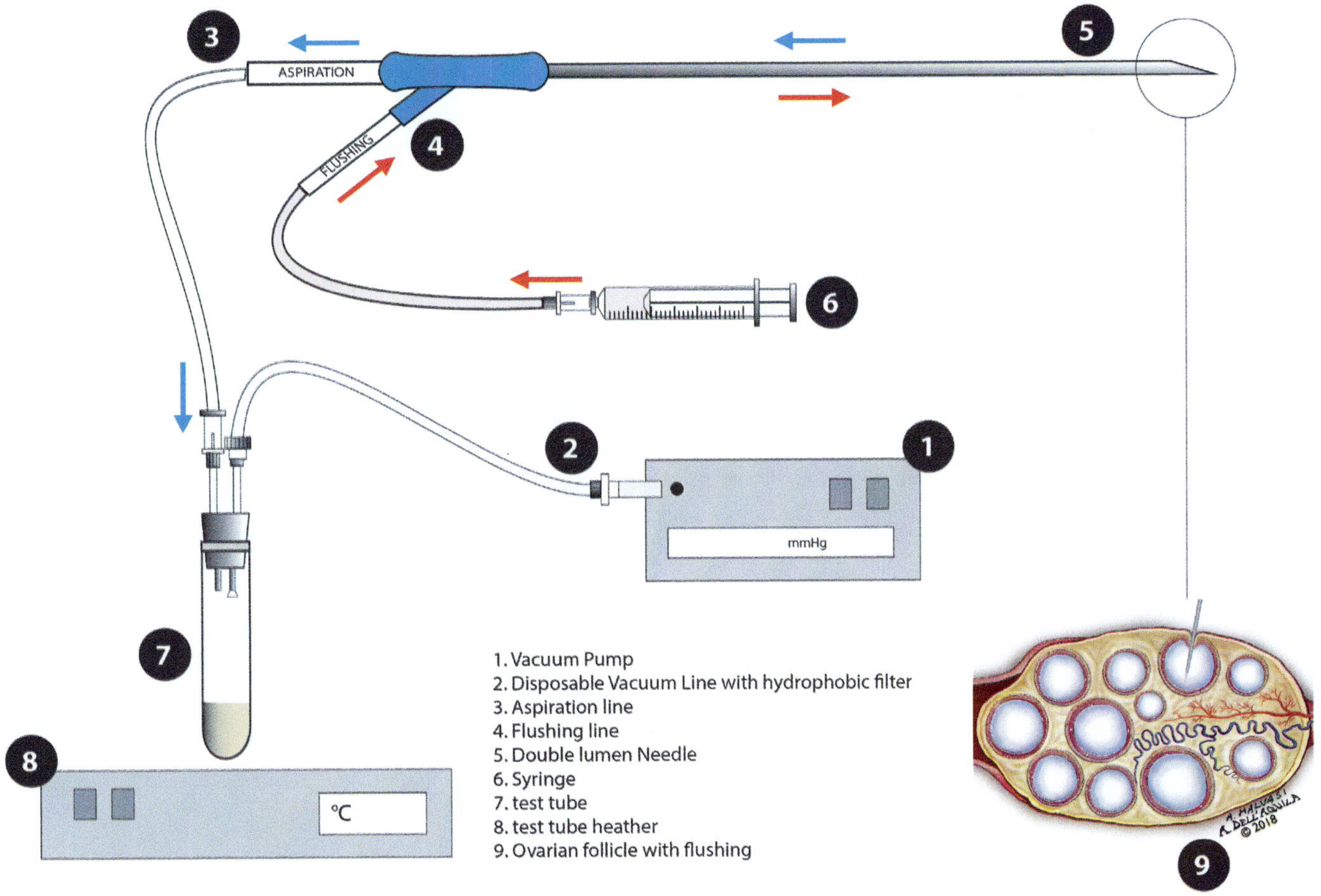

1. Vacuum Pump
2. Disposable Vacuum Line with hydrophobic filter
3. Aspiration line
4. Flushing line
5. Double lumen Needle
6. Syringe
7. test tube
8. test tube heather
9. Ovarian follicle with flushing

Fig. 12.6 Aspiration set with double lumen needle for flushing

disadvantages include longer procedure time with more anesthetics and more tissue handling, with, the possibility to remove also the follicular cells important for endocrine luteal support function.

In IVM oocytes are embedded in a granulosa cell matrix instead of free floating in follicular fluid, so the data on flushing in conventional IVF cannot be applied given the small volume of fluid in antral follicles and the large dead space in most single lumen needles; so flushing antral follicles using single lumen needle makes no sense (Tables 12.1 and 12.3).

A double lumen needle or a pseudo-double lumen needle (Steiner-Tan) is required for flushing. If a double lumen needle is used, the diameter of the aspiration channel is reduced, and pressure at the aspiration machine needs to be increased to maintain the desired velocity at the tip; this mechanism can originate turbulence that can potentially free the oocyte. Such turbulence could also enhance factors leading to damage of the COC.

Fluid can easily be injected into the ovary outside of the follicle, theoretically losing an oocyte from the follicle and also leading to impaired visualization.

Fry et al. conducted studies on the benefit of flushing in bovine models with a 17-gauge double lumen needle and compared it to a single lumen needle: they aspirated 1500 fol-licles using 50 mmHg of pressure with and without flushing and found no difference in the oocyte recovery rate. Rose and Laky compared use of the 19-gauge Cook immature oocyte aspiration needle without flushing to the Steiner-Tan needle with flushing and found no difference in the number of oocytes retrieved [7]. Another concern is that standard approach in IVM of removing the needle to flush it and having to pass it into the vagina and ovary several times makes an IVM retrieval more traumatic than a conventional IVF retrieval [5]. Flushing enables the surgeon to leave the needle in the ovary and not remove it until all follicles have been aspirated.

12.5 Retrieval Technique

Speaking about the techniques of retrieval, we must underline that a great discussion is about needle insertion, needle rotation, and timing to apply vacuum pressure, although some gynecologists prefer to use the double-needle technique (Fig. 12.7).

Needle insertions into biological tissues can be viewed as a first boundary displacement of the tissue followed by a planar crack of the follicle.

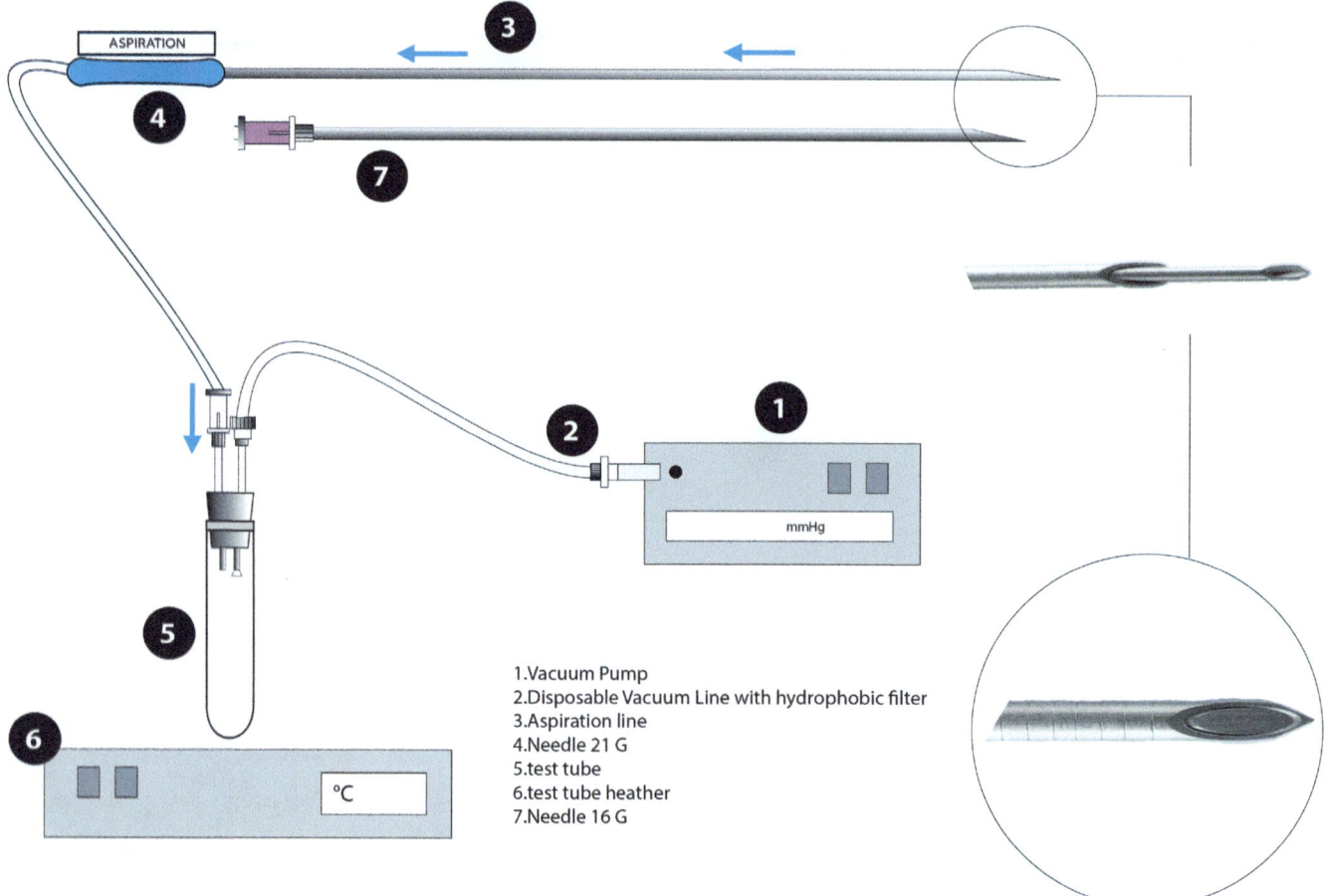

Fig. 12.7 Aspiration set with double needle

When a needle pressures the boundary if the object being entered is not fixed (like the ovary), the force applied to the needle can be transferred into motion of that object increasing displacement without resulting in puncture, so that insufficient axial vector force increases just tissue distortion. Multiple experimental studies show that the puncture force required decreases as the insertion velocity of the needle increases,: in fact kinetic energy at the tip increases [23, 24] with square of the velocity (kinetic energy = 0.5 × mass × velocity squared); thus a 25% increase in needle velocity should increase the energy available at the tip to induce puncture by 50%.

These observations suggest that it is desirable to insert a needle into the follicle with as much velocity as safely possible.

In IVM (Fig. 12.8), Dr. Lim believes that the best way to undertake retrieval is to grasp the needle with the surgeon's fingertips (like a pencil) and advance it using an "overhand motion." Advancing the needle using the muscles of the fingers and wrist increases the velocity of needle insertion while maintaining control. The alternative and more common aspiration approach is to keep the table lower and advance the needle with an "underhand" motion using the muscles of the wrist and forearm.

As the needle crosses the boundary, the load at the needle point decreases and a planar crack is created in the follicle wall. The crack is enlarged as the tip fully enters the follicle: a larger crack could increase the potential of an oocyte being lost from the follicle.

Some surgeons enter and aspirate the follicle without moving the needle; others advocate that the needle should be rotated and moved up and back slightly for scraping or curetting the wall of the follicle.

For conventional IVF, Dahl et al. showed that rotating the needle in a follicle during aspiration increased the number of oocytes obtained [25] (Fig. 12.9). One clear benefit of gentle needle rotation is decreasing the likelihood of the needle lumen becoming prematurely blocked by a collapsing follicle wall or large debris. Rotation and axial movement may also help keep the tip of the needle inside the follicle. Needle movement is likely to make the needle's

Fig. 12.8 Recruitable
follicles pool for IVM

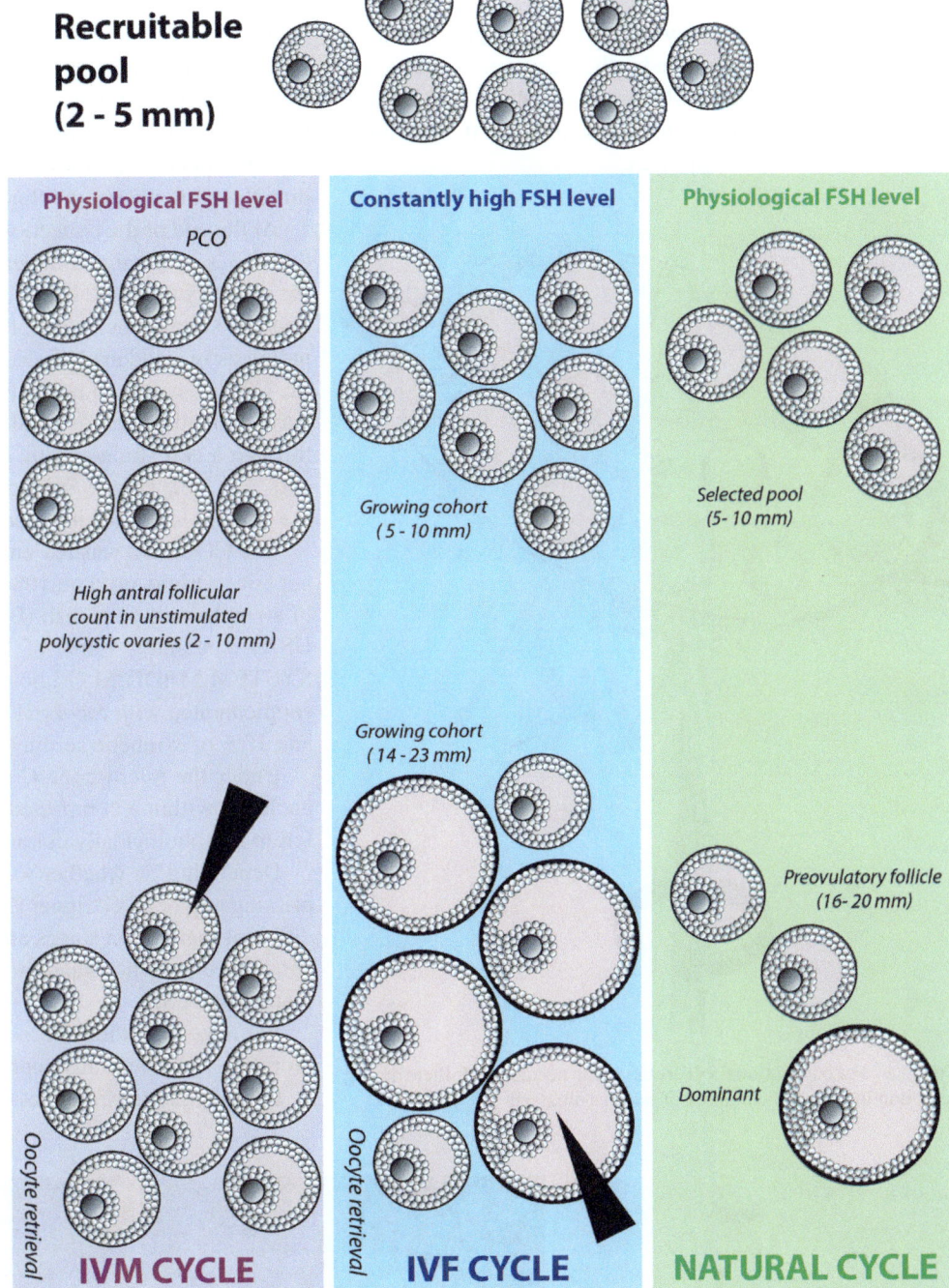

ultrasound markings easier to see, and thus, it will enhance the surgeon's visualization. Finally, rotating the needle may enhance penetration into a follicle that has only partially been entered and whose wall stretches under the slow advancement of the needle.

The last topic is the correct timing of applying pressure to the follicle; the commonest technique is to apply vacuum pressure just before entering each follicle to reduce the loss of free fluid created by the puncture into the ovary [15].

After the fluid has been aspirated from a follicle and the aspiration pressure has been released, it is possible for negative pressure to pull an oocyte back into a follicle because the aspiration system returned to atmospheric pressure.

Otherwise, pulling the needle out of the ovary and vagina while continuing to apply vacuum pressure could cause a massive spike of pressure within the needle with high-speed turbulent flow that can damage the COC.

12.6 Oocyte Management

In our department the oocyte retrieval was performed by transvaginal ultrasound-guided follicle aspiration with a single lumen aspiration needle (Gynetics cod. 4551-E2 17-gauge 35 cm, Belgium) connected to a vacuum pump (Craft Pump-Rocket UK, pressure 80 mmHg).

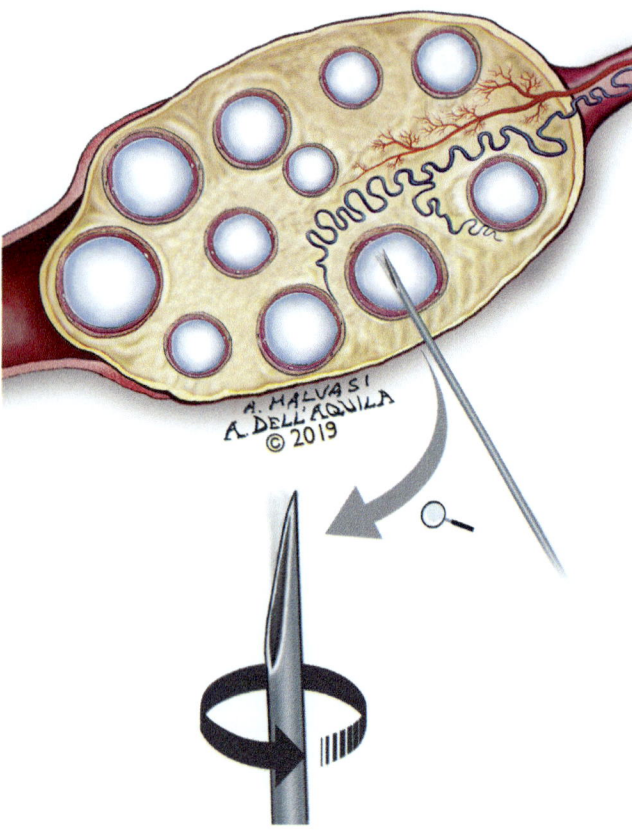

Fig. 12.9 For conventional IVF, rotating the needle in a follicle during aspiration increased the number of oocytes obtained

The follicular aspirates, containing cumulus–oocyte complexes (COCs), are collected in a single bottle (tissue culture flask, 50 mL) instead of classical tubes, containing 15 mL pre-warmed flushing medium with heparin (Origio, Denmark). This strategy has been applied in order to avoid the "stop and go" in aspiration (Fig. 12.10a–c). Using this trick the doctor can move from one follicle to another one directly, without stop the fluid aspiration.

At the end of the collection, the follicular fluid containing the COCs is examined under the stereomicroscope looking for the oocytes (Figs. 12.11, 12.12, and 12.13). This may be done by simply pouring the fluid into a petri dish for examination as in standard IVF. However, due to the small size of the COCs because of a diminished cumulus mass, the better way to identify them is to filter the follicular fluid aspirated through a cell strainer with 70 μm of pore size (BD Falcon cod. 352,350, USA). Subsequently it is necessary to wash the strainer with flushing medium.

The COCs are washed once in flushing medium without heparin (Origio prod.no.10840125, Denmark), then placed in a single-well petri dish (Becton Dickinson, Falcon 3037, USA) containing 1 mL of IVM medium (vial 2 of IVM SYSTEM MEDIUM Origio prod. no. 82214010, Denmark) supplemented with rec–FSH 0.075 IU/mL, hCG 0.1 IU/mL, and 10% of synthetic serum (Irvine, USA).

Under the microscope COCs appear smaller than usual, enclosed within a compacted cumulus complex or with different morphologically cumulus oophorus.

Depending on whether women are exposed to mild FSH priming and/or hCG trigger [26], oocytes may be collected at different maturation stages and therefore may require different culture conditions and times of maturation before insemination by ICSI.

We have classified the oocytes based on two variables: morphology of cumulus oophorus and stage of maturation.

In particular they are classified as follow:

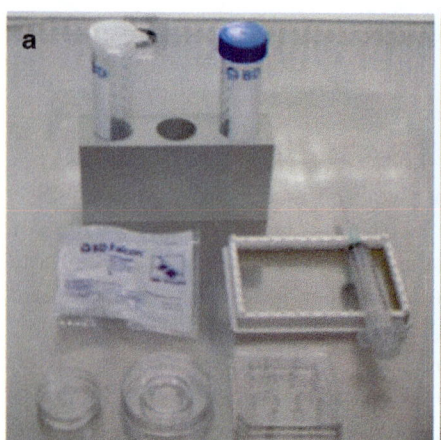
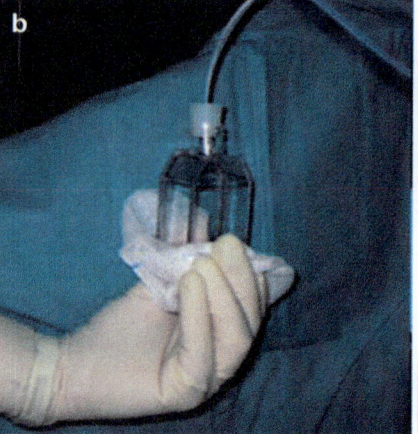
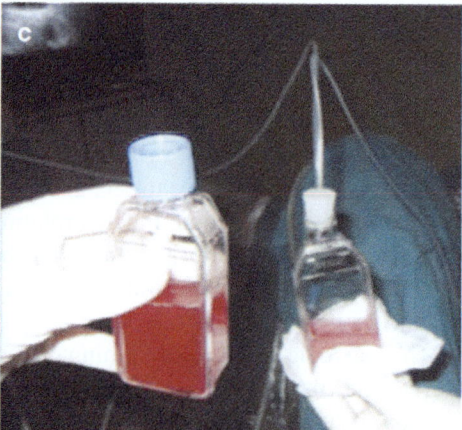

Fig. 12.10 (**a**) Disposable tube and Petri dishes for classical IVF. (**b**) and (**c**) Disposable 50 mL bottles to collect follicular fluid in IVM

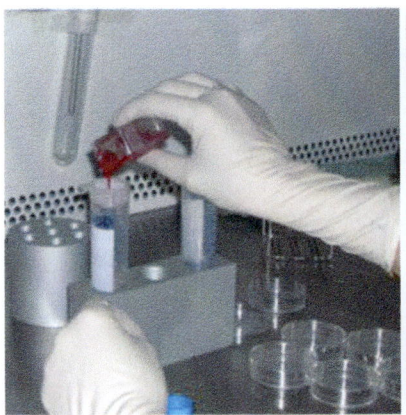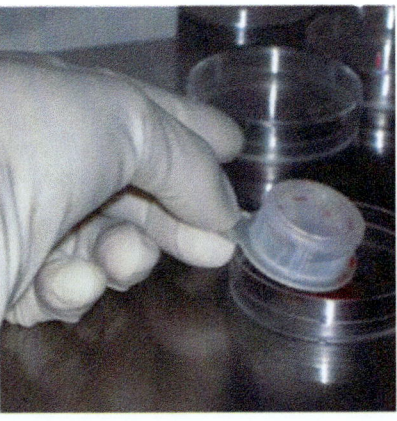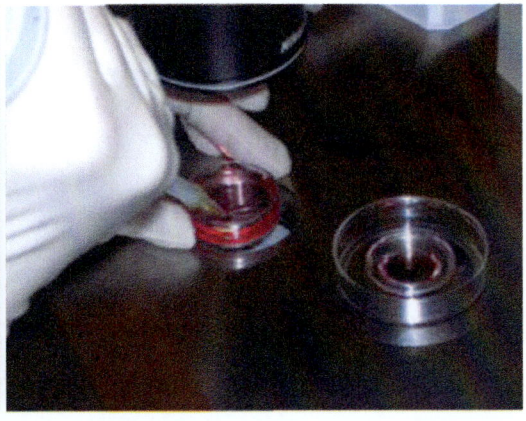

Fig. 12.11 At the end of the collection, the follicular fluid containing the COCs is examined under the stereomicroscope looking for the oocytes. This may be done by simply pouring the fluid into a petri dish for examination as in standard IVF. However, due to the small size of the COCs because of a diminished cumulus mass, the better way to identify them is to filter the follicular fluid aspirated through a cell strainer with 70 μm of pore size (BD Falcon cod. 352,350, USA). Subsequently it is necessary to wash the strainer with flushing medium

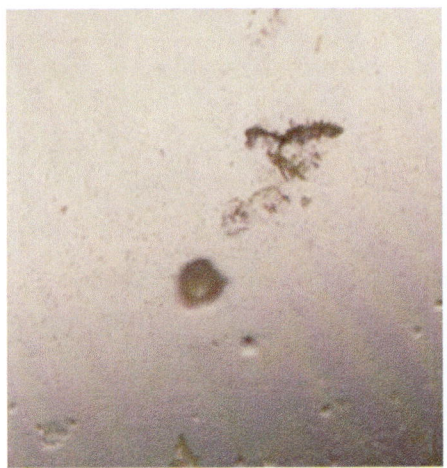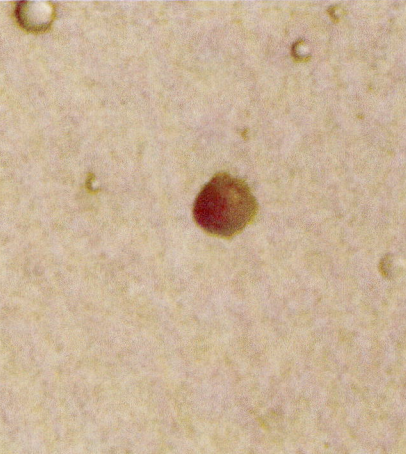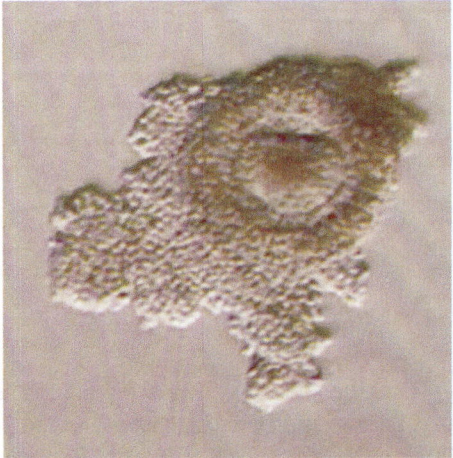

Fig. 12.12 Cumulus-oocyte complexes taken from antral follicles (<12 mm). Observation performed on the stereomicroscope with 6× magnification

- *COMPACT CUMULUS (CC)*
- *EXPANDED CUMULUS (EC)*
- *MATURE EXPANDED CUMULUS (EC-MII)*
- *NUDE OR ATRETIC* [27].

The *compact cumulus* (CC) includes immature oocyte (GV) with a full or partial compact multilayer cumulus around constituted by cubical and strictly compact granulosa cells, defined as "full or sparse" depending on the presence of complete or partial multilayer of granulosa cells.

The *expanded cumulus* (EC) includes immature oocyte (GV or MI) with a slack and fluffy multilayer cumulus of granulosa cells all around. The COC usually shows a dark corona radiata. To check the maturation stage is necessary "to spread" them under microscope.

The *expanded cumulus metaphase-II* (EC-MII) includes mature oocyte (metaphase II) with a slack and fluffy, abundant multilayer cumulus all around. They usually show an expanded corona radiata and an oocyte with the first polar body (1 PB) extruded, whose presence can be confirmed by spreading of cumulus cells or total removal with mechanical/enzymatic system.

Immature oocytes without any granulosa cells around are classified as nude and degenerated oocytes as atretic. These oocytes are usually GV stage, and they are immediately discarded.

The different types of COCs should be cultured separately as soon as they are identified and collected from the follicular fluid.

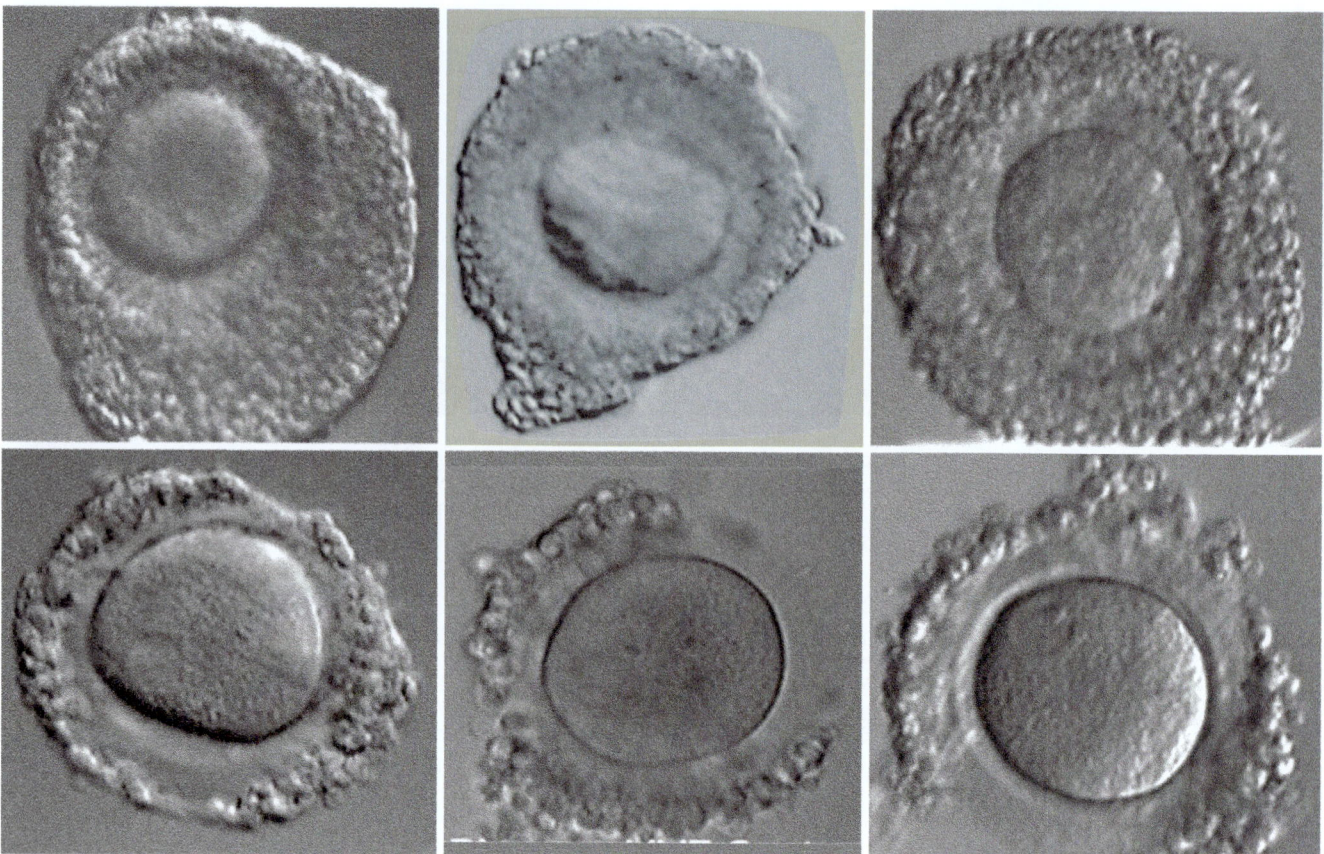

Fig. 12.13 Cumulus-oocyte complexes taken from antral follicles (<12 mm). Observation performed on the invertomicroscope with 20× magnification

The immature oocytes with compacted cumulus cells (CC) are stored in an incubator at 37 °C and 5% CO_2 in a humidified atmosphere for 30 h. The oocytes with expanded and slack cumulus cells (EC) are cultured for 3 h and are investigated again under microscope to identify the presence of the germinal vesicle following the spreading technique. The oocytes with GV signal are placed again into the maturation medium without removal of cumulus complex. If no signal of GV is observed, the cumulus-oocyte complexes are treated with hyaluronidase solution 80 IU/mL (Sage Media, USA) in order to remove the cumulus complex. Only oocytes with the first polar body (metaphase II stage) are used for the insemination the same day.

Oocytes that still appear immature after the removal of granulosa cells are discarded. After 30 h of culture all the cumulus-oocyte complexes remained are treated with hyaluronidase solution 80 IU/mL (Sage Media, USA) in order to remove the cumulus complex.

All the MII oocytes, selected according to cytoplasmic characteristics (homogeneous or with granularity, presence of vacuoles or smooth endoplasmic reticulum aggregates or presence of dark zona), were fertilized only by ICSI.

Following insemination, the oocytes are transferred into a standard IVF culture medium and treated exactly as in normal IVF and ICSI procedures. Fertilization is assessed 16–18 h after injection by the presence of two pronuclei. The embryo cleavage is evaluated 48 h after injection.

The embryo transfers should be carried out on day 2, day 3, or at blastocyst stage.

References

1. Rose BI. Approaches to oocyte retrieval for advanced reproductive technology cycles planning to utilize in vitro maturation: a review of the many choices to be made. J Assist Reprod Genet. 2014;31(11):1409–19.
2. Dessole S, Rubattu G, Ambrosini G, Miele M, Nardelli GB, Cherchi PL. Blood loss following noncomplicated transvaginal oocyte retrieval for in vitro fertilization. Fertil Steril. 2001;76:205–6.
3. Liberty G, Hyman JH, Eldar-Geva T, Latinsky B, Gal M, Margalioth EJ. Ovarian hemorrhage after transvaginal ultrasonographically guided oocyte aspiration: a potentially catastrophic and not so rare complication among lean patients with polycystic ovary syndrome. Fertil Steril. 2010;93:874–9.
4. Awonuga A, Waterstone J, Oyesanya O, Curson R, Nargund G, Parsons J. A prospective randomized study comparing needles of

different diameters for transvaginal ultrasound-directed follicle aspiration. Fertil Steril. 1996;65(1):109–13.

5. Seyhan A, Ata B, Son W-Y, Dahan MH, Tan S-L. Comparison of complication rates and pain scores after transvaginal ultrasound guided oocyte pickup procedures for in vitro maturation and in vitro fertilization cycles. Fertil Steril. 2014;101:705–9.

6. Van Gerwin DJ, Dankelman J, van den Dobbelsteen JJ. Needle-tissue interaction forces-a survey of experimental data. Med Eng Phys. 2012;34:665–80.

7. Rose BI, Laky DC. A comparison of the cook single lumen immature ovum IVM needle to the Steiner-Tan pseudo double lumen flushing needle for oocyte retrieval for IVM. J Assist Reprod Genet. 2013;30:855–60.

8. Horne R, Bishop CJ, Reeves G, Wood C, Kovacs GT. Aspiration of oocytes for in vitro fertilization. Hum Reprod Update. 1996;2:77–85.

9. Wikipedia. Needle gauge comparison chart. http://en.wikipedia.org/wiki/Needle_gauge_comparison_chart. Assessed 25 Apr 2014.

10. Trounson A, Wood C, Kausche A. In vitro maturation and the fertilization and developmental competence of oocytes recovered from untreated polycystic ovarian patients. Fertil Steril. 1994;62:353–62.

11. Fry RC, Niall EM, Simpson TL, Squires TJ, Reynolds J. The collection of oocytes from bovine ovaries. Theriogenology. 1997;47:977–87.

12. Bols PEJ, Van Soom A, Vandenheede JMM, de Kruif A. Effects of aspiration vacuum and needle diameter on cumulus oocyte complex morphology and developmental capacity of bovine oocytes. Theriogenology. 1995;45:1001–14.

13. Lowe B, Osborn JC, Fothergill DJ, Lieberman BA. Factors associated with accidental fractures of the zona pellucida and multipronuclear human oocytes following in-vitro fertilization. Hum Reprod. 1988;3(7):901–4.

14. Goud PT, Goud AP, Qian C, Laverge H, Van der Elst J, De Sutter P, Dhont M. In-vitro maturation of human germinal vesicle stage oocytes: role of cumulus cells and epidermal growth factor in the culture medium. Hum Reprod. 1998;13(6):1638–44.

15. Lopata A, Johnston IW, Leeton JF, Muchnicki D, Talbot J, Wood C. Collection of human oocytes at laparoscopy and laparotomy. Fertil Steril. 1974;25:1030–8.

16. Hashimoto S, Fukuda A, Murata Y, et al. Effect of aspiration vacuum on the developmental competence of immature human oocytes using a 20-gauge needle. Reprod Biomed Online. 2007;14:444–9.

17. Wynn P, Picton HM, Krapez JA, Rutherford AJ, Balen AH, Gosden RH. Pretreatment with follicle stimulating hormone promotes the numbers of human oocytes reaching metaphase II in in-vitro maturation. Hum Reprod. 1998;13:3132–8.

18. Levy G, Hill MJ, Ramirez CI, Correa L, Ryan ME, DeCherney AH, et al. The use of follicle flushing during oocytes retrieval in assisted reproductive technologies: a systemic review and meta-analysis. Hum Reprod. 2012;27:2373–9. 29.

19. Wongtra-Ngan S, Vutavanich T, Brown J. Follicular flushing during oocyte retrieval in assisted reproductive techniques. Cochrane Database Syst Rev. 2010;(9):CD004634.

20. Roque M, Sampaio M, Geber S. Follicular flushing during oocyte retrieval: a systematic review and meta-analysis. J Assist Reprod Genet. 2012;29:1249–54.

21. Waterstone JJ, Parsons JH. A prospective study to investigate the value of flushing follicles during transvaginal ultrasound-directed follicle aspiration. Fertil Steril. 1992;57(1):221–3.

22. Bols PEJ, Ysebaert MT, Van Soom A, de Kruif A. Effects of needle tip bevel and aspiration procedure on the morphology and developmental capacity of bovine compact cumulus oocyte complexes. Theriogenology. 1997;47:1221–36.

23. Aziz N, Biljan MM, Taylor CT, Manasse PR, Kingsland CR. Effect of aspirating needle caliber on outcome of in-vitro fertilization. Hum Reprod. 1993;8:1098–100.

24. Mahvash M, Dupont PE. Fast needle insertion to minimize tissue deformation and damage. IEEE Int Conf Robot Autom. 2009;2009:3097–102.

25. Dahl SK, Cannon S, Aubuchon M, Williams DB, Robins JC, Thomas MA. Follicle curetting at the time of oocyte retrieval increases the oocyte yield. J Assist Reprod Genet. 2009;26:335–9.

26. Fadini R, Dal Canto MB, Mignini Renzini M, Brambillasca F, Comi R, Fumagalli D, Lain M, Merola M, Milani R, De Ponti E. Effect of different gonadotrophin priming on IVM of oocytes from women with normal ovaries: a prospective randomized study. Reprod Biomed Online. 2009;19(3):343–51.

27. Dal Canto MB, Brambillasca F, Mignini Renzini M, Coticchio G, Merola M, Lain M, De Ponti E, Fadini R. Cumulus cell-oocyte complexes retrieved from antral follicles in IVM cycles: relationship between COCs morphology, gonadotrophin priming and clinical outcome. J Assist Reprod Genet. 2012;29(6):513–9.

Oocyte Retrieval in Egg Donation

13

Antonio Pellicer and Victor Hugo Gomez

Contents

Today, it has become well established and successful representing approximately 14% of all ART treatments in Spain (according to the national registry of the Spanish Society of Fertility, SEF, available at http://www.registrosef.com) and 10% in the USA [1, 2]. Its use has been steadily increasing due to sociological changes that resulted in a delayed age of motherhood in modern society which nowadays is often desired at ages where women are less fertile. This leads to a lower number of pregnancies per woman. For this reason, women attending infertility clinics nowadays tend to be from more advanced age, and oocyte donation is currently the only available option to achieve pregnancy [2, 3].

Oocyte donation is defined as an assisted reproductive technique (ART) in which the female gamete is provided by a different woman than the one who will receive the oocyte or the resulting embryo. It offers the highest success rates for pregnancy, and it is the best treatment option for those women with previous failed in vitro fertilization (IVF) treatment using their own oocytes or for those who, due to other medical or physiological conditions, are unable to undergo such treatment [4].

A. Pellicer · V. H. Gomez (✉)
Reproductive Medicine Unit IVIRMA, Valencia, Spain
e-mail: apellicer@ivirma.com; VictorHugo.Gomez@ivirma.com

© Springer Nature Switzerland AG 2020
A. Malvasi, D. Baldini (eds.), *Pick Up and Oocyte Management*, https://doi.org/10.1007/978-3-030-28741-2_13

Table 13.1 The oocytes donors must have an absolutely problem-free medical history

Characteristics of oocyte donors
• *Between the age of 18 and 35*
• *Good physical and mental health*
• *Negative history for genetically transmissible medical disease*
• *Negative history for sexually transmitted disease such: toxoplasmosis, rubella, chlamydia, gonorrhoea*
• *Negative* **HIV**, *syphilis,* **HCV**, **HBV**

After the report of the first pregnancy achieved through this technique by the Australian team of Trounson and Wood in 1983 [5] and the first successful pregnancy achieved after oocyte donation 1 year later in 1984, described by Lutjen et al., the technique has not ceased to increase and the results have improved over the years, largely due to a substantial improvement of laboratory practice, which has led to an improvement of embryo quality. At present, it is the assisted reproductive technology that provides the best outcomes, offering the best live birth rates in IVF practice. This allows us to achieve a pregnancy in nearly every woman, regardless of her age, absence of ovaries, or ovarian impairment [6, 7]. The reason for such success is due to the selection of young, healthy donors. This suggests that uterine receptivity plays a secondary role [8–10], and embryo quality seems to be the most important parameter to achieve pregnancy (Table 13.1).

13.1 Characteristics of Oocyte Donors

There are certain criteria and some screening procedures to become an oocyte donor. According to the current Spanish legislation, donors must be between the ages of 18 and 35 and in good physical and mental health. They must have a negative history for genetically transmissible medical diseases and sexually transmitted diseases such as syphilis, toxoplasmosis, rubella, gonorrhoea, chlamydia, hepatitis B virus, hepatitis C virus and HIV [11]. At IVI clinics, donors get their karyotype checked, and they must have a normal 46, XX karyotype to be included in our Oocyte Donation Programme. Donors are limited to only six live births, and these must be registered in the national register of donors.

13.2 Ovarian Stimulation Protocols in Oocyte Donor Cycles

Donor stimulation protocols should be simple, safe, and convenient to the patient. Nowadays, the GnRH antagonist protocol is clearly the best protocol, which involves the use of

GnRH analogues in ovulation induction. This reduces the risk of developing ovarian hyperstimulation syndrome (OHSS) [12, 13], as reported by Griesinger et al. in a meta-analysis published in 2006 [14].

This new approach, most widely accepted actually, was validated in 2009, when consensus was reached by a group of experts who met in Copenhagen to evaluate the existing evidence on the use of GnRHa to trigger final oocyte maturation in in vitro fertilization/intracytoplasmic sperm injection (IVF/ICSI), specifically in oocyte donor cycles.

They suggested that it was time to change the usual protocols and that it was unacceptable to put donors at risk when there was an efficient way to reduce the risk of ovarian hyperstimulation.

The group of experts concluded that the stimulation protocols involving the use of antagonists and ovarian induction with GnRH analogues should be recommended for oocyte donor cycles [15, 16].

Furthermore, for oocyte donors, this approach will shorten the length of luteal phase (4–6 days), and the earlier onset of withdrawal bleeding reduce ovarian volumes and diminish abdominal distension, and avoidance of estradiol monitoring during stimulation which altogether might substantially decrease the burden of treatment for oocyte donors [12, 17–19].

13.3 Ovulation Induction

Ovarian pickup (OPU) is scheduled when there are >3 follicles of sizes >17 mm or at least one follicle 20 mm, provided that the total number of follicles measuring >14 mm is ≥8 follicles [20].

Concerning the optimal dosage interval and type of analogue for triggering of final oocyte maturation could be from 0.2 to 0.5 mg of subcutaneous triptorelin or leuprorelin, or, alternatively, administering 200 μg of nasal buserelin. Identical results after oocyte collection have been obtained when compared to the use of 0.1 mg of triptorelin (in one bolus) [21, 22].

Oocyte retrieval must be scheduled with great precision: oocyte maturation is completed at 25–30 h. After the preovulatory LH surge (or hCG injection or GnRH agonist administration). Follicular rupture occurs on average within 37 h. Following hCG administration, the earliest follicular rupture is about 39 h and the latest is about 41 h [23, 24].

13.4 Oocyte Retrieval

Transvaginal oocyte retrieval is the most common method of oocyte collection in IVF cycles. It consists of the aspiration of follicular fluid, and it is performed using

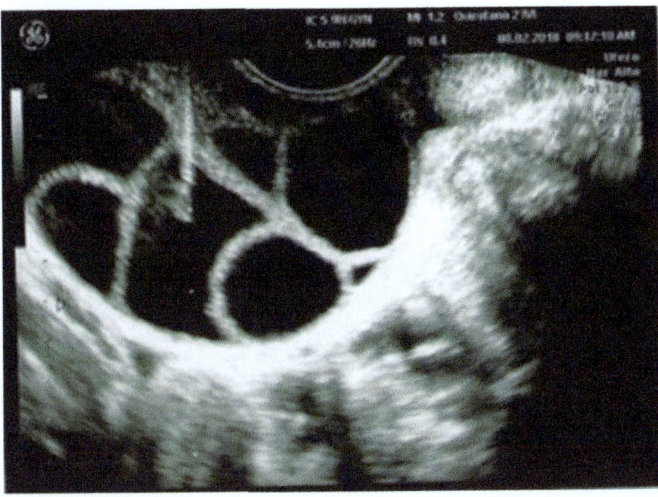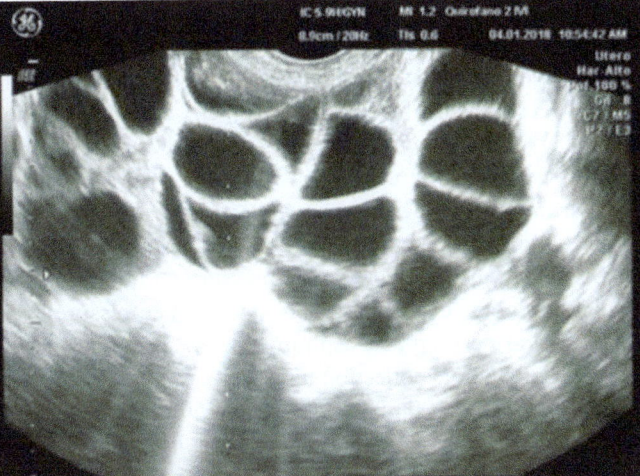

Fig. 13.1 Transvaginal ultrasound-guided follicle aspiration

Fig. 13.2 Oocyte retrieval

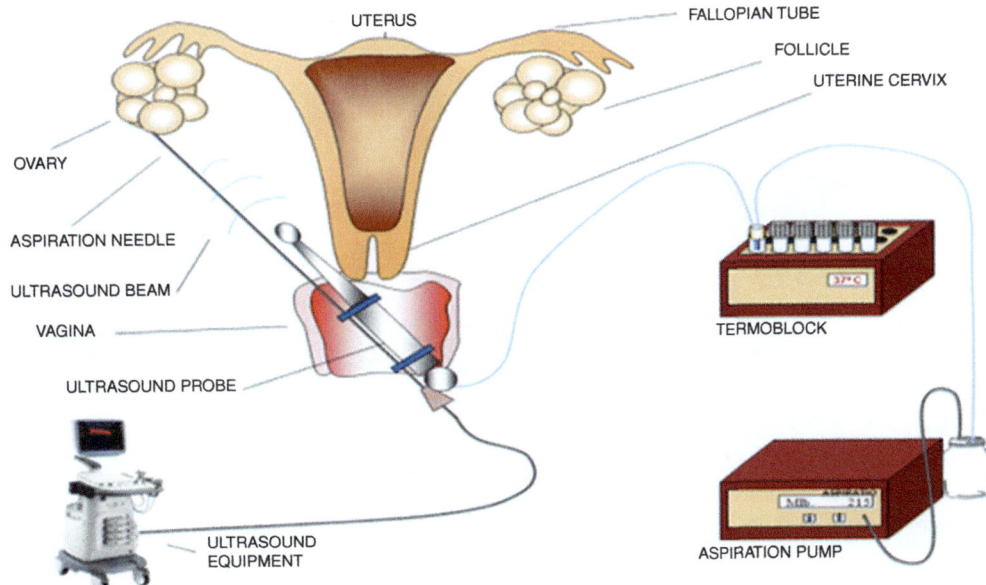

transvaginal ultrasonography. It is focused on obtaining the maximum number of oocytes to be fertilized after they have reached in vivo nuclear and cytoplasmic maturation, before follicle rupture. This technique was first introduced in 1981 [25–28], and since then, the technique has been used worldwide, as it is minimally invasive, thus replacing laparoscopic approach that had been previously performed. It has now become the gold standard for IVF therapy [29–31] (Fig. 13.1).

The success of the technique depends not only on the inherent characteristics of the oocyte, which might be influenced by the actual process of oocyte collection, but also on other factors such as the length of the ovarian stimulation phase, the type of anaesthesia used (local, sedation or general), the type of aspiration needle, aspiration alone or aspiration with follicular flushing, and the experience and skills of the clinician [32] (Fig. 13.2 and Table 13.2).

Table 13.2 The advantage of ultrasound transvaginal many compared to another type of retrieval

Advantages
Transvaginal oocyte retrieval offers the following advantages: • The distance to reach the ovary is shorter • Higher-resolution pictures enable the identification of the ovaries and the aspiration of follicles • No risk of skin damage • The procedure can be conveniently performed in the outpatient setting • Lower cost than other techniques • Fewer staff is required • Easy to learn thanks to the use of ultrasound guidance • All follicles can be visualized and punctured, even in case of severe pelvic adhesions • It gives more precision than the abdominal approach • Analgesia can be achieved by local anaesthesia, under paracervical block, sedation, or general anaesthesia • It is well accepted by patients

13.5 Materials

Ultrasound equipment with multi-frequency, transvaginal (5–7.5 MHz) probe, which must be correctly configured. The transducer, equipped with a needle guide and crosshairs that must be seen on the screen (Fig. 13.3).

Aspiration pump/Vacuum pump with adjustable suction power control (Labotect Aspirator 3) with a negative pressure of 160 mmHg, however the actual pressure on the tip of the needle does not exceed 160 mmHg since some pressure loss is caused. Furthermore, the aspiration needle is connected to a 14 mL polystyrene collection tube (Falcon® 17 × 100 mm), 17 mm gauge and 100 mm length, and a 50 cm long Teflon line, via a silicone stopper. Another catheter is attached to the aspiration needle, and it is used to connect another Teflon flexible catheter of 1.2 mm diameter (Fig. 13.4).

Oocyte Pickup Needle: It should cause minimal tissue injury when passing through the vagina and ovary and

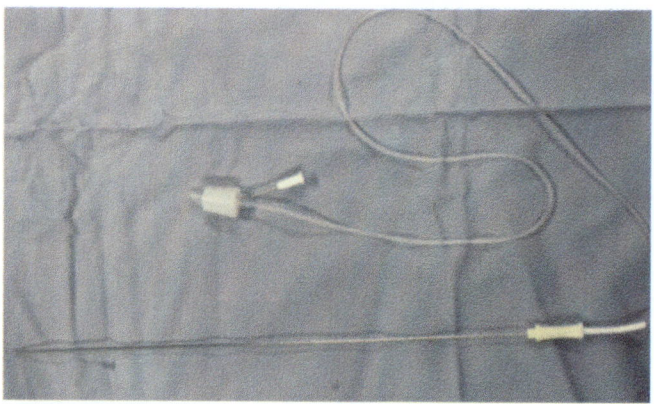

Fig. 13.5 Oocyte pickup needle

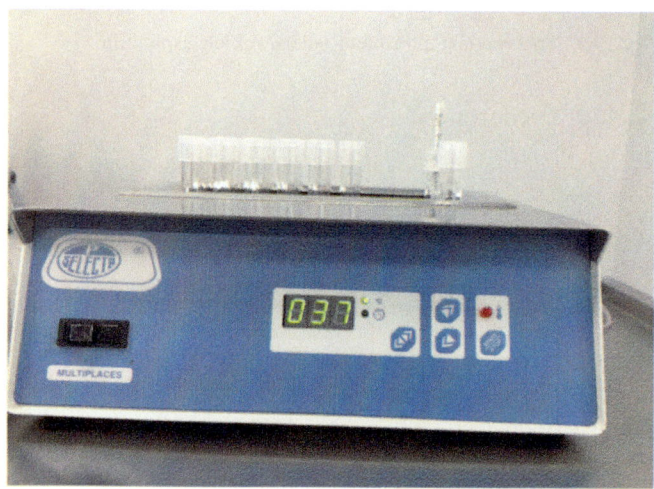

Fig. 13.6 Thermoblock

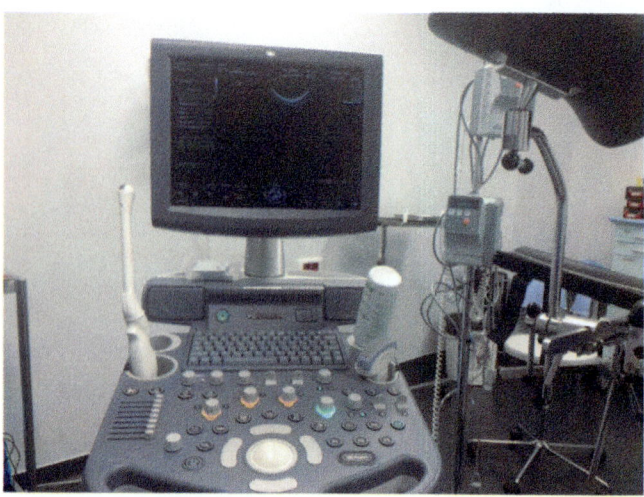

Fig. 13.3 Ultrasound equipment

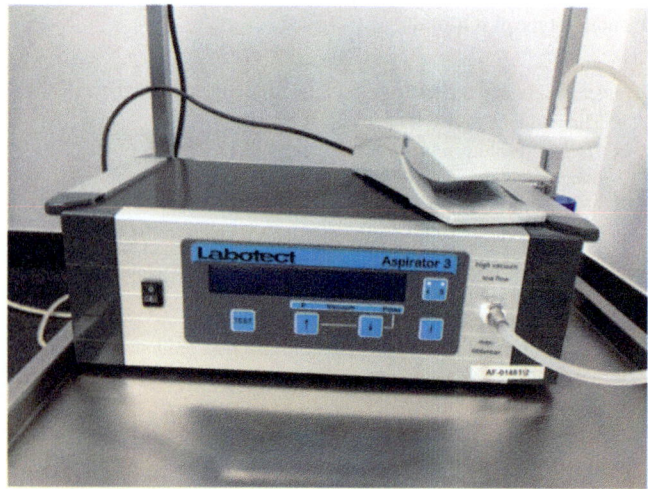

Fig. 13.4 Aspiration pump

guarantee high visibility for the correct approach to the follicle by the clinician. There are today many different needles for oocyte aspiration. The ones commonly used at IVI clinics have a length of 350 mm, with an aspiration system with 800 mmHg pressure and 19-g diameters and with embossed echogenic marked tips (Fig. 13.5).

13.5.1 Thermoblock/Heating Block Thermostat

For storing the aspiration tubes and maintain a constant temperature in follicular fluid aspirates at 37 °C. (Fig. 13.6).

13.6 Ovum Pickup Technique for the Collection of Oocytes

Ovum pickup should be performed at exactly 36 h after the administration of the ovulation trigger. For donor cycles, ovulation is induced with 0.2 mg of triptorelin acetate

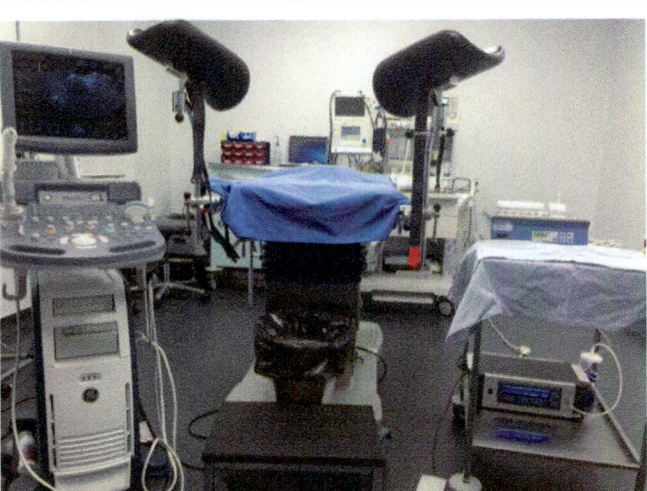

Fig. 13.7 Theatre of an IVF

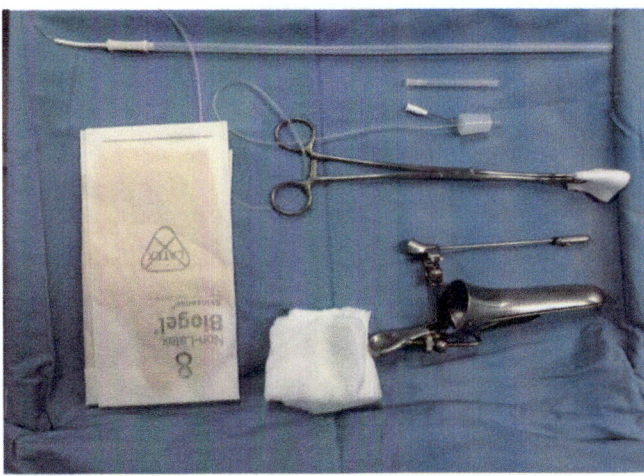

Fig. 13.8 OPU instruments

(Decapeptyl®; IpsenPharma, Barcelona, Spain) [12, 17, 19, 33]. Antibiotic prophylaxis is recommended the night before oocyte retrieval with a single dose of 1 g of oral azithromycin (Zitromax® Pfizer, S.A, Madrid, Spain) [34].

Oocyte retrieval is a surgical procedure that usually occurs in the theatre of an IVF clinic (Fig. 13.7), under general or local anaesthesia. Before starting the surgery, the team will check the surgical equipment and flush the aspiration system, and then the needle is rinsed with flushing media for removal of potential debris or contaminations inside the needle. The vacuum pressure is verified as higher pressure could affect oocyte integrity, thus decreasing their quality and increasing the proportion of oocytes without zona pellucida.

At least one operator (gynaecologist) and one assistant (nurse) are needed to perform this technique. While one is performing the follicle aspiration, the assistant will be changing the tubes for each of the follicles aspirated. The transducer tip of the ultrasound probe is covered with an ultrasound gel, and it is then covered with a protective sterile rubber sheath (or number 8 glove). A guide is attached to the probe and a disposable 19-gauge aspiration needle is used (Kitazato Medical, Tokyo, Japan).

Observing strict rules of sterility through the exclusive use of sterile supplies (namely needle guides, vaginal probe covers, patient drapes) (Fig. 13.8) has become the standard practice during these procedures. Disinfection of the vaginal probe in between usages has also been advocated to reduce bacterial contaminations resulting from unidentified probe cover defects.

Most commonly, the approach is vaginal and performed under ultrasound guidance. General intravenous anaesthesia is administered, the patient is placed in a gynaecological position and the procedure is begun, once the patient is asleep; before the procedure is started, the patient is advise to empty her bladder, in order to reduce the risk of urinary bladder injury and facilitate the access to the ovaries during transvaginal oocyte retrieval (TVOR).

A vaginal speculum is then placed, and saline solution (at 35–37 °C) [35] or non-cytotoxic antiseptic agents (such as chlorhexidine) are flushed to clean the area. It is not advisable to use iodide agents since they can be potentially cytotoxic but to use gauze pads and Foerster ring forceps [36, 37].

The transvaginal probe must be carefully inserted, and an ultrasound scan is made in order to visualize the pelvic area to confirm the number and size of follicles according to previous follicle tracking scans. The uterus is located and examined, together with the ovaries and pelvic vessels in order to determine the best way to approach the ovaries and assess any potential risks (full bladder, retrouterine ovaries, cysts, endometrial fibroids, uterine fibroids, etc.) that could hinder oocyte recovery. If the bladder is full, it must be emptied using a urinary probe. Then, the gloves must be changed, and if possible, powder-free gloves should be used. As it is shown in Fig. 13.9, it is recommended to use the left hand to hold the transducer and the right hand to hold the needle when aspirating the left ovary, and the other way around, when aspirating the right ovary.

Once the most accessible ovary is selected, the needle is penetrated through the vaginal fornix into the follicle, by applying a steady inwards pressure, with the vaginal probe, in order to directly access as closer as possible to the ovary (1–3 cm distance), immobilize the ovaries and avoid movements, reduce the risk of intraoperative rupture of the ovarian capsule, and keep bowel loops away.

Before penetrating the tissue, the probe should be rotated to 90° from the midsagittal plane in order to reduce the risk of lesions of the vessels of the vaginal wall. Also Doppler ultrasound guidance (Fig. 13.10) can be used to avoid vascular injury.

When the biggest follicle is visualized on the ultrasound screen, once the needle is inserted (Fig. 13.11), a controlled

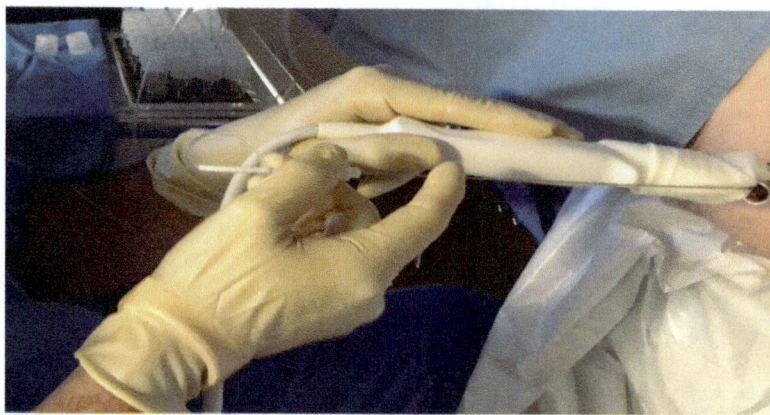
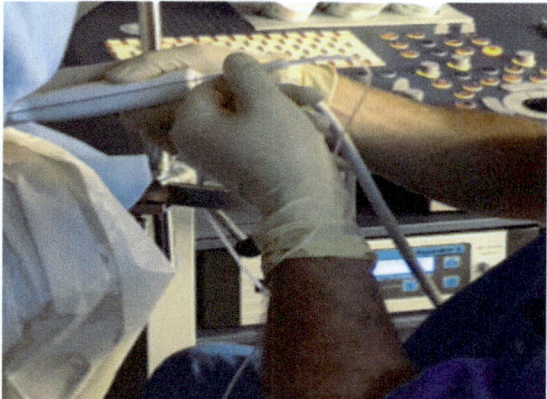

Fig. 13.9 Follicle aspiration using both hands

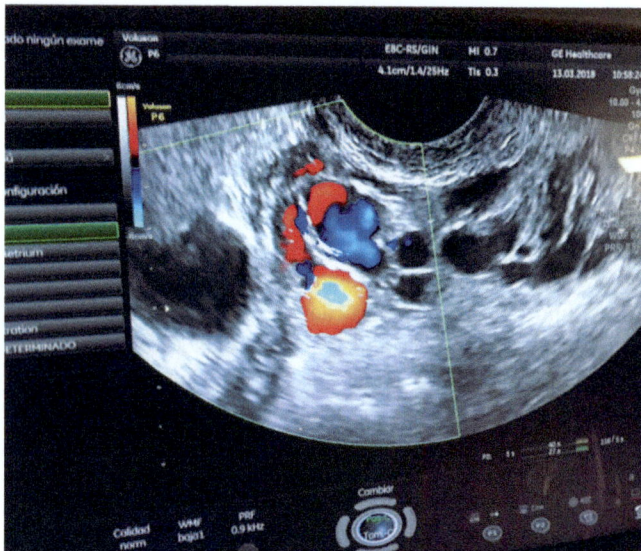

Fig. 13.10 Use colour Doppler to identify pelvic vessels

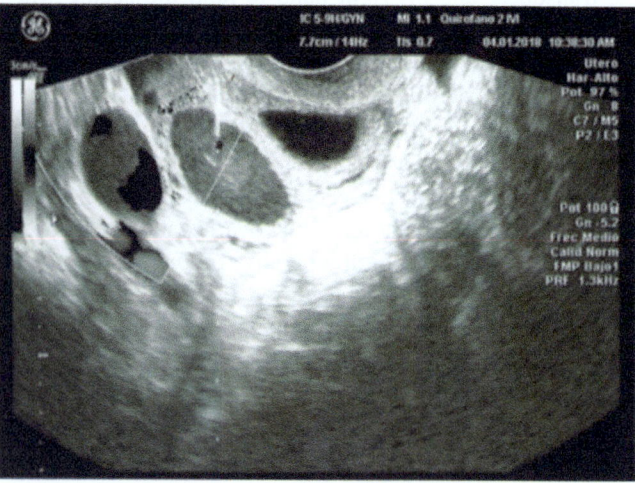

Fig. 13.11 Follicular aspiration with needle

Table 13.3 A review of complications following transvaginal oocyte retrieval for in vitro-fertilization [42]

Safety measures should be taken during ovum pick-up, such as:
• When inserting the needle, use colour Doppler ultrasound guidance
• The tip of the needle must be visualized at all times in order to prevent injury to the adjacent pelvic structures
• Aspirate completely the follicle before changing to another follicle
• Do not make any sudden or lateral movements once the ovary has been punctured
• Do not rotate the needle once in place as this could cause injury to the ovary
• Once the needle has entered the ovarian cortex, follicles should be punctured in a fan-shaped manner starting from the entering point. Puncture the follicle where the biggest diameter is found

vacuum is applied to the needle and the follicular fluid is aspirated from the ovary and aspiration of the other follicles is performed without removing the needle from the ovary, following the same approach (Table 13.3).

Whenever possible, a single puncture of each ovary is performed, and, once inserted, puncture the remaining follicles [38]. Bleeding often occurs in the ovarian capsule after puncture; therefore, the number of punctures should be limited to reduce the risk of post-retrieval bleeding.

Oocyte aspiration is often completed at the end of the procedure, aspirating thick and viscous fluid (granulosa cells of the corona radiata and cumulus).

Therefore, the aspiration should be continued until the last drop of fluid is aspirated. In order to do so, the long bevelled needle should be rotated 90° in a clockwise and counterclockwise fashion inside the follicle after complete aspiration of the follicular fluid, followed by one 2-mL flush solution that can be changed several times. This procedure is reserved for cases of low oocyte recovery [38, 39].

Aspiration pressure may be different depending on the type and length of the needle; there is a lack of studies

Table 13.4 Recommended pressure for needle Kitazato

Gauge and length of the needle	Aspiration pressure (mmHg)
17G × 35 cm	130
18G × 35 cm	170
19G × 35 cm	200–230
20G × 30 cm	300
20G × 35 cm	200–230
21G × 30 cm	350–400

describing the effect of aspiration pressure on oocyte quality and pregnancy outcomes. A few studies have quoted using aspirating pressures ranging between 150 and 200 mmHg, or occasionally, even lower [40].

At IVI clinics, disposable 19-gauge aspiration needles are used with 160 mmHg aspiration pressure. (Kitazato Medical, Tokyo, Japan) (Table 13.4).

If flushing is interrupted, the needle must be rotated 45° to restore the flow of liquid (this can happen when the tip of the aspiration needle is attached to the follicular wall). Alternatively, increasing the aspiration pressure should help restore the flow. The needle could also be removed from the ovary in order to flush the aspiration system if we suspect of any potential occlusion caused by blood clots and/or ovarian tissue before continuing with the procedure [40, 41].

Intuitively, careful ultrasound visualization of all round-shaped translucent structures in both longitudinal and transverse axes is recommended practice for distinguishing vessels and avoiding misidentification of ovarian follicles during needle advancement.

Once the aspiration of follicles in one ovary is completed, the other ovary is punctured. This second ovary is usually more accessible after having punctured the first ovary. The aspiration needle must be removed and flushed with wash media. The vaginal transducer probe is then rotated and the position of the needle on the screen changes.

The same procedure is performed.

Regarding the proportion of oocytes recovered by this surgical approach, at least 80% of the oocytes are collected [42]. Several studies have compared the effectiveness of aspiration alone with aspiration with follicular flushing, showing higher proportion of recovered oocytes when aspiration alone was performed, compared to those where aspiration and follicular flushing were made. The later reported longer operation times and an increased used of analgesics. This was concluded after the literature review of Cochrane in 2010, which was later followed by a meta-analysis in 2012 [43–45] best placed in the thermal block set at 37 °C. Once three quarters of the tube is full, it is transferred to the IVF lab in a thermoblock in order to maintain the temperature. The lab is then informed of the change of collection tube and ovary and the ovum pick-up is completed. Follicular fluid obtained is analysed by the biologists under the microscope, who will confirm the presence and number of oocytes.

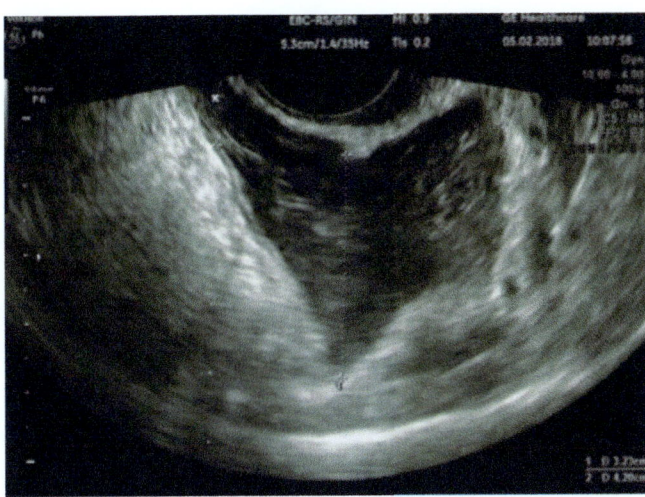

Fig. 13.12 Liquid in the pouch of Douglas

After the puncture of both ovaries, the pelvic cavity is assessed with the transvaginal probe in order to confirm the absence of bleeding.

Accumulation of liquid in the pouch of Douglas oocyte is frequently found after oocyte retrieval, up to 100 mL is normal [46, 47]. The liquid is removed before finishing the surgical procedure (Fig. 13.12); this routine helps to reduce postoperative pain caused by peritoneal irritation.

If an active bleeding point is suspected, ultrasound evaluation of the patient must be performed before the patient is discharged from hospital.

Visual examination of the posterior fornix and cervix for lesions and/or bleeding is performed. Flush the vagina with 0.9% saline solution. Press firmly for a few seconds with a swab to stop bleeding [35, 48]. Remove vaginal speculum.

In the IVF laboratory, the oocytes are recovered from the follicular fluid in order to be washed and placed in the incubator maintaining a 5% CO_2 at 37 °C until insemination or ICSI. For oocytes that will be vitrified and not donated, new screening tests for HIV Ag/Ab and HCV Ab are performed within 40 days.

13.7 Post Oocyte Retrieval Follow-Up

One of the main aspects of post oocyte retrieval care is the management of pain, which is although difficult to evaluate and might be influenced by many factors, such as fear of pain, anxiety, surgical skills of the doctor, operation time and other technical factors, such as needle diameter and the sharpness during ovum-pickup (OPU) [49].

After OPU, 3% of patients experienced severe to very severe pain and 2% of patients were still suffering from severe pain 2 days after the procedure [31, 34, 35, 48]. Intraoperative analgesia should be indicated and routine postoperative analgesic regime should be given in order to minimize postoperative pain.

After ovum pickup, the patient rests 2 h at the clinic under observation to discard circulatory complications and determine the need of further analgesia. The patient is then discharged if there are no complications.

For donors who yielded >20 oocytes or presented high serum estradiol levels (E2 > 3500 pg/mL) or in the event of difficult oocyte retrieval or patients who report any symptoms, a follow-up visit is scheduled.

Clear postoperative instructions are given to the patients, along with information on emergency contact telephone numbers (24 h) in case of bleeding, temperature, feeling of weakness, dizziness or poor general condition.

13.8 Other Approaches to Oocyte Recovery

The technique of oocyte retrieval has evolved thanks to the use and the improvements of ultrasonography; using ultrasound guidance, various methods of oocyte retrieval included percutaneous [50], transvesical [25, 50], per-urethral [51] and transvaginal follicle aspiration [52].

Several studies have found that both patient and clinician preference for transvaginal ultrasound over abdominal ultrasound for follicular monitoring and aspiration. Hence, gynaecologists care by many are often more skilled in transvaginal ultrasound due to the frequency of use.

As such, transvaginal ultrasound-guided aspiration has become the standard of care in women undergoing oocyte retrieval during IVF [29, 53]. Problems arise when the ovaries are not accessible transvaginally. Historically, in these cases laparoscopy was performed for oocyte retrieval, or these women were not considered candidates for IVF.

An alternative retrieval method is the transabdominal ultrasound-guided retrieval in women whose ovaries were not accessible by transvaginal ultrasonography, in cases in which ultrasonographic follicular monitoring was feasible only transabdominally or in those cases where vaginal access to the ovary was not possible, in either one or both ovaries, despite the usual technique of applying abdominal pressure to push the ovaries into the pelvis [30].

Due to decreased elasticity of the abdominal skin, each ovary typically required multiple punctures, which has the potential for increased patient discomfort and scarring of the skin. However, it has been shown that transabdominal aspiration of one or both ovaries can be done without sacrificing safety or efficacy. Although a slight decrease in the total number of oocytes retrieved transabdominally has been reported, this did not translate into fewer mature oocytes or fewer embryos. Furthermore, no increase in damage to the oocytes was observed [29].

13.9 Factors Influencing Oocyte Retrieval

13.9.1 Inaccessible Ovaries at Oocyte Retrieval

Inaccessibility of the ovaries transvaginally is uncommon; it ranges from 0.4 [29] to 1.7% of cases where one or both ovaries may be inaccessible at transvaginal oocyte retrieval (TVOR) [54] (Figs. 13.13 and 13.14).

It is more common in patients with previous pelvic surgery, uterine adhesions, which may distort the pelvic anatomy and the normal ovarian location, including endometriosis, uterine fibroids or congenital anomalies of the genital tract, such as Müllerian anomaly can make the procedure almost impossible. Those patients with previous history of inaccessible ovaries at transvaginal oocyte retrieval might be more prone to have this problem; however, it should not be relied upon to accurately predict their occurrence.

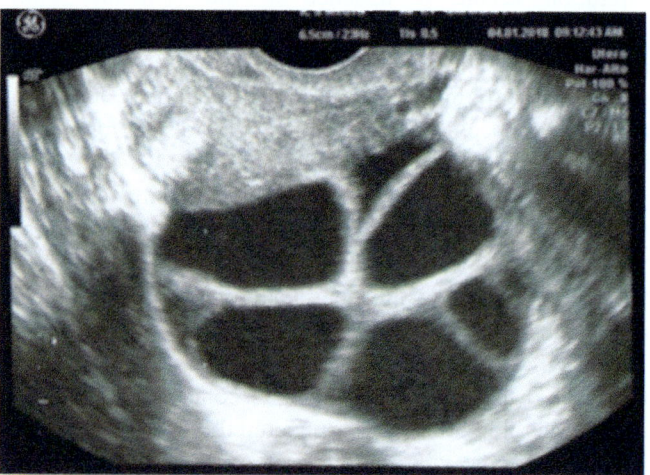

Fig. 13.13 Retrouterine ovary

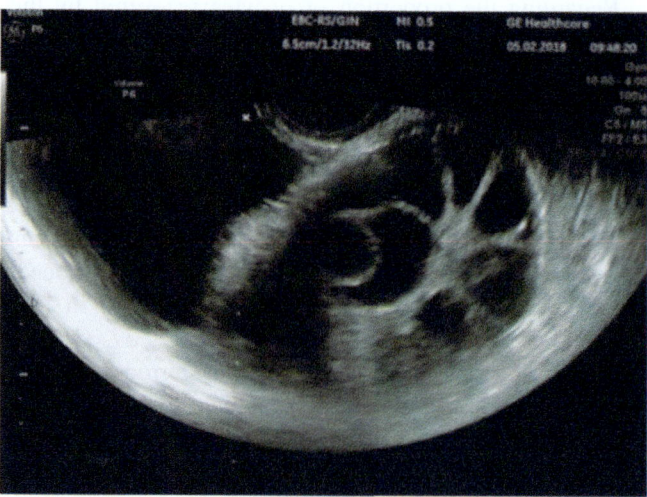

Fig. 13.14 Inaccessible ovary due to full bladder

Fig. 13.15 Procedure when inaccessible ovaries at oocyte retrieval

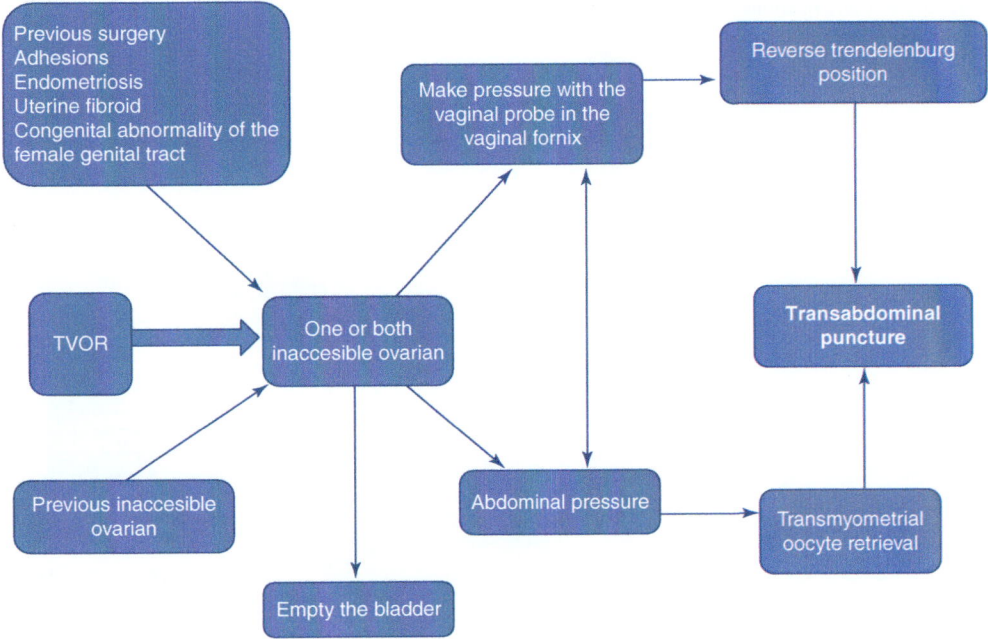

It is important to identify such factors, paying special attention to the position of ovaries and the vaginal accessibility during transvaginal follicular monitoring at the ovarian stimulation stage in order to identify those patients at high risk of transvaginally inaccessible ovaries. This information should be documented in the patient's record, most of the times, the professional performing the scan might not be the same one carrying out the OPU.

In order to access the ovaries, patients should be asked to completely empty the bladder before OPU, even they do not feel the urge to urinate. Intraoperatively, if one or both ovaries are found to be inaccessible and the bladder is full, a disposable catheter should be used to empty the bladder as this can bring the ovaries closer to the vagina and render them accessible. Another management option is the use of appropriate pressure, with or without concomitant abdominal pressure, in order to bring an inaccessible ovary closer to the vaginal wall. Sometimes, reverse Trendelenburg position and lateral table tilt can also help (Fig. 13.15).

Sometimes the ovary is firmly fixed behind the uterus and, despite various manoeuvers, the only way transvaginally would be through the uterus, transmyometrially in order to aspirate the follicles of a retroverted ovary [54].

If all transvaginal attempts fail, then transabdominal ultrasound-guided oocyte retrieval could be used on one or both ovaries without sacrificing safety or efficacy and is useful in cases where vaginal access to the ovaries is denied [30].

13.10 Complications Following Oocyte Retrieval

Short-term complications are usually divided into two categories (Fig. 13.16).

13.10.1 Complications Arising from Ovarian Stimulation

The main known complication arising from ovarian stimulation is ovarian hyperstimulation syndrome (OHSS), which is nowadays a rare event in oocyte donors, thanks to the use of the GnRH antagonist protocol followed by induction with GnRH analogue [18, 55, 56].

13.10.2 Complications Following Oocyte Retrieval

Complications related to the oocyte retrieval procedure, either by the procedure itself or by the venous blood areas, appear to be more important, since they may lead to haemorrhage, pelvic infections (occurring in 0.01–0.6%), ovarian torsion (occurring in 0.08–0.13%) injuries of the adjacent organs, mainly.

There is a low risk of complications noted in oocyte retrievals involving oocyte donors (<0.5%) [57]. Although not all of them have been reported in the literature, some studies have determined their occurrence. These studies have

Fig. 13.16 Complications
following oocyte retrieval

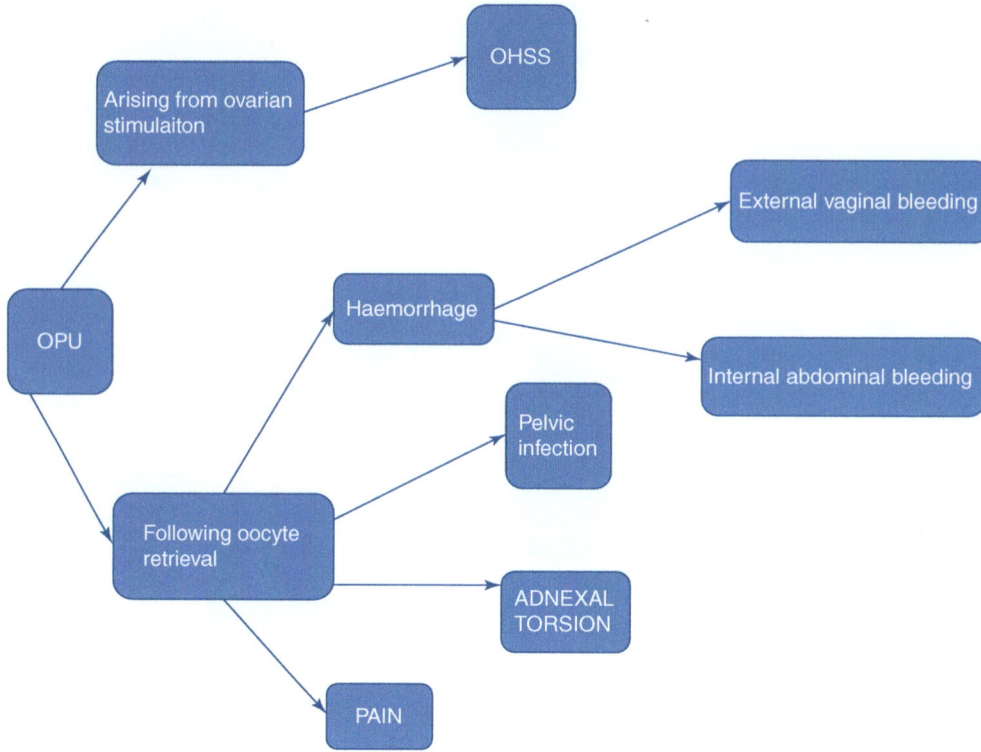

Fig. 13.17 Procedure when
haemorrhage during OPU

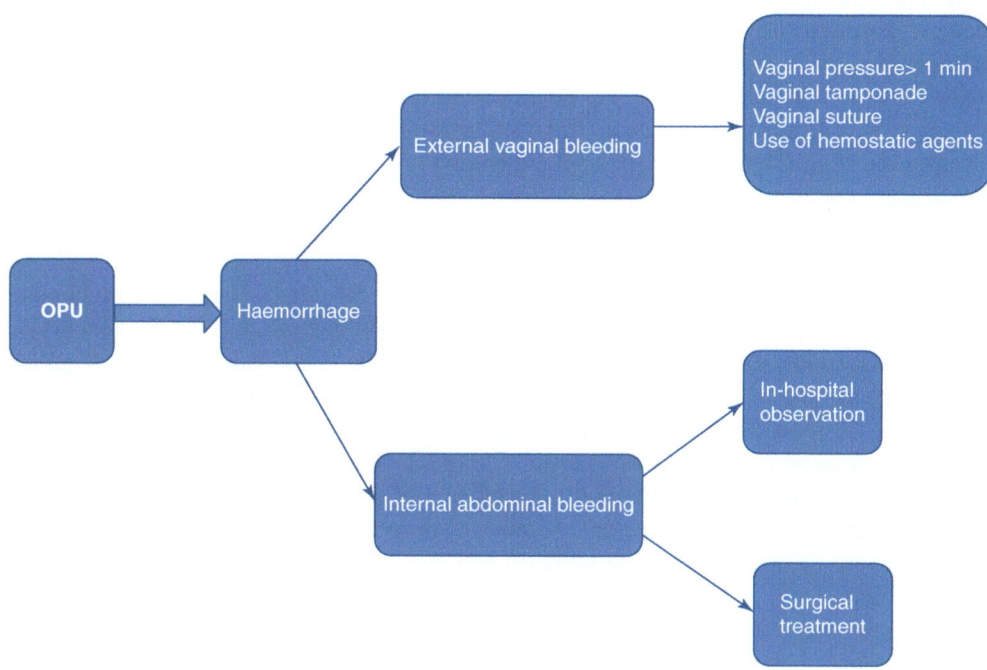

shown risks and complications are similar to those experienced by women undergoing IVF [58].

The potential surgical hazards associated with oocyte retrieval include risks of bleeding, pelvic infection, pain, ovarian torsion and injury to adjacent pelvic organs [34, 35, 48].

However, because of the possible health risks for these patients, it is prudent to limit the number of stimulated cycles for a given donor to 6 [1].

13.10.3 Haemorrhage

Bleeding events probably remain one of the most frequent complications following OPU. In fact, bleeding is a reasonable consequence of the process of needle insertion through vascularized tissues and could manifest either as external or as internal abdominal bleeding (Fig. 13.17).

13.10.4 External Vaginal Bleeding

The most common complication associated with oocyte retrieval is the external vaginal bleeding, which has been reported an incidence of 8.6%. However, the definition and quantification of vaginal bleeding remain unclear; to date, there is no consensus as to whether bleeding is abnormal or not.

In their prospective cohort study on more than 1000 procedures, Ludwig et al. reported the occurrence of vaginal wall bleeding requiring local compression of >1 min in 2.7% of cases, significant bleeding occurred in 0.1% of cases and required tamponade for 3 h, and no cases necessitating vaginal suturing were reported. Other studies [59] have reported cases of minor vaginal bleeding which requiring local vaginal pressure of 1–2 min. In more severe cases, the use of haemostatic agents and/or suturing may be required to control local bleeding.

It has been estimated that the risk of vaginal bleeding during OPU may be increased by the presence of predisposing factors, such as the number of vaginal wall punctures, needle diameter and poor operator's technique. Reducing the number of vaginal wall entries by aligning multiple ovarian follicles for aspiration during a single needle pass may therefore be desired. The choice of smaller diameter needles could have an additional impact on reducing the amount and likelihood of bleeding, despite the lack of supportive scientific evidence. It has also been suggested that the application of firm inwards pressure on the vaginal wall during needle entry decreases tissue thickness, hence hypothetically reducing the likelihood of bleeding. Avoidance of lateral displacement of the needle during oocyte retrieval away from its original path further reduces the incidence of vaginal wall tears requiring suturing. In the event of increased pelvic varicosities or in the case of a retroverted uterus, careful ultrasound visualization of the paravaginal and paracervical vascular plexus before needle advancement is highly advisable to reduce the frequency and intensity of vaginal bleeding.

13.10.5 Internal Abdominal Bleeding

Internal abdominal bleeding following TVOR is an event, which occurs at a much higher frequency than is clinically recognized, and can be caused by needle injury to the ovarian pedicle, uterine arteries, iliac vessels, median sacral arteries and visceral organs.

Bodri et al. [34, 48] assessed the complication rate in oocyte donation cycles through the analysis of 4052 oocyte retrievals. In this series, the authors reported a 0.35% rate of hospital admissions for bleeding, where 0.12% required laparoscopy to repair the complications.

In the prospective study of Ludwig et al., no clinically significant abdominal bleeding events were recorded following 1058 OPU procedures. In retrospective studies, the incidence of clinically significant internal abdominal bleeding has been reported to range from 0.08 to 0.2%. Aragona et al. [45, 46] observed severe peritoneal bleeding requiring surgical treatment in 0.06% of 7098 cases, all of whom manifested as hemodynamic instability and abdominal pain as late as 12 h following the procedure. About 750–1000 mL of fluid was detected in the abdominal cavity by ultrasound pelvic scanning. In a retrospective review of 3241 procedures, Liberty et al. further reported the incidence of clinically significant internal abdominal bleeding to be 0.2%, all originating from injury to the ovaries [60].

The amount of blood loss did not appear to correlate with the number of follicles aspirated, oocytes collected, preovulatory estradiol levels and/or duration of the procedure.

Thorough monitoring of vital signs and recording of pain symptoms following the procedure should determine the need for an extended postoperative observational period or prompt the initiation of a more involved investigation. The pattern of pain distribution may also be helpful in refining diagnostic accuracy.

Accurate diagnosis and management play an important role in safeguarding patient's well-being and impacting recovery. A good surgical technique may also reduce the risks of internal abdominal bleeding. Careful ultrasound visualization of all round-shaped translucent structures in both longitudinal and transverse axes is the recommended practice for distinguishing vessels and avoiding misidentification of ovarian follicles during needle advancement. The immobilization of the ovary by the application of steady inward pressure by the ultrasound probe may reduce organ slippage and minimize the risk of lacerations to the ovarian capsule. In addition, avoidance of lateral needle movements away from the original needle path is likely to reduce the incidence of lacerations to the outer capsule and inner stroma of the ovary.

At the end of OPU, ultrasound inspection of the pelvis prior to vaginal probe withdrawal is considered good practice to evaluate the rate of fluid accumulation in the posterior pouch of Douglas and/or the presence of significant fluid turbulence indicative of active bleeding [61]. Some investigators have also proposed an additional ultrasound examination at the time of patient discharge, which is about 1–2 h later.

13.10.6 Pelvic Infection

Pelvic infection is the second most commonly reported complication following transvaginal oocyte retrieval (TVOR). It is a well-documented complication among infertile women submitted to in vitro fertilization treatments as compared with oocyte donors, where data is scarce [46].

Fig. 13.18 Procedure when
pelvic infection following
OPU

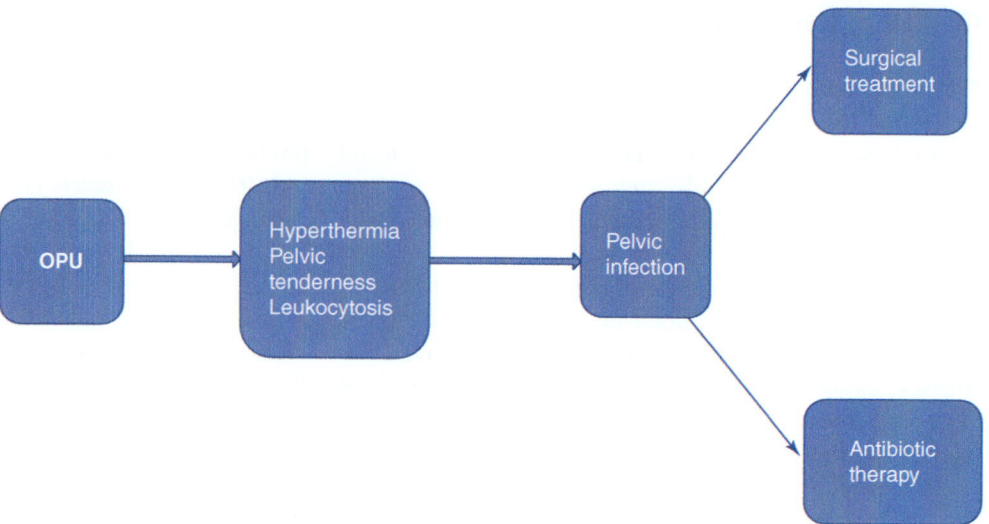

It is a rare but potentially serious complication. The severity of infection ranges from a minor infection with pyrexia, leucocytosis and abdominal pain, to a major medical event such as pelvic abscess formation or sepsis [59].

Several etiological mechanisms have been suggested to contribute to the relatively high rate of pelvic infections following OPU; one of them may be the direct inoculation of vaginal microorganisms through the needle path from the vagina into the peritoneal cavity during the procedure. Another possible route of infection can be the reactivation of a latent pelvic infection due to a previous pelvic inflammatory disease (PID) or unintentional bowel puncture during TVOR [62, 63].

Although an overall incidence of 0.03–0.6% for pelvic infections and tubo-ovarian abscesses has been reported in the medical literature, limited evidence is available regarding predisposing factors, the need for prophylactic antibiotics and the most appropriate means of preoperative vaginal preparation [64].

Weinreb et al. [63] reported in a retrospective study comparing 526 oocyte donors who received prophylactic antibiotics for oocyte retrieval with a comparable group of 625 who did not the incidence of infection after retrieval was reduced from 0.4 to 0% in the group receiving antibiotics. Although the results obtained were not statistically significant, the data suggested that prophylactic antibiotics at retrieval should be considered to minimize the risk of infection, since the benefit of minimizing the incidence of pelvic infection outweighs the risk of allergy, discomfort or bacterial resistance resulting from antibiotic use.

Ludwig et al. [35] described the use of isotonic saline solution to soak the vagina when no preventive antibiotics were used; however, the study did not analyse the clinical evidence of pelvic infection among these women.

In their prospective study of 2670 TVOR, Bennett et al. reported fever, leucocytosis and pelvic tenderness in 0.3% of

cases, which were managed by subsequent antibiotic therapy.

Aragona et al. [46] reported two cases of ovarian abscess (0.03%) among 7098 IVF cycles, regardless of the use of prophylactic antibiotics and negative culture for vaginal infections.

In their retrospective study of 4052 donor oocyte retrievals, Bodri et al. reported no cases of pelvic infection when prophylactic azithromycin was given on the evening before and during the procedure, and when the vagina was disinfected using chlorhexidine followed by abundant washing with isotonic saline solution.

One has to avoid the puncture of endometrioma as well as hydrosalpinx in order to reduce the risk of infection [65, 66].

The universal use of antibiotic prophylaxis and the common adoption of aseptic techniques to reduce OPU procedure-associated infections [46, 59, 67] e-associated infections remains an unsettled dilemma. Pelvic abscesses continue to occur despite their use [46, 59, 67].

In view of this, it is expected that oocyte donors have a low incidence of pelvic infections, since donors, by definition, are young and healthy with no potential risk factor of infection following oocyte retrieval, as already shown (Fig. 13.18).

13.10.7 Adnexal Torsion

Adnexal torsion (Fig. 13.19) is a rare but serious complication to ovarian hyperstimulation. The risk is increased due to the presence of predisposing factors such as enlarged and at the same time mobile ovaries.

Patients with ovarian hyperstimulation syndrome (OHSS) seem to be associated with an increased risk of complications, since large cysts and the presence of fluid in the pelvic ascites

Fig. 13.19 Adnexal torsion
after OPU

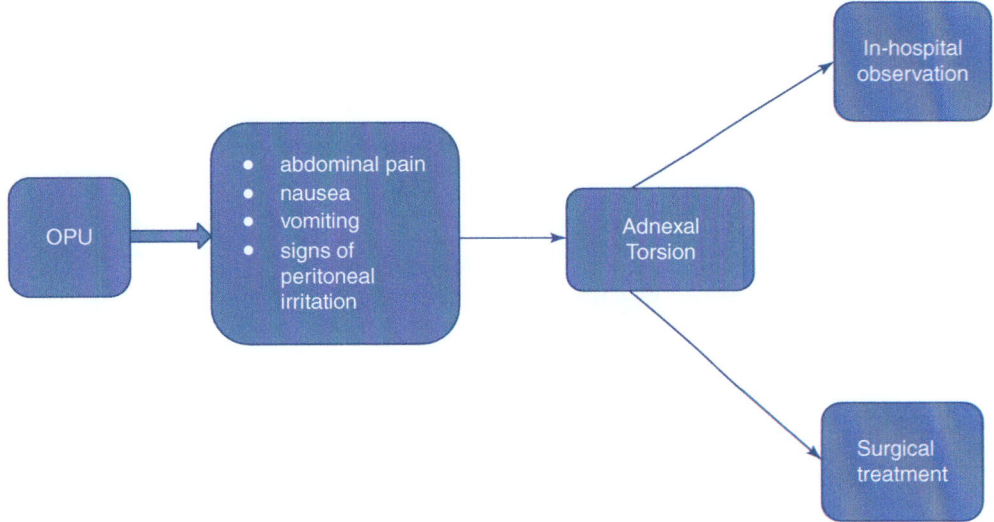

facilitate twisting on the vascular pedicle. The incidence of ovarian torsion ranges from 0.8% in all IVF cycles to 7.5% in patients with OHSS [68, 69].

The etiopathogensis of ovarian torsion refers to the rotation of the ovarian vascular pedicle at the infundibulo-pelvic ligament and causes obstruction to venous outflow, lymphatic circulation and arterial inflow. It may lead to gangrene and haemorrhagic necrosis, which may result in infection. If untreated, then peritonitis and death may ultimately result.

The diagnosis of ovarian torsion is based on the patient's clinical picture detailing acute onset of abdominal pain, and a history of nausea and vomiting and signs of peritoneal irritation. Additional clinical findings may include anorexia, fever, leucocytosis and a palpable mass. Maintaining a high degree of suspicion is important, especially in infertility patients who have been submitted to ovarian stimulation and present the symptoms already enumerated.

Although the diagnosis of ovarian torsion is difficult, careful analysis of presenting symptoms is critical to avoid irreversible ischemia and infarction. Distinguishing ovarian torsion from mild hyperstimulation can be challenging, both clinically and radiologically. Both entities may manifest with abdominal pain, nausea, and vomiting. However, the diagnosis should be made based on clinical findings, since sonography is not reliable in the diagnosis or exclusion of ovarian torsion and Doppler examination still has a limited role. Laparoscopy is the gold standard for its diagnostic evaluation [70, 71]. In conclusion, ovarian torsion is often difficult to diagnose and requires immediate surgery, preferably by laparoscopic detorsion of the twisted ovary, regardless of the ischemic appearance of the adnexa, to restore the blood supply and avoid adnexectomy.

13.10.8 Pain

It is difficult to evaluate pain experience after OPU, because many factors can have an influence such as fear of pain, anxiety, the number of oocytes retrieved, the number of punctures to the vaginal wall, the operation time, the clinician's skill and technical factors including needle diameter [49] and the difficulties found during the oocyte retrieval process. For most cases, some pain is unavoidable. After the procedure, only 2–3% of the patients described their pain as severe, and. 0.4% as the worst pain they had ever experienced [31, 72]; however, even when only a single follicle is punctured, oocyte retrieval can be painful.

Pain during oocyte retrieval is caused by the aspirating needle puncturing the vaginal skin and ovarian capsule, as well as its manipulation within the ovary during the procedure. General anaesthesia may be used for this procedure, but since that has significant resource requirements, many IVF units use conscious sedation and analgesia [73].

During OPU several options are available for pain relief including general anaesthesia, regional anaesthesia and conscious sedation. Conscious sedation is administered alone or together with paracervical block or acupuncture [73, 74].

However, more and more patients request anaesthesia or sedation when OPU is performed. Anaesthesia during OPU and the usage of analgesics straight away following the surgery help patients find less pain caused by multiple punctures in the vagina [72, 75].

Bodri et al. [34] conducted a retrospective study to evaluate the complications related to ovarian stimulation and oocyte retrieval in 4052 oocyte donor cycles, where only two patients experienced severe pain and required hospital admission.

Ludwig et al. [35] conducted a study where they asked patients to rank their amount of pain 2 h after OPU. About

Fig. 13.20 Pain after OPU

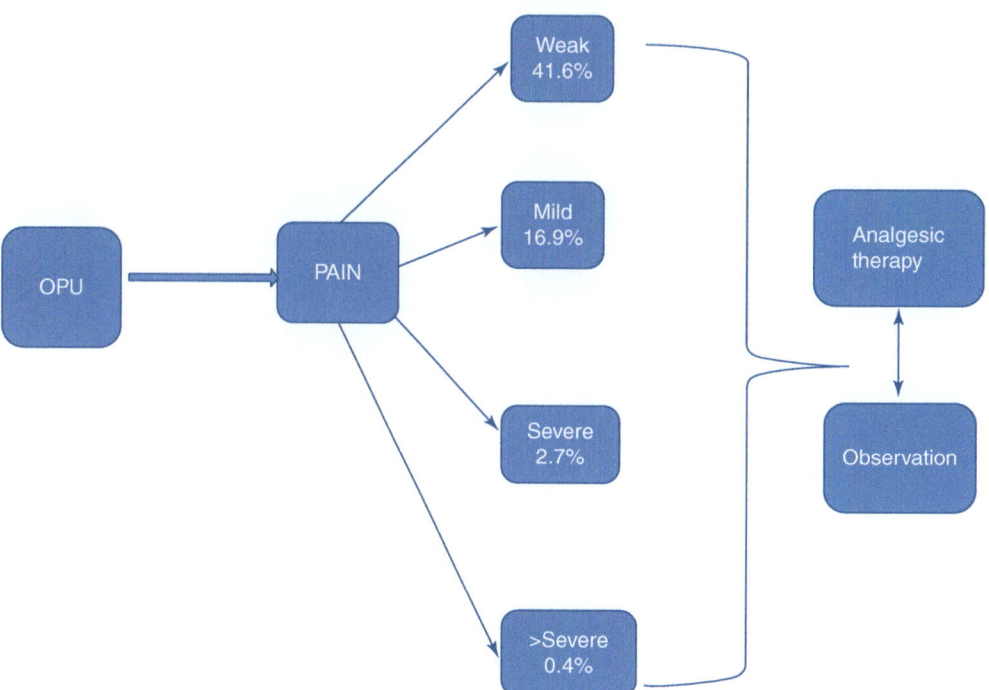

38.5% of patients had no pain 2 h after OR, 41.6% had mild pain, whereas 16.9% of patients recorded medium pain, 2.7% severe pain and 0.4% very severe pain. Ten percent of patients were still suffering from pain 2–3 days after the procedure.

It is important, however, not to underestimate the intensity of post-egg retrieval pain in oocyte donors, especially the persistent pattern of pelvic pain following TVOR, as it may be indicative of a more serious underlying condition warranting further investigation in order to intercept signs and symptoms of the complications described above (Fig. 13.20).

References

1. Practice Committee of the American Society for Reproductive Medicine; and Practice Committee of the Society for Assisted Reproductive Technology. Repetitive oocyte donation: a committee opinion. Fertil Steril. 2014;102(4):964–6. ISSN 1556-5653; 0015-0282.
2. Laws PJ, Tracy SK, Sullivan EA. Perinatal outcomes of women intending to give birth in birth centers in Australia. Birth (Berkeley, Calif.). 2010;37(1):28–36. ISSN 1523-536X; 0730-7659.
3. ESHRE Capri Workshop Group. Failures (with some successes) of assisted reproduction and gamete donation programs. Hum Reprod Update. 2013;19(4):354–65. ISSN 1460-2369; 1355-4786.
4. Budak E, et al. Improvements achieved in an oocyte donation program over a 10-year period: sequential increase in implantation and pregnancy rates and decrease in high-order multiple pregnancies. Fertil Steril. 2007;88(2):342–9. ISSN 1556-5653; 0015-0282.
5. Trounson A, et al. Pregnancy established in an infertile patient after transfer of a donated embryo fertilised in vitro. Br Med J. 1983;286(6368):835–8. ISSN 0267-0623; 0267-0623.

6. Yeh JS, et al. Pregnancy rates in donor oocyte cycles compared to similar autologous in vitro fertilization cycles: an analysis of 26,457 fresh cycles from the Society for Assisted Reproductive Technology. Fertil Steril. 2014;102(2):399–404. ISSN 1556-5653; 0015-0282.
7. Centers for Disease Control and Prevention, American Society for Reproductive Medicine, Society for Assisted Reproductive Technology. Assisted reproductive technology success rates: national summary and fertility clinic reports. 2010 ed. Atlanta: Department of Health and Human Services; 2008.
8. Wang YA, Farquhar C, Sullivan EA. Donor age is a major determinant of success of oocyte donation/recipient programme. Hum Reprod. 2012;27(1):118–25. ISSN 1460-2350; 0268-1161.
9. Borini A, et al. Oocyte donation programs: strategy for improving results. Ann N Y Acad Sci. 2011;1221:27–31. ISSN 1749-6632; 0077-8923.
10. Gupta P, et al. A study of recipient related predictors of success in oocyte donation program. J Hum Reprod Sci. 2012;5(3):252–7. ISSN 0974-1208; 1998-4766.
11. Guidelines for gamete donation: 1993. The American Fertility Society. Fertil Steril. 1993;59, 2(Suppl 1):1S–9S. ISSN 0015-0282; 0015-0282.
12. Vuong TN, et al. Gonadotropin-releasing hormone agonist trigger in oocyte donors co-treated with a gonadotropin-releasing hormone antagonist: a dose-finding study. Fertil Steril. 2016;105(2):356–63. ISSN 1556-5653; 0015-0282.
13. Melo M, et al. GnRH agonist versus recombinant HCG in an oocyte donation programme: a randomized, prospective, controlled, assessor-blind study. Reprod Biomed Online. 2009;19(4):486–92.. ISSN 1472-6491; 1472-6483
14. Griesinger G, et al. GnRH agonist for triggering final oocyte maturation in the GnRH antagonist ovarian hyperstimulation protocol: a systematic review and meta-analysis. Hum Reprod Update. 2006;12(2):159–68. ISSN 1355-4786; 1355-4786.
15. Humaidan P. Agonist trigger: what is the best approach? Agonist trigger and low dose hCG. Fertil Steril. 2012;97(3):529–30. ISSN 1556-5653; 0015-0282.

16. Prapas N, et al. GnRH agonist versus GnRH antagonist in oocyte donation cycles: a prospective randomized study. Hum Reprod. 2005;20(6):1516–20. ISSN 0268-1161; 0268-1161.

17. Humaidan P, et al. GnRH agonist for triggering of final oocyte maturation: time for a change of practice? Hum Reprod Update. 2011;17(4):510–24. ISSN 1460-2369; 1355-4786.

18. Castillo JC, Humaidan P, Bernabeu R. Pharmaceutical options for triggering of final oocyte maturation in ART. BioMed Res Int. 2014;2014:580171. ISSN 2314-6141.

19. Hernandez ER, Gomez-Palomares JL, Ricciarelli E. No room for cancellation, coasting, or ovarian hyperstimulation syndrome in oocyte donation cycles. Fertil Steril. 2009;91(4 Suppl):1358–61. ISSN 1556-5653; 0015-0282.

20. Bodri D, et al. Triggering with human chorionic gonadotropin or a gonadotropin-releasing hormone agonist in gonadotropin-releasing hormone antagonist-treated oocyte donor cycles: findings of a large retrospective cohort study. Fertil Steril. 2009;91(2):365–71. ISSN 1556-5653; 0015-0282.

21. Kolibianakis EM, et al. Fixed versus flexible gonadotropin-releasing hormone antagonist administration in in vitro fertilization: a randomized controlled trial. Fertil Steril. 2011;95(2):558–62. ISSN 1556-5653; 0015-0282.

22. Castillo JC, Garcia-Velasco J, Humaidan P. Empty follicle syndrome after GnRHa triggering versus hCG triggering in COS. J Assist Reprod Genet. 2012;29(3):249–53. ISSN 1573-7330; 1058-0468.

23. Andersen AG, et al. Time interval from human chorionic gonadotrophin (HCG) injection to follicular rupture. Hum Reprod. 1995;10(12):3202–5. ISSN 0268-1161; 0268-1161.

24. Taymor ML, et al. Ovulation timing by luteinizing hormone assay and follicle puncture. Obstet Gynecol. 1983;62(2):191–5. ISSN 0029-7844; 0029-7844.

25. Lenz S, Lauritsen JG, Kjellow M. Collection of human oocytes for in vitro fertilisation by ultrasonically guided follicular puncture. Lancet. 1981;1(8230):1163–4. ISSN 0140-6736; 0140-6736.

26. Gembruch U, et al. Transvaginal sonographically guided oocyte retrieval for in-vitro fertilization. Hum Reprod. 1988;3 Suppl 2:59–63. ISSN 0268-1161; 0268-1161.

27. Wiseman DA, et al. Oocyte retrieval in an in vitro fertilization-embryo transfer program: comparison of four methods. Radiology. 1989;173(1):99–102. ISSN 0033-8419; 0033-8419.

28. Wikland M, Enk L, Hamberger L. Transvesical and transvaginal approaches for the aspiration of follicles by use of ultrasound. Ann N Y Acad Sci. 1985;442:182–94. ISSN 0077-8923; 0077-8923.

29. Barton SE, et al. Transabdominal follicular aspiration for oocyte retrieval in patients with ovaries inaccessible by transvaginal ultrasound. Fertil Steril. 2011;95(5):1773–6. ISSN 1556-5653; 0015-0282.

30. Roman-Rodriguez CF, et al. Comparing transabdominal and transvaginal ultrasound-guided follicular aspiration: a risk assessment formula. Taiwan J Obstet Gynecol. 2015;54(6):693–9. ISSN 1875-6263; 1028-4559.

31. Ozaltin S, Kumbasar S, Savan K. Evaluation of complications developing during and after transvaginal ultrasound—guided oocyte retrieval. Ginekol Pol. 2018;89(1):1–6. ISSN 0017-0011; 0017-0011.

32. Leung AS, Dahan MH, Tan SL. Techniques and technology for human oocyte collection. Expert Rev Med Devices. 2016;13(8):701–3. ISSN 1745-2422; 1743-4440.

33. Bodri D, et al. Comparison between a GnRH antagonist and a GnRH agonist flare-up protocol in oocyte donors: a randomized clinical trial. Hum Reprod. 2006;21(9):2246–51. ISSN 0268-1161; 0268-1161.

34. Bodri D, et al. Complications related to ovarian stimulation and oocyte retrieval in 4052 oocyte donor cycles. Reprod Biomed Online. 2008;17(2):237–43. ISSN 1472-6491; 1472-6483.

35. Ludwig AK, et al. Perioperative and post-operative complications of transvaginal ultrasound-guided oocyte retrieval: prospective study of >1000 oocyte retrievals. Hum Reprod. 2006;21(12):3235–40. ISSN 0268-1161; 0268-1161.

36. Hannoun A, et al. Effect of betadine vaginal preparation during oocyte aspiration in in vitro fertilization cycles on pregnancy outcome. Gynecol Obstet Investig. 2008;66(4):274–8.. ISSN 1423-002X; 0378-7346

37. van Os HC, et al. Vaginal disinfection with povidon iodine and the outcome of in-vitro fertilization. Hum Reprod. 1992;7(3):349–50. ISSN 0268-1161; 0268-1161.

38. Rose BI, Laky D. A comparison of the cook single lumen immature ovum IVM needle to the steiner-tan pseudo double lumen flushing needle for oocyte retrieval for IVM. J Assist Reprod Genet. 2013;30(6):855–60. ISSN 1573-7330; 1058-0468.

39. Von Horn K, et al. Randomized, open trial comparing a modified double-lumen needle follicular flushing system with a single-lumen aspiration needle in IVF patients with poor ovarian response. Hum Reprod. 2017;32(4):832–5. ISSN 1460-2350; 0268-1161.

40. Mok-Lin E, et al. Follicular flushing and in vitro fertilization outcomes in the poorest responders: a randomized controlled trial. Hum Reprod. 2013;28(11):2990–5. ISSN 1460-2350; 0268-1161.

41. Seyhan A, et al. Comparison of complication rates and pain scores after transvaginal ultrasound-guided oocyte pickup procedures for in vitro maturation and in vitro fertilization cycles. Fertil Steril. 2014;101(3):705–9. ISSN 1556-5653; 0015-0282.

42. El-Shawarby S, et al. A review of complications following transvaginal oocyte retrieval for in-vitro fertilization. Hum Fertil. 2004;7(2):127–33. ISSN 1464-7273; 1464-7273.

43. Kumaran A, et al. Oocyte retrieval at 140-mmHg negative aspiration pressure: a promising alternative to flushing and aspiration in assisted reproduction in women with low ovarian reserve. J Hum Reprod Sci. 2015;8(2):98–102. ISSN 0974-1208; 1998-4766.

44. Roque M, Sampaio M, Geber S. Follicular flushing during oocyte retrieval: a systematic review and meta-analysis. J Assist Reprod Genet. 2012;29(11):1249–54. ISSN 1573-7330; 1058-0468.

45. Wongtra-Ngan S, Vutyavanich T, Brown J. Follicular flushing during oocyte retrieval in assisted reproductive techniques. Cochrane Database Syst Rev. 2010;(9):CD004634. ISSN 1469-493X; 1361-6137.

46. Aragona C, et al. Clinical complications after transvaginal oocyte retrieval in 7,098 IVF cycles. Fertil Steril. 2011;95(1):293–4. ISSN 1556-5653; 0015-0282.

47. Ragni G, et al. Blood loss during transvaginal oocyte retrieval. Gynecol Obstet Investig. 2009;67(1):32–5. ISSN 1423-002X; 0378-7346.

48. Siristatidis C, et al. Clinical complications after Transvaginal oocyte retrieval: a retrospective analysis. J Obstet Gynaecol. 2013;33(1):64–6. ISSN 1364-6893; 0144-3615.

49. Nakagawa K, et al. The effect of a newly designed needle on the pain and bleeding of patients during oocyte retrieval of a single follicle. J Reprod Infertil. 2015;16(4):207–11. ISSN 2228-5482; 2228-5482.

50. Lenz S, Lauritsen JG. Ultrasonically guided percutaneous aspiration of human follicles under local anesthesia: a new method of collecting oocytes for in vitro fertilization. Fertil Steril. 1982;38(6):673–7. ISSN 0015-0282; 0015-0282.

51. Parsons J, et al. Oocyte retrieval for in-vitro fertilisation by ultrasonically guided needle aspiration via the urethra. Lancet. 1985;1(8437):1076–7. ISSN 0140-6736; 0140-6736.

52. Dellenbach P, et al. Transvaginal sonographically controlled follicle puncture for oocyte retrieval. Fertil Steril. 1985;44(5):656–62. ISSN 0015-0282; 0015-0282.

53. Sauer MV, Kavic SM. Oocyte and embryo donation 2006: reviewing two decades of innovation and controversy. Reprod Biomed Online. 2006;12(2):153–62. ISSN 1472-6483; 1472-6483.

54. Davis LB, Ginsburg ES. Transmyometrial oocyte retrieval and pregnancy rates. Fertil Steril. 2004;81(2):320–2. ISSN 0015-0282; 0015-0282.

55. Donoso P, Devroey P. Low tolerance for complications. Fertil Steril. 2013;100(2):299–301. ISSN 1556-5653; 0015-0282.

56. Sismanoglu A, et al. Ovulation triggering with GnRH agonist vs. hCG in the same egg donor population undergoing donor oocyte cycles with GnRH antagonist: a prospective randomized cross-over trial. J Assist Reprod Genet. 2009;26(5):251–6. ISSN 1573-7330; 1058-0468.

57. Maxwell KN, Cholst IN, Rosenwaks Z. The incidence of both serious and minor complications in young women undergoing oocyte donation. Fertil Steril. 2008;90(6):2165–71. ISSN 1556-5653; 0015-0282.

58. Sauer MV. Defining the incidence of serious complications experienced by oocyte donors: a review of 1000 cases. Am J Obstet Gynecol. 2001;184(3):277–8. ISSN 0002-9378; 0002-9378.

59. Bennett SJ, et al. Complications of transvaginal ultrasound-directed follicle aspiration: a review of 2670 consecutive procedures. J Assist Reprod Genet. 1993;10(1):72–7. ISSN 1058-0468; 1058-0468.

60. Liberty G, et al. Ovarian hemorrhage after transvaginal ultrasonographically guided oocyte aspiration: a potentially catastrophic and not so rare complication among lean patients with polycystic ovary syndrome. Fertil Steril. 2010;93(3):874–9. ISSN 1556-5653; 0015-0282.

61. Risquez F, Confino E. Can Doppler ultrasound-guided oocyte retrieval improve IVF safety? Reprod Biomed Online. 2010;21(4):444–5. ISSN 1472-6491; 1472-6483.

62. Dicker D, et al. Severe abdominal complications after transvaginal ultrasonographically guided retrieval of oocytes for in vitro fertilization and embryo transfer. Fertil Steril. 1993;59(6):1313–5. ISSN 0015-0282; 0015-0282.

63. Weinreb EB, et al. Should all oocyte donors receive prophylactic antibiotics for retrieval? Fertil Steril. 2010;94(7):2935–7. ISSN 1556-5653; 0015-0282.

64. Tsai YC, et al. Vaginal disinfection with povidone iodine immediately before oocyte retrieval is effective in preventing pelvic abscess formation without compromising the outcome of IVF-ET. J Assist Reprod Genet. 2005;22(4):173–5. ISSN 1058-0468; 1058-0468.

65. Romero B, et al. Pelvic abscess after oocyte retrieval in women with endometriosis: a case series. Iran J Reprod Med. 2013;11(8):677–80. ISSN 1680-6433; 1680-6433.

66. Garcia-Velasco JA, Somigliana E. Management of endometriomas in women requiring IVF: to touch or not to touch. Hum Reprod. 2009;24(3):496–501. ISSN 1460-2350; 0268-1161.

67. Andersen AN, et al. Assisted reproductive technology in Europe, 2001. Results generated from European Registers by ESHRE. Hum Reprod. 2005;20(5):1158–76. ISSN 0268-1161; 0268-1161.

68. Roest J, et al. The incidence of major clinical complications in a Dutch transport IVF programme. Hum Reprod. 1996;2(4):345–53. ISSN 1355-4786; 1355-4786.

69. Baron KT, et al. Emergent complications of assisted reproduction: expecting the unexpected. Radiographics. 2013;33(1):229–44. ISSN 1527-1323; 0271-5333.

70. Pena JE, et al. Usefulness of Doppler sonography in the diagnosis of ovarian torsion. Fertil Steril. 2000;73(5):1047–50. ISSN 0015-0282; 0015-0282.

71. Bar-On S, et al. Emergency laparoscopy for suspected ovarian torsion: are we too hasty to operate? Fertil Steril. 2010;93(6):2012–5. ISSN 1556-5653; 0015-0282.

72. Hildebrandt NB, Host E, Mikkelsen AL. Pain experience during transvaginal aspiration of immature oocytes. Acta Obstet Gynecol Scand. 2001;80(11):1043–5. ISSN 0001-6349; 0001-6349.

73. Kwan I, et al. Pain relief for women undergoing oocyte retrieval for assisted reproduction. Cochrane Database Syst Rev. 2013;(1):CD004829. ISSN 1469-493X; 1361-6137.

74. Singhal H, et al. Patient experience with conscious sedation as a method of pain relief for transvaginal oocyte retrieval: a cross sectional study. J Hum Reprod Sci. 2017;10(2):119–23. ISSN 0974-1208; 1998-4766.

75. Baldini D, et al. The safe use of the transvaginal ultrasound probe for transabdominal oocyte retrieval in patients with vaginally inaccessible ovaries. Front Women Health. 2018;3(2):1–3.

Oocytes Retrieval in Metabolic Syndrome

14

Daniele De Viti, Assunta Stragapede, Elena Pacella, and Domenico Baldini

Contents

14.1 Introduction

Pregnancy-related cardiovascular complications are rare clinical conditions that can lead to significant maternal morbidity and mortality. With the implementation of infertility treatment, a new selected population of woman can experience pregnancy. Women with multiple medical problems and women near or beyond menopause are now able to conceive.

D. De Viti (✉)
Department of Cardiology, Santa Maria Hospital, GVM Care and Research, Bari, Italy

A. Stragapede
Department of Emergency and Organ Transplantation, Section of Internal Medicine, Endocrinology, Andrology and Metabolic Diseases, University of Bari, Bari, Italy

E. Pacella
Ophthalmology Section the Department of Sense Organs, Faculty of Medicine and Dentistry, Sapienza University of Rome, Rome, Italy
e-mail: elena.pacella@uniroma1.it

D. Baldini
Center for Medically Assisted Procreation, MOMO' fertiLIFE, Bisceglie, Italy

Despite many unanswered questions, clinicians should be prepared for the challenges and potential cardiovascular complications related to patients who are epidemiologically different than those seen in the past.

As a consequence of the combined effect of social changes and medical progress, interventions for infertility have greatly increased in number and sophistication; medical complications of infertility interventions can be direct effects of related drugs and technologies and indirect consequences of the induced pregnancy, multiple gestation, or associated medical condition.

An Italian prospective study conduct in a tertiary university maternity hospital between 2005 and 2016 [1] was done to assess whether risk of severe maternal morbidity at delivery differs for women who conceived using assisted reproductive technology (ART) compared to those with a spontaneous conception using the World Health Organization criteria for potentially life-threatening conditions and near miss maternal mortality. The incidence of near miss in the entire cohort was 3.3 cases per 1000 births (95% confidence interval 2.6–4.1). The crude prevalences of potentially life-threatening conditions and maternal near miss were higher among ART than non-ART deliveries (27.1% vs. 5.7% and

2.6% vs. 0.3%, respectively). The cardiovascular dysfunction requiring vasoactive drugs was one of the three most common causes of maternal near miss cases.

Therefore it is essential to assess whether risk of severe maternal cardiovascular morbidity differs for women who conceives using ART compared to those with a spontaneous conception in order to define qualitative and quantitative strategies to improve patient care, especially in the prevention of severe cardiovascular complications.

14.2 Advanced Maternal Age

Motherhood at or beyond the edge of reproductive age is a new aspect of what clinicians previously referred to as pregnancy in the "older gravida" [2]. In the United States alone, the 2001 rates for births to women aged 35–39, 40–44, and 45–49 years rose 30, 47, and 190% compared with 1990. Specifically, there were about 5000 births to women ≥ 45 years. Some complications may occur more frequently in older mothers as a result of accumulated prior diseases. Hypertension is the most common modifiable risk factor for cardiovascular disease, the leading cause of death in both men and women. The prevalence and severity of hypertension rise markedly with age, and blood pressure control becomes more difficult with aging in both genders, particularly in women [3]. Hypertension is a major risk factor for cardiovascular disease (CVD) in pregnant women. Hypertensive disorders in pregnancy include chronic hypertension, gestational hypertension, pre-eclampsia, and eclampsia. All of these have been associated with maternal, fetal, and neonatal morbidity and mortality. The recent European Society of Hypertension/European Society of Cardiology guidelines for the management of arterial hypertension [4] recommend drug treatment of severe hypertension in pregnancy (>160/110 mmHg, Class I; Level of Evidence C) and consideration of drug treatment in pregnant women with persistent elevation of BP 150/95 mmHg and in those with BP 140/90 in the presence of gestational hypertension (with or without pre-existing hypertension), asymptomatic organ damage, or symptoms at any time during pregnancy (Class IIb; Level of Evidence C).

Hypertension occurs in about 8% of women of reproductive age. There are remarkable differences in the prevalence of hypertension between racial/ethnic groups. Obesity is a risk factor of particular importance in this population because it affects over 30% of young women in the USA, is associated with more than fourfold increased risk of hypertension, and is potentially modifiable [5].

Using NHANES from 1999 to 2008, in women 20–44 years old hypertension estimated to complicate up to 5% of the estimated four million pregnancies in the United States each year [6] is a major source of maternal and fetal morbidity. Between 10 and 25% of women with chronic hypertension will develop superimposed pre-eclampsia [7].

The prevalence of hypertension increased significantly with age, from 2.7% in women age 20–34 to 18.4% in women age 40–44. The increased prevalence of hypertension with advanced age may explain the increased cardiovascular risk for some pregnancy complications in women of advanced maternal age. The problem of chronic hypertension in pregnancy is likely to become more common as the number of mothers of advanced age increases, in particular for women who conceive using ART compared to those with a spontaneous conception. Approximately 5% of women of reproductive age took antihypertensive medications. Futhermore, in most epidemiologic studies of women in reproductive age, is defined the upper age limit for statistical analysis of population at 44 years old, but women older than this can become pregnant through assisted reproduction, and hypertension is likely even more prevalent in this group.

Many clinical studies show that the ART singleton pregnancies had a significantly increased risk of pregnancy-induced hypertension [8].

In a meta-analysis of Qin [8], 50 cohort studies comprising 161,370 ART and 2,280,224 spontaneously conceived singleton pregnancies were identified to determine whether there are any increases in pregnancy-related complications and adverse pregnancy outcomes in singleton pregnancies after ART compared with those conceived naturally. The ART singleton pregnancies had a significantly increased risk of pregnancy-induced hypertension (relative risk [RR] 1.30, 95% confidence interval [CI] 1.04–1.62; $I(2) = 79\%$), gestational diabetes mellitus (RR 1.31, 95% CI 1.13–1.53; $I(2) = 6\%$), and other adverse pregnancy outcomes. These results are largely related to the increased gestational age of ART pregnancies women. A retrospective cohort study was done in 2015 to determine whether there are differences in adverse pregnancy outcomes in very advanced maternal age (vAMA) women (a total of 472 women aged ≥45 years) who conceived with ART compared with spontaneous conceptions [9]. For singleton pregnancies, vAMA women who conceived with ART were significantly older (47.0 ± 2.3 vs. 45.6 ± 0.1 years), more likely to be white (88.1% vs. 75.6%), and less parous (0.4 ± 0.9 vs. 1.2 ± 1.8) than vAMA women who conceived spontaneously. Rates of cardiovascular maternal complications were similar in the two populations.

The majority of the published studies have been unanimous about the special caution attitude required for the older mother, especially those women who experience pregnancy after ART.

14.3 Metabolic Disorders

Metabolic disorders are a major problem for overweight women seeking pregnancy (Fig. 14.1).

Women with a history of fertility problems have a higher risk of gestational diabetes mellitus (GDM) than women without a history of fertility problems (Fig. 14.2).

The association between fertility problems and risk of GDM is attenuated with increasing age and is more pronounced among primiparous women and women with polycystic ovary syndrome [10].

In the Danish National Patient Registry during 2004–2010 among women with fertility problems ($n = 49,616$) and women without fertility problems ($n = 323,061$), after

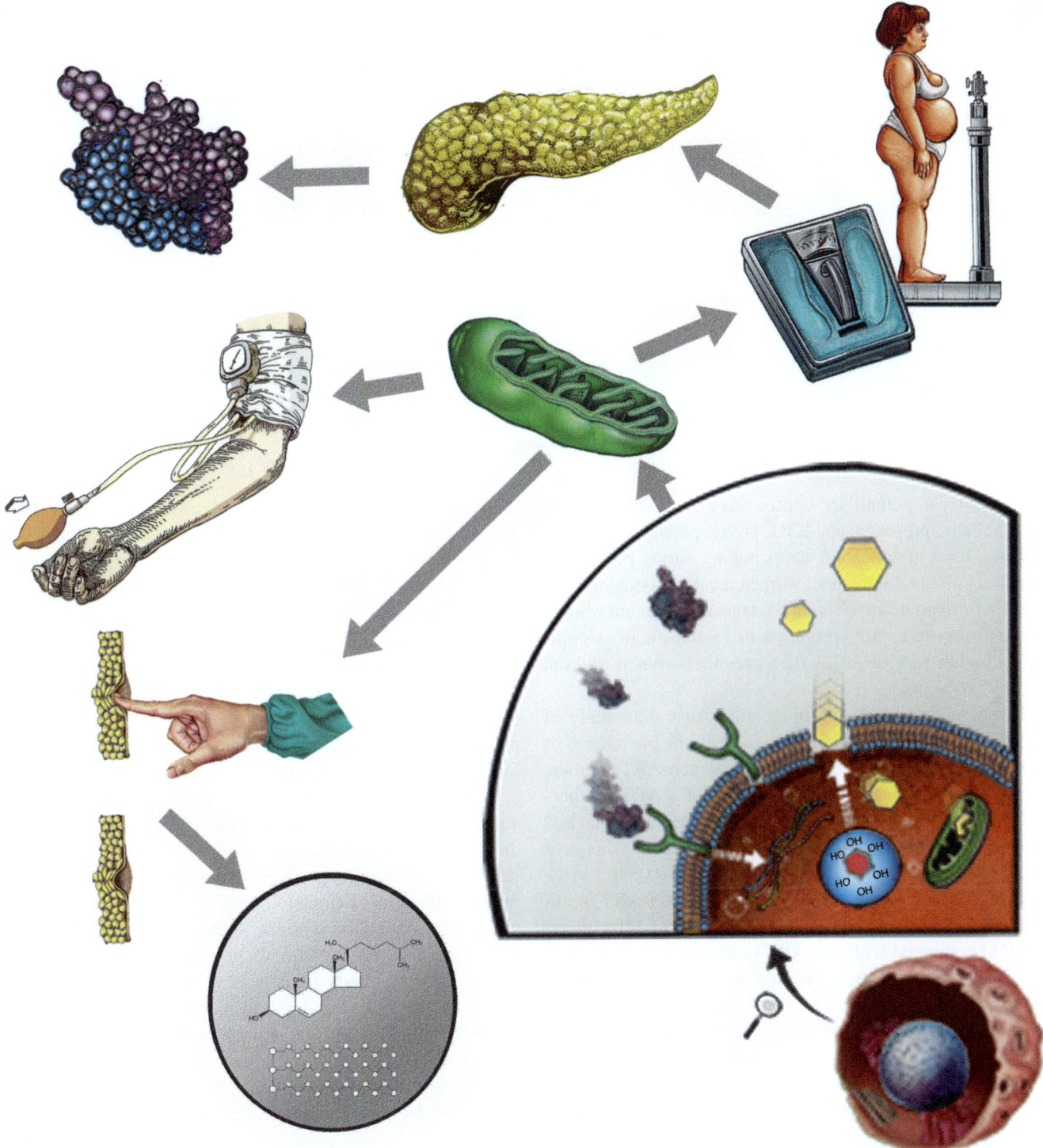

Fig. 14.1 Metabolic disorders are a major problem for overweight women seeking pregnancy

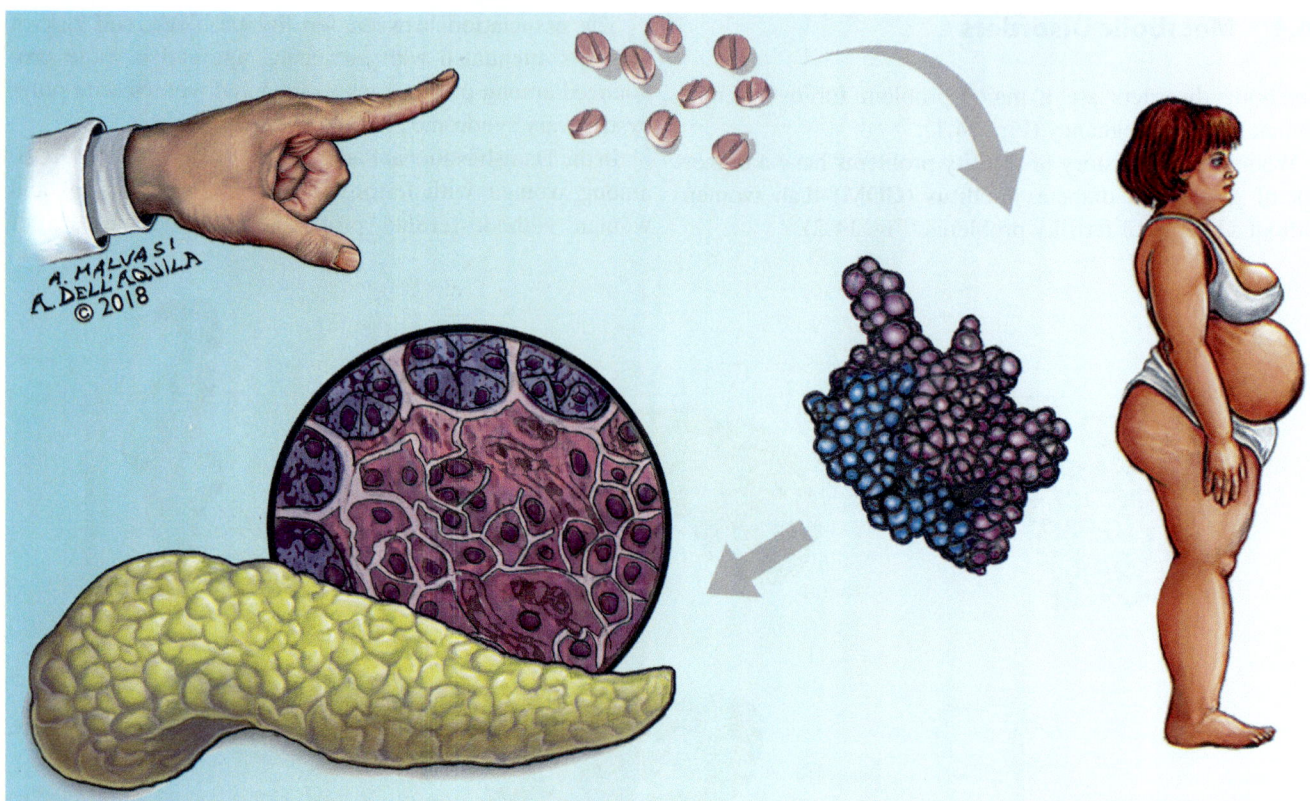

Fig. 14.2 An alteration in insulin secretion is typical of diabetic patients

adjustment for potentially confounding factors, including maternal age, prepregnancy BMI, parity, parental history of diabetes, level of education, and smoking during pregnancy, a total of 7433 (2%) pregnant women received a diagnosis of GDM. Multivariate analysis showed that the pregnant women with a history of fertility problems had a statistically significantly higher risk of GDM than pregnant women without fertility problems.

In a population retrospective cohort Australian study of 400,392 mothers between 2007 and 2009, the prevalence of GDM was compared between ART and non-ART mothers [11]. The prevalence of GDM was 7.6% for ART mothers and 5.0% for non-ART mothers ($P < 0.01$). Mothers who had twins had higher prevalence of GDM than those who gave births to singletons (8.8 versus 7.5%, $P = 0.06$ for ART mothers; and 7.3 versus 5.0%, $P < 0.01$ for non-ART mothers). Overall, ART mothers had a 28% increased likelihood of GDM compared with non-ART mothers (AOR 1.28, 95% CI 1.20–1.37). Of mothers who had singletons, ART mothers had higher odds of GDM than non-ART mothers (AOR 1.26, 95% CI 1.18–1.36). There was no significant difference in the likelihood of GDM among mothers who had twins between ART and non-ART (AOR 1.18, 95% CI 0.94–1.48). For mothers aged <40 years, the younger the maternal age,

the higher the odds of GDM for ART singleton mothers compared with non-ART singleton mothers. It was not possible to investigate which ART procedure is associated with increased risk of GDM and how the risk could have been minimized.

Women after ART constitute a high-risk group for critical obstetric states not only in the nearest time period but also long after ART. When pregnancy terms exceeded 22 weeks after ART, the percentage of pre-eclampsia and gestation pancreatic diabetes increases, whereas bleeding is the main factor in spontaneously conceived pregnancies [12].

It is uncertain if the increased risk of pregnancy cardiovascular complications related with ART is caused by ART directly or is an association of the underlying factors causing infertility. In a retrospective database analysis of 50,381 women delivering a singleton pregnancy in four public hospital obstetric units in western Sydney [13] (1727 pregnancies followed ART; 48,654 spontaneous conceptions), adjusted for age, body mass index, and smoking, ART was associated with increased risk of hypertension and diabetes. In a selected cohort of 508 women receiving ART in whom the cause of infertility was known, ovulatory dysfunction was present in 145 women and 336 had infertility despite normal ovulatory function. Ovulatory dysfunction was associated with increased risk of diabetes (OR 2.94, 95% CI 1.72–5.02) and hypertension (OR 2.40, 95% CI 1.15–5.00) compared to women with normal ovulatory function. The risk of cardiovascular complications rests predominantly when ovulatory dysfunction is the cause of infertility. Such disorders probably predispose towards diabetes and hypertension, which is then exacerbated by pregnancy. Ovulatory disorders are an independent risk factor for GDM and hypertension in women receiving assisted reproduction treatments [14]. Strong risk factors for GDM are age, body mass index, mode of ART (major in IVF/ICSI than in IUI pregnant) [15], and progesterone use during pregnancy.

The impact of ovulation induction and ovarian stimulation on the risk of GDM and hypertension requires further study. In a large French cohort to evaluate the role of ovarian stimulation procedures on the risk of pregnancy-induced hypertension and GDM, spontaneous pregnancies (group A), pregnancies achieved after mild ovarian ovulation induction without other ART procedures (group B), pregnancies after mild ovarian stimulation and ART procedures (group C), and pregnancies after multi (>2) follicular stimulation with gonadotropin therapy and ART procedures (group D) were selected [16]. The incidence rates of pregnancy-induced hypertension are 2.7, 11.6, 4.2, and 2.5% in groups A, B, C, and D, respectively ($P = 0.004$). The high incidence of pregnancy-induced hypertension in pregnancies following ovulation induction was driven by polycystic ovarian syndrome (PCOS) per se. In other case, a significant contribution of IVF compared to conception with ovulary induction drugs without IVF was significant only for pre-eclampsia [17].

The exogenous sex hormones, GnRH-a and gonadotropin may affect the sex hormones secretion through hypothalamic-pituitary-gonadal axis and other mechanism, so the hormone-related complications like GDM and pre-eclampsia may occur. Most reports haven't done the systematic research and could not reveal the correlation between controlled ovarian hyperstimulation (COH), exogenous progesterone treatment, and pregnancy complications.

In a Chinese prospective population-based cohort study [18], the use of Gn was a risk factor in GDM and PE and, as shown in Table 14.1, there was a significant correlation between the dosages of Gn and the incidence of GDM and PE whether adjusted with maternal age, ethnicity, and body mass index. There was not a significant correlation between the exogenous progesterone treatment and the incidence of GDM and PE whether adjusted with maternal age, ethnicity, and body mass index.

14.4 Peripartum Cardiomyopathy

Peripartum cardiomyopathy (PPCM) is a type of dilated cardiomyopathy of unknown origin that occurs in previously healthy women in the final month of pregnancy and up to 5 months after delivery. The reported incidence of PPCM varies because the diagnosis is not always consistent and a comparison with age-matched nonpregnant women does not exist. Although the incidence is low—less than 0.1% of pregnancies—morbidity and mortality rates are high at 5–30% [19–21].

Table 14.1 Correlations between the dosages of Gn and pregnancy complications

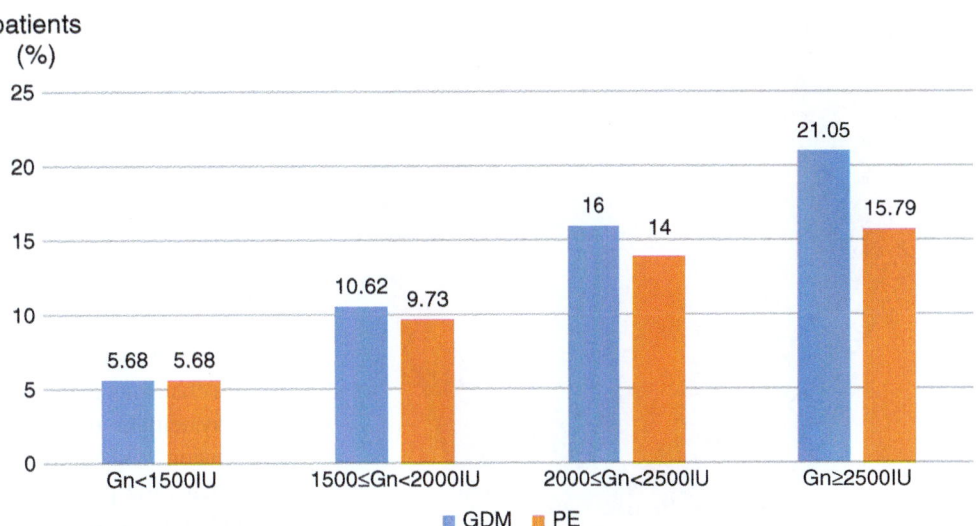

GDM gestational diabetes mellitus, PE pre-eclampsia

Several risk factors predispose a woman to PPCM, including increased maternal age, multiparity, multiple pregnancies, and pregnancies complicated by pre-eclampsia and gestational hypertension [22]. Precise mechanisms that lead to PPCM remain poorly defined. During pregnancy, blood volume and cardiac output increase, increase metabolic demands, and afterload decreases because of relaxation of vascular smooth muscle. These changes cause a brief, and reversible, hypertrophy of the left ventricle to meet the needs of the mother and fetus (Figs. 14.3 and 14.4). This transient left ventricular dysfunction during the third trimester and early postpartum period resolves shortly after birth in a normal pregnancy. PPCM might be due, in part, to an exaggerated decrease in left ventricular function when these hemodynamic changes of pregnancy occur. Thus, the onset of PPCM

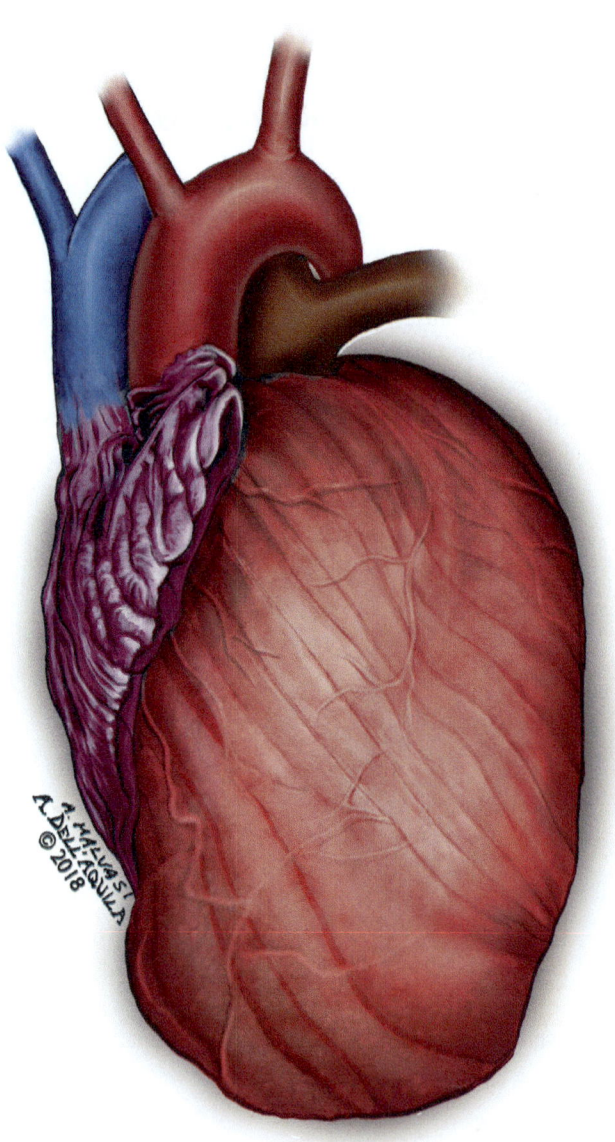

Fig. 14.3 Left ventricular dilatation is typical in hypertensive patients

can easily be masked and missed because the manifestations can mimic those of mild heart failure. Women with PPCM most commonly have dyspnea, dizziness, chest pain, cough, neck vein distension, fatigue, and peripheral edema. Women can also have arrhythmias, embolic events due to the dilated dysfunctional left ventricle. They can also have other indications typical of heart failure: hypoxia, jugular venous distention, gallop, rales, and hepatomegaly.

PPCM is a diagnosis of exclusion, and the definitive diagnosis of PPCM depends on echocardiographic identification of new-onset heart failure during a limited period around parturition. A diagnosis of PPCM requires the exclusion of other causes of heart failure: myocardial infarction, sepsis, severe pre-eclampsia, pulmonary embolism, valvular diseases, and other forms of cardiomyopathy.

In PPCM, the electrocardiogram may be normal or may show left ventricular hypertrophy, ST-T wave abnormalities, dysrhythmias, Q-waves in the anteroseptal precordial leads, and prolonged PR and QRS intervals.

Data on clinical outcomes and natural history of PPCM are variable. Most of the women recover completely, but a few develop progressively worsening HF and, ultimately, death.

The prognosis is best when PPCM is diagnosed and treated early. Recommended echocardiographic criteria for diagnosis of PPCM include an ejection fraction (EF) <45% and fractional shortening <30% with a left ventricular end-diastolic measurement of 4.8 cm/m^2 of body surface area [23].

Functional atrioventricular regurgitation may also be present secondary to ventricular dilatation. Women who recovered early have significantly higher ejection fractions on last follow-up compared with women who has late or partial recovery.

Given that the disease is rare and the symptoms such as dyspnea, dizziness, fatigue, and peripheral edema can be masked and missed, echocardiography is essential for diagnosis (Table 14.2). In a high number of studies reported in literature, the majority of those patients were diagnosed in the postpartum period [23].

The role of hypertension in PPCM has been unclear; some consider it a risk factor for development of PPC. Pre-eclampsia is often cited as a risk factor for the development of PPCM and recent research suggests that PE and PPCM share mechanisms that contribute to their pathobiology [24].

In a systematic review to identify prevalence rates of PE, hypertension, and multiple gestations in women diagnosed with PPCM, the pooled prevalence of 22% was more than quadruple the 5% average worldwide background rate of PE in pregnancy ($P < 0.001$). The rates of hypertension during pregnancy (37% [95% CI: 29–45%]) and multiple gestations (9% [95% CI: 7–11%]) were also elevated. In another 2015

Fig. 14.4 Echocardiographic view in a pregnant woman with hypertension and obesity. Note the presence of larger left ventricular end-diastolic diameter values and increased thickness of the interventricular septum

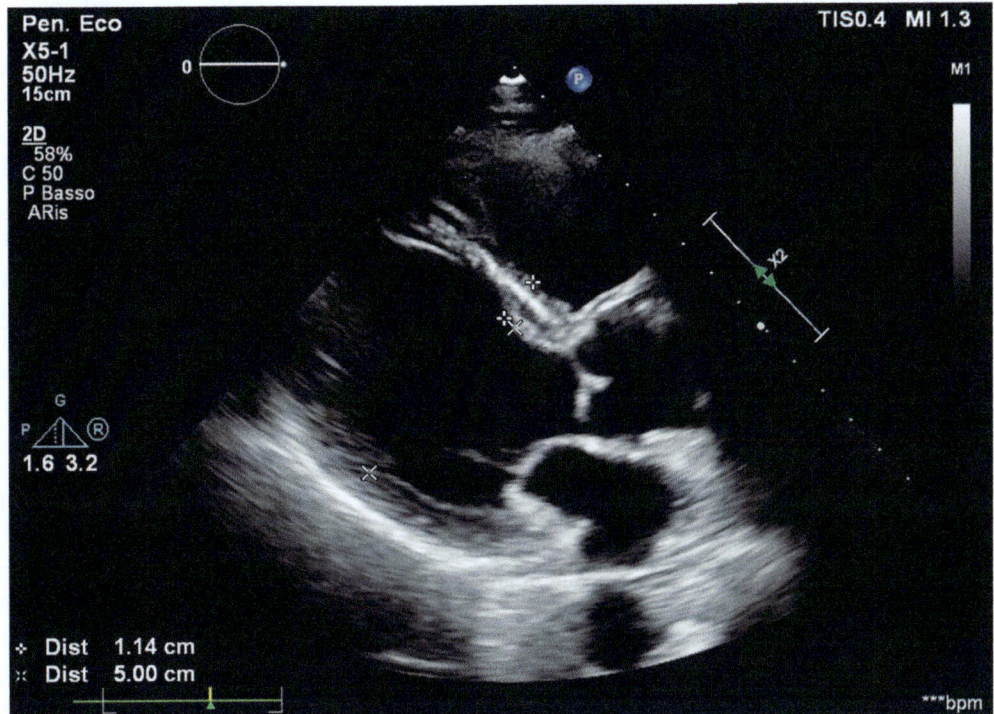

Table 14.2 Peripartum cardiomyopathy echocardiographic characteristics and mortality in various studies

Author	McNamara	Ntusi	Biteker	Cooper	Sliwa	Mishra
LVEF (%) at entry	35 ± 10	24 ± 8	26 ± 6	27 ± 7	30 ± 9	31 ± 7
LVEF (%) at follow-up	53 ± 10	31	–	45 ± 14	50 ± 14	43 ± 8
LVEDD at entry, cm	5.5 ± 0.1	7.4 ± 1.1	6.6 ± 0.6	–	5.6 ± 0.6	6.4 ± 1.2
LVEDD at follow-up, cm	–	–	–	–	5 ± 0.9	5 ± 0.7
Recovered LVEF (%)	72	20	48	82	–	–
Mortality (%)	4	17	24	0	28	23

LVEDD left ventricular end-diastolic diameter, *LVEF* left ventricular ejection fraction

retrospective study [25], women diagnosed with PPCM were older than controls. A significantly higher proportion were primiparous (63.9%), carried multifetal pregnancies (33.3%) and had hypertensive pregnancy complications (38.9%). Even if there are no data on direct association between PPCM and ART, 36% of PPCM patients of this population conceived with in vitro fertilization, and six of them received ovum donation. Thus risk factors for peripartum cardiomyopathy include primiparity, hypertension, and multifetal pregnancies; ART are not independently associated with PPCM but rather through other risk factors for PPCM.

Controlled ovarian stimulation by exogenous gonadotropins is a key procedure during the in vitro fertilization cycle to obtain a sufficient number of oocytes in humans. Although generally safe, more studies demonstrated that repeated superovulation had deleterious effects on the ovaries. However, whether repeated superovulation adversely affects on heart function remains unclear. In a 2018 study by Zhang et al., the role of long-term repeated superovulation in ovar-

ian aging and especially in associated disorders such as cardiovascular diseases was investigated [26]. This study used mice as the study model to evaluate the structure and function of ovaries that have previously received ten cycles of repeated superovulation treatments. Heart function was detected by ultrasonography, and heart ejection fraction significantly decreased in the repeated superovulation group mice. These results suggest that repeated superovulation may increase the risk of cardiovascular diseases by accelerating ovarian aging.

OHSS may involve, according to its grade of severity, elevated or decreased levels of growth factors, cytokines, mediators, changes in hormones, renin-angiotensin and kinin-kallikrein system [27]. Reports of high concentration of tumor necrosis factor-α (TNF-α), interferon-γ, interleukin-6, C-reactive protein (CRP), and Fas/apoptosis antigen 1 (Apo-1) in peripartum cardiomyopathy [28] suggest an underlying inflammatory process for the pathophysiologic development of PPCM.

14.5 Management of PPCM: Compensated Heart Failure

No randomized clinical trials have been done to evaluate therapies specifically in PPCM. So management of PPCM is similar to standard treatment for heart failure; careful attention should be paid to fetal safety and to excretion of drug during breastfeeding after delivery. The first aim is to improve symptoms through conventional pharmacologic therapies and, if necessary, nonpharmacologic therapies. The second aim is to effect a cure through the administration of targeted therapies. Treatment focuses on reducing preload and afterload and increasing cardiac inotropy [29]. Polypharmacy may be required for optimal management [30]. Medications should be continued until evidence indicates improved and/or resolved left ventricular dysfunction. Preload reduction is accomplished by administration of vasodilators, such as nitrates, most of which are safe during pregnancy and breastfeeding.

Diuretics are important for management of signs and symptoms; diuretics reduce preload and treat pulmonary congestion or peripheral edema. Both hydrochlorothiazide and furosemide are safe during pregnancy and lactation. However, diuretic-induced dehydration can cause uterine hypoperfusion and maternal metabolic acidosis, so bicarbonate monitoring and management with acetazolamide are needed. Potassium-sparing diuretic spironolactone has been used successfully to treat heart failure [31], but the insufficiency of data regarding its use in pregnancy means that cautious administration is warranted for preload reduction, although caution is warranted in antepartum women because rapid changes in intravascular volume can lead to a decrease in blood supply to the uterus and therefore the fetus [32]. Restriction of dietary sodium is also helpful in preload reduction. Bed rest was once standard care but is no longer recommended because of the increased risk of thromboembolism [33].

Angiotensin-modulating agents are considered first-line drugs for heart-failure management. Angiotensin-converting enzyme inhibitors and angiotensin receptor blockers improve survival but are contraindicated in pregnancy because of their teratogenicity [34, 35]. Also, since they are secreted in breast milk, breastfeeding must be stopped before commencing therapy. Safe alternatives during pregnancy include hydralazine and nitrates [36]. Hydralazine is safe during pregnancy and is the primary vasodilator drug antepartum. More severe cases warrant the use of intravenous nitroglycerin starting at 10–20 µg/min and continuing up to 200 µg/min. Nitroprusside is not recommended because of the potential for cyanide toxicity [37].

β-Blockers are crucial for long-term management of systolic dysfunction. Although safe during pregnancy, β1-selective blockers are preferred over nonselective β-blockers to avoid anti-tocolytic action induced by β2-receptor blockade [38]. Carvedilol combined with a blockade to restrict peripheral vasoconstriction has been shown to be effective in peripartum cardiomyopathy. However, β-blockers should not be given in the early stages of PPCM because they can decrease perfusion in the acute decompensated phase of the disease.

Digoxin, an inotropic and dromotropic agent, is safe to use during pregnancy and calcium channel blockers (dihydropyridines, such as amlodipine) have been shown to successfully reduce interleukin-6 levels in heart-failure patients [39, 40], but concomitant uterine hypoperfusion requires cautious use of these agents.

14.5.1 Decompensated Heart Failure

In pregnant women with acute decompensating heart failure, management begins with the ABCs (airway, breathing, circulation). Women with impending respiratory failure from pulmonary edema require rapid initiation of supported ventilation; however, attempts involving noninvasive ventilation may obviate intubation [41]. Breathing is supported with supplemental oxygen to relieve signs and symptoms related to hypoxemia and is assessed via continuous pulse oxymetry.

Women with acute heart failure benefit from intravenous administration of positive inotropic agents such as dobutamine and milrinone, none of which are contraindicated in pregnancy. Positive inotropic agents improve cardiac performance, facilitate diuresis, preserve end-organ function, and promote clinical stability [42]. Milrinone has vasodilating properties for both the systemic and the pulmonary circulation, a mechanism that may be a marked benefit over other inotropic agents. In women with systolic blood pressure less than 90 mmHg, dobutamine may be preferred over milrinone. Inotropic agents are of greatest value in women who have relative hypotension and an intolerance or no response to vasodilators and diuretics.

Medical therapy can be unsuccessful in women with PPCM, and mechanical cardiovascular support with an intra-aortic balloon pump or ventricular assist devices may be required [43, 44]. Use of short-term extracorporeal membrane oxygenation has also been of benefit in women with PPCM whose heart failure was refractory to medical therapy and who had persistent pulmonary edema with hypoxemia.

In conclusion, PPCM is a rare but serious cause of cardiac failure. All women having clinical features suggestive of PPCM in late pregnancy and early puerperium should be evaluated using echocardiography and should be followed in order to receive optical medical therapy; those with persistent sign and symptoms associated to persistent ventricular dysfunction should be hospitalized and the pregnancy should be managed in multidisciplinary units as some cases may require intensive care management due to severe cardiac decompensation.

14.6 ART in Patients with Heart Disease

The incidence of pregnancy in women with cardiovascular disease is rising, primarily due to the increased number of women with congenital heart disease reaching reproductive age and the changing demographics associated with advancing maternal age related to ART treatment. Furthermore, many of these women are delaying pregnancy until later in life when they may be exposed to a greater number of complications from their heart disease. A relatively high proportion of these women will pursue fertility treatment to achieve a pregnancy; consequently, the management of subfertile woman with heart disease is of growing importance. It is also important to consider that fertility therapy failure is anyway associated with an increased risk of long-term adverse cardiovascular events [45]. Women with heart disease have an increased baseline risk of these obstetric and perinatal complications [46, 47]. They may not tolerate additional risks imposed by ART. Although most cardiac conditions are well tolerated during pregnancy and women can deliver safely with favorable outcomes, there are some cardiac conditions that have significant maternal and fetal morbidity and mortality.

Cardiac disease affects approximately 2% of pregnancies in the Western world [48]. Anemia occurs because plasma volume increases more rapidly than does red blood cell mass. Enlargement of left ventricular mass and volume manifests itself as cardiomegaly on chest radiography and as left-axis deviation on electrocardiography. Higher cardiac output is caused early (during the first trimester) by increased stroke volume, and late (after week 20 of gestation) by a rise in heart rate. Fetal compression of the inferior vena cava (when the mother is in the supine position) can diminish cardiac output and thereby contribute to a hypercoagulable state. During labor, cardiac output can increase by 80% (compared with 25% during caesarian section), which leads to fluctuations of blood pressure and venous return. In the Western world, congenital heart disease (such as left to right shunts, left ventricular outflow tract obstruction, Marfan syndrome, hypertrophic cardiomyopathy, unrepaired and repaired cyanotic heart disease) accounts for approximately 80% of cardiac disease during pregnancy. In developing countries, rheumatic heart disease remains the most common cardiac disease during pregnancy (75%), whereas congenital heart disease is much less common (15%). In the United States, hypertensive disorders are the most frequent cardiovascular events, complicating approximately 7% of pregnancies [47]. Acute coronary syndrome [49] is rare (1–2/35,000 pregnan-

cies) but carries a mortality rate of up to 10%. Spontaneous coronary artery dissection, thought to be related to the effects of progesterone, is one manifestation.

Because of thromboembolism, mechanical heart valves are a significant cause of morbidity and—in up to 15% of affected patients—of death. Anticoagulation options include unfractionated heparin or low-molecular-weight heparin as a bridge to warfarin, which has a dose-dependent embryopathy rate of <10%.

Contraindications to pregnancy include pulmonary hypertension, severe systemic ventricular dysfunction (or residual dysfunction from peripartum cardiomyopathy), severe left-sided obstructive lesions, or a dilated aortic root (45 mm with Marfan syndrome or 50 mm with bicuspid aortic valve). Cyanosis with a baseline oxygen saturation level of <85% carries a >85% chance that pregnancy will not result in a live birth. Conversely, a baseline oxygen saturation level of >90% enables a >90% chance of a live birth.

The important question in these patients is does fertility treatment increase the risk of cardiovascular events? However, complications in pregnant women with heart disease treated with ART have not been described, despite parallel trends of delayed childbearing and increasing prevalence of heart disease among reproductive-aged women.

In medical records of women followed in the Pregnancy and Heart Disease Program, the first report of pregnancy outcomes in women with heart disease conceiving by ART [50], the 68% of pregnancies were in women with a congenital heart defect, and 32% in women with acquired heart disease. Most pregnancies were first births (nulliparity, 64%), and 9% were multiples.

All pregnancies resulted in live births, except 1 that was electively terminated at 17 weeks due to fetal omphalocele. Overall, 73% of pregnancies were associated with at least 1 complication. Adverse cardiac maternal outcomes (27% vs. 13%) and fetal or neonatal outcomes (45% vs. 20%) were more common in pregnant women with heart disease conceiving with ART series compared with pregnant women with heart disease not conceiving with ART [46]. Prematurity also was more common among infants in this series compared with infants in a reference ART population (32% vs. 13%) [51]. This report highlights the complex medical issues facing modern maternal demographics. ART-treated women with vulnerable heart lesions are at risk of OHSS and thromboembolism. OHSS is a potentially serious complication of ART that may result in fluid shifts, maternal hypotension, thromboembolism, and death. Even mild forms of OHSS may be poorly tolerated in women with ventricular dysfunction, left ventricular outflow tract obstruction, Fontan circulation, or pulmonary arterial hypertension.

Multiple gestations, a further important aspect in ART, remain a significant risk of gonadotropin treatment. Multiple gestations in ART pregnancies are associated with a higher cardiac output compared with single pregnancies. This increased hemodynamic burden can be problematic in women with significant left-sided obstructive valve lesions (such as aortic stenosis) or left ventricular systolic dysfunction. Multiple pregnancies have higher rates of pre-eclampsia and other morbidities that are poorly tolerated in the setting of pre-existing heart disease.

To reduce the risk of multiple pregnancies associated with ART, the number of embryos replaced should be carefully evaluated, according to characteristic such as patient's heart defect, maternal age, and grade of embryos.

The management of women with heart disease conceiving with ART needs a risk stratification with a thorough cardiovascular history and examination, 12-lead ECG, and accurate echocardiographic evaluation (Fig. 14.5) [52].

In counseling should be considered the underlying cardiac lesion (especially ventricular function, pulmonary pressure, severity of obstructive lesions, persistence of shunts, and presence of hypoxemia), maternal functional status most often defined by New York Heart Association (NYHA) functional class, the possibility of further palliative or corrective surgery, additional associated risk factors, and the risk of congenital heart disease in offspring. The risk of recurrence of congenital heart disease in offspring should be evaluated, in particular for women conceiving with ART.

Left heart obstructive lesions have a higher recurrence rate. Certain conditions such as Marfan syndrome are autosomal dominant, conferring a 50% risk of recurrence in an offspring.

Patients with congenital heart disease who reach reproductive age should be offered genetic counseling so that they are fully informed of the mode of inheritance and recurrence risk as well as the prenatal diagnosis. Women with inherited cardiac conditions who have an identified genetic mutation may wish to explore the option of pre-implantation genetic screening.

However, more information is urgently needed to help guide medical and obstetric management of women with heart disease treated with ART.

The additional potential risks conferred by ART in conjunction with cardiac-specific maternal and fetal risks must be weighed against the desire for pregnancy. Modified ART protocols and close antenatal surveillance at a center with

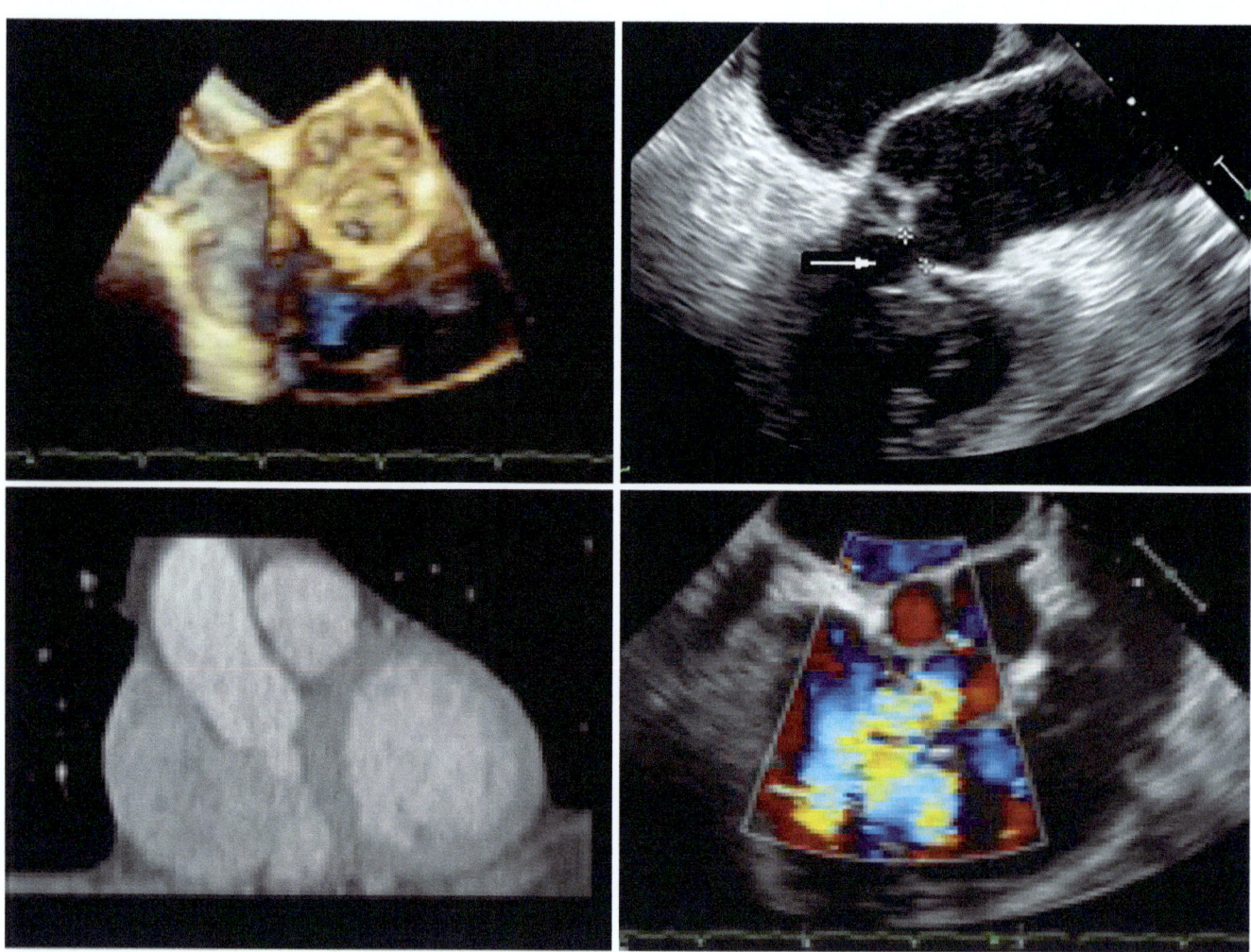

Fig. 14.5 Two-dimensional transesophageal echocardiography showing a significant congenital fistula from the aorta into the right ventricular outflow tract

expertise in pregnancy and heart disease are recommended because of high complication rates.

14.7 Polycystic Ovarian Syndrome and Metabolic Syndrome

Polycystic ovarian syndrome (PCOS) is complex disorder, affecting approximately 5–10% of the women in reproductive age group [53, 54]. It is characterized by chronic anovulation, hyperandrogenism, and polycystic ovaries (Figs. 14.6, 14.7, and 14.8).

The other metabolic abnormalities associated with PCOS are obesity, dyslipidemia, insulin resistance, glucose intolerance, and hypertension, which confer an increased risk of long-term health consequences due to the high prevalence of insulin resistance, impaired glucose tolerance, type 2 diabetes, dyslipidemia, and numerous cardiovascular risk factors [55].

Most of these metabolic features are also shared by the metabolic syndrome (MBS), which is defined according to the guidelines of National Cholesterol Education Program Adult Treatment Panel (NCEP ATP III) 2005 as having three or more of the following abnormalities [56]:

- Waist circumference in females >88 cm
- Fasting serum glucose ≥100 mg/dL
- Fasting serum triglycerides ≥150 mg/dL
- Serum HDL-C

MBS is associated with atherosclerosis, hypertension, dyslipidemia, coronary artery disease, and diabetes. Some of the factors affecting the prevalence of MBS are age [57, 58], obesity [57], insulin resistance [59], and underlying PCOS [60, 61]. Many of the metabolic abnormalities of PCOS patients overlap with components of MS (Table 14.3) [62].

The prevalence rates of MS in PCOS women vary among different countries and ethnicities as follows: 43–46% in America [63, 64], 37.9% in India [65], 35.3% in Thailand [66], 28.4% in Brazil [67], 16.8% in China [68], 14.5% in Korea [69], 11.6% in Turkey [70], and 8.2% in Southern Italy [71].

It is important to know these epidemiological aspects because PCOS is the most common endocrinopathy among women of reproductive age and many infertile women who need ART presented with PCOS. The most frequently presented feature associated with PCOS is primary infertility in about 70% of the patients [72]. The presence of PCOS and MBS increases the risk of the in vitro fertilization (IVF) procedure and is also associated with increased obstetric risk and even death. The potential risks for women with MBS who undergo ART procedures increased with age. More adverse cardiovascular risk profiles of women with PCOS have been demonstrated in several studies [73, 74]. Pathogenetic mechanisms of these impairments are not completely clarified yet, but insulin resistance (IR) appears

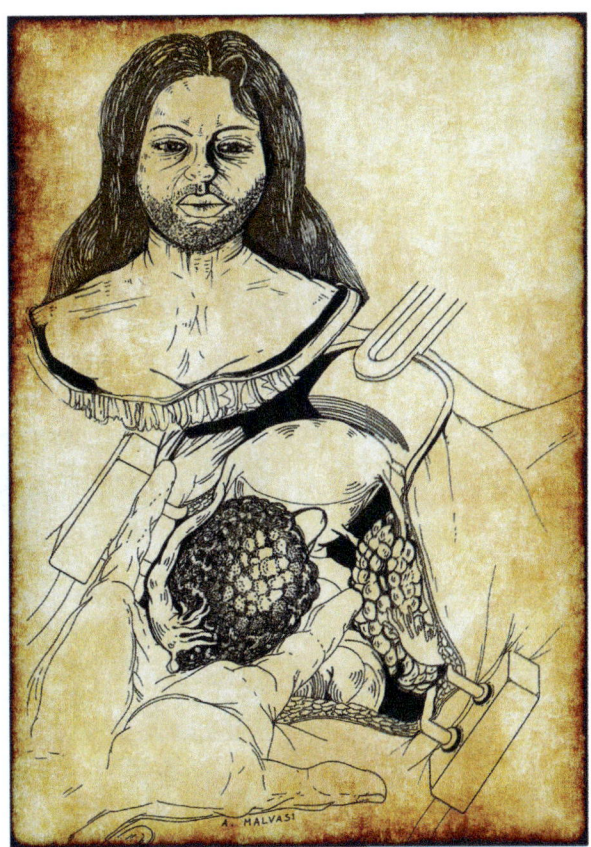

Fig. 14.6 Story picture of patient with PCOS

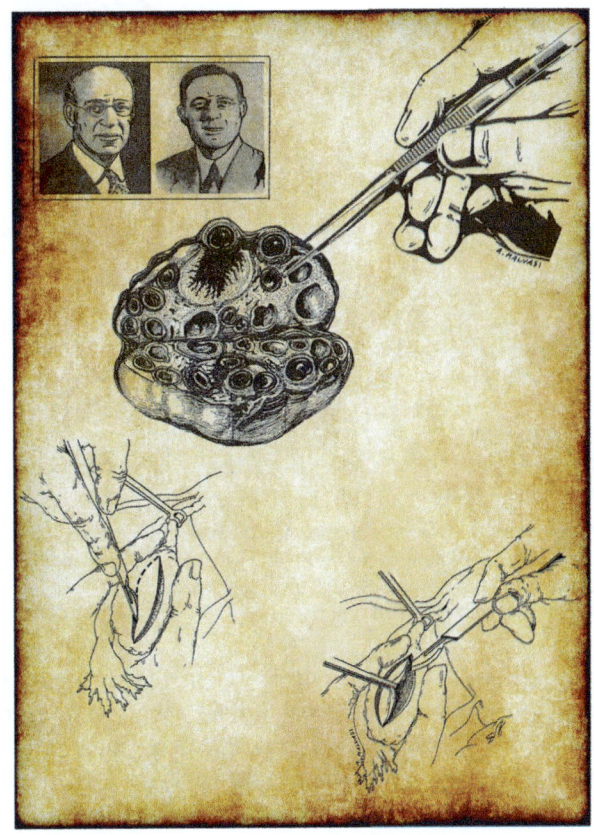

Fig. 14.7 Dr. Irving Freil Stein and Dr. Michael Leventhal; 80 years ago described the polycystic ovaries

Fig. 14.8 Echographic aspect typical of micropolycystic ovaries

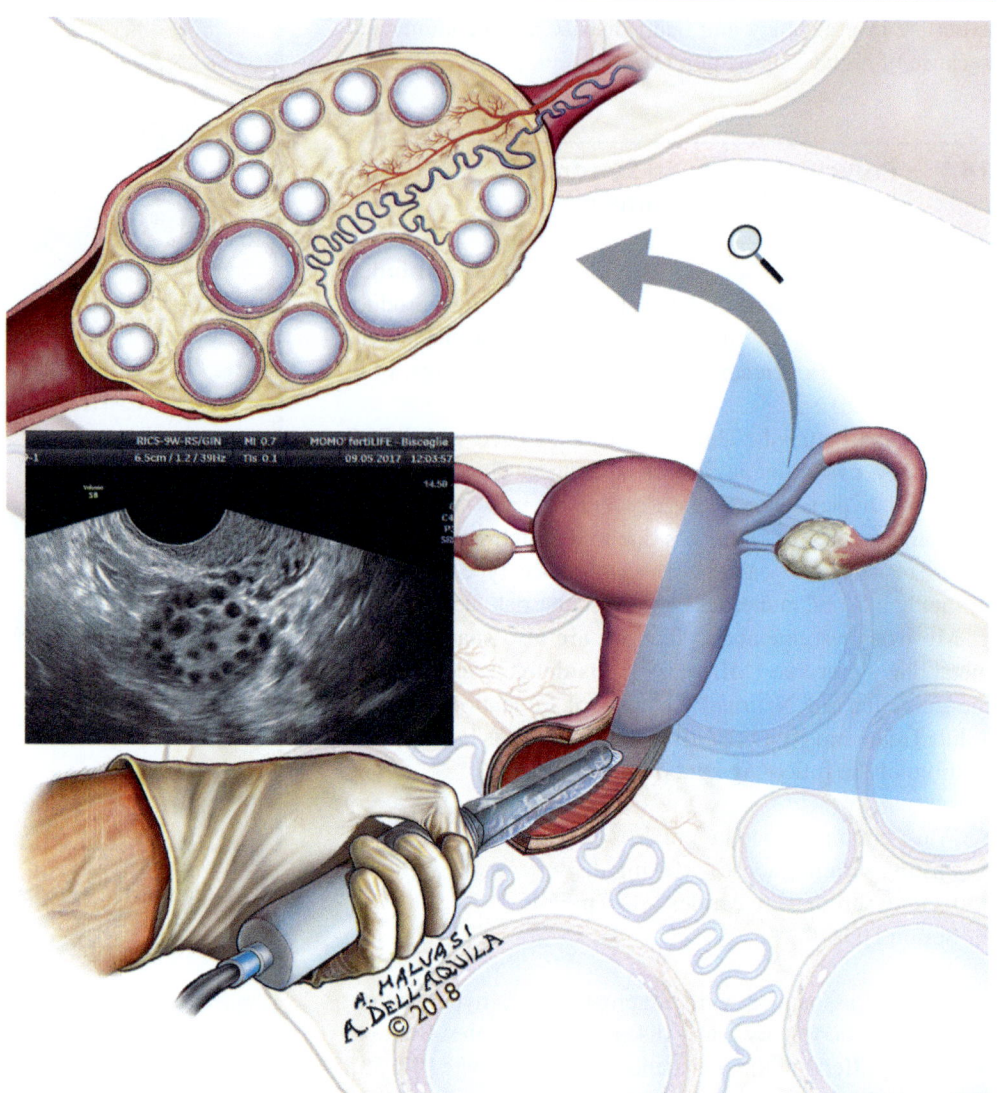

Table 14.3 Prevalence of metabolic syndrome components[a] in 624 patients with PCOS

	Prevalence %(n)		
MS components	MS ($n = 123$)	Without MS ($n = 501$)	Total ($n = 624$)
HDL-C < 50 mg/dL	92.8 (114)	66.3 (332)	71.5 (446)
WC ≥ 88	82.9 (102)	22.8 (114)	34.6 (216)
TG ≥ 150 mg/dL	70.7 (87)	15 (75)	26 (162)
FG ≥ 100 mg/dL	43.9 (54)	5.6 (28)	13.1 (82)
BP ≥ 130/85 mmHg	8.1 (10)	0.8 (4)	2.2 (14)

PCOS polycystic ovary syndrome, *MS* metabolic syndrome, *HDL-C* high-density lipoprotein cholesterol, *WC* waist circumference, *TG* triglycerides, *FG* fasting glucose, *BP* blood pressure
[a]According to NCEP ATPIII criteria

to play a critical role, such as the key factor linking hypertension, glucose intolerance, obesity, lipid abnormalities, and coronary artery disease. Several PCOS women present abdominal adiposity (visceral fat) with a level of IR, similar to that present in women with type 2 diabetes, in association with an increased incidence of impaired glucose tolerance [75]. All markers of insulin resistance are abnormal in women with PCOS with metabolic syndrome compared with those without metabolic syndrome. The serum triglyceride/high-density lipoprotein cholesterol (TG/HDL-C) ratio correlates with insulin resistance and a serum TG/HDL-C > 3.2 has a high sensitivity and specificity for the detection of metabolic syndrome in women with PCOS [76].

PCOS is a risk factor for type 2 diabetes (T2DM) but the magnitude of risk is uncertain, fasting plasma glucose is an inadequate screening test for T2DM in this population and the oral glucose tolerance test is superior; the identification of women with PCOS for diabetes screening is constrained by current diagnostic criteria for PCOS. Women with PCOS represent a unique group of women at high risk for the development of coronary heart disease [77, 78]. Danish population women with PCOS and no previous diagnosis of cardiovascular disease were recently studied; the main study outcome was cardiovascular events including hypertension and dyslipidemia. The total event rate of cardiovascular event was 22.6 per 1000 patient years in PCOS vs. 13.2 per 1000 patient years in controls; the median age at diagnosis of cardiovascular event was 35 (28–42) years in PCOS vs. 36 (30–43) years in controls. Obesity, diabetes and infertility, and previous use of oral contraceptives were associated with increased risk of development of cardiovascular event in PCOS [79].

Several cardiovascular risk factors are often related to structural alterations, such as endothelial dysfunction, oxidative stress, and low-grade chronic inflammation, that are present even at early age in PCOS women. Farther the presence of OHSS, a possible effect of ART treatment, may involve elevated levels of cytokines and inflammatory markers.

Numerous studies have suggested the importance of various different cytokines (IL-1, IL-11, LIF, IL-12, and IL-18) in infertility and recurrent miscarriage, with particular emphasis on the role that endometrial cytokines may play [80]. In obese women with PCOS, adipocytes are the source of many compounds of the endocrine activity and some of them are also markers and mediators of inflammation. Increased levels of proinflammatory cytokines in blood can promote insulin resistance atherosclerosis. IL-18, TNF, IL-6, and hs-CRP are often elevated in patient with polycystic ovary syndrome [81]. Interleukin-18 (IL-18) is considered as a strong marker of inflammation and insulin resistance; cardiovascular risk is significantly higher in PCOS patient compared to controls [82]. Elevated serum IL-18 levels are associated with increased carotid intima-media wall thickness that is an early predictor of atherosclerosis and a strong independent predictor of the occurrence of major cardiovascular events. Every 0.1 mm increase in carotid intima-media wall thickness has been estimated to increase the risk of a myocardial infarction by 15% and the risk of stroke by 18% [83, 84]. The prognostic events that define the severity of PCOS and involvement of cardiovascular risk in PCOS include endothelial dysfunction and upregulation of oxidative stress. In PCOS women, the circulating biomarkers of oxidative stress are in abnormal levels that are independent of overweight; the plasma levels of NO and H_2O_2 and the arginine bioavailability are reduced. In addition, hyperglycemia per se promotes reactive species generation in PCOS [85, 86]. The women with PCOS had significantly higher serum advanced oxidation protein products than control women [87], and plasma levels of pregnancy-associated plasma protein-A (PAPP-A) are often elevated [88]. PAPP-A is a high molecular weight that is associated with vulnerable plaque and may be a predictor of cardiovascular disease and mortality [89].

Ischemic heart disease during pregnancy or the early postpartum period is a rare condition but has been shown to be associated with poor maternal as well as fetal outcome. There is no evidence that ART treatment increases the risk of ischemic heart events although information related to ischemic heart disease in pregnancy is derived from case reports and small series. It is unclear from the literature whether the incidence of myocardial infarction (MI) is increasing or more cases are being reported. The main contributing factor could be a higher prevalence of the metabolic syndrome. The changes in the obstetrics practice may have altered or even increased the incidence of MI. Thus, for example, the use of tocolytics (ritodrine), prostaglandins (PGE2) and the increase of multiple pregnancies in the population as a consequence of ART may all have contributed to the apparent increased incidence of MI [90]. A review published by Roth shows that MI occurs more commonly in multigravidas (66%), and the majority of patients (72%) are older than 30 years, frequent characteristics in patient undergoing ART [91]. A recent series on pregnancy-associated spontaneous coronary artery dissection, reported between 2000 and 2015, included 120 cases; 94 of the women (81%) were >30 years and 47 (40.5%) were >35 years; use of hormonal therapy before pregnancy ($n = 38$) was reported in 7 women (18.5%), 4 used oral contraceptives, and 3 were hormonally treated for infertility [92, 93]. With the continuing trend of childbearing at older ages and advances in reproductive technology enabling many older women to conceive, it may be expected that its occurrence will increase.

The different diagnostic criteria used for the diagnosis of PCOS for the past two decades create several phenotypes of PCOS that differed metabolically (Table 14.4) [94].

There are three definitions for PCOS: one adopted in 1990 (classical PCOS with phenotypes A and B), an other in 2003 (Rotterdam criteria with four phenotypes A–D), a wider definition including the 1990 phenotypes, and the Androgen Excess (AE) and PCOS Society (AE-PCOS) criteria proposed in 2006 [94, 95]. The different diagnostic criteria create several phenotypes of PCOS. It is even suggested that these subgroups differ metabolically [96]. One extensive review by Moran and Teede sought to compare the metabolic profiles among these different reproductive phenotypes (Table 14.5) [97–99].

Most studies conclude that women with NIH PCOS (phenotypes A and B) present with more adverse metabolic profiles (including higher IR, increased prevalence of metabolic syndrome, and more adverse lipid profiles) than those with non-NIH PCOS (phenotypes C and D). Phenotypes C and D are not actually related to increased CVD risk, and thus screening for CVD risk factors of intervening for primary CVD prevention in young women is not cost-effective. There is an increasing number of suggestions to return to the 1990

Table 14.4 PCOS diagnostic criteria

NIH 1990	Rotterdam 2003	AE-PCOS Society 2006
Both of the following[a]: 1. Chronic anovulation, documented by oligo- or amenorrhea 2. Clinical and/or biochemical signs of hyperandrogenism (with exclusion of other etiologies, e.g., congenital adrenal hyperplasia) with or without PCO on ultrasound	At least two of the following[a]: 1. Chronic anovulation, documented by oligo- or amenorrhea 2. Clinical and/or biochemical signs of hyperandrogenism 3. Polycystic ovaries by ultrasound	Clinical and/or biochemical signs of hyperandrogenism and at least one of the following[a]: 1. Ovarian dysfunction (oligo/anovulation) 2. Polycystic ovarian morphology by ultrasound

[a]After exclusion of the other diseases that can produce a similar clinical picture

Table 14.5 Diagnostic phenotypes of PCOS

Phenotype A NIH PCOS: hyperandrogenism and oligo/anovulation with PCO

Phenotype B NIH PCOS: hyperandrogenism and oligo/anovulation without PCO

Phenotype C Non-NIH PCOS: hyperandrogenism with PCO but with normal ovulation

Phenotype D Non-NIH PCOS: no hyperandrogenism but with oligo/anovulation and with PCO

Adapted from Moran and Teede [97]

criteria plus some metabolic parameters to identify real CVD risk in this population. However, such a strategy needs verification by large, prospective studies.

Obesity plays a role in the expression of metabolic features and other clinical manifestations of PCOS [100, 101] and it is linked with worse biotechnological and clinical in vitro fertilization outcome [102]. Obese PCOS women have a ten-fold increase in their risk of suffering from DM2 and a seven-fold increase of IGT compared with normal weight PCOS women [103]. An accelerated rate of conversion from IGT to DM2 is strongly dependent upon BMI [104]. The patient's risk of developing cardiovascular disease increases with increasing BMI. In PCOS and non-PCOS women, levels of TNF-α [105, 106], IL-6, and CRP [106] correlate directly with BMI, but overweight and obese PCOS women in some studies have presented with significantly higher levels of these inflammatory markers than their BMI-matched non-PCOS counterparts [106, 107] (Fig. 14.9). Dyslipidemia is the most common metabolic abnormality in PCOS [100]. Elevated LDL [108–110] and VLDL [109] in PCOS are further elevated when excess adiposity is present, but, as confirmed by a recent meta-analysis, the higher levels occur in PCOS independently of obesity [111].

Despite small changes in lipid profiles in PCOS, most women with PCOS are young and have normal blood pres-

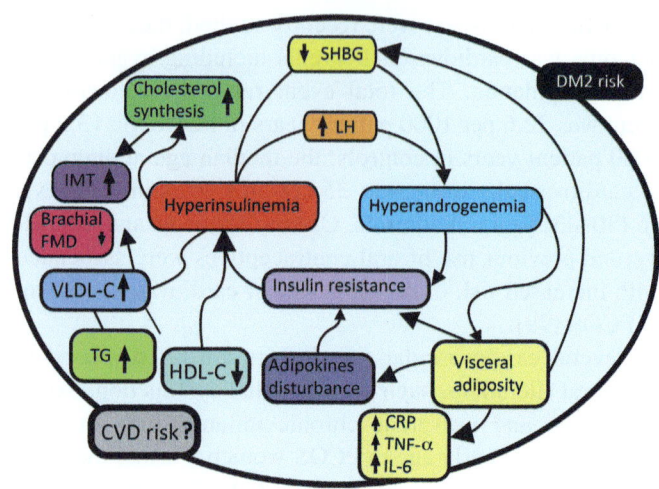

Fig. 14.9 Pathophysiology of metabolic disturbances in PCOS. *CVD* cardiovascular disease, *TG* triglycerides, *HDL-C* high-density lipoprotein cholesterol, *VLDLC* very-low-density lipoprotein cholesterol, *CRP* C-reactive protein, *TNF-α* tumor necrosis factor-alpha, *IL-6* interleukin-6, *FMD* flow-mediated dilatation, *IMT* intima-media thickness, *SHBG* sex hormone binding globulin, *LH* luteinizing hormone, *DM* diabetes mellitus

sure and do not qualify for primary prevention of cardiovascular disease [100]. Nevertheless, performing at least one measurement of lipid profiles in PCOS in conjunction with an assessment for other cardiovascular risk factors such as smoking and family history of CVD is suggested [100]. It is estimated that 80–90% of women reporting menstrual irregularity have PCOS [100]. The subgroup of PCOS women reporting a history of very irregular menses most frequently refer to ART. An investigation followed 82,439 women aged 20–35 for 14 years [112]. Compared with women reporting a history of regular menses, women reporting a history of very irregular menses had a significantly higher risk of nonfatal and fatal cardiovascular disease, even after adjustment for BMI, age, menopausal status, and smoking [112]. Furthermore, a recent meta-analysis indicated a two-fold increased risk of coronary heart disease (CHD) and stroke for patients with PCOS relative to women without PCOS [113].

In conclusion, obese women with PCOS should be targeted for aggressive treatment and prevention of cardiovascular disease, and a careful screening of all PCOS women should include OGTT; more frequent screenings are required for those with other DM2 risk factors, such as a family history of DM2. Early diagnosis and treatment of PCOS in adolescents are essential in ensuring adulthood health [114, 115]; in adolescent girls with PCOS, hyperandrogenemia is a risk factor of MBS independent of obesity and insulin resistance [116, 117]. The patients with PCOS should be counseled to reduce cardiovascular risk factors through weight control, exercise, lifestyle intervention, and/or pharmacologic interventions. Treatment of the associated cardiovascular risk factors, including insulin resistance, hypertension, and dyslipidemia, should be incorporated into the routine PCOS patient wellness care program [118]. Assessment of the concentrations of inflammatory markers may become a very useful test in evaluating the risk of developing atherosclerosis and cardiovascular disease, long before their clinical manifestation. Further evaluation and treatment should follow to ensure the safety of ART procedures and of ensuing pregnancies.

References

1. Cromi A, Marconi N, Casarin J, Cominotti S, Pinelli C, Riccardi M, Ghezzi F. Maternal intra and postpartum near-miss following assisted reproductive technology: a retrospective study. BJOG. 2018;125:1569–78.
2. Blickstein I. Motherhood at or beyond the edge of reproductive age. Int J Fertil Womens Med. 2003;48(1):17–24.
3. Hage FG, Mansur SJ, Xing D, Oparil S. Hypertension in women. Kidney Int Suppl. 2013;3:352–6.
4. Mancia G, Fagard R, Narkiewicz K, Redon J, Zanchetti A, Böhm M, et al. 2013 ESH/ESC guidelines for the management of arterial hypertension: the task force for the management of arterial hypertension of the European Society of Hypertension (ESH) and of the European Society of Cardiology (ESC). Eur Heart J. 2013;34(28):2159–219.
5. Bateman BT, Shaw KM, Kuklina EV, Callaghan WM, Seely EW, Hernández-Díaz S. Hypertension in women of reproductive age in the United States: NHANES 1999–2008. PLoS One. 2012;7(4):e36171.
6. Sibai BM. Chronic hypertension in pregnancy. Obstet Gynecol. 2002;100:369–77.
7. Sibai BM, Lindheimer M, Hauth J, Caritis S, VanDorsten P, et al. Risk factors for preeclampsia, abruption placentae, and adverse neonatal outcomes among women with chronic hypertension. National Institute of Child Health and Human Development network of maternal-fetal medicine units. N Engl J Med. 1998;339:667–71.
8. Qin J, Liu X, Sheng X, Wang H, Gao S. Assisted reproductive technology and the risk of pregnancy-related complications and adverse pregnancy outcomes in singleton pregnancies: a meta-analysis of cohort studies. Fertil Steril. 2016;105(1):73–85.
9. Jackson S, Hong C, Wang ET, Alexander C, Gregory KD, Pisarska MD. Pregnancy outcomes in very advanced maternal age pregnancies: the impact of assisted reproductive technology. Fertil Steril. 2015;103(1):76–80.
10. Holst S, Kjær SK, Jørgensen ME, Damm P, Jensen A. Fertility problems and risk of gestational diabetes mellitus: a nationwide cohort study. Fertil Steril. 2016;106(2):427–34.
11. Wang YA, Nikravan R, Smith HC, Sullivan EA. Higher prevalence of gestational diabetes mellitus following assisted reproduction technology treatment. Hum Reprod. 2013;28(9):2554–61.
12. Bashmakova NV, Davydenko NB, Malgina GB, Putilova NV. Epidemiology of critical states during pregnancy after assisted reproductive technologies. Gynecol Endocrinol. 2016;32(sup2):47–51.
13. Barua S, Hng TM, Smith H, Bradford J, McLean M. Ovulatory disorders are an independent risk factor for pregnancy complications in women receiving assisted reproduction treatments. Aust N Z J Obstet Gynaecol. 2017;57(3):286–93.
14. Stern JE, Luke B, Tobias M, Gopal D, Hornstein MD, Diop H. Adverse pregnancy and birth outcomes associated with underlying diagnosis with and without assisted reproductive technology treatment. Fertil Steril. 2015;103(6):1438–45.
15. Ashrafi M, Gosili R, Hosseini R, Arabipoor A, Ahmadi J, Chehrazi M. Risk of gestational diabetes mellitus in patients undergoing assisted reproductive techniques. Eur J Obstet Gynecol Reprod Biol. 2014;176:149–52.
16. Carbillon L, Gronier H, Cedrin-Durnerin I, Pharisien I, Nguyen MT, Valensi P, Cosson E. The impact of ovulation induction and ovarian stimulation on the risk of pregnancy-induced hypertension and on neonatal outcomes: a case/control study. Eur J Obstet Gynecol Reprod Biol. 2017;217:137–43.
17. Chaveeva P, Carbone IF, Syngelaki A, Akolekar R, Nicolaides KH. Contribution of method of conception on pregnancy outcome after the 11–13 weeks scan. Fetal Diagn Ther. 2011;30:9–22.
18. Jie Z, Yiling D, Ling Y. Association of assisted reproductive technology with adverse pregnancy outcomes. Iran J Reprod Med. 2015;13(3):169–80.
19. Hibbard JU, Lindheimer M, Lang RM. A modified definition for peripartum cardiomyopathy and prognosis based on echocardiography. Obstet Gynecol. 1999;4(2):311–5.
20. Tidswell M. Peripartum cardiomyopathy. Crit Care Clin. 2004;20:777–88.
21. Sliwa K, Skudicky D, Bergemann A, Candy G, Puren A, Sareli P. Peripartum cardiomyopathy: analysis of clinical outcome, left ventricular function, plasma levels of cytokines and Fas/APO-1. J Am Coll Cardiol. 2000;35(3):701–5.
22. Pearson G, Veille J, Rahimtoola S, et al. Peripartum cardiomyopathy: National Heart, Lung, and Blood Institute and Office of Rare Diseases (National Institutes of Health) workshop recommendations and review. JAMA. 2000;283(9):1183–8.
23. Asad ZUA, Maiwand M, Farah F, Dasari TW. Peripartum cardiomyopathy: a systematic review of the literature. Clin Cardiol. 2018;41(5):693–7.
24. Bello N, Rendon ISH, Arany Z. The relationship between pre-eclampsia and peripartum cardiomyopathy: a systematic review and meta-analysis. J Am Coll Cardiol. 2013;62(18):1715–23.
25. Shani H, Kuperstein R, Berlin A, Arad M, Goldenberg I, Simchen MJ. Peripartum cardiomyopathy—risk factors, characteristics and long-term follow-up. J Perinat Med. 2015;43(1):95–101.
26. Zhang J, Lai Z, Shi L, Tian Y, Luo A, Xu Z, Ma X, Wang S. Repeated superovulation increases the risk of osteoporosis and cardiovascular diseases by accelerating ovarian aging in mice. Aging (Albany NY). 2018;10(5):1089–102.
27. Binder H, Dittrich R, Einhaus F, Krieg J, Müller A, Strauss R, Beckmann MW, Cupisti S. Update on ovarian hyperstimulation syndrome: part 1—incidence and pathogenesis. Int J Fertil Womens Med. 2007;52(1):11–26.
28. Bhattacharyya A, Basra SS, Sen P, Kar B. Peripartum cardiomyopathy: a review. Tex Heart Inst J. 2012;39(1):8–16.
29. Williams J, Mozurkewich E, Chilimigras J, Van De Ven C. Critical care in obstetrics: pregnancy specific conditions. Best Pract Res Clin Obstet Gynaecol. 2008;22(5):825–46.
30. Heart Failure Society of America. Executive summary: HFSA 2006 comprehensive heart failure practice guideline. J Card Fail. 2006;12(1):10–38.
31. Lampert MB, Hibbard J, Weinert L, Briller J, Lindheimer M, Lang RM. Peripartum heart failure associated with prolonged tocolytic therapy. Am J Obstet Gynecol. 1992;168(2):493–5.
32. Egan DJ, Bisanzo MC, Hutson HR. Emergency department evaluation and management of peripartum cardiomyopathy. J Emerg Med. 2009;36(2):141–7.
33. Moioli M, Menada MV, Bentivoglio G, Ferrero S. Peripartum cardiomyopathy. Arch Gynecol Obstet. 2010;281(2):183–8.
34. Sliwa K, Hilfiker-Kleiner D, Petrie MC, et al.; Heart Failure Association of the European Society of Cardiology Working Group on Peripartum Cardiomyopathy. Current state of knowledge on aetiology, diagnosis, management, and therapy of peri-

partum cardiomyopathy: a position statement from the Heart Failure Association of the European Society of Cardiology Working Group on Peripartum Cardiomyopathy. Eur J Heart Fail. 2010;12(8):767–778.

35. Pyatt JR, Dubey G. Peripartum cardiomyopathy: current understanding, comprehensive management review and new developments. Postgrad Med J. 2011;87(1023):34–9.

36. Ro A, Frishman W. Peripartum cardiomyopathy. Cardiol Rev. 2006;14(1):35–42.

37. Lata I, Gupta R, Sahu S, Singh H. Emergency management of decompensated peripartum cardiomyopathy. J Emerg Trauma Shock. 2009;2(2):124–8.

38. Arnold JM, Liu P, Demers C, et al.; Canadian Cardiovascular Society. Canadian Cardiovascular Society consensus conference recommendation on heart failure 2006: diagnosis and management. Can J Cardiol. 2006;22(1):23–45.

39. Jahns BG, Stein W, Hilfiker-Kleiner D, Pieske B, Emons G. Peripartum cardiomyopathy—a new treatment option by inhibition of prolactin secretion. Am J Obstet Gynecol. 2008;199(4):e5–6.

40. De Jong JS, Rietveld K, van Lochem LT, Bouma BJ. Rapid left ventricular recovery after cabergoline treatment in a patient with peripartum cardiomyopathy. Eur J Heart Fail. 2009;1(2):220–2.

41. Gavaert S, van Belleghem Y, Bouchez S, et al. Acute and critically ill peripartum cardiomyopathy and "bridge to" therapeutic options: a single center experience with intra-aortic balloon pump, extracorporeal membrane oxygenation and continuous flow left ventricular assist devices. Crit Care. 2011;15(2):R93.

42. Abboud J, Murad Y, Chen-Scarabelli C, Saravolatz L, Scarabelli TM. Peripartum cardiomyopathy: a comprehensive review. Int J Cardiol. 2007;118(3):295–303.

43. Keogh A, Macdonald P, Spratt P, Marshman D, Larbalestier R, Kaan A. Outcome in peripartum cardiomyopathy after heart transplantation. J Heart Lung Transplant. 1994;13(2):202–7.

44. Smith IJ, Gillham MJ. Fulminant peripartum cardiomyopathy rescue with extracorporeal membranous oxygenation. Int J Obstet Anesth. 2009;18(2):186–8.

45. Udell JA, Lu H, Redelmeier DA. Failure of fertility therapy and subsequent adverse cardiovascular events. CMAJ. 2017;189:E391–7.

46. Siu SC, Sermer M, Colman JM, et al. Prospective multicenter study of pregnancy outcomes in women with heart disease. Circulation. 2001;104:515–21.

47. Drenthen W, Boersma E, Balci A, et al. Predictors of pregnancy complications in women with congenital heart disease. Eur Heart J. 2010;31:2124–32.

48. Lam W. Heart disease and pregnancy. Tex Heart Inst J. 2012;39(2):237–9.

49. Roth A, Elkayam U. Acute myocardial infarction associated with pregnancy. J Am Coll Cardiol. 2008;52(3):171–80.

50. Dayan N, Laskin CA, Spitzer K, et al. Pregnancy complications in women with heart disease conceiving with fertility therapy. J Am Coll Cardiol. 2014;64(17):1862–4.

51. Sazonova A, Redelmeier DA. Long term cardiovascular risk in women prescribed fertility therapy. J Am Coll Cardiol. 2013;62:1704–12.

52. De Viti D, et al. Congenital aorto-right ventricular fistula associated with pulmonary hypertension in an old female patient. J Cardiovasc Echogr. 2018;28(2):141–2.

53. Knochenhauer ES, Key TJ, Kahsar-Miller M, Waggoner W, Boots LR, Azziz R. Prevalence of the polycystic ovary syndrome in unselected black and white women of the southeastern United States: a prospective study. J Clin Endocrinol Metab. 1998;83:3078–82.

54. Azziz R, Woods KS, Reyna R, Key TJ, Knochenhauer ES, Yildiz BO. The prevalence and features of the polycystic ovary syndrome in an unselected population. J Clin Endocrinol Metab. 2004;89:2745–9.

55. Vignesh JP, Mohan V. Polycystic ovary syndrome: a component of metabolic syndrome? J Postgrad Med. 2007;53:128–34.

56. Grundy SM, Cleeman JI, Daniels SR, Donato KA, Eckel RH, Franklin BA, et al. Diagnosis and management of the metabolic syndrome: an American Heart Association/National Heart, Lung, and Blood Institute scientific statement. Circulation. 2005;112:2735–52.

57. Park YW, Zhu S, Palaniappan L, Heshka S, Carnethon MR, Heymsfield SB. The metabolic syndrome: prevalence and associated risk factor findings in the US population from the Third National Health and Nutrition Examination Survey, 1988–1994. Arch Intern Med. 2003;163:427–36.

58. Alvarez Cosmea A, López Fernández V, Suárez García S, Arias García T, Prieto Díaz MA, Díaz González L. Differences in the prevalence of metabolic syndrome according to the ATP-III and WHO definitions. Med Clin (Barc). 2005;124:368–70.

59. Seidell JC. Obesity, insulin resistance and diabetes—a worldwide epidemic. Br J Nutr. 2000;83(Suppl 1):S5–8.

60. Lobo RA, Carmina E. The importance of diagnosing the polycystic ovary syndrome. Ann Intern Med. 2000;132:989–93.

61. Sharma S, Majumdar A. Prevalence of metabolic syndrome in relation to body mass index and polycystic ovarian syndrome in Indian women. J Hum Reprod Sci. 2015;8(4):202–8.

62. Madani T, Hosseini R, Ramezanali F, Khalili G, et al. Metabolic syndrome in infertile women with polycystic ovarian syndrome. Arch Endocrinol Metab. 2016;60(3):199–204.

63. Glueck CJ, Papanna R, Wang P, Goldenberg N, Sieve-Smith L. Incidence and treatment of metabolic syndrome in newly referred women with confirmed polycystic ovarian syndrome. Metabolism. 2003;52(7):908–15.

64. Apridonidze T, Essah PA, Iuorno MJ, Nestler JE. Prevalence and characteristics of the metabolic syndrome in women with polycystic ovary syndrome. J Clin Endocrinol Metab. 2005;90(4):1929–35.

65. Bhattacharya SM. Prevalence of metabolic syndrome in women with polycystic ovary syndrome, using two proposed definitions. Gynecol Endocrinol. 2010;26(7):516–20.

66. Weerakiet S, Bunnag P, Phakdeekitcharoen B, Wansumrith S, Chanprasertyothin S, Jultanmas R, et al. Prevalence of the metabolic syndrome in Asian women with polycystic ovary syndrome: using the International Diabetes Federation criteria. Gynecol Endocrinol. 2007;23(3):153–60.

67. Soares EM, Azevedo GD, Gadelha RG, Lemos TM, Maranhão TM. Prevalence of the metabolic syndrome and its components in Brazilian women with polycystic ovary syndrome. Fertil Steril. 2008;89(3):649–55.

68. Ni RM, Mo Y, Chen X, Zhong J, Liu W, Yang D. Low prevalence of the metabolic syndrome but high occurrence of various metabolic disorders in Chinese women with polycystic ovary syndrome. Eur J Endocrinol. 2009;161(3):411–8.

69. Park HR, Choi Y, Lee HJ, Oh JY, Hong YS, Sung YA. The metabolic syndrome in young Korean women with polycystic ovary syndrome. Diabetes Res Clin Pract. 2007;77(Suppl):S243–6.

70. Vural B, Caliskan E, Turkoz E, Kilic T, Demirci A. Evaluation of metabolic syndrome frequency and premature carotid atherosclerosis in young women with polycystic ovary syndrome. Hum Reprod. 2005;20(9):2409–13.

71. Carmina E, Napoli N, Longo RA, Rini GB, Lobo RA. Metabolic syndrome in polycystic ovary syndrome (PCOS): lower prevalence in southern Italy than in the USA and the influence of criteria for the diagnosis of PCOS. Eur J Endocrinol. 2006;154(1):141–5.

72. Bilal M, Haseeb A, Rehman A. Relationship of polycystic ovarian syndrome with cardiovascular risk factors. Diabetes Metab Syndr. 2018;12(3):375–80.

73. Talbott EO, Zborowskii JV, Boudraux MY. Do women with polycystic ovary syndrome have an increased risk of cardiovascular disease? Review of the evidence. Minerva Ginecol. 2004;56(1):27–39.

74. Sukalich S, Guzick D. Cardiovascular health in women with polycystic ovary syndrome. Semin Reprod Med. 2003;21(3):309–15.

75. Orio F, Vuolo L, Palomba S, Lombardi G, Colao A. Metabolic and cardiovascular consequences of polycystic ovary syndrome. Minerva Ginecol. 2008;60(1):39–51.

76. Dokras A, Bochner M, Hollinrake E, Markham S, Vanvoorhis B, Jagasia DH. Screening women with polycystic ovary syndrome for metabolic syndrome. Obstet Gynecol. 2005;106(1):131–7.

77. Tomlinson J, Millward A, Stenhouse E, Pinkney J. Type 2 diabetes and cardiovascular disease in polycystic ovary syndrome: what are the risks and can they be reduced? Diabet Med. 2010;27(5):498–515.

78. Talbott EO, Zborowskii JV, et al. Do women with polycystic ovary syndrome have an increased risk of cardiovascular disease? Review of the evidence. Minerva Ginecol. 2004;56(1):27–39.

79. Glintborg D, Rubin KH, et al. Cardiovascular disease in a nationwide population of Danish women with polycystic ovary syndrome. Cardiovasc Diabetol. 2018;17(1):37.

80. Laird SM, Tuckerman EM, Li TC. Cytokine expression in the endometrium of women with implantation failure and recurrent miscarriage. Reprod Biomed Online. 2006;13(1):13–23.

81. Marciniak A, Nawrocka Rutkowska J, et al. Cardiovascular system disease in patient with polycystic ovary syndrome—the role of inflammation process in this pathology and possibility of early diagnosis and prevention. Ann Agric Environ Med. 2016;23(4):537–41.

82. Dawood A, Alkafrawy N, et al. The relationship between IL-18 and atherosclerotic cardiovascular risk in Egyptian lean women with polycystic ovary syndrome. Gynecol Endocrinol. 2018;34(4):294–7.

83. Kaya C, Pabuccu R, et al. Plasma interleukin-18 levels are increased in the polycystic ovary syndrome: relationship of carotid intima-media wall thickness and cardiovascular risk factors. Fertil Steril. 2010;93(4):1200–7.

84. Meyer ML, Malek AM, Wild RA, Korytkowski MT, Talbott EO. Carotid artery intima-media thickness in polycystic ovary syndrome: a systematic review and meta-analysis. Hum Reprod Update. 2012;18(2):112–26.

85. Hyderali BN, Mala K. Oxidative stress and cardiovascular complications in polycystic ovarian syndrome. Eur J Obstet Gynecol Reprod Biol. 2015;191:15–22.

86. Krishna MB, Joseph A, et al. Impaired arginine metabolism coupled to a defective redox conduit contributes to low plasma nitric oxide in polycystic ovary syndrome. Cell Physiol Biochem. 2017;43(5):1880–92.

87. Kaya C, Erkan AF, Cengiz SD, Dünder I, Demirel OE, Bilgihan A. Advanced oxidation protein products are increased in women with polycystic ovary syndrome: relationship with traditional and nontraditional cardiovascular risk factors in patients with polycystic ovary syndrome. Fertil Steril. 2009;92(4):1372–7.

88. Ozturk M, Oktem M, et al. Elevated PAPP-A levels in lean patient with polycystic ovary syndrome. Taiwan J Obstet Gynecol. 2018;57(3):394–8.

89. Bonaca MP, Scirica BM, et al. Prospective evaluation of pregnancy-associated plasma proteina and outcomes in patients with acute coronary syndromes. J Am Coll Cardiol. 2012;60(4):332–8.

90. Bondagji NS. Ischaemic heart disease in pregnancy. J Saudi Heart Assoc. 2012;24(2):89–97.

91. Roth A, et al. Acute myocardial infarction associated with pregnancy. J Am Coll Cardiol. 2008;52(3):171–80.

92. Havakuk O, Goland S, Mehra A, Elkayam U. Pregnancy and the risk of spontaneous coronary artery dissection: an analysis of 120 contemporary cases. Circ Cardiovasc Interv. 2017;10(3).

93. Karadag B, Roffi M. Postpartal dissection of all coronary arteries in an in vitro-fertilized postmenopausal woman. Tex Heart Inst J. 2009;36(2):168–70.

94. Teede H, Deeks A, Moran L. Polycystic ovary syndrome: a complex condition with psychological, reproductive and metabolic manifestations that impacts on health across the lifespan. BMC Med. 2010;8:41.

95. Baldani DP, Skrgatic L, Ougouag R. Polycystic ovary syndrome: important underrecognised cardiometabolic risk factor in reproductive-age women. Int J Endocrinol. 2015;2015: 786362.

96. Diamanti-Kandarakis E, Dunaif A. Insulin resistance and the polycystic ovary syndrome revisited: an update on mechanisms and implications. Endocr Rev. 2012;33(6):981–1030.

97. Moran L, Teede H. Metabolic features of the reproductive phenotypes of polycystic ovary syndrome. Hum Reprod Update. 2009;15(4):477–88.

98. Kauffman RP, Baker TE, et al. Endocrine and metabolic differences among phenotypic expressions of polycystic ovary syndrome according to the 2003 Rotterdam consensus criteria. Am J Obstet Gynecol. 2008;198(6):670.

99. Daskalopoulos GN, Karkanaki A, Karagiannis A, Mikhailidis DP, Athyros VG. Is the risk for cardiovascular disease increased in all phenotypes of the polycystic ovary syndrome? Angiology. 2011;62(4):285–90.

100. Randeva HS, Tan BK, Weickert MO, et al. Cardiometabolic aspects of the polycystic ovary syndrome. Endocr Rev. 2012;33(5):812–41.

101. Baldani DP, Skrgatic L, Goldstajn MS, Vrcic H, Canic T, Strelec M. Clinical, hormonal and metabolic characteristics of polycystic ovary syndrome among obese and nonobese women in the Croatian population. Coll Antropol. 2013;37(2):465–70.

102. Ciepiela P, Baczkowski T, Brelik P, et al. Biotechnological and clinical outcome of in vitro fertilization in non-obese patients with polycystic ovarian syndrome. Folia Histochem Cytobiol. 2007;45(Suppl 1):s65–71.

103. Norman RJ, Masters L, Milner CR, Wang JX, Davies MJ. Relative risk of conversion from normoglycaemia to impaired glucose tolerance or non-insulin dependent diabetes mellitus in polycystic ovarian syndrome. Hum Reprod. 2001;16(9):1995–8.

104. Ehrmann DA, Barnes RB, Rosenfield RL, Cavaghan MK, Imperial J. Prevalence of impaired glucose tolerance and diabetes in women with polycystic ovary syndrome. Diabetes Care. 1999;22(1):141–6.

105. Gonzalez F, Thusu K, Abdel-Rahman E, Prabhala A, Tomani M, Dandona P. Elevated serum levels of tumor necrosis factor alpha in normal-weight women with polycystic ovary syndrome. Metab Clin Exp. 1999;48(4):437–41.

106. Samy N, Hashim M, Sayed M, Said M. Clinical significance of inflammatory markers in polycystic ovary syndrome: their relationship to insulin resistance and body mass index. Dis Markers. 2009;26(4):163–70.

107. Escobar-Morreale HF, Luque-Ramírez M, González F. Circulating inflammatory markers in polycystic ovary syndrome: a systematic review and metaanalysis. Fertil Steril. 2011;95(3):1048.

108. Legro RS, Kunselman AR, Dunaif A. Prevalence and predictors of dyslipidemia in women with polycystic ovary syndrome. Am J Med. 2001;111(8):607–13.

109. Graf MJ, Richards CJ, Brown V, Meissner L, Dunaif A. The independent effects of hyperandrogenaemia, hyperinsulinaemia, and obesity on lipid and lipoprotein profiles in women. Clin Endocrinol. 1990;33(1):119–31.

110. Talbott E, Clerici A, Berga SL, et al. Adverse lipid and coronary heart disease risk profiles in young women with polycystic ovary syndrome: results of a case-control study. J Clin Epidemiol. 1998;51(5):415–22.

111. Wild RA, Rizzo M, Clifton S, Carmina E. Lipid levels in polycystic ovary syndrome: systematic review and meta-analysis. Fertil Steril. 2011;95(3):1073.

112. Solomon CG, Hu FB, Dunaif A, et al. Menstrual cycle irregularity and risk for future cardiovascular disease. J Clin Endocrinol Metab. 2002;87(5):2013–7.

113. de Groot PCM, Dekkers OM, Romijn JA, Dieben SWM, Helmerhorst FM. PCOS, coronary heart disease, stroke and the influence of obesity: a systematic review and meta-analysis. Hum Reprod Update. 2011;17(4):495–500.

114. Otto-Buczkowska E, et al. Early metabolic abnormalities-insulin resistance, hyperinsulinemia, impaired glucose tolerance and diabetes, in adolescent girls with polycystic ovarian syndrome. Przegl Lek. 2006;63(4):234–8.

115. Tsikouras P, Spyros L, et al. Features of polycystic ovary syndrome in adolescence. J Med Life. 2015;8(3):291–6.

116. Coviello AD, Legro RS, Dunaif A. Adolescent girls with polycystic ovary syndrome have an increased risk of the metabolic syndrome associated with increased androgen levels independent of obesity and insulin resistance. J Clin Endocrinol Metab. 2006;91(2):492–7.

117. Aydin Y, Hassa H, et al. What is the risk of metabolic syndrome in adolescents with normal BMI who have polycystic ovary syndrome? J Pediatr Adolesc Gynecol. 2015;28(4):271–4.

118. Alexander CJ, Tangchitnob EP, Lepor NE. Polycystic ovary syndrome: a major unrecognized cardiovascular risk factor in women. Rev Cardiovasc Med. 2009;10(2):83–90.

Oocyte Quality

15

Pierre Boyer, Patricia Rodrigues, Marie Boyer,
and Giovanni Vizziello

Contents

Routine harvesting oocytes for in vitro fertilization (IVF) started in the early 1980s.

Only then gynecologists and scientist had the opportunity to study the human female gamete, until this time all the knowledge of this extraordinary cell was inferred from animal models.

The day of oocyte retrieval, also known as oocyte pick-up, is the start of all IVF process. In early 1960s, collection of the precious egg was the main concern of every gynecologist. Thanks to doctor Patrick Steptoe and his collaboration with doctor Bob Edwards oocyte recovery succeeded, and Louise Brown was born 40 years ago [1].

The success of IVF depends on oocyte pick-up. Despite age, major impact factor on oocyte quality, ovarian stimulation, and oocyte pick-up also influence oocyte quality. Here we will revisit oocyte pick-up: how it is done and its influence in oocyte quality. We will go through the complete process from triggering to oocyte management in vitro.

P. Boyer (✉) · M. Boyer
Service de Médecine et Biologie de la Reproduction,
Hôpital Saint-Joseph, Marseille, France
e-mail: pboyer@hopital-saint-joseph.fr;
mboyer@hopital-saint-joseph.fr

P. Rodrigues
Life Sciences Department—School of Psychology and Life Sciences, Lusófona University Lisbon, Lisbon, Portugal

Centro de Médico de Assistência à Reprodução—CEMEARE, Lisbon, Portugal
e-mail: patricia.rodrigues@ulusofona.pt

G. Vizziello
IVF Lab MOMO' fertiLIFE, Bisceglie, Italy

15.1 Oocyte Pick-Up

15.1.1 Ovarian Stimulation and Oocyte Pick-Up

Ovarian stimulation is fundamental for IVF; without it there is no oocytes to pick-up. Triggering ovulation with exogenous gonadotropins and gonadotropin-releasing hormone (GnRH) agonist or antagonist (to suppress pituitary)

© Springer Nature Switzerland AG 2020
A. Malvasi, D. Baldini (eds.), *Pick Up and Oocyte Management*, https://doi.org/10.1007/978-3-030-28741-2_15

avoiding premature ovulation is essential for the cumulus to detach itself from the wall of the follicle [2]. Oocyte pick-up occurs after final stages of oocyte maturation (when the female gamete is ready to be fertilzed), but before follicular rupture or the oocyte will be lost [3]. The classic pick-up schedule is 36 h post luteinizing hormone (LH) triggering injection. After using hCG 5000 units, urinary extraction of chorionic gonadotropin, its recombinant form is currently the only one available on the market. Agonist release using their flare-up action is also possible in pituitary-controlled ovarian stimulation by GnRH antagonists.

The time of collection is wider than 36 h after triggering. There is almost no follicular rupture before 40 h as we can observe during gamete intrafallopian transfer (GIFT) procedure.

15.1.2 From Laparoscopy to Ultrasound-Guided Puncture

Initially, oocyte pick-up was done by laparoscopy [4].

After having first identified the occurrence of the LH peak by iterative dosing, Steptoe and Edwards proposed a laparoscopic intervention to recover the oocytes. This procedure was used between 1978 and 1986 with more than 30% failure of collection [4]. The high rate of failure was not satisfactory; the number of pregnancies and children born per year of activity was low.

Some of the disadvantages of laparoscopic method lie in the necessary use of general anesthesia, the limitation of access to adherent or covered ovaries and its common postoperative abdominal discomfort and hospitalization stay of 6–24 h. But most importantly, its ineffectiveness compared to the echo guided collection. With laparoscopy it is only possible to access the most prominent follicles on the surface of the ovary, which limits the results.

Together with the mastery of ovulation trigger fundamentally changed the prognosis and ensured development of teams capable of intervening in most countries. A newer and more efficient method for oocyte recovery had to be developed and that was when ultrasound-guided oocyte collection was described [5, 6]. This method brought reliability and reproducibility to this long-standing random act [7]. Initially, the number of oocytes was not significantly higher, but the method was much simpler and with time became more efficient [7, 8].

While using laparoscopic oocyte collection was possible to check follicular fluids, the mature follicle wall became more and more translucent allowing the fluid to be visible. Puncture had to be carried out perpendicular to the follicle to avoid rupture with oocyte loss. Unlike today's guided ultrasound puncture, the needle had to be in a particular angle at the ovary to puncture the follicle. Whereas today, it is the needle that will search each follicle [7].

The collection of human oocytes for IVF by ultrasound-guided percutaneous follicular puncture was first described in 1981 [5]. This was a natural development based on the previous knowledge of ultrasound-guided punctures of other abdominal organs. Filling the urinary bladder with a volume of 300–500 mL gave better visualization and was routinely used. This transvesical aspiration route utilized an abdominal transducer equipped with an attached needle guide. Its main disadvantages lie in the difficulty of performing this procedure with local anesthesia since the bladder wall remains sensitive in many cases to needle puncture, and filling of the bladder with up to 500 mL, which usually causes a significant degree of patient discomfort. This method requires a degree of training and experience in ultrasound techniques by the operator before satisfactory oocyte collection rates can be achieved. For these reasons, another ultrasound-guided method emerged—the transvaginal route with endovaginal probes [6, 9]. This method remains in use until today [7, 8].

Transvaginal ultrasound-guided aspiration is done with a puncture needle with diameters between −16 and −17 gauge, to avoid damage the oocyte with the suction force [10]. It can be done with a 10–20 mL syringe controlled by hand, and a higher volume causes a higher suction force which can damage the oocyte during aspiration towards the needle [10]. An increased diameter ratio of the puncture needle and the higher volume syringe may be responsible for increasing the suction force. Instead of using a syringe, oocyte pick-up can also be done by using an aspiration device, where the puncture needle is coupled to the ultrasound guide, as in the syringe method, but the other end is connected with an aspirator which is then connected to a tube to which the follicular fluid is aspirated. The suction/aspiration force should be controlled to avoid oocyte damage [10].

15.1.3 Follicle Aspiration

While follicular fluid is aspirated it is possible to see within the tube, cellular elements from the granulosa attesting the follicular puncture. In case of cystic follicles aspiration, the aspirated fluid is citric yellow. The fluid is bloodier if small follicles are aspirated, which is responsible for difficult cumulus-oocyte complexes isolation. For that it has been suggested to rinse with a heparinized medium to avoid clotting. Ideally, a puncture is a little bloody leaving an orange color liquid or the cellular elements are visible to the naked eye, indicating the aspiration of mature follicles.

Follicular flushing after follicle aspiration should maximize the number of oocytes recovered [10]. However, no study really proved the increased number of oocytes using flushing, and due to its disadvantages: longer procedures, more anesthetics, possibility of cell removal with potential important endocrine luteal support, flushing is not routinely used [10].

Identification of collection tubes at the site of follicular puncture is a key point to identity-vigilance and traceability for clinical-biological transmission. Oocyte pick-up is done in an operating room, which ideally communicates with the IVF laboratory. However, it may not be the case, so transport to the laboratory should be organized in order to maintain oocyte survival and traceability-security conditions [11, 12].

In the beginning of the establishment of IVF centers, the embryology teams were often located away from the puncture sites. This situation still remains current in some cases. The quality of transportation could explain the differences in results from one team to another, even within the same laboratory. Pre-heated blocks should be used to transport the tubes with the follicular fluid, ensuring a temperature as stable as possible at 36.5 ± 1 °C. Temperature regulation is required during transport, with heat input which can be autonomous or connected to a vehicle-type cigarette lighter transport device. Several tube types can be used for collection of follicular fluids, the most common are sterile 14 mL tubes [11].

15.1.4 Abnormalities Related to Oocyte Pick-Up

There is no risk of deterioration of oocyte quality related to the collection, the conditions are today controlled from the physical point, depression of 100 mmHg, physiological fluids tested for rinses, absence of toxicity like gaseous anesthetics. The risk of damaging the oocyte exists in case of pressure vacuum on the suction pump. The examination then shows the distended corona and the broken oocyte with cytoplasm separated into two (Fig. 15.1a and b), or simply a complete damaged oocyte, which will be excluded from any technique (Fig. 15.1c).

15.2 Oocyte Isolation In Vitro

15.2.1 Follicular Fluids Examination

Follicular aspirated fluids examination should be performed in strict aseptic conditions, under a vertical laminar flow hood, and with the least heat loss possible [11]. The search for the cumulus-oocyte complexes (COCs) can be performed with the naked eye in backlighting for better cell refraction.

The spreading of the fluid in a large petri dish makes it possible to locate the oocyte within the cumulus and the cells of corona radiata. Isolation is then done under a stereomicroscope with a heated stage to maintain the oocyte temperature near 37 °C. Exposure to light and exterior environment should be minimal, and sample analysis must be quick [11]. Particularly, if follicular fluid is bloody, the fastest analysis lowers risks for coagulation. The storage conditions must also be controlled to ensure maintenance of the physicochemical parameters such as temperature and heat the most stable as possible. Again, the speed of the operator is important because prolonged exposure of the oocyte to the follicular fluid will have an impact on oocyte quality. Therefore, it is recommended to choose a close buffer medium, like HEPES to maintain pH stable, when working under the hood, instead of a bicarbonate buffer medium which needs to be kept at 5–6% CO_2 [11].

Following isolation and morphological evaluation, oocytes are placed in an appropriate medium in an incubator at 37 °C with 5–6% CO_2 until IVF sperm insemination and/or Intra-Cytoplasmic Sperm Injection (ICSI) denudation and microinjection (Fig. 15.2).

Timing for insemination and microinjection is important to oocyte quality and/or embryo development, every species oocyte has a fertilization window, and in humans that window is between 24 and 36 h post-LH surge [13]. Afterwards, an aging process of in vitro of human oocyte will initiate, and this includes a slow migration of the spindle away from the cortex and an increased susceptibility to abnormal egg activation, apoptosis, and aneuploidy [13]. Usually, insemination or microinjection of mature

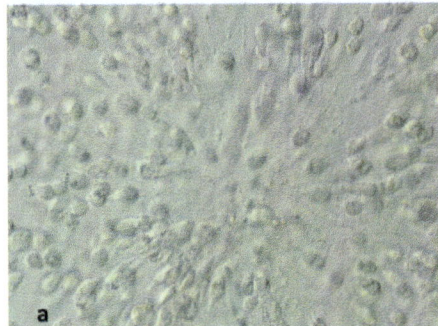 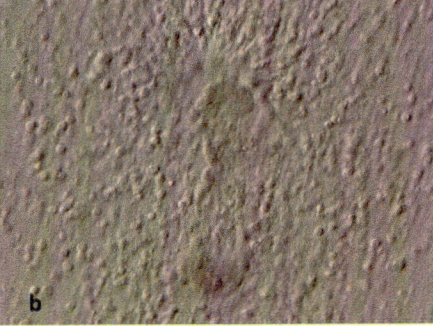 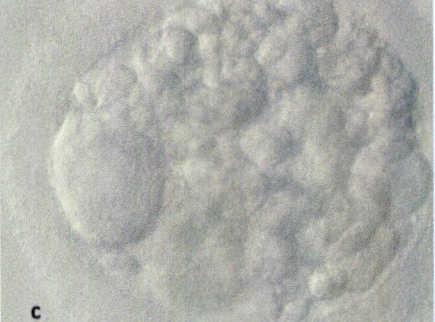

Fig. 15.1 Occurrence of abnormalities due to hyper aspiration pressure during oocyte collection: (**a**) corona without oocyte; (**b**) separation of the oocytes into two; (**c**) oocyte in fragmentation

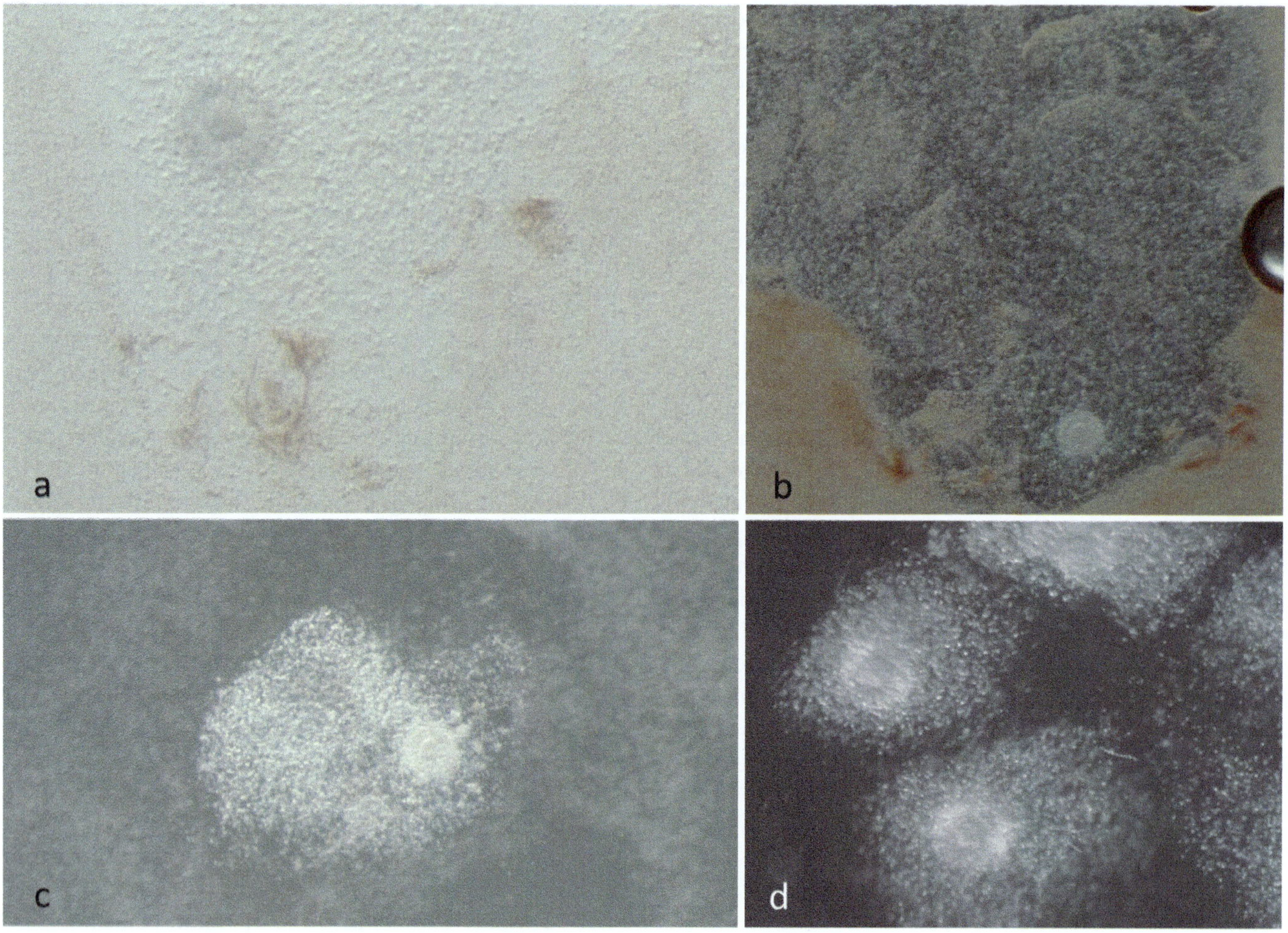

Fig. 15.2 Oocyte sampling: often in bloody follicular fluid the COCs present traces of blood (**a**) magnification 5× and (**b**) magnification 8×; (**c**, **d**) regular appearance of COCs while waiting for insemination (IVF) or denudation (ICSI)

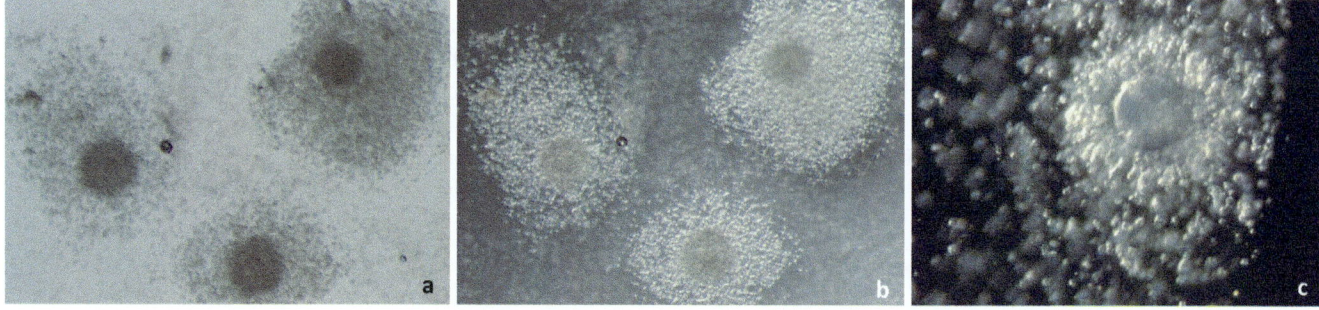

Fig. 15.3 Oocyte isolation: (**a**, **b**) alternating backlighting allows for more clear sampling the maturity of cumulus cells; (**c**) at higher magnification (20×) with the black underground it is possible to observe the expanded cumulus cells indicative of maturation

oocytes is done approximately within 4 h after oocyte pick-up. For the same reasons, if freezing instead of fertilizing the oocytes, the same precautions should be used (Fig. 15.3).

15.2.2 Oocyte Evaluation

Embryo morphology assessment is a key element in any IVF laboratory, but interestingly the morphology assessment of the

recovered oocytes is not [14]. In case of ICSI, a quick evaluation is performed after denudation, providing superficial information of which meiotic stage the oocytes are: germinal vesicle (GV—Fig. 15.1a), metaphase I (MI—Fig. 15.1b), or metaphase II (MII—Fig. 15.1c), in order to select oocytes to microinject [14]. Oocyte quality is of upmost importance for which female fertility is totally dependent on [15]. A better knowledge of what governs oocyte quality is important, due to the fact that this initial evaluation could give the embryologist a prediction of oocyte developmental potential, and ultimately embryo development [15].

Nevertheless, there are very few signs of egg quality on the day of collection. Historically, it is the expansion of the cumulus that is associated with its growth and served as a maturity assessor. However, in conventional IVF, this relationship between cumulus and meiosis resume does not predict fertilization, and all oocytes collected are usually inseminated without further evaluation. It is denudation 24 h afterwards that confirms oocyte maturity by the presence of a polar body (PB) and eventual fertilization if two pronuclei (PN) are also present. This observation is imperfect because we can attest to meiosis resume, but nothing certifies that it was the case at the time of contact with the spermatozoa. If there is a fertilization failure, it is easily explained when we encounter the oocytes in GV or MI stage or if intra-cytoplasmic smooth endoplasmic reticulum (sER) sacculi are present [13], uncertainties remain in the case of MII fail to fertilize, which still affects about 30% of oocytes, including those of ICSI [16]. The presence of smooth endoplasmic reticulum (sER) clusters in the MII ooplasm is associated with low pregnancy rates [17–19]. In IVF, it is also associated with failure of fertilization that must be overpassed by using ICSI.

Oocyte maturation is a complex event, which implies synchronism of nuclear and cytoplasmic maturation. Resume of meiosis is initiated with the LH surge, and oocyte meiosis from prophase (PI) of meiosis I, and it arrests again in metaphase II and awaits sperm entry and fertilization [3].

Nevertheless, these are morphological features, which may not represent the very true nature of the oocyte quality. The same quality can be compromised by many other factors as it has been mentioned. There are still more studies needed to truly access oocyte quality during IVF procedures (Fig. 15.4).

15.2.3 Oocyte Maturation

Oocyte maturation consists in the progression from diplotene of prophase I (PI) to MII of the second meiosis division [3]. This step of oocyte maturation prior to fertilization is very fast and crucial, and it occurs just prior to ovulation and after the LH surge [3, 20]. This progression occurs at nuclear and cytoplasmic level; without it the oocyte will not recognize the spermatozoid and will not fertilize. All of these mechanisms depend on the bi-directional communication between the oocyte and cumulus cells [20, 21]. In human, this process takes about 30 h [19] (Fig. 15.5).

The cumulus cells communicate with the oocyte, and vice versa, through transzonal projections (TZPs) that extend from the cumulus cells traversing the zona pellucida (ZP) into the ooplasm of the oocyte [22]. The factors exchanged between the oocyte and the somatic cells are responsible for maintaining meiotic arrest and cytoplasm stockpiling of molecules and organelles, which will be the maternal contribution to maturation, fertilization, and embryo development [3, 15]. Table 15.1 summarizes nuclear and cytoplasmic aspects of oocyte maturation.

Nuclear maturation will occur spontaneously if the oocyte is released from the follicle [23]. However, the objective is to have a MII oocyte at the time of oocyte pick-up (Fig. 15.1c). The quiescent immature oocyte has its nucleus arrested in diplotene of PI of first meiotic division, also known as GV (Fig. 15.1a). Following the hCG dose 36 h before oocyte pick-up, the GV initiates breakdown (germinal vesicle breakdown—GVBD) and start forming the MI spindle (Fig. 15.1b). In human, it forms in center of the oocyte, having to relocate to the oocyte cytoplasmic membrane, so that the asymmetrical cytokinesis occurs with the extrusion the first PB (Fig. 15.1c) [3].

When cultured in vitro, human oocyte maturation is observed 24–48 h in culture with no hCG stimulation, and in 30 h if the patient was treated with hCG [23]. The relocation

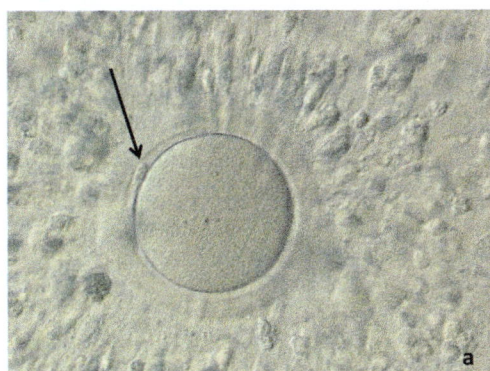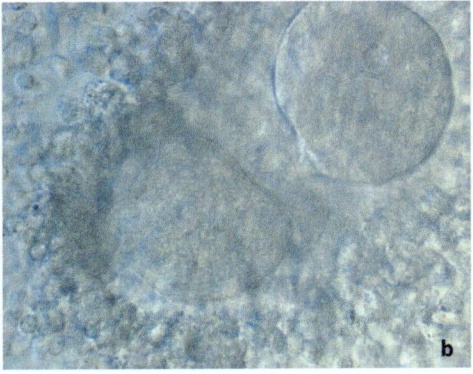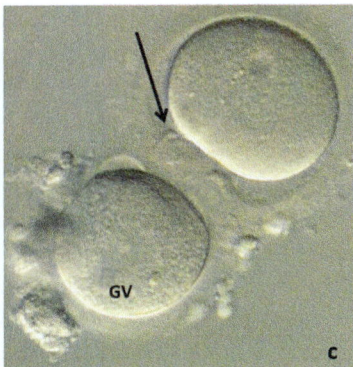

Fig. 15.4 Oocyte evaluation: (**a**) sometimes the cumulus cells in the COC are so well expanded that allow to visualize the presence of the PB (arrow), confirming nuclear maturation, magnification 10×; (**b**, **c**) rare sighting of two oocytes within the same corona cells, but each oocyte has its own zona pellucida (ZP); (**c**) interestingly and despite being subjected to same hormone dosage, after denudation the oocytes were in different stages of meiosis—GV and MII (arrow in the PB), magnification 15×

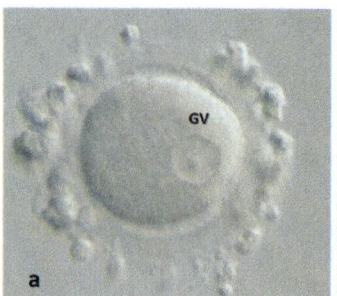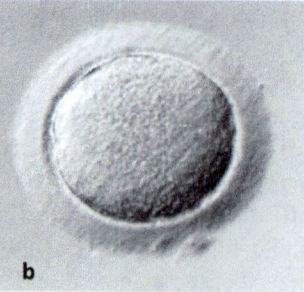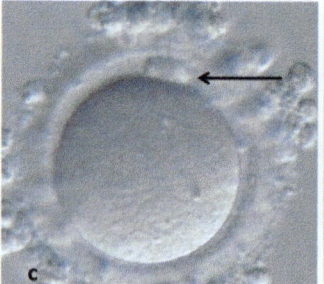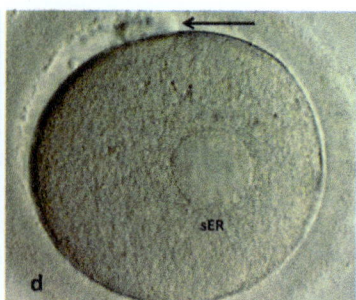

Fig. 15.5 Oocyte maturity stages: (**a**) germinal vesicle (GV); (**b**) metaphase I (MI); (**c**) metaphase II (MII) presence of a polar body (PB—arrow); (**d**) MII oocyte exhibiting a sER in the cytoplasm, sign of immature cytoplasm

Table 15.1 Oocyte maturation: from PI to MII

	Prophase I	Metaphase I	Metaphase II
Nuclear	GV centrally located in the cytoplasm	MI spindle centrally located	MII spindle under the oolemma and PB extruded
Cytoplasm			
• Cortical granules • Mitochondria • Endoplasmic reticulum	Distributed widely through the cytoplasm Sparse Organized in network from cortex to the interior of the cytoplasm	Distributed widely through the cytoplasm Sparse Grouped near the MI spindle Similar distribution as in prophase I	Underneath the oolemma Underneath the oolemma Clusters throughout the cell, including around the MII spindle

oocyte cytoplasm [3]. The ER is the intercellular calcium (Ca2+) store for the necessary Ca2+ oscillations for triggering meiotic maturation to MII and meiotic completion at fertilization [3]. ER is well organized and distributed throughout the cytoplasm in prophase I and metaphase I; however, in metaphase II the ER forms clusters throughout the cytoplasm including around the MII spindle [3]. The cortical granules are secretory organelles that prevent more than one spermatozoid to fertilize the oocyte (polyspermy prevention) [3]. These vesicles are dispersed through the cytoplasm during prophase I and metaphase I, clustering underneath the oolemma in MII. Cortical granules are activated by the Ca2+ oscillation at fertilization [3]. Cytoplasmic maturation is accomplished through massive intracellular reorganization of the organelles, induced by cell cycle kinases in response to LH triggering [21].

of the MI spindle is driven by cytoplasmic streaming which pushes the MI spindle closest to the oocyte membrane. The relocation leads also to the formation of a thick layer of F-actin in the cortex just above the spindle. This highly polarized configuration of the oocyte is necessary for a cytokinesis to occur with the less amount of cytoplasm possible to ensure oocyte/embryo quality [3].

Regarding cytoplasmic maturation, as in other somatic cells, the oocyte cytoplasm is composed of several organelles; among them is the endoplasmic reticulum (ER), Golgi complex (GC), lysosomes, ribosomes, mitochondria, and annulated lamellae.

However, oocytes have two other organelles that are oocyte exclusive: cortical granules (CG) and Balbiani's body [24]. Mitochondria are the energy source for maturation, fertilization, and embryo development, and also are involved in oocyte aging due to reduced efficiency in managing the free radicals [24]. This organelle is abundant throughout the cytoplasm during meiosis I until MI spindle forms when it locates in the surrounding of the spindle; just before cytokinesis it relocates to the spindle pole farthest of the oocyte membrane, ensuring that the oocyte energy reserve is kept within the

15.2.4 Oocyte Denudation and ICSI Timing: Impact on Oocyte Quality

The success of ART depends upon oocyte quality, hence avoiding long oocyte manipulations is very important. The oocyte competence is predicted by oocyte nuclear and cytoplasmic maturation [25]. This is particularly important due to the oocyte ability to fertilize, even after it loses its capacity to develop into viable embryo [26]. Age is an important factor in oocyte quality and is usually assumed that oocytes collected from younger women may hold longer periods of incubation than those of older women [25]. However, longer incubation periods before ICSI or vitrification can age even young oocytes, inducing detrimental outcomes, as shown in mice oocyte aged in culture; the same calcium oscillations induced apoptosis instead of fertilization [27, 28]. Timing matters at all female ages.

Results are still inconsistent regarding what is the best time to denudate oocytes, but the timing between denudation and ICSI or vitrification is consensual [11, 25]. It should be short because denuded oocytes are more vulnerable to any external changes [11, 25, 27, 29].

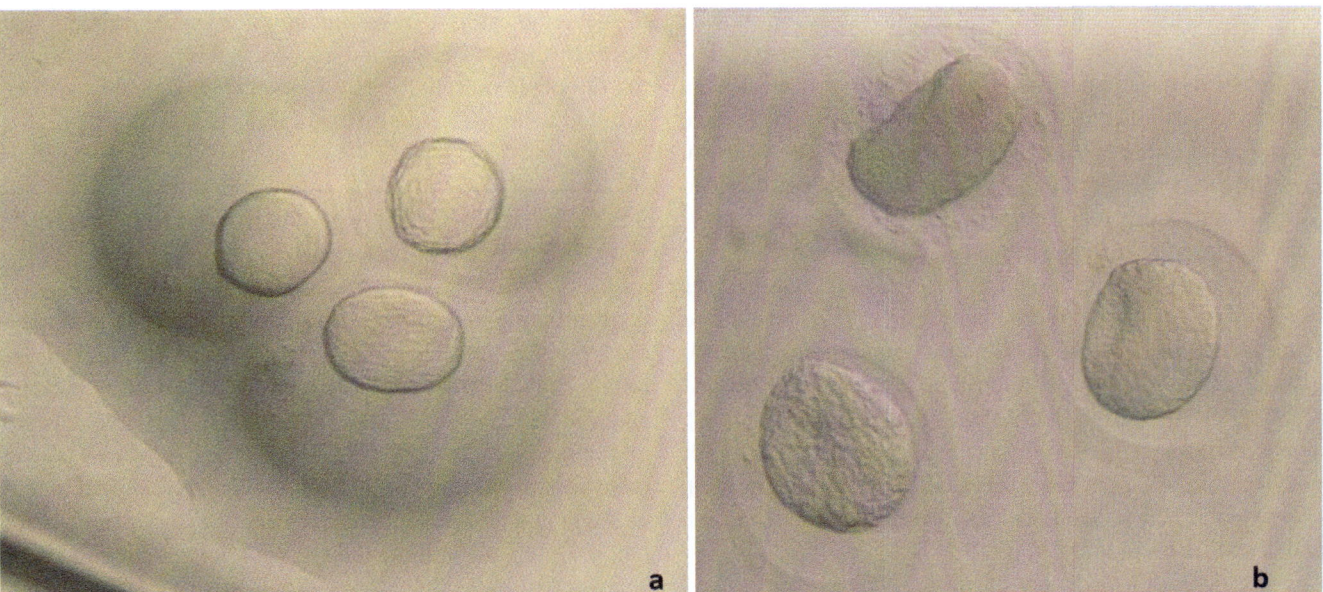

Fig. 15.6 Oocyte vitrification: a group of three oocytes (**a**) in vitrification solution; (**b**) recovering post-thawing

Pre-incubate cumulus-oocyte complexes (COCs) before denudation may not increase the number of mature oocytes but may allow for those already in MII to complete cytoplasmic maturation [14, 29]. Even though this is a nonconsensual subject, it is consensual to everyone that excessive incubation time decreases oocyte quality [29].

It was demonstrated that after warmed the MII oocyte spindle integrity starts to decline after 2–3 h in culture before ICSI, and oocyte had been cryopreserved 2–3 h prior to pick-up [29]. It has been shown that performing ICSI 2–3 h post oocyte pick-up or 38–39 h post hCG triggering has a good impact on implantation rates [25]. Whereas, earlier other authors suggested 37–41 h post hCG triggering for better implantation rates [30].

Independently of the differences, these results demonstrate that we have at least a 3 h window to perform ICSI or to vitrify the oocytes after pick-up without compromising the oocytes quality.

15.2.5 Oocyte Vitrification

Oocyte vitrification in the context of in vitro fertilization has to be considered today as part of the daily life in an ART laboratory [31]. This technical advance is responsible for oocyte quality and survival after freezing/warming. The vitrification of mature oocytes is an alternative to freezing embryos and the difficulties that this represents for some couples and certain situations such as the preservation of female fertility [32]. Vitrification only maintains the qualitative potential of the oocyte collected.

The success rates of this technique are very good, both oocyte survival post-thawing and fertilization rates, which are indicative of how well the oocyte quality is preserved, allowing for a personalized approach in patient care [32]. For example, if a patient is in risk of ovarian hyperstimulation syndrome (OHSS) a "freeze all" approach can be chosen with the same security as freeze all embryos [32]. It can also be used safely in poor-responder patients as a strategy to accumulate oocytes [33].

Taking into consideration the timing of culture prior to execution of the technique, and how harmful it can be to the oocyte quality, an ART laboratory should adjust their work to the requirements of this technique. It is therefore recommended that this task should be assigned to an experienced embryologist with no other assignments, for better results (Fig. 15.6).

15.2.6 Limitation of Oocyte Quality Evaluation

Oocyte quality evaluation is mostly morphological, with the exception of denuded oocytes for ICSI, the majority of the retrieved oocytes are evaluated superficially for cumulus overall size, coloration, and expansion [14]. In case of ICSI, however, due to denudation it is possible to assess the developmental stage (GV/MI/MII), and some degenerative signs of cytoplasm, PB, and/or zona pellucida (ZP) [14]. Nevertheless, this evaluation is still quite insufficient for predicting higher oocyte fertilization rate and embryo quality.

Spindle imaging using a polscope (polarized light microscope) was proposed in addition to PB observation for better oocyte maturity assessment [34]. Their investigation showed that the presence of the meiotic spindle was a good additional morphological parameter for oocyte quality evaluation [34]. However, it is not feasible for most ART clinics to have a polarized light imaging system. Polscope has been shown, in some cases of spindle abnormalities, to be inefficient to assess spindle and predict oocyte quality [35]. It is still, however, a valid noninvasive method to evaluate oocytes.

The variety of oocyte and embryo classification tables used by the different professionals may also contribute to more inadequate evaluation. With the intention to standardize and develop a more efficient evaluation of oocytes and embryos in 2011, it was published a global consensus [36]. This consensus suggested the inclusion in the evaluation of oocyte morphology: COCs, ZP, perivitelline space (PVS), PB, cytoplasm, and vacuolization, based on expert opinion and scientific literature.

Note should be made that one of the major limitations of these evaluation parameters is the inability to determine cytoplasmic maturity (oocyte is prepared for activation, fertilization, and development), which might not be synchronous with nuclear maturation (resumption of meiosis and progression to MII—extruded PB) [37].

The most important factor in the success of an in vitro fertilization is the number of oocytes available for a patient. Ovarian reserve evaluation with antral follicular count and AMH dosage reflects what the patient can expect as a response to the treatment.

Ultrasound allows to follow up ovarian stimulation, by visualizing and measuring the number of liquid structures (follicles), which are growing in the ovary. Despite the strong correlation between ultrasound images and the number of oocytes isolated when looking for COCs, this number must always be confirmed on the day of oocyte retrieval. The knowledge of the results of ultrasound and hormonal level is useful to the biologist in charge of the analysis of the pick-up product.

There is a direct correlation between the number of oocyte and the pregnancy rate [38]. When oocyte numbers are too high, there is a reverse reflection on pregnancy rate [38]. The maximum probability of success is reached on 15 oocytes; beyond 15 oocytes the qualitative effect turns against the results in pregnancy, increasing the possibility of hyperstimulation, which has a negative effect on pregnancy results [37]. In addition to impaired quality due to the large number of oocytes, the risk of bleeding may endanger the life of the patient.

Due to law 40/2004 in Italy, drastic oocyte selection was imposed to select only three oocytes after pick-up. It led to an increased oocytes research programs but when we look closely to the results on National register for patients, there has been no change in results [32].

Nevertheless, oocyte examination or its environment still needs further investigation to reach a better predictive potential of oocyte morphology evaluation. This objective will be fulfilled by transcriptomic research in cumuli cells [39].

15.3 Oocyte Quality to Support Embryonic Early Development

A quantifiable link between oocyte observations and embryonic development has not yet been found, despite all the efforts [14]. Microscopic observations of cellular elements taken separately do not allow to establish a reliable correlation either with development or implantation. Several oocyte structures including: meiotic spindle, ZP, presence of vacuoles, PB and oocyte shape, PVS, central cytoplasmic granulation, COCs maturation show no predictive value to better characterize developmental competence of the oocytes. Further studies are necessary to have a predictive potential of embryo quality based on morphological observations of the oocyte [14].

Regarding patient information of their success rate, if no infertility cause diagnosed, age has the most impact on the outcome of the attempt. The age of the oocyte is most important for the quality of the embryo designed [24]. Oocyte's age can be measured in maternal age (years) and/or time after collection (h). Pregnancy rates are directly related to maternal age, which is validated by the oocyte donation model. The oocyte provides all the elements for embryonic development with the exception of half of the nuclear material, and even after the awakening of the embryonic genome, until implantation, the embryo uses and exhausts all the reserves and resources of the oocyte [21, 24]. An important factor to keep in mind is that the intra-pellucidal volume of the oocyte and that of the embryo until day 5 are identical, whereas the exponential multiplication of cell divisions decreases the nucleus-cytoplasmic ratio. An implanting blastocyst retrospectively confirms the good quality of an oocyte.

15.4 Conclusions

No clear tendency in recent publications to a general increase in predictive value of morphological features has been described [14]. Day 0 or pick-up day is one of the more stressing days in the IVF procedure due to the unknown before follicular fluid examination. Even when oocyte number is confirmed, the uncertainty remains if associated with maternal age. We can only predict a statistical value correlated to the maternal age with the information after pick-up. If we keep in mind that female fertility preservation started with oocytes and oocyte numbers, the quality is of upmost importance in women whose health is in danger. Whether if it is for fertilization or freezing it is only possible to evaluate oocyte quality after pick-up, but only a few parameters are still available with real prognostic value for this first day. No doubt this is a subject under development, and we wait expectant for newer guidelines.

References

1. Steptoe PC, Edwards RG. Birth after the implantation of human embryo. Lancet. 1978;312(8085):366. https://doi.org/10.1016/S0140-6736(78)92957-4.
2. Sighinolfi G, Sunkara SK, La Marca A. New strategies of ovarian stimulation based on the concept of ovarian follicular waves: from conventional to random and double stimulation. RBMOnline. 2018;37(4):489–97. https://doi.org/10.1016/J.RBMO.2018.07.006.
3. McGinnis LK, Rodrigues P, Limback D. Structural aspects of oocyte maturation in encyclopedia of reproduction. 2nd edition in references in biomedical sciences. Elsevier; 2018. https://doi.org/10.1016/B978-0-12-801238-3.64445-8.
4. Steptoe PC, Edwards RG. Laparoscopic recovery of preovulatory human oocytes after priming of ovaries with gonadotrophins. Lancet. 1970;295(7649):683–9. https://doi.org/10.1016/S0140-6736(70)90923-2.
5. Lenz S, Lauritsen JG, Kjellow M. Collection of human oocytes for in vitro fertilisation by ultrasonically guided follicular puncture. Lancet. 1981;1:1163–4.
6. Wikland M, Nilsson L, Hansson R, Hamberger L, Janson JO. Collection of human oocytes by the use of sonography. Fertil Steril. 1983;39(5):603–8.
7. Flood JT, Muasher SJ, Simonetti S, Kreiner D, Acosta AA, Rosenwaks Z. Comparison between laparoscopically and ultrasonographically guided transvaginal follicular aspiration methods in an in vitro fertilization program in the same patient using the same stimulation protocol. J In Vitro Fert Embryo Transf. 1989;6(3):180–5.
8. Tanbo T, Henriksen T, Mangus Ø, Abyholm T. Oocyte retrieval in an IVF program: a comparison of laparoscopic and transvaginal ultrasound-guided follicular puncture. Acta Obstet Gynecol Scand. 1988;67(3):243–6.
9. Dellenbach P, Nisband I, Moreau L, Feger B, Plumere C, Gerlinger P, Brun B, Rumpler Y. Transvaginal sonographically controlled ovarian follicle puncture for egg retrieval. Lancet. 1984;1(8392):1467.
10. Leung ASO, Dahan MH, Tan SL. Techniques and technology for human oocyte collection. Expert Rev Med Devices. 2016;13(8):701–3.
11. Santos MJ, Apter S, Coticchio G, Debrocks S, Lundin K, Plancha CE, Prados F, Rienzi L, Verheyen G, Woodwards B, Vermeulen N. Committee of the Special Interest Group on Embryology. Revised guidelines for good practice in IVF laboratories. Hum Reprod. 2016;31(4):685.
12. Rienzi L, Bariani F, Dalla Zarza M, Albani E, Benini F, Chamayou S, Minasi MG, Parmegiani L, Restelli L, Vizziello G, Costa AN. Comprehensive protocol of traceability during IVF: the result of a multicentre failure mode and effect analysis. Hum Reprod. 2017a;32(8):1612–20.
13. McGinnis LK, Pelech S, Kinsey WH. Post-ovulatory aging of oocytes disrupts kinase signaling pathways and lysosome biogenesis. Mol Reprod Dev. 2014;81:928–45.
14. Rienzi L, Vajta G, Ubaldi F. Predictive value of oocyte morphology in human IVF: a systematic review of the literature. Hum Reprod Update. 2011;17(1):34–45.
15. Gilchrist RB, Lane M, Thompson JG. Oocyte-secreted factors: regulators of cumulus cell function and oocyte quality. Hum Reprod Update. 2008;14(2):159–77.
16. Swain JE, Pool TB. ART failure: oocyte contributions to unsuccessful fertilization. Hum Reprod Update. 2008;14(5):431–46.
17. Otsuki J, Okada A, Marimoto K, Kubo H. The relationship between pregnancy outcome and smooth endoplasmic reticulum clusters in MII human oocytes. Hum Reprod. 2004;19(7):1591–7.
18. Ebner T. Prognosis of oocytes showing aggregation of smooth endoplasmic reticulum. RBMOnline. 2008;16(1):113–7.
19. Coticchio G, Canto MD, Fadini R, Renzini MM, Guglielmo MC, Miglietta S, Palmerini MG, Macchiarelli G, Nottola SA. Ultrastructure of human oocytes after in vitro maturation. Mol Hum Reprod. 2016;22(2):110–8.
20. Li R, Albertini DF. The road to maturation: somatic cell interaction and self-organization of mammalian oocyte. Nat Rev Mol Cell Biol. 2013;14(3):141–52.
21. Gosden R, Lee D. Portrait of an oocyte: our obscure origin. J Clin Invest. 2010;120(4):973–83.
22. Albertini DF, Combelles CM, Benecchi E, Carabatsos MJ. Cellular basis for paracrine regulation of ovarian follicle development. Reproduction. 2001;121:647–53.
23. Trouson. Biology and Pathology of the Oocyte, second edition. Cambridge Ed: A. Trounson, R. Gosden & UEichenlaub-Ritter. 2013.
24. Albertini DF. The mammalian oocyte. Chapter 2 in Knobil and Neill's physiology of reproduction. In: Part 1 gametes, fertilization and embryologenesis. 4th ed. vol. I. Elsevier; 2015. pp. 59–97.
25. Bárcena P, Rodríguez M, Obradors A, Vernaeve V, Vassena R. Should we worry about the clock? Relationship between time to ICSI and reproductive outcomes in cycles with fresh and vitrified oocytes. Hum Reprod. 2016;31(6):1182–91.
26. Lundin K, Sjogren A, Hamberger L. Reinsemination of one-day-old oocytes by use of intracytoplasmic sperm injection. Fertil Steril. 1996;66:1130–5.
27. Patrat C, Kaffel A, Delaroche L, Guibert J, Jouannet P, Epelboin S, de Ziegler D, Wolf J-P, Fauque P. Optimal timing for oocyte denudation and intracytoplasmic sperm injection. Obstet Gynecol Int. 2011;2012:1–7.
28. Cohen Y, Malcov M, Schwartz T, Mey-Raz N, Carmon A, Cohen T, Lessing JBL, Amit A, Azem F. Spindle imaging: a new marker for optimal timing of ICSI? Hum Reprod. 2004;19(3):649–54.
29. Bromfield JJ, Coticchio G, Hutt K, Sciajno R, Borini A, Albertini DF. Meiotic spindle dynamics in human oocytes following slow-cooling cryopreservation. Hum Reprod. 2009;24(9):2114–23.
30. Dozortsev D, Nagy P, Abdelmassih S, Oliveira F, Brasil A, Abdelmassih V, Diamond M, Abdelmassih R. The optimal time for intracytoplasmic sperm injection in the human is from 37 to 41 hours after administration of human chorionic gonadotropin. Fertil Steril. 2004;82(6):1492–6.
31. Boyer P, Rodrigues P, Tourame P, Silva M, Barata M, Perez-Alzaa J, Gervoise-Boyer M. Third millennium assisted reproductive technologies: the impact of oocyte vitrification. In: Friedler S, editor. In vitro fertilization—innovative clinical and laboratory aspects. Ed Open Access editions: InTech; 2012. p 123–136. https://doi.org/10.5772/38596.
32. Rienzi L, Gracia C, Maggiulli R, LaBarbera AR, Kaser DJ, Ubaldi FM, Vanderpoel S, Racowsky C. Oocyte, embryo and blastocyst cryopreservation in ART: systematic review and meta-analysis comparing slow-freezing versus vitrification to produce evidence for the development of global guidance. Hum Reprod Update. 2017b;23(2):139–55.
33. Cobo A, Garrido N, Crespo J, José R, Pellicer A. Accumulation of oocytes: a new strategy for managing low-responder patients. Reprod Biomed Online. 2012;24:424–32.

34. Coticchio G, Sciajno R, Hutt K, Bromfield J, Borini A, Albertini DF. Comparative analysis of the metaphase II spindle of human oocytes through polarized light and high-performance confocal microscopy. Fertil Steril. 2010;93(6):20156–2064.

35. Alpha Scientists in Reproductive Medicine and ESHRE Special Interest Group of Embryology. The Istanbul consensus workshop on embryo assessment: proceeding of an expert meeting. Hum Reprod. 2011;26(6):1270–80. https://doi.org/10.1093/humreprod/der037.

36. Ebner T, Moser M, Tews G. Is oocyte morphology prognostic of embryo development potential after ICSI? Reprod Biomed Online. 2006;12(4):442–6.

37. Sunkara SK, Khalafi Y, Maheshwari A, Seed P, Coomarasamy A. Association between response to ovarian stimulation and miscarriage following IVF: an analysis of 124 351 IVF pregnancies. Hum Reprod. 2014;29(6):1218–24.

38. Assou S, Al-Edani T, Haouzi D, Philippe N, Lecellier CH, Piquemal D, Commes T, Ait-Ahmed O, Dechaud H, Hamamah S. MicroRNAs: new candidates for the regulation of human cumulus-oocyte complex. Hum Reprod. 2013;28(11):3038–49.

39. Gordo AC, Rodrigues P, Kurokawa M, Jellerette T, Exley GE, Warner C, Fissore R. Intracellular calcium oscillations signal apoptosis rather than activation in in vitro aged mouse eggs. BOR. 2002;66(6):1828–37.

Relevance of Oocyte Morphology on ICSI Outcomes

16

Claire O'Neill, Stephanie Cheung, Alessandra Parrella, Derek Keating, Philip Xie, Zev Rosenwaks, and Gianpiero D. Palermo

Contents

The observation of the oocyte has always been at the base of the embryological evaluation since the inception of in vitro insemination procedures [1]. However, the identification of oocyte characteristics and/or ooplasm dysmorphism under an inverted microscope (Fig. 16.1) have mostly been carried out after the exposure of the oocyte-cumulus complex to the inseminating spermatozoa. Therefore, the evaluation of oocyte complexion was carried out mostly on oocytes that had failed to undergo fertilization. This led to the work of some investigators who attempted to describe these anomalies and concluded that dysmorphic oocytes were not capable of undergoing fertilization and if ever they would, they would not be able to develop into viable embryos [2].

The advent of ICSI requiring removal of the cumulus cells (Fig. 16.2) has changed this assessment and has allowed embryologists to characterize oocyte morphology prior to sperm injection and therefore define specific morphological patterns mainly in terms of oocyte shape, nuclear attributes, cytoplasmic traits, and the zona pellucida features [3]. These patterns appear as a consequence of a specific superovulation protocol or to the response of a particular patient to a standard drug regimen [4].

Interestingly, even the use of LH-containing drugs has been linked to a high recurrence of a particular oocyte dysmorphism, therefore leading to the debate on the role of urinary gonadotropins, native or purified, versus the recombinant FSH drugs [5, 6]. These oocyte characterizations evidenced an array of defects affecting its ability to undergo fertilization or to support the development of the resulting conceptus, albeit in an inconsistent manner.

Indeed, several investigations that probed the causative effect of oocyte morphology on embryo development and implantation have led to the debate ignited by studies identifying certain ooplasmic features significantly impairing fertilization and embryo quality [7] with other studies finding no correlation between clinical outcome and this particular attribute [8–10]. Furthermore, specific oocyte defects such as a dark ooplasmic area and a granular cytoplasm were described as being associated with poor embryo developmental quality [11, 12] (Fig. 16.3). A meta-analysis on the effect of oocyte morphological characteristics in relation to clinical outcome concluded that based on the data from eligible studies, metaphase-II oocytes with a large polar body, large perivitelline space, refractile bodies, or vacuoles were associated with an impaired fertilization rate; however, these phenomenon did not, for any of these defects, significantly affect embryo quality [13]. This lack of causation of oocyte dysmorphism on embryo quality was also corroborated by a systematic review published during the same year that in addition failed to evidence a correlation of oocyte features with its ability to undergo fertilization [3].

C. O'Neill · S. Cheung · A. Parrella · D. Keating · P. Xie
Z. Rosenwaks · G. D. Palermo (✉)
The Ronald O. Perelman and Claudia Cohen Center for Reproductive Medicine, Weill Cornell Medicine, New York, NY, USA
e-mail: zrosenw@med.cornell.edu; gdpalerm@med.cornell.edu

Fig. 16.1 Identification of oocyte characteristics and/or ooplasm dysmorphism under an inverted microscope

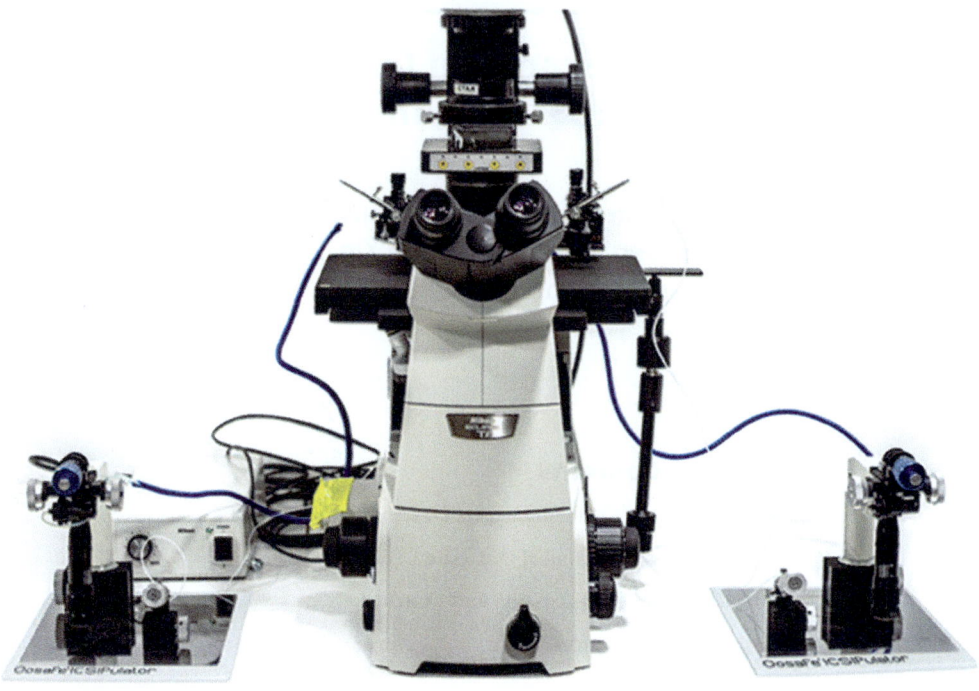

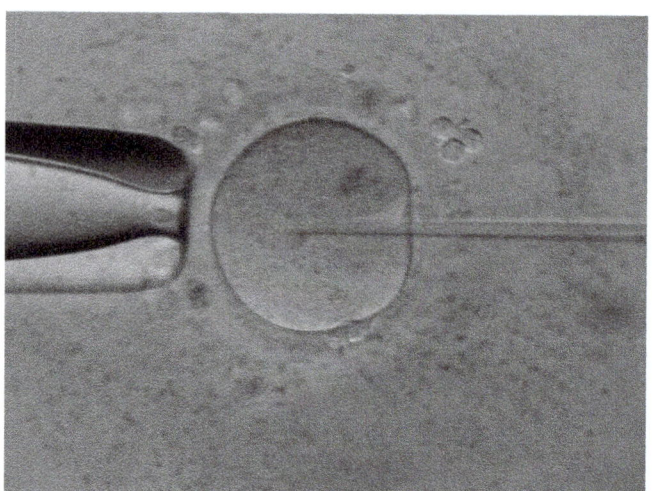

Fig. 16.2 The advent of ICSI requiring removal of the cumulus cells has changed this assessment and has allowed embryologists to characterize oocyte morphology

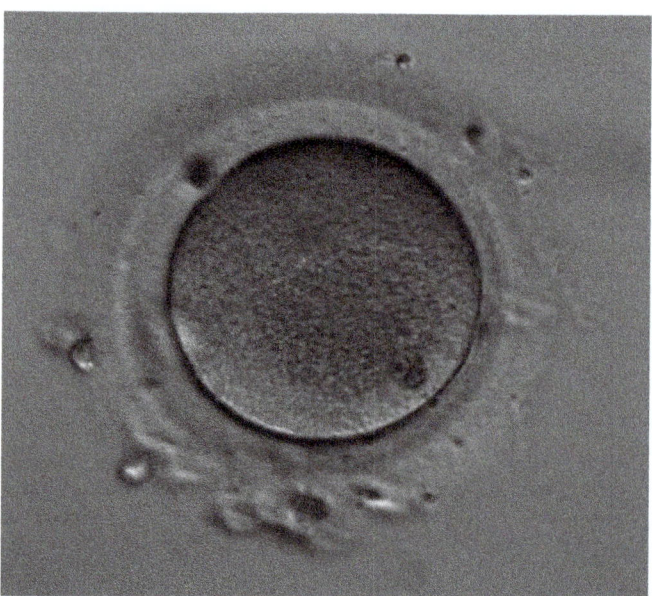

Fig. 16.3 Granular cytoplasm

Here we plan to revisit the occurrence and variety of specific ootid anomalies detected at the time of ICSI, in our own setting and population, to evaluate the eventual ability of these eggs to be fertilized, and to measure the competence of the resulting conceptus to implant. To control for a subtle effect inferred by ooplasmic dysmaturity, the data were analyzed in couples where at least 70% of the oocytes retrieved were at metaphase-II. Finally, in order to control for oocyte aneuploidy, the analysis was then carried out on couples with a female partner ≤35 years old.

16.1 Morphological Description

The terminology to describe oocyte morphology has generally found a consensus among the different laboratories with only small differences in nomenclature. For the purpose of analyzing the significance of each feature in relation to the oocyte function, we have categorized them into four groups: nuclear, cytoplasmic, zona pellucida, and shape/size. When assessing metaphase-II oocytes at the time of ICSI (carried out at a magnification of 400×), annotations were typically made for each individual oocyte detailing any dysmorphism observed by the ICSI operator. A normally developed metaphase-II oocyte should have a spherical zona pellucida enclosing a clear ooplasm and a distinct first polar body [14]. In a cohort of 129,412 oocytes assessed at our center over a 10-year period, of all the morphological features, the top three most represented aberrations were a granular cytoplasm (6.07%), dark central granularity (5.76%), and a large perivitelline space (4.72%).

Among the functional categories, the nuclear defects were the least prevalent occurring at 0.3% of all oocytes assessed. **Nuclear defects** entail any irregularity of the first polar body such as a fragmented polar body, an abnormally large polar body, or an extrusion of more than one polar body (Table 16.1, numbers 1–3).

The **cytoplasmic dysmorphic** patterns (Figs. 16.4, 16.5, 16.6, 16.7, 16.8, 16.9, and 16.10) are instead among the most prevalent, with 19.7% of oocytes presenting with a distinctive ooplasmic characteristic. The cytoplasm can present inclusions, refractile bodies, smooth endoplasmic reticulum, a central granulation referred to as dark center, vacuoles, granular cytoplasm, and mottled cytoplasm, i.e., a heterogenous, marked patterns of granularity that are not uniform (Table 16.1, numbers 4–10).

The next most recurrent category at 8.1% concerns **irregularities related to the zona pellucida** such as a large perivitelline space, perivitelline debris, a dark zona pellucida, a thin zona pellucida, an abnormally shaped zona pellucida, and a bi-layered zona pellucida (Table 16.1, numbers 11–16).

The last category, **shape/size** at the frequency of 1.4%, entails irregularities of contour of the oocyte defined as irregular, oval, or in size, characterized by a large cytoplasmic volume. Although the shape of the oocyte has not been found to be linked to fertilization or day 3 embryo quality [3, 15], giant oocytes (Fig. 16.11), verisimilarly generated by the fusion of two prophase-I oocytes and often characterized by the presence of two polar bodies, have been

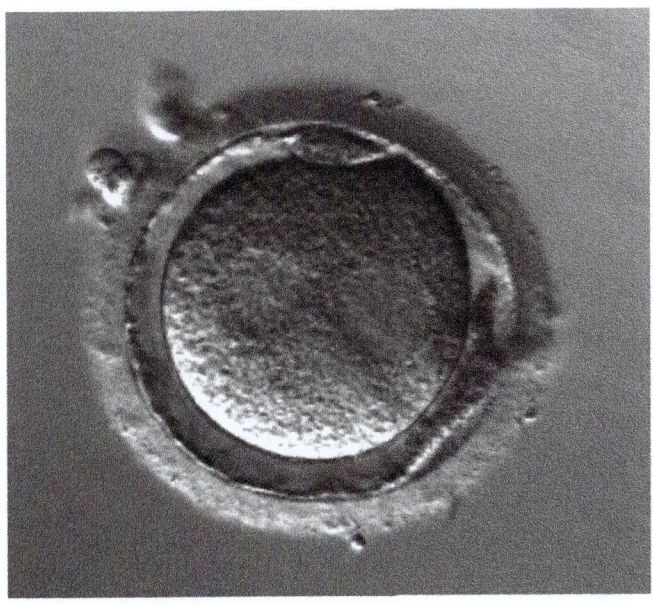

Fig. 16.4 Granular cytoplasm and vacuoles

Table 16.1 Cytoplasmic dysmorphic patterns

Nuclear	1. Fragmented PB		285 (0.22%)
	2. Large polar body		19 (0.01%)
	3. Two polar bodies		61 (0.04%)

(continued)

Table 16.1 (continued)

Cytoplasmatic	4.	Inclusions		3602 (2.8%)
	5.	Refractile bodies		1545 (1.2%)
	6.	Smooth endoplasmic reticulum		1454 (1.1%)
	7.	Central granulation/dark center		7452 (5.8%)
	8.	Vacuoles		3483 (2.7%)
	9.	Granular cytoplasm		7852 (6.1%)
	10.	Mottled cytoplasm		56 (0.04%)

Table 16.1 (continued)

Zona Pellucida	11.	Expanse of the perivitelline space		6106 (4.7%)
	12.	Debris within perivitelline space		2288 (1.8%)
	13.	Dark zona pellucida		1149 (0.9%)
	14.	Thin zona pellucida		184 (0.1%)
	15.	Abnormal zona pellucida		653 (0.5%)
	16.	Bi-layered zona		40 (0.03%)
Shape/Size	17.	Oocyte irregular in shape		783 (0.6%)
	18.	Oval oocyte		859 (0.7%)
	19.	Giant oocyte		234 (0.2%)

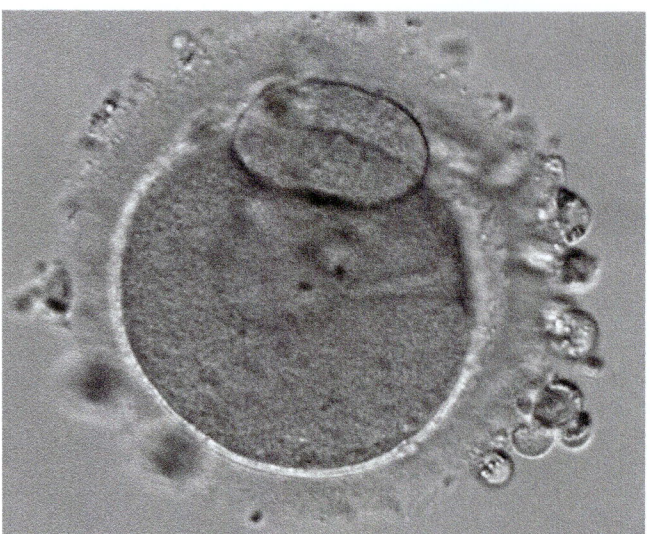

Fig. 16.5 Large polar body

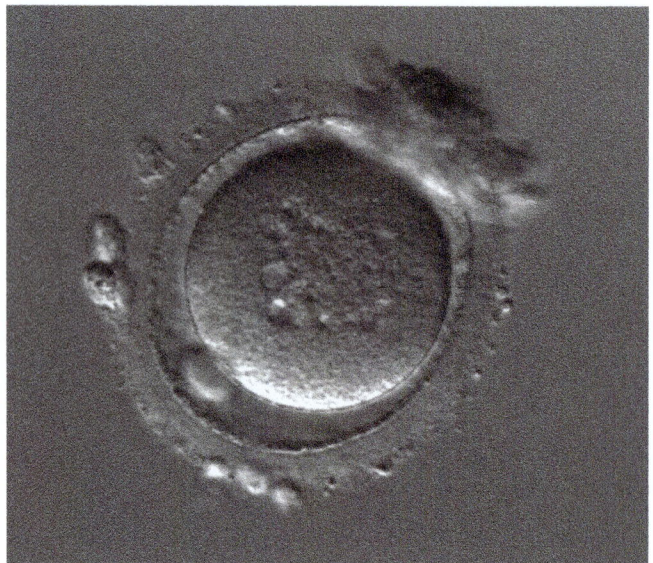

Fig. 16.6 Cytoplasmatic vacuoles

found to have a higher incidence of aneuploidy and/or multiple-ploidy [16, 17].

16.2   Clinical Outcome

From October 2008 to May 2018, a total of 10,329 patients were treated in 12,580 ICSI cycles with at least five oocytes injected were included in the analysis with an average male partner age of 39.7 ± 7 years and a female partner 37.3 ± 5 years. Of these cycles, 58.6% had at least one oocyte with a morphological defect. Cycles that had inadequate ejaculated sperm parameters for ICSI (<1 million/mL) or that used surgically retrieved spermatozoa were excluded.

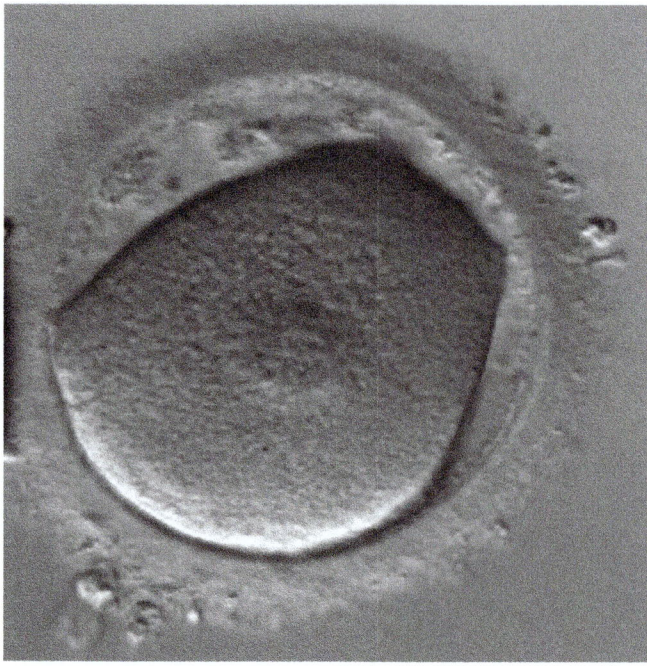

Fig. 16.7 Large perivitelline space with oocyte dysmorphism

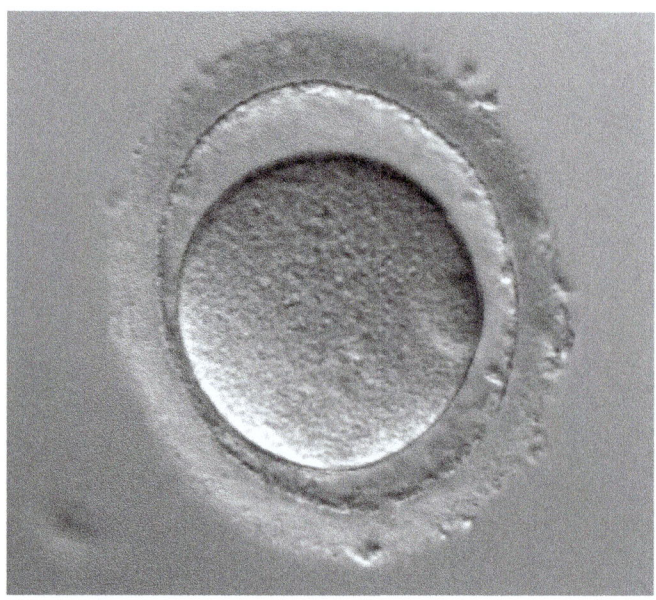

Fig. 16.8 Large perivitelline space

Superovulation was carried out by considering multiple factors such as patient weight, age, serum anti-mullerian hormone (AMH) level, antral follicular count, and any history of previous response to stimulation protocols. Patients were super-ovulated with gonadotropins daily (Gonal F, EMD Serono, Geneva, Switzerland; Menopur, Ferring Pharmaceuticals Inc., Parsippany, NJ, USA; and/or Follistim, Merck, Kenilworth, NJ, USA). Suppression of pituitary gland function was achieved by administering either a GnRH-antagonist (Ganirelix acetate, Merck, Kenilworth,

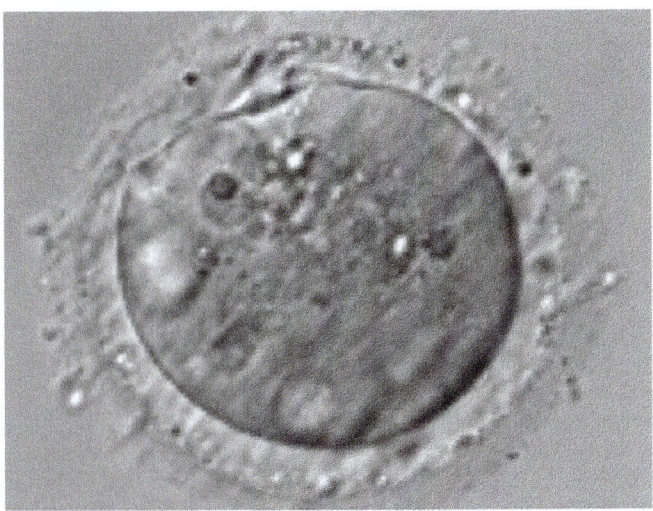

Fig. 16.9 Refractile bodies

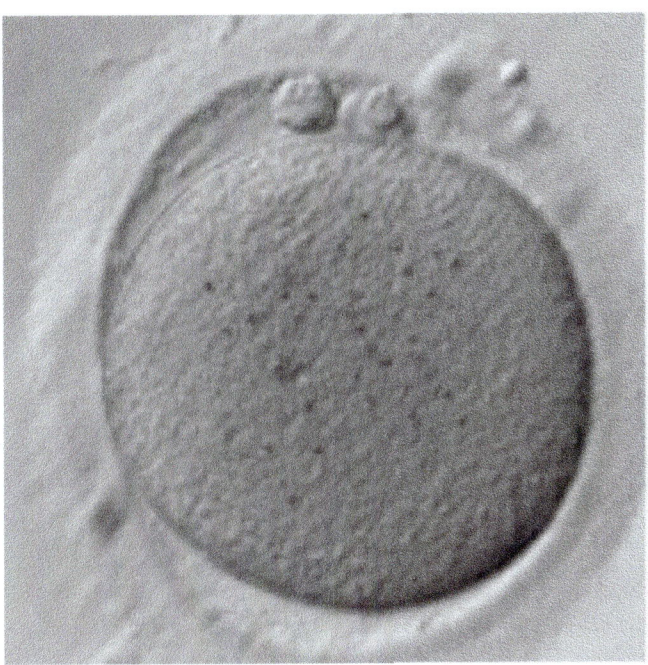

Fig. 16.11 Giant oocyte

We found that the fertilization, clinical pregnancy, and implantation rates progressively decreased as the cycles increased in the percentage of oocytes with a dysmorphism ($P < 0.00001$), particularly in the groups of 75–100% (Table 16.2). The delivery and ongoing rates progressively decreased with the increasing proportion of dysmorphic oocytes ($P < 0.00001$). The inverse occurred with the pregnancy loss ($P < 0.05$) when the oocyte defects appeared at a rate over 25% (Table 16.2).

We then attempted to control for an effect of maturity rate by including only cycles that had at least 70% metaphase-II oocyte maturity. The effect of oocyte morphology on fertilization ($P < 0.00001$), clinical pregnancy rate ($P < 0.00001$), and implantation ($P < 0.00001$) remained significant (Table 16.3). The delivery and ongoing decreased over 25% of morphologic anomalies ($P < 0.00001$) but no difference was noted for the pregnancy losses.

We then repeated the analysis with the intent to control for an oocyte aneuploidy confounder and therefore we included cycles with a female partner of ≤ 35 years old. This resulted in a significant impairment of fertilization ($P < 0.001$) for the group 75–100%, while the implantation appeared to decrease ($P < 0.05$) over 25% of oocyte characteristics (Table 16.4).

Interestingly, when we performed an analysis that controlled concurrently for an adequate proportion of metaphase-II as well as oocyte aneuploidy, the comparison failed to evidence any effect of any proportion of oocyte dysmorphism on clinical outcome (Table 16.5).

Furthermore, we assessed within the younger women cohort, the clinical outcome taking into consideration the morphological categories focused on oocyte function such as

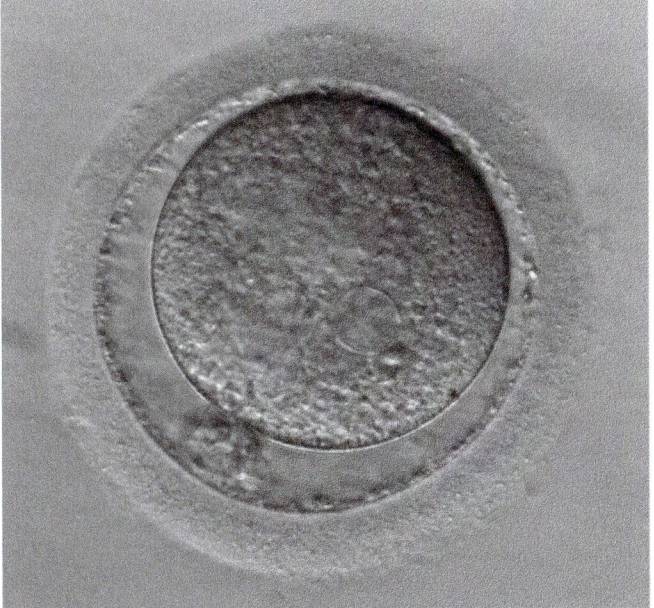

Fig. 16.10 Smooth endoplasmatic reticulum

NJ, USA; or Cetrotide, EMD-Serono Inc., Rockland, MA, USA) or GnRH-agonists (leuprolide acetate, Abbott Laboratories, Chicago, IL, USA). Ovulation was triggered with human chorionic gonadotropin (hCG, Ovidrel, EMD Serono) once the two lead follicles were at least 17 mm in diameter. Oocyte retrieval was performed 35–37 h posttrigger under conscious sedation [18].

We stratified these cases according to the percentage of oocytes displaying morphological anomalies in quartiles ranging from 0–24%, 25–49%, 50–74%, and 75–100% of oocytes having an annotation regarding a particular morphological feature. Clinical outcome including fertilization, clinical pregnancy, implantation, deliveries, and pregnancy loss were recorded and compared.

Table 16.2 Characteristics and clinical outcome of couples according to the proportion of oocytes with dysmorphic features

Dysmorphic oocytes (%)	0–24	25–49	50–74	75–100
No. of patients	5658	1928	1533	1210
No. of cycles	7362	2150	1702	1366
Male age (mean ± SD)	40.0 ± 7	40.1 ± 7	40.1 ± 7	40.6 ± 7
Female age (mean ± SD)	37.6 ± 5	38.0 ± 5	38.1 ± 5	38.4 ± 5
Fertilization (mean % ± SD)	77.5 ± 19[a]	78.0 ± 18[b]	76.7 ± 20[c]	72.7 ± 22[d]
Clinical pregnancy (%)	2325/4766 (48.8)[e]	613/1363 (45.0)[f]	474/1094 (43.3)[g]	338/932 (36.3)[h]
Implantation (%)	3007/14116 (21.3)[i]	797/4291 (18.6)[j]	612/3485 (17.6)[k]	420/3030 (13.9)[l]
Miscarriage (%)	213/2325 (9.2)[m]	77/613 (12.6)[n]	54/474 (11.4)[o]	44/338 (13.0)[p]
Delivery and ongoing (%)	2112/4766 (44.3)[q]	536/1363 (39.3)[r]	420/1094 (38.4)[s]	294/932 (31.5)[t]

a vs. b, c, d: ANOVA (two-tailed), 3 df, effect of oocyte morphology on fertilization rates, $P < 0.00001$

e vs. f, g, h: χ^2, 2 × 4, 3 df, effect of oocyte morphology on clinical pregnancy rates, $P < 0.00001$

i vs. j, k, l: χ^2, 2 × 4, 3 df, effect of oocyte morphology on implantation rates, $P < 0.00001$

m vs. n, o, p: χ^2, 2 × 4, 3 df, effect of oocyte morphology on miscarriage rates, $P < 0.05$

q vs. r, s, t: χ^2, 2 × 4, 3 df, effect of oocyte morphology on delivery and ongoing pregnancy rates, $P < 0.00001$

Table 16.3 Characteristics and clinical outcome of couples according to the proportion of oocytes with dysmorphic features and a maturity rate ≥70% at the time of insemination

Dysmorphic oocytes (%)	0–24	25–49	50–74	75–100
No. of patients	5660	1490	1132	788
No. of cycles	4541	1628	1234	846
Male age (mean ± SD)	40.0 ± 7	40.3 ± 7	40.7 ± 7	40.7 ± 7
Female age (mean ± SD)	37.8 ± 5	38.1 ± 5	38.6 ± 5	38.5 ± 5
Fertilization (mean % ± SD)	78.8 ± 18[a]	78.9 ± 18[b]	78.5 ± 18[c]	75.4 ± 19[d]
Clinical pregnancy (%)	1884/3663 (51.4)[e]	480/1031 (46.6)[f]	368/799 (46.1)[g]	231/568 (40.7)[h]
Implantation (%)	2450/10945 (22.4)[i]	621/3305 (18.8)[j]	476/2539 (18.7)[k]	292/1938 (15.1)[l]
Miscarnage (%)	170/1884 (9.0)	59/480 (12.3)	44/368 (12.0)	27/231 (11.7)
Delivery and ongoing (%)	1714/3663 (46.8)[q]	421/1031 (40.8)[r]	324/799 (40.6)[s]	204/568 (35.9)[t]

a vs. b, c, d: ANOVA (two-tailed), 3 df, effect of oocyte morphology on fertilization rates, $P < 0.00001$

e vs. f, g, h: χ^2, 2 × 4, 3 df, effect of oocyte morphology on clinical pregnancy rates, $P < 0.00001$

i vs. j, k, l: χ^2, 2 × 4, 3 df, effect of oocyte morphology on implantation rates, $P < 0.00001$

q vs. r, s, t: χ^2, 2 × 4, 3 df, effect of oocyte morphology on delivery and ongoing pregnancy rates, $P < 0.00001$

Table 16.4 Characteristics and clinical outcome of couples according to the proportion of oocytes with dysmorphic features and a female partner ≤35 years of age

Dysmorphic oocytes (%)	0–24	25–49	50–74	75–100
No. of patients	1970	615	440	309
No. of cycles	2403	647	480	336
Male age (mean ± SD)	35.3 ± 6	35.5 ± 6	34.8 ± 4	35.0 ± 5
Female age (mean ± SD)	32.1 ± 3	32.3 ± 3	32.1 ± 3	32.2 ± 3
Fertilization (mean % ± SD)	77.5 ± 19[a]	78.0 ± 18[b]	76.7 ± 20[c]	72.7 ± 22[d]
Clinical pregnancy (%)	904/1610 (56.1)	236/426 (55.4)	164/314 (52.2)	117/231 (50.6)
Implantation (%)	1148/3446 (33.3)[e]	304/956 (31.8)[f]	204/707 (28.9)[g]	152/529 (28.7)[h]
Miscarriage (%)	65/904 (7.2)	20/236 (8.5)	9/164 (5.5)	7/117 (6.0)
Delivery and ongoing (%)	839/1610 (52.1)	216/426 (50.7)	155/314 (49.4)	110/231 (47.6)

a vs. b, c, d: ANOVA (two-tailed). 3 df, effect of oocyte morphology on fertilization rates, $P < 0.001$

e vs. f, g, h: χ^2, 2 × 4, 3 df, effect of oocyte morphology on implantation rates, $P < 0.05$

Table 16.5 Characteristics and clinical outcome of couples according to the proportion of oocytes with dysmorphic features with a maturation rate ≥70% at the time of insemination and a female partner ≤35 years of age

Dysmorphic oocytes (%)	0–24	25–49	50–74	75–100
No. of patients	1803	454	333	203
No. of cycles	1838	474	355	211
Male age (mean ± SD)	35.34 ± 6	35.5 ± 6	35.1 ± 4	34.9 ± 5
Female age (mean ± SD)	32.1 ± 3	32.3 ± 3	32.3 ± 3	32.2 ± 3
Fertilization (mean % ± SD)	80.5 ± 17	80.7 ± 17	80.6 ± 17	78.3 ± 16
Clinical pregnancy (%)	722/1242 (58.1)	176/317 (55.5)	130/241 (53.9)	79/141 (56.0)
Implantation (%)	921/2630 (35.0)	225/694 (32.4)	161/526 (30.6)	104/327 (31.8)
Miscarriage (%)	56/722 (7.8)	12/176 (6.8)	6/130 (4.6)	3/79 (3.8)
Delivery and ongoing (%)	656/1242 (53.6)	164/317 (51.7)	124/241 (51.5)	76/141 (53.9)

nuclear, cytoplasmic, zona pellucida, or shape/size. These morphological functional features were compared to a control cohort of cycles with a matched female age with no dysmorphic annotations on any of the injected oocytes.

This analysis evidenced a clear effect of the nuclear categories of defects that appeared to significantly affect fertilization that decreased from 78.6 to 74.0% ($P < 0.05$, Fig. 16.12). This effect of the nuclear category remained true for the clinical pregnancy rate that decreased from 56.5 to 42.7% ($P < 0.05$, Fig. 16.13). While a similar trend was

Fig. 16.12 Fertilization rate by oocyte dysmorphism category, females ≤35

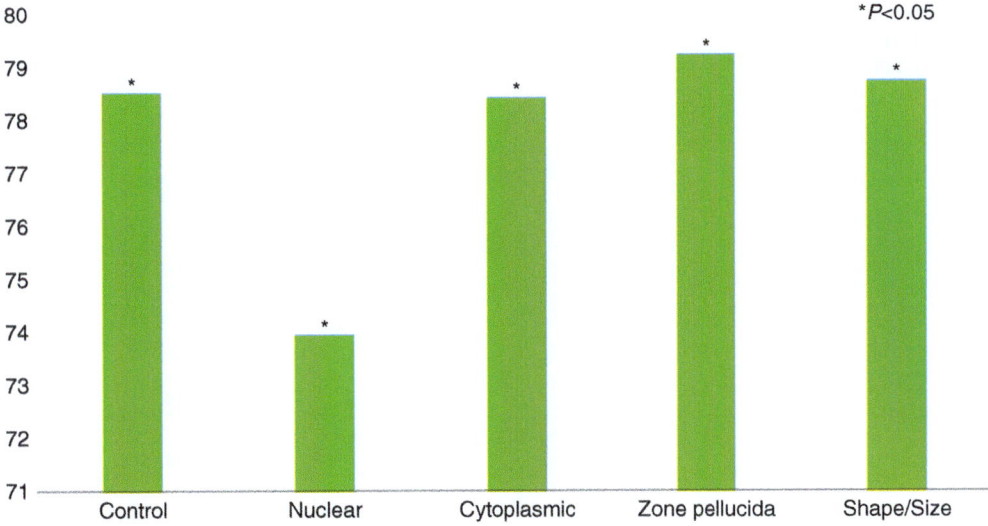

Fig. 16.13 Clinical pregnancy rate by oocyte dysmorphism category, females ≤35

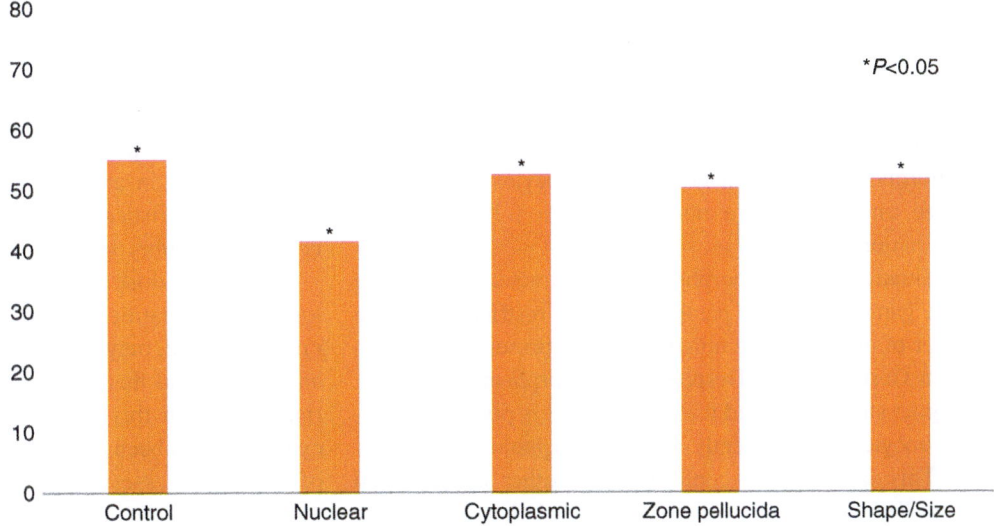

noted for this category of abnormalities in relation to the pregnancy loss, it did not reach statistical significance (Fig. 16.14).

16.3 Discussion and Conclusions

The assessment of oocyte morphology is embedded into the embryological evaluation since its inception and indeed, oocyte with morphological defects appeared to fertilize poorly with standard in vitro insemination. The advent of ICSI, which requires the removal of the cumulus cells, has allowed visualization of oocyte characteristics prior to insemination and is also helpful in overcoming fertilization failure of these featured oocytes, therefore providing higher chances for a subsequent embryo selection and successful outcome. It has long been debated the role of these morphological features on the oocyte's ability to be fertilized and generate competent embryos. Moreover, particular cytoplasmic features may interfere with the proper placement of the spermatozoon during ICSI insemination.

It has been indicated that the stimulation protocol and particularly the gonadotropin preparation may affect the appearance of ooplasmic abnormalities. Indeed, one study showed that highly purified FSH seems to grant more mature oocytes, a lower incidence of dark center and cytoplasmic granularity [16]. The findings were confirmed in a more recent Turkish study that also linked cytoplasmic dysmorphism to an impaired embryo development with a higher rate of zona pellucida abnormalities [19]. An earlier study from Austria concluded that outer layer abnormalities lead to a higher oocyte degeneration rate following ICSI [20]. In our experience, only oolemma characteristics are linked to a higher occurrence of degeneration rate [21, 22].

Fig. 16.14 Pregnancy loss by oocyte dysmorphism category, females ≤35

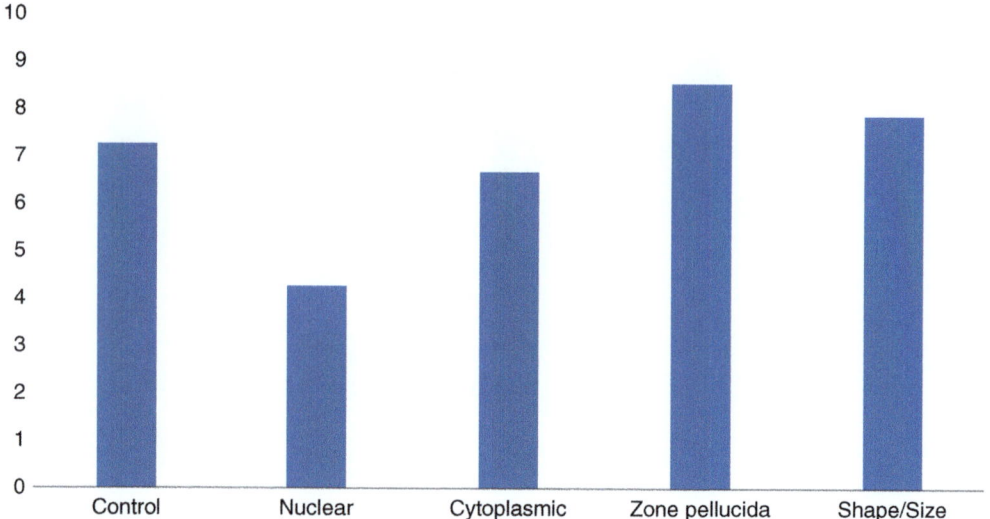

An interesting study from the UK indicated that the morphological characteristics of oocytes are multifactorial, and they depend on the ovarian superovulation protocol or the hormonal environment generated by the effects of these drugs. However, this study evidenced that, independently of the morphological characteristics, the oocytes appeared to fertilize and generate a normal embryo following ICSI insemination [10].

Evaluation of the morphological characteristics of the female gamete becomes paramount when restrictions on the number of oocytes to be utilized are also present, such as in Italy or Germany [23]. Despite the dysmorphisms observed, a Belgian study indicated that with ICSI it is possible to fertilize oocytes independently of their morphological quality [24]. This data was also confirmed by another study carried out in Turkey that specifically evidenced that a centrally located granular cytoplasm did not affect the fertilization rates nor the embryo quality [25].

A study that utilizes similar characterizations of the oocyte dysmorphic features such as the ones described in our study was a meta-analysis carried out in Italy and formulated a detailed scrutiny of the literature on the different dysmorphic aspects such as nuclear, cytoplasmic, zona pellucida, and shape/size defects. This study condensed the findings of 50 papers published in a 15-year span about the predictive value of the non-invasive parameters of metaphase-II oocytes. Their findings were inconclusive, and the authors suggested more coordinated research to generate a consensus [3].

A paper from Naples by the Brian Dale group, in addition to the oocyte morphological characteristics such as oocyte granularity, added the oolemma behavior during the actual ICSI procedure. The authors found that the oocytes with "top quality" yielded a higher fertilization rate versus those with "lowest quality." Although there was no difference on embryo quality once fertilized, "top quality" oocytes led to a superior clinical pregnancy rate [26].

Among all the attributes assessed in our study, nuclear abnormalities appear the most relevant in impairing fertilization and clinical pregnancy rates. However, this finding was not confirmed in an Italian study that examined the polar body characteristics but without identifying any effect on consequent embryo development [27].

Early work done at Cornell found that combined morphological abnormalities, although may not affect fertilization or pregnancy rate, may indeed carry an association with oocyte aneuploidy and therefore an increase in chances of miscarriage [28]. On this subject, a centrally located granulated cytoplasm has been shown to lead to aneuploidy in over half of the oocytes assessed [25].

In conclusion, while a variety of features have been described and may influence the ultimate embryo selection method, particularly with the advent of time-lapse observation (Fig. 16.15), it is still not clear the impact that these morphological traits have on clinical outcome. In fact, these characteristics present unpredictably within the same patient in repeated ART superovulation cycles. Nonetheless, they may recur in the same patient in a later cycle.

Therefore, it is not clear if it is due to a particular hormonal milieu generated by a specific superovulation protocol or by the response of a particular patient to ovarian superovulation. Fortunately, the presence of these oocyte dysmorphic traits is limited most of the time to a few oocytes within the retrieved cohort to be inseminated and therefore, the effect on clinical outcome can be mitigated by an adequate number of metaphase-II oocytes and auspiciously a younger female partner.

This, however, does not preclude a causative effect of the specific morphological aberration on impairing the

Fig. 16.15 Device for time-lapse observation

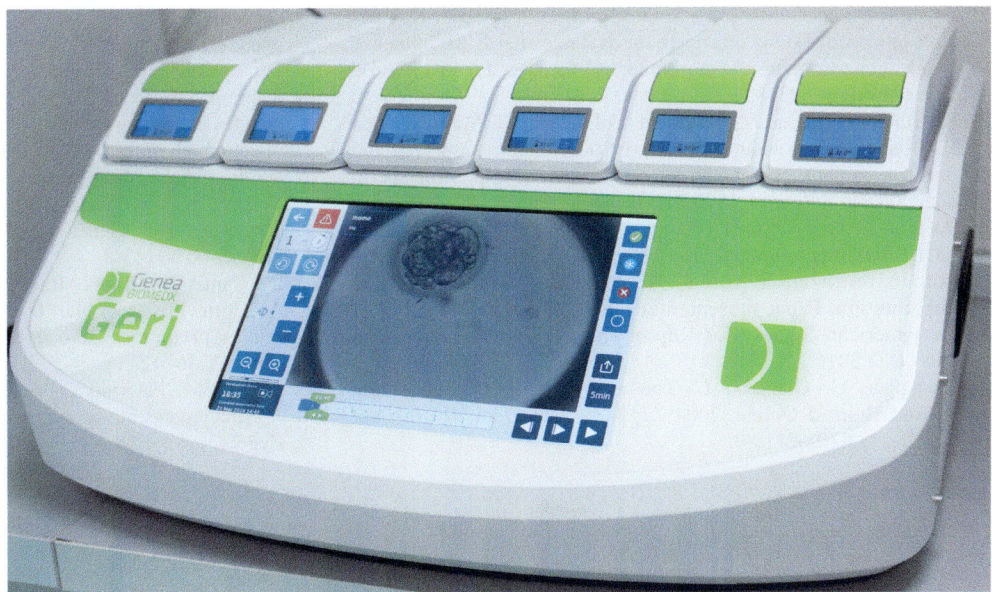

ability of that particular oocyte to be fertilized and generate an embryo.

The whole argument about the evaluation of the female gamete has reached new heights since the implementation of ICSI, which has allowed a clear assessment of oocyte characteristics prior to insemination and at the same time helps to overcome fertilization failure of these featured oocytes, therefore providing higher chances for a subsequent embryo selection and successful outcome.

References

1. Veeck LL. Oocyte assessment and biological performance. Ann N Y Acad Sci. 1988;541:259–74.
2. Van Blerkom J. Occurrence and developmental consequences of aberrant cellular organization in meiotically mature human oocytes after exogenous ovarian hyperstimulation. J Electron Microsc Tech. 1990;16:324–46. https://doi.org/10.1002/jemt.1060160405.
3. Rienzi L, Vajta G, Ubaldi F. Predictive value of oocyte morphology in human IVF: a systematic review of the literature. Hum Reprod Update. 2011;17:34–45. https://doi.org/10.1093/humupd/dmq029.
4. Swain JE, Pool TB. ART failure: oocyte contributions to unsuccessful fertilization. Hum Reprod Update. 2008;14:431–46. https://doi.org/10.1093/humupd/dmn025.
5. Cheon KW, Byun HK, Yang KM, Song IO, Choi KH, Yoo KJ. Efficacy of recombinant human follicle-stimulating hormone in improving oocyte quality in assisted reproductive techniques. J Reprod Med. 2004;49:733–8.
6. Imthurn B, Macas E, Rosselli M, Keller PJ. Nuclear maturity and oocyte morphology after stimulation with highly purified follicle stimulating hormone compared to human menopausal gonadotrophin. Hum Reprod. 1996;11:2387–91.
7. Xia P. Intracytoplasmic sperm injection: correlation of oocyte grade based on polar body, perivitelline space and cytoplasmic inclusions with fertilization rate and embryo quality. Hum Reprod. 1997;12:1750–5.
8. Balaban B, Urman B, Sertac A, Alatas C, Aksoy S, Mercan R. Oocyte morphology does not affect fertilization rate, embryo quality and implantation rate after intracytoplasmic sperm injection. Hum Reprod. 1998;13:3431–3. https://doi.org/10.1093/humrep/13.12.3431.
9. Esfandiari N, Burjaq H, Gotlieb L, Casper RF. Brown oocytes: implications for assisted reproductive technology. Fertil Steril. 2006;86:1522–5. https://doi.org/10.1016/j.fertnstert.2006.03.056.
10. Serhal PF, Ranieri DM, Kinis A, Marchant S, Davies M, Khadum IM. Oocyte morphology predicts outcome of intracytoplasmic sperm injection. Hum Reprod. 1997;12:1267–70.
11. Merviel P, et al. Impact of oocytes with CLCG on ICSI outcomes and their potential relation to pesticide exposure. J Ovarian Res. 2017;10:42. https://doi.org/10.1186/s13048-017-0335-2.
12. Ten J, Mendiola J, Vioque J, de Juan J, Bernabeu R. Donor oocyte dysmorphisms and their influence on fertilization and embryo quality. Reprod Biomed Online. 2007;14:40–8.
13. Setti AS, Figueira RC, Braga DP, Colturato SS, Iaconelli A Jr, Borges E Jr. Relationship between oocyte abnormal morphology and intracytoplasmic sperm injection outcomes: a meta-analysis. Eur J Obstet Gynecol Reprod Biol. 2011;159:364–70. https://doi.org/10.1016/j.ejogrb.2011.07.031.
14. Alpha Scientists in Reproductive Medicine and ESHRE Special Interest Group of Embryology. The Istanbul consensus workshop on embryo assessment: proceedings of an expert meeting. Hum Reprod. 2011;26:1270–83. https://doi.org/10.1093/humrep/der037.
15. Halim B, Lubis HP, Novia D, Thaharuddin M. Does oval oocyte have an impact on embryo development in in vitro fertilization? JBRA Assist Reprod. 2017;21:15–8. https://doi.org/10.5935/1518-0557.20170005.
16. Balakier H, Bouman D, Sojecki A, Librach C, Squire JA. Morphological and cytogenetic analysis of human giant oocytes and giant embryos. Hum Reprod. 2002;17:2394–401.
17. Rosenbusch B, Schneider M, Glaser B, Brucker C. Cytogenetic analysis of giant oocytes and zygotes to assess their relevance for the development of digynic triploidy. Hum Reprod. 2002;17:2388–93.
18. Irani M, et al. Blastocyst development rate influences implantation and live birth rates of similarly graded euploid blastocysts. Fertil Steril. 2018;110:95–102.e101. https://doi.org/10.1016/j.fertnstert.2018.03.032.
19. Balaban B, Urman B. Effect of oocyte morphology on embryo development and implantation. Reprod Biomed Online. 2006;12:608–15.

20. Ebner T, Yaman C, Moser M, Sommergruber M, Jesacher K, Tews G. A prospective study on oocyte survival rate after ICSI: influence of injection technique and morphological features. J Assist Reprod Genet. 2001;18:623–8.

21. Palermo GD, Alikani M, Bertoli M, Colombero LT, Moy F, Cohen J, Rosenwaks Z. Oolemma characteristics in relation to survival and fertilization patterns of oocytes treated by intracytoplasmic sperm injection. Hum Reprod. 1996;11:172–6.

22. Pereira N, Cozzubbo T, Cheung S, Rosenwaks Z, Palermo GD. Revisiting oolemma characteristics during ICSI in relation to fertilization patterns and embryo development and implantation. Paper presented at the 72nd Annual Meeting of the American Society for Reproductive Medicine, Salt Lake City, UT; 2016.

23. Benagiano G, Gianaroli L. The new Italian IVF legislation. Reprod Biomed Online. 2004;9:117–25. https://doi.org/10.1016/S1472-6483(10)62118-9.

24. De Sutter P, Dozortsev D, Qian C, Dhont M. Oocyte morphology does not correlate with fertilization rate and embryo quality after intracytoplasmic sperm injection. Hum Reprod. 1996;11:595–7.

25. Kahraman S, et al. Relationship between granular cytoplasm of oocytes and pregnancy outcome following intracytoplasmic sperm injection. Hum Reprod. 2000;15:2390–3.

26. Wilding M, Di Matteo L, D'Andretti S, Montanaro N, Capobianco C, Dale B. An oocyte score for use in assisted reproduction. J Assist Reprod Genet. 2007;24:350–8. https://doi.org/10.1007/s10815-007-9143-8.

27. De Santis L, Cino I, Rabellotti E, Calzi F, Persico P, Borini A, Coticchio G. Polar body morphology and spindle imaging as predictors of oocyte quality. Reprod Biomed Online. 2005;11:36–42.

28. Alikani M, Palermo G, Adler A, Bertoli M, Blake M, Cohen J. Intracytoplasmic sperm injection in dysmorphic human oocytes. Zygote. 1995;3:283–8.

Endometriosis, Infertility, and Oocyte Quality

Andrea Tinelli, Ceana H. Nezhat, Farr R. Nezhat,
Ospan A. Mynbaev, Radmila Sparic, Ioannis P. Kosmas,
Renata Beck, and Antonio Malvasi

Contents

17.1   **Introduction**.. 266
17.1.1 Infertility and Endometriosis.. 266
17.1.2 Endometriosis-Related Infertility.. 270
17.1.3 Peritoneal Fluid of Patient with Endometriosis...................................... 273
17.1.4 The Oocyte Quality... 274
17.1.5 Impact of Endometriosis on Oocyte Quality.. 276

17.2   **Transvaginal Ultrasound-Guided Oocyte Retrieval in Patients with Endometriosis**............ 285

References.. 286

A. Tinelli (✉)
Division of Experimental Endoscopic Surgery, Imaging,
Technology and Minimally Invasive Therapy, Department
of Obstetrics and Gynecology, Vito Fazzi Hospital, Lecce Italy

Laboratory of Human Physiology, Phystech BioMed School,
Faculty of Biological and Medical Physics, Moscow Institute
of Physics and Technology (State University), Dolgoprudny,
Russia

C. H. Nezhat
Minimally Invasive Surgery Fellowship Program,
Nezhat Medical Center, Atlanta, GA, USA

Training and Education Program, and Minimally Invasive Surgery
and Robotics, Northside Hospital, Atlanta, GA, USA

Department of Gynecology and Obstetrics, School of Medicine,
Emory University, Atlanta, GA, USA

Society of Reproductive Surgeons, Birmingham, AL, USA
e-mail: ceana@nezhat.com

F. R. Nezhat
Department of Obstetrics and Gynecology, Weill Cornell Medical
College of Cornell University, New York, NY, USA

Division of Minimally Invasive Gynecologic Surgery, Department
of Obstetrics and Gynecology, NYU-Winthrop University
Hospital, State University of New York at Stony Brook,
College of Medicine, New York, NY, USA
e-mail: farr@farrnezhatmd.com

O. A. Mynbaev
Laboratory of Human Physiology, Phystech BioMed School,
Faculty of Biological and Medical Physics,

Moscow Institute of Physics and Technology (State University),
Dolgoprudny, Russia

Division of Molecular Technologies, Research Institute
of Translational Medicine, N. I. Pirogov Russian National
Research Medical University, Moscow, Russia

Institute of Numerical Mathematics, RAS, Moscow, Russia

R. Sparic
Clinic of Gynecology and Obstetrics, Clinical Center of Serbia,
Belgrade, Serbia

School of Medicine, University of Belgrade, Belgrade, Serbia
e-mail: radmila@rcub.bg.ac.rs

I. P. Kosmas
Laboratory of Human Physiology, Phystech BioMed School,
Faculty of Biological and Medical Physics, Moscow Institute
of Physics and Technology (State University), Dolgoprudny, Russia

Department of Obstetrics and Gynecology, Ioannina State General
Hospital G. Hatzikosta, Ioannina, Greece

R. Beck
Department of Anesthesia, Santa Maria Hospital, GVM Care and
Research, Bari, Italy

A. Malvasi
Laboratory of Human Physiology, Phystech BioMed School,
Faculty of Biological and Medical Physics, Moscow Institute
of Physics and Technology (State University), Dolgoprudny, Russia

Department of Obstetrics and Gynecology, GVM Care
and Research Santa Maria Hospital, Bari, Italy

© Springer Nature Switzerland AG 2020
A. Malvasi, D. Baldini (eds.), *Pick Up and Oocyte Management*, https://doi.org/10.1007/978-3-030-28741-2_17

265

Abbreviations

ART	Assisted reproductive technique
COH	Controlled ovarian hyperstimulation
COS	Controlled ovarian stimulation
COX-2–PGE2	Cyclooxygenase-2 prostaglandin-2
FF	Follicular fluid
GM-CSF	Granulocyte macrophage-colony stimulator factor
GPx	Glutathione peroxidase
GR	Glutathione reductase
ICSI	Intracytoplasmatic sperm injection
IFN-α	Interferon-α
IL-1	Interleukin-1
IL-12	Interleukin-12
IL-2	Interleukin-2
IL-4	Interleukin-4
IL-6	Interleukin-6
IL-8	Interleukin-8
IVF	In vitro fertilization
LPO	Lipid peroxidation
MCP-1	Monocyte chemotactic protein-1
MCs	Mast cells
MMPs	Matrix metalloproteinases
NK	Natural Killer
NO	Nitric oxide
OFF	Ovarian follicular fluid
OS	Oxidative stress
PCR	Polymerase chain reaction
PDGF	Platelet-derived growth factor
PF	Peritoneal fluid
PG	Prostaglandin
PP	Peripheral plasma
ROL	Retinol
ROS	Reactive oxygen species
SOD	Superoxide dismutase
SOD1	Superoxide dismutase 1
TAC	Total antioxidant capacity
TEM	Transmission electron microscopy
TGF-β	Transforming growth factor-β
TNF-α	Tumor necrosis factor-α
VEGF	Vascular endothelial growth factor 3

17.1 Introduction

Endometriosis is an inflammatory disease affecting till the 10% of reproductive-aged women, linked to infertility in almost half of the patients. Unfortunately, the pathogenesis of endometriosis and its associated infertility is unknown, even if there are some theories [1].

Literature demonstrated that patients suffering endometriosis have genetic, biochemical, or immunological dysfunction that prevents the removal of the tissue from the peritoneal cavity and rather facilitates tissue adhesion to peritoneal structures [2].

The dysfunctional immune system of patient with endometriosis generally have dysregulated a multitude of immune cell types, including neutrophils, macrophages, dendritic cells, natural killer cells, T helper cells, and B cells [3] (Fig. 17.1).

A part the oxidative stress and oocyte quality, as possible ethiopathogenic mechanisms for endometriosis (Fig. 17.2), the cytokines and the chemokines involved in inflammation process, angiogenesis, and tissue growth are increased in the plasma and peritoneal fluid (PF) of women with endometriosis. This process is suspected to stimulate symptoms commonly presented including pain and infertility [4].

Statistical reports showed that 35–50% patients affected by endometriosis experienced infertility and 25–50% of infertile women have endometriosis [5].

If in healthy couples the monthly fecundity rate, which is a couple's probability of conceiving in 1 month, is 15–20%, on the contrary, women with endometriosis have a monthly fecundity rate of 2–10% [6].

Endometriosis is a heritable condition influenced by multiple genetic and environmental factors, with an overall heritability estimated at approximately 50%. Authors investigated whether single nucleotide polymorphisms (SNPs) rs7521902, rs10859871, and rs11031006 mapping to WNT4, VEZT, and FSHB genetic loci, respectively, are associated with risk for endometriosis in a Greek population. Genotyping of the rs7521902, rs10859871, and rs11031006 SNPs was performed with Taqman primer/probe sets. A significant association was detected with the AC genotype of rs7521902 (WNT4) in patients with stage III and IV disease only. Evidence for association with endometriosis was also found for the AC genotype of the rs10859871 of VEZT. Notably, a significant difference in the distribution of the AG genotype and the minor allele A of FSHB rs11031006 SNP was found between the patients with endometriosis and controls. They found a genetic association between rs11031006 (FSHB) SNP and endometriosis. WNT4 and VEZT genes constitute the most consistently associated genes with endometriosis. In the present study, an association of rs7521902 (WNT4) and rs10859871 (VEZT) was confirmed in women with endometriosis at the genotypic but not the allelic level [7].

17.1.1 Infertility and Endometriosis

Almost 50% of adolescents with intractable dysmenorrhea or pelvic pain are diagnosed with endometriosis, but it is not yet clear why only certain women develop the condition.

Fig. 17.1 Pathogenesis and risk factors

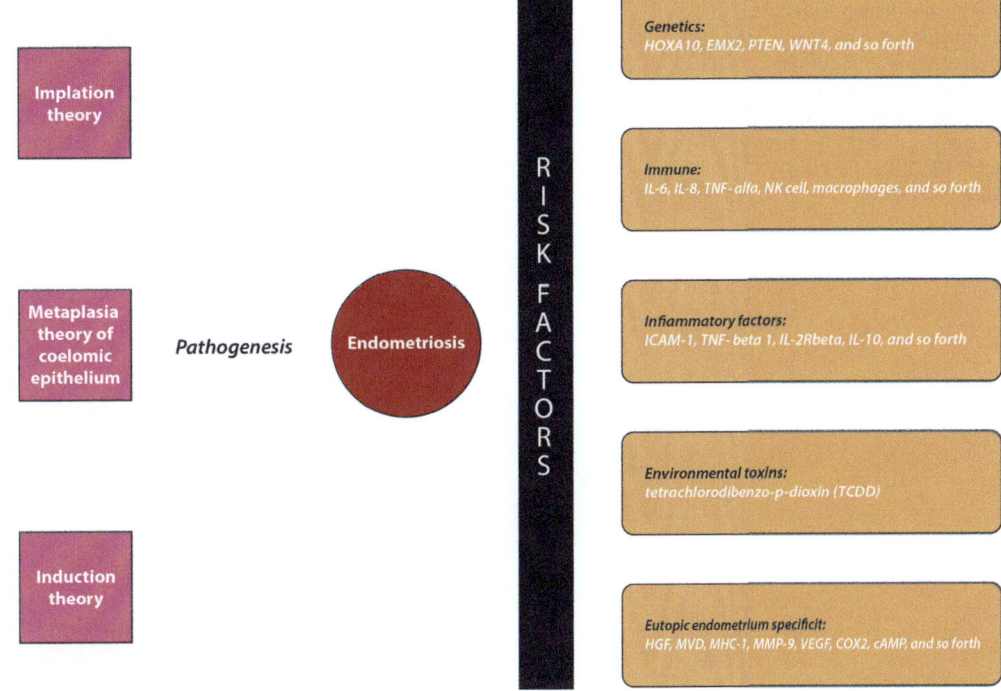

The monthly fecundity rate in normal couples of reproductive age is known to be 15–20%, whereas the rate in infertile women with endometriosis ranges from 2 to 10% [8].

A meta-analysis proposed that the chance of achieving pregnancy was lower for patients with endometriosis compared to those with tubal factor infertility (OR 0.56; 95% CI, 0.44–0.70) [9].

However, the association between infertility and early-stage disease, from minimal endometriosis [stage I] and mild endometriosis [stage II], according to the ASRM score (Fig. 17.3), in which no substantial pelvic anatomical changes are identified, remains controversial [10].

The improvement of Controlled Ovarian Hyperstimulation (COH) with GnRH-a downregulation and the application of ICSI technology may suppress some negative influences of endometriosis on pregnancy [11, 12].

Dong et al. investigated the impact of endometriosis on the IVF/ICSI outcomes, comparing ovarian stimulation parameters and IVF/ICSI outcomes. Patients with stage I-II and stage III-IV endometriosis required higher dosage and longer duration of gonadotropins, but had lower day 3 high-quality embryos rate, when compared to patients with tubal infertility. In addition, the number of oocytes retrieved, the number of obtained embryos, the number of day 3 high-quality embryos, serum E2 level on the day of hCG, and fertilization rate were lower in patients with stage III-IV endometriosis than those in tubal factors group. Except reduced implantation rate in stage III-IV endometriosis group, no differences were found in other pregnancy parameters. This study concluded that IVF/ICSI yielded similar pregnancy outcomes in patients with different stages of endometriosis and patients with tubal infertility [13].

Barbosa et al. evaluated whether the presence or severity of endometriosis affects the outcome of ART in a systematic review, investigating all studies comparing the outcome of ART in women with and those without endometriosis, or at different stages of the disease. Women with endometriosis undergoing ART have practically the same chance of achieving clinical pregnancy and live birth as do women with other causes of infertility. No relevant difference was observed in the chance of achieving clinical pregnancy and live birth following ART when comparing stage-III/IV with stage-I/II endometriosis [14].

In a recent review, Tanbo and Fedorcsak affirmed that medical or hormonal treatment alone has little or no effect and should only be used in conjunction with ART. Of the various methods of ART, intrauterine insemination, due to its simplicity, can be recommended in women with minimal or mild peritoneal endometriosis, even though insemination may yield a lower success rate than in women without endometriosis. IVF is an effective treatment option in less-advanced disease stages, and the success rates are similar to the results in other causes of infertility. However, women with more advanced stages of endometriosis have lower success rates with IVF [15].

How endometriosis affect infertility? The most widely accepted theory, which was developed by Sampson, holds that that endometrial tissue refluxed to the fallopian tubes fails to be

268

A. Tinelli et al.

Fig. 17.2 Oxidative stress and oocyte quality: possible ethiopathogenic mechanism involved in minimal/mild endometriosis-related infertility. *ROS* reactive oxygen species, *PF* peritoneal fluid, *FF* follicular fluid, *CC* cumulus cells

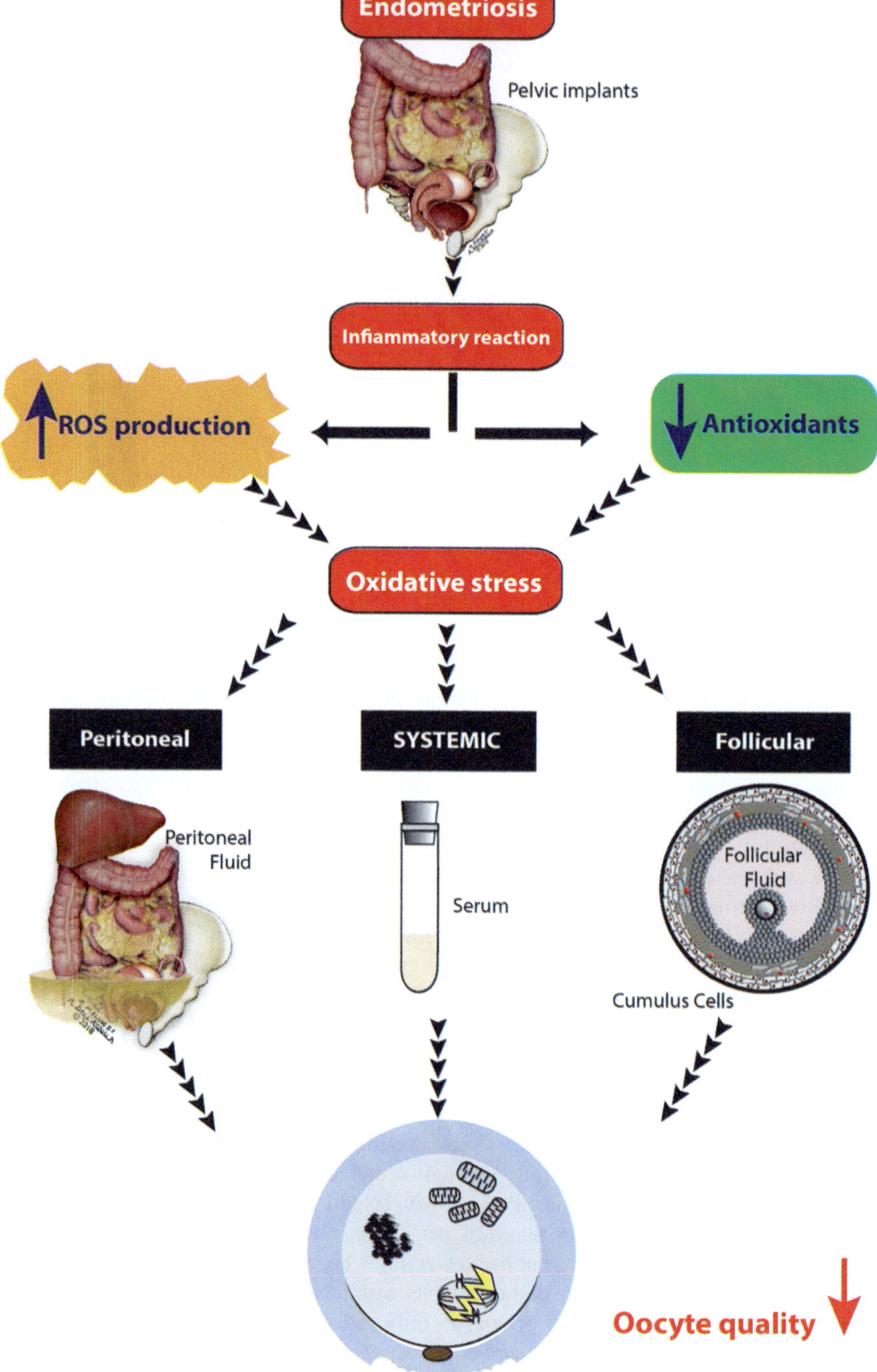

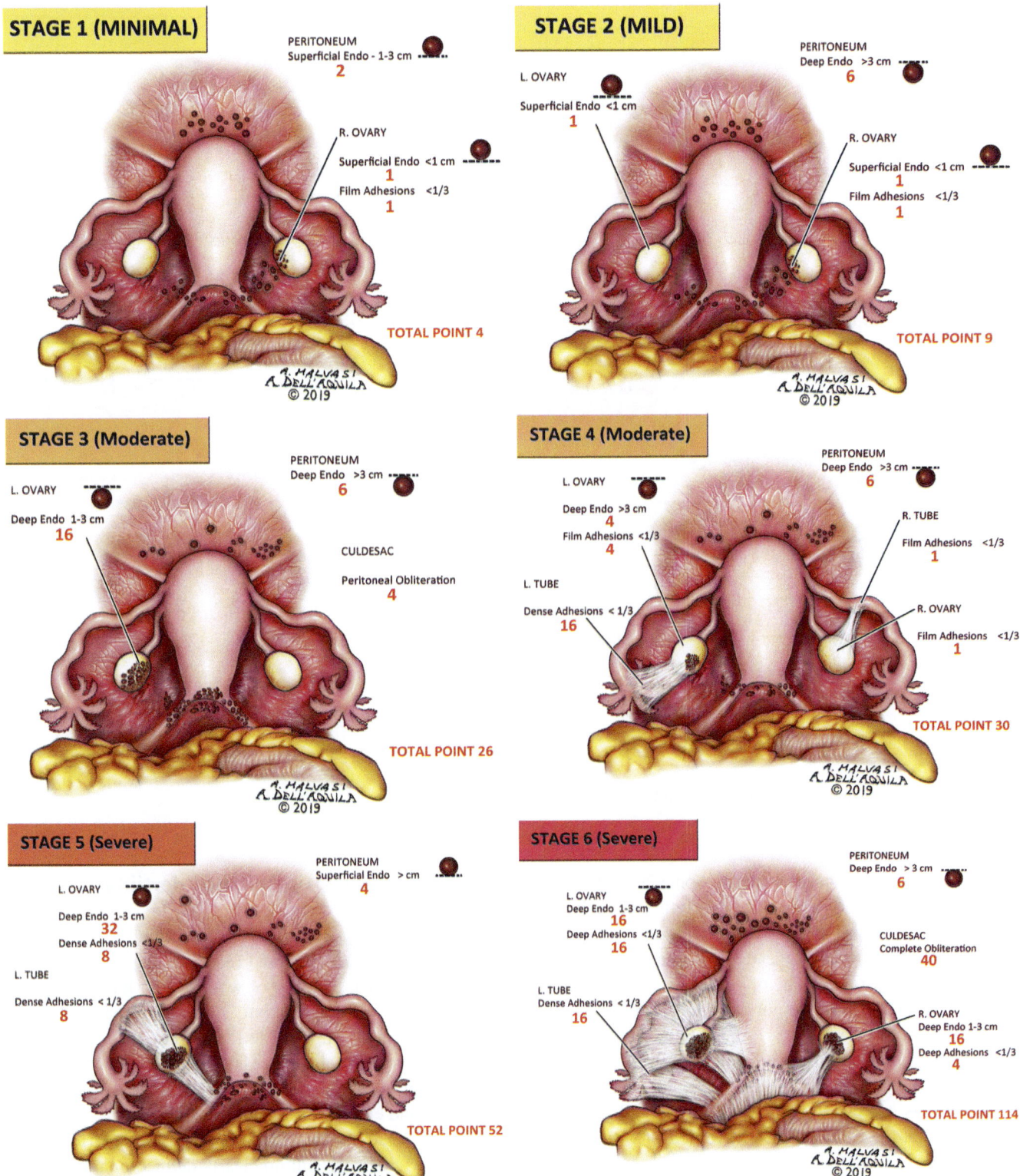

Fig. 17.3 ASRM staging criteria for endometriosis

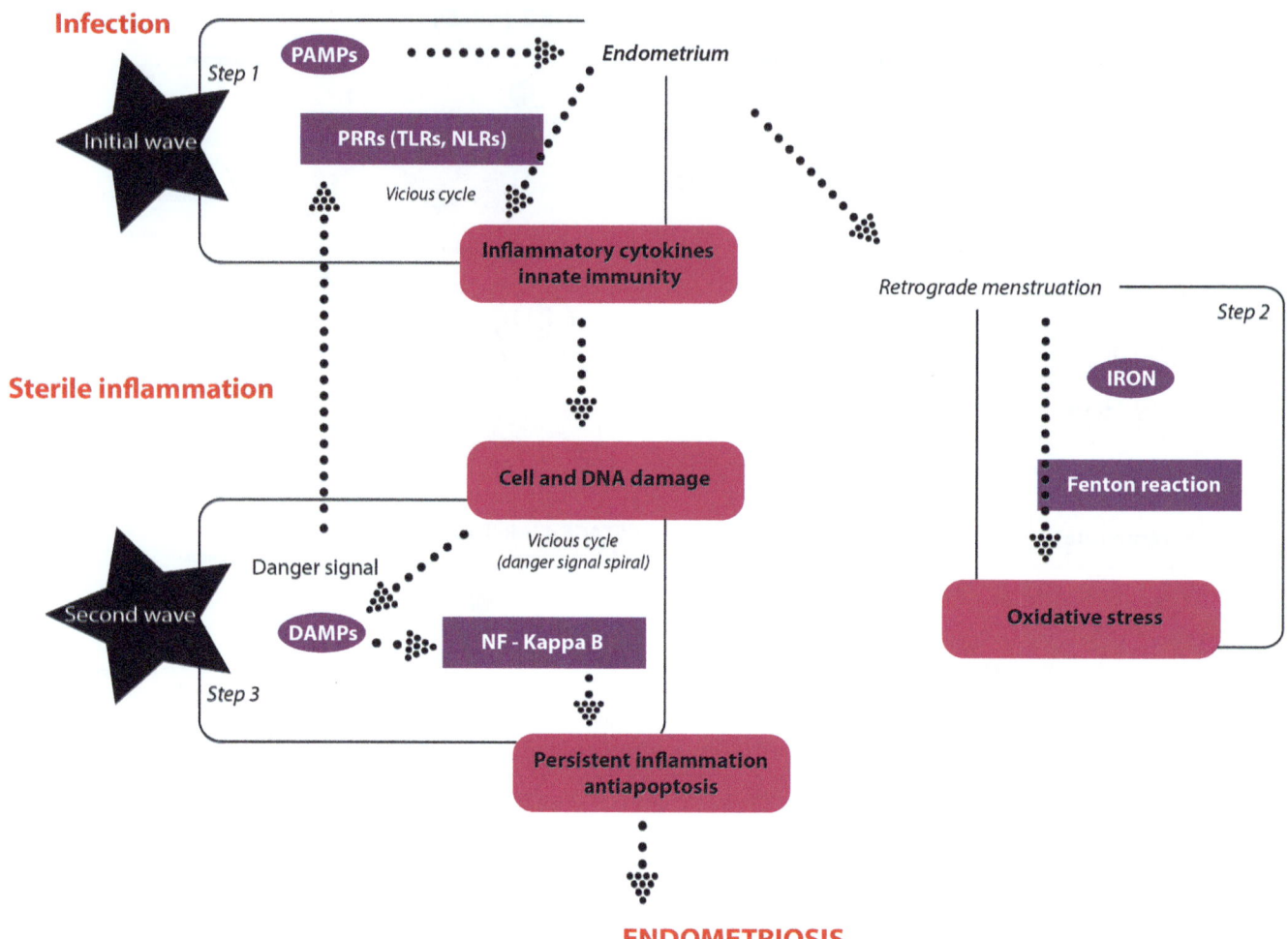

Fig. 17.4 Pathogenetic mechanisms of endometriosis

cleared and attaches to the peritoneum. Some 70% of women who menstruate regularly exhibit bleeding reflux, but only 10% develop endometriosis [16] (Figs. 17.4, 17.5, and 17.6).

Recently, it has been suggested that abnormal immune function and dysregulation of immune mediators are responsible for the poor response to treatment, and poor clearance, of ectopic endometrium. Immune status is now considered to play an important role in the initiation and progression of endometriosis. Several studies have shown that the levels of activated macrophages, T cells, B cells, and inflammatory cytokines are increased in women with endometriosis [17, 18].

Reductions in NK cell cytotoxic function have been observed in the peritoneal fluid (PF) of patients with endometriosis implying that a defect in NK cell cytotoxic function, preventing elimination of endometrial cells from ectopic sites, may cause endometriosis [19, 20].

17.1.2 Endometriosis-Related Infertility

Endometriosis may contribute to infertility by impairing ovarian and tubal function and reducing uterine receptivity (Fig. 17.6); in fact, 35–50% of women with infertility have endometriosis [10], and about 30–50% of patients with endometriosis have impaired fertility [21].

Endometriosis is also associated with a reduced rate of pregnancy after IVF, which may be due to the poor qualities of oocytes and embryos [22].

Despite the advances in the research of endometriosis role in infertility, there are still no clearly defined treatment protocols. Low pregnancy rates after IVF are observed in patients with endometriosis, compared to those with tubal factor of infertility. The detrimental impact, if any, of endometriosis on IVF outcome would be expected to be on embryo "quality" and/or endometrial receptivity [23].

Fig. 17.5 Pathogenetic theory of menstrual reflux

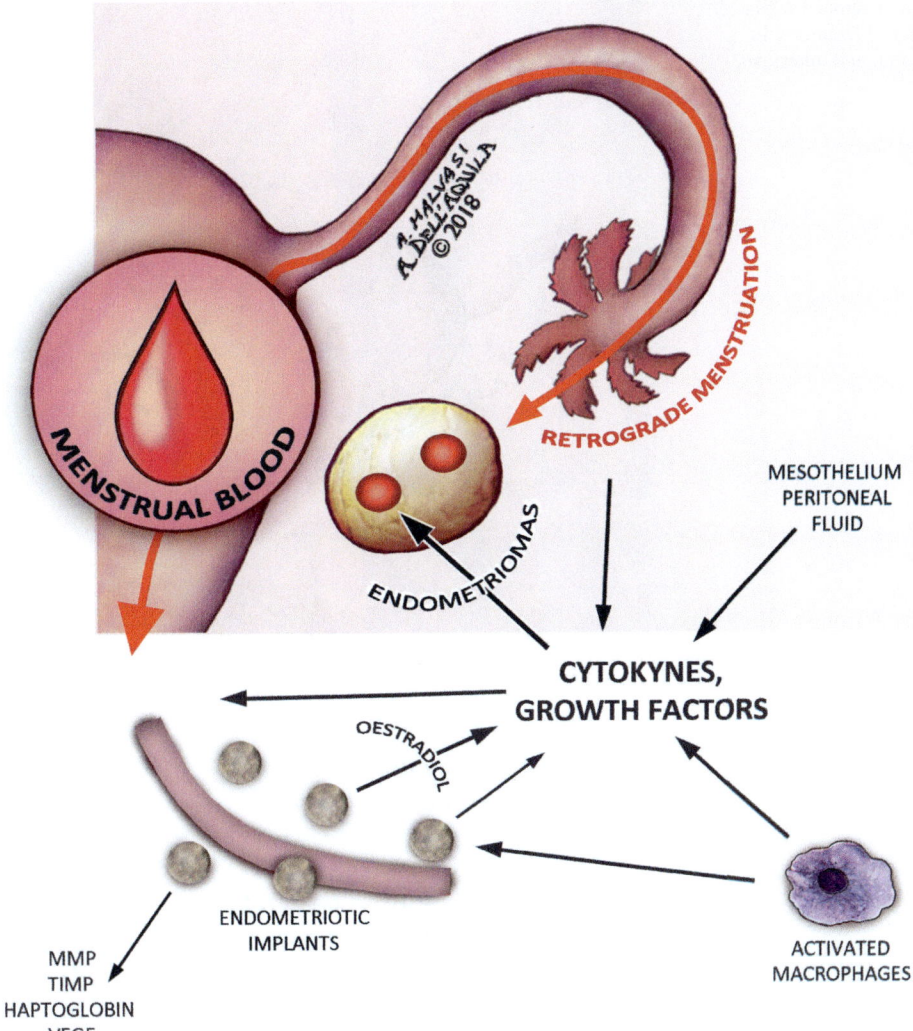

Analyzing retrospective studies on in vitro fertilization (IVF) and oocyte donation programs showed that women with endometriosis have significantly reduced pregnancy rates per cycle and per transfer as well as reduced implantation rates. Moreover, studies reported that healthy ovum donation to patients with endometriosis produces the same rate of implantation and pregnancy compared to controls [23].

Retrospective and prospective clinical trials on IVF success rate have shown decreased oocyte and embryo quality and low ovarian reserves in women with endometriosis compared to controls [24].

Nevertheless, human studies indicate poor oocyte and embryo quality and lower pregnancy rates in women with endometriosis, addressing the problem on pro-inflammatory cytokines and chemokines that negatively interact with the oocyte and embryo, with damage to the oocyte and embryo [25].

In fact, intrafollicular levels of IL-8, IL-12, and adrenomedullin are elevated in women with endometriosis under-

going IVF and are indicators of impaired embryo and oocyte quality [26].

Poor oocyte quality was observed and measured, in retrospective IVF studies, by diminished blastomere cleavage rates, increased numbers of arrested embryos, and impaired cytosolic events [27].

In addition, reports also suggest that other etiological factors, such as in utero exposure to diethylstilbestrol, environmental exposure to endocrine disrupting agents, low birth weight, and dietary choices may play significant roles in the development of endometriosis [28].

Outcomes of in vitro fertilization cycles in women with endometriosis are significantly worse than in patients without this condition. The impact of endometriosis on ovarian reserve and the quality of retrieved oocytes seems evident. Lower implantation rates, however, raise the question whether this finding is purely the consequence of lower number and poorer quality of embryos, or whether it also reflects compromised endometrial receptivity [29].

Fig. 17.6 Factors associated with reduced fecundity in women with endometriosis

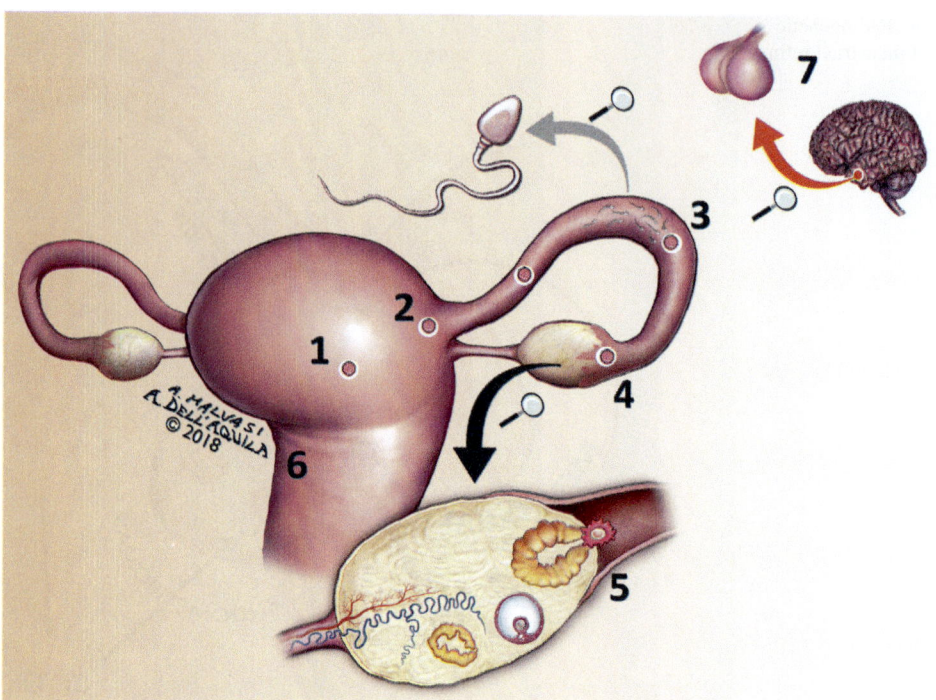

1. **IMPLANTATION:**
-Reduced uterine receptivity;
-Altered hormone regulation.

2. **PREIMPLANTATION EMBRYO:**
-Poor embryo quality;
-Early embryo arrest.

3. **FERTILIZATION:**
-Oocyte-linked reduced fertilization rate;
-Poor sperm binding;
-Reduced sperm mobility.

4. **OVULATION:**
-Fewer oocytes;
-Altered oocyte quality;
-Luteinized Unruptered
Follicle Syndrome.

5. **OVARY:**
-Impaired folliculogenesis;
-Fewer follicles;
-Luteal defect;
-Altered steroidogenesis.

6. **PREGNANCY:**
-Increased pre-term loss;
-Recurrent miscarriages.

7. **PITUITARY:**
-Altered pituitary-ovarian axis;
-Altered LH surge.

Accumulating evidence indicates that endometriosis is associated with aberrant transcriptional profiles in the eutopic endometrium of women and baboons resulting in dysregulation of critical signaling pathways [30].

Endometriosis is known to be associated with several deregulated molecules related to the pathogenesis of the disease, such as cyclooxygenase-2 (COX-2) and aromatase. The COX-2 enzyme, encoded by the PTGS2 gene (prostaglandin–endoperoxide synthase 2), is naturally induced by aromatase and is involved in the conversion of arachidonic acid into prostaglandins, which, in turn, regulate aromatase levels in endometriotic tissue [31].

In the endometrial tissue of patients with endometriosis, aberrant aromatase is induced via cyclooxygenase-2 prostaglandin-2 (COX-2–PGE2) pathway deregulation, with a positive feedback cycle. It is also related to proliferative and inflammatory properties of ectopic implants [32].

The PTGS2 gene, which encodes cyclooxygenase 2 (COX-2), is deregulated in endometriotic lesions and plays a crucial role in the acquisition of oocyte competence [33].

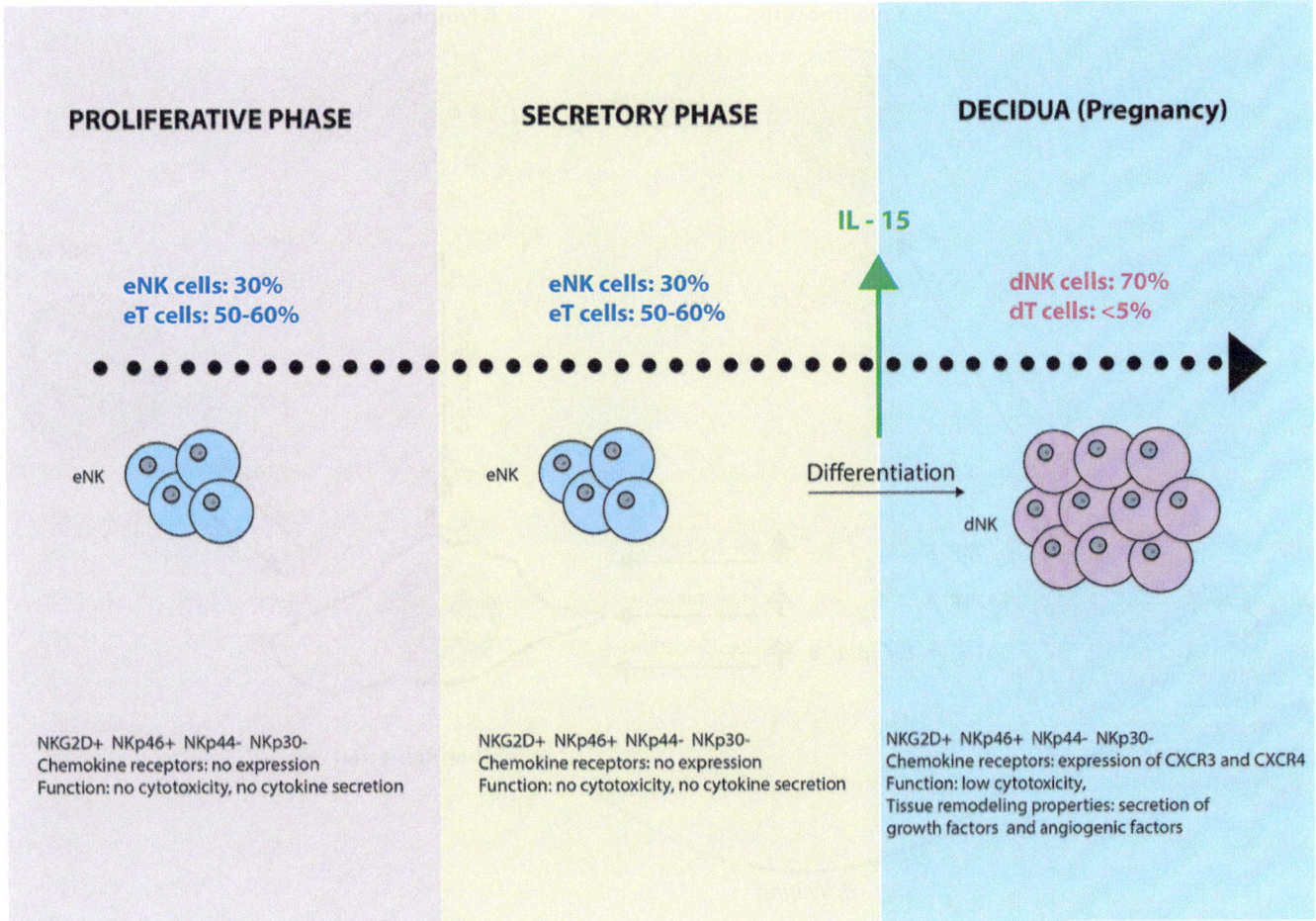

Fig. 17.7 Expression of NK cells in the endometrium

17.1.3 Peritoneal Fluid of Patient with Endometriosis

Endometrial fragments refluxed during menstruation induce inflammation within the peritoneal cavity [34].

Normally, neutrophils and macrophages are among the first immune cells (Fig. 17.7) to be recruited to this area and, both, are primary contributors to the elevations in pro-inflammatory and chemotactic cytokine levels found in the peritoneal fluid (PF) [35].

In addition to encouraging the growth of peritoneal implants, macrophages are a major source of angiogenic mediators, including TNF-α and IL-8 [36].

Endometriosis also involves significant disarray in the production and metabolism of nitric oxide (NO), a ubiquitous free radical in the oocyte microenvironment that plays a vital role in virtually every step of oocyte development, including meiotic maturation, fertilization, embryonic cleavage, and implantation [37].

Authors demonstrated a significant role of NO in delaying oocyte aging and maintaining the integrity of the spindle apparatus.

Decreased bioavailability of NO under certain pathologic conditions could therefore result in abnormalities in oocyte viability and developmental capacity [38].

Further, sperm, travelling through the uterus and fallopian tubes, also interact with inflammatory cytokines in the PF and similarly encounter damage.

Moreover, endometriosis is linked to the Natural Killer (NK) cells dysfunction; NK cells comprise 15% of all circulating lymphocytes, particularly those of the innate immune system, and protect against tumor development and viral infections.

Most studies have found that the numbers of cytotoxic NK cells are functionally defective and reduced in the PF and peripheral blood of patients with endometriosis and that this is accompanied by an overall decrease in NK cell activity [16] (Fig. 17.8).

In such patients, the populations of NK cells (CD32CD56+) are significantly decreased, whereas the proportions of immature NK cells (CD272CD11b2) among CD32CD56+ NK cells are increased in the PF. Functional impairment and diminished cytotoxicity of NK cells within the peritoneal cavity have also been well documented in such patients [39].

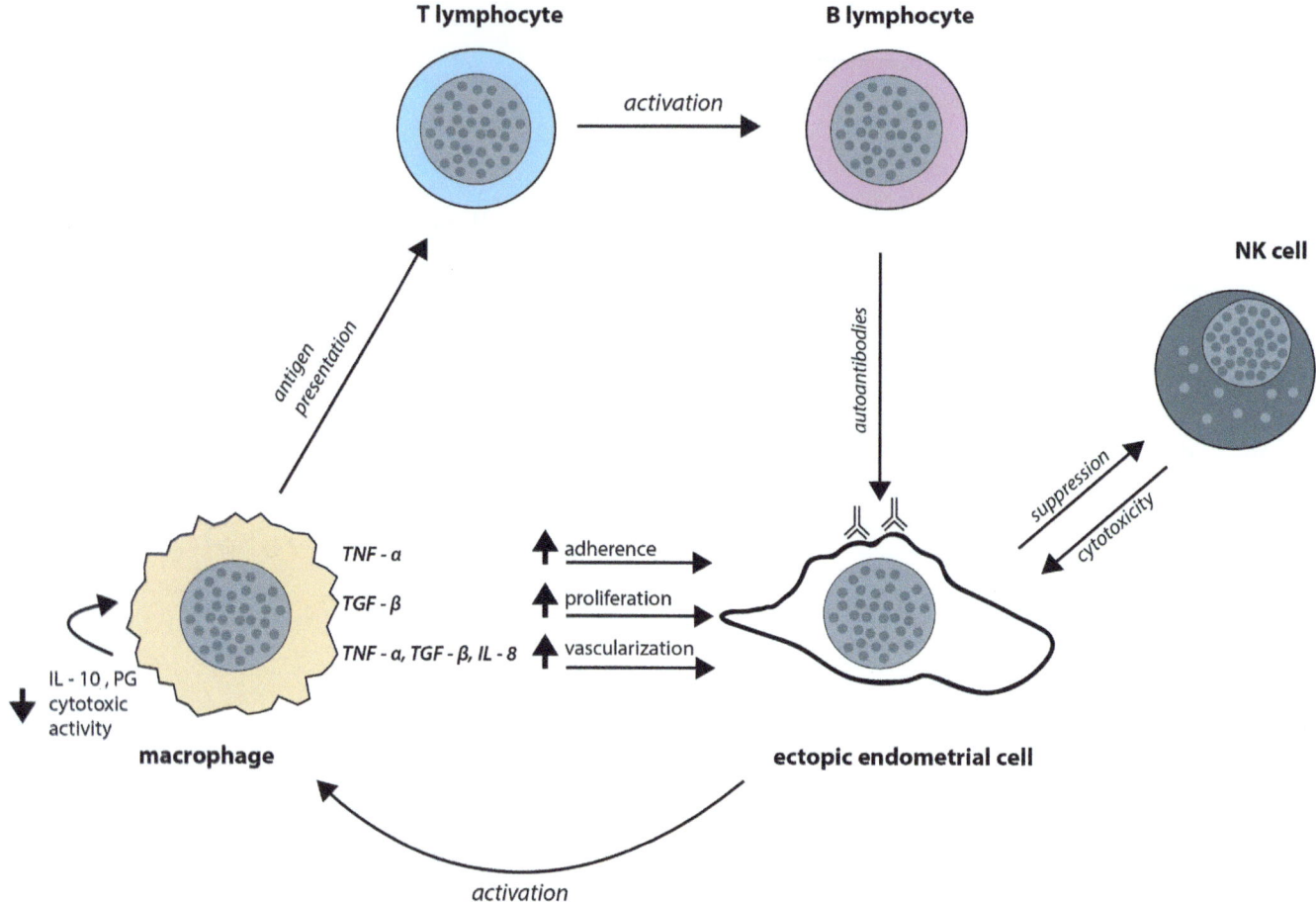

Fig. 17.8 Interaction between immune cells and ectopic endometrial cells in the peritoneal cavity

In addition, the levels of the inflammatory cytokines IL-6, IL-8, IL-1b, IFN-γ, and TNF-α increase in the PF of patients with endometriosis, which is consistent with the elevated levels noted in the serum [16].

Inflammatory cytokines including TNF-α and oxidative stress has been shown to directly hinder sperm motility [25, 26].

Similarly, murine embryos incubated in the PF from women with endometriosis have shown diminished growth rates of embryos, increased rates of apoptosis, DNA fragmentation, and increased number of embryos arrested in development [40].

Dexamethasone reduced the observed embryotoxic effect of the PF from women with endometriosis-associated infertility. Dexamethasone is a glucocorticoid that has been shown to reduce the expression of prostaglandins and other inflammatory mediators dysregulated in endometriosis [41].

Additionally, inhibiting TNF-α reduces embryotoxic effect on mouse embryos incubated with PF from infertile women with endometriosis [42].

Collectively, these studies link inflammation in the PF, specifically TNF-α, with embryo toxicity. Studying the toxicity of PF from women with endometriosis is limited by ethical constraints as interfering with human embryos vio-

lates moral and ethical considerations. However, this murine model provides a convincing argument to suggest the PF from women with endometriosis produces a damaging effect on the embryo [40].

17.1.4 The Oocyte Quality

Patients with endometriosis continue to pose difficulties in achieving pregnancy. Studies have shown lower implantation rates in non-endometriotic patients who received oocytes from women with endometriosis, whereas healthy donated oocytes have proven to contribute to a pregnancy with similar chances in women without the disease. The question still to be answered is whether this situation applies for natural cycles or whether it is the use of gonadotropin-releasing hormone analogs and hormonal replacement therapy used for endometrial priming in oocyte recipients that reestablishes an adequate uterine environment [29].

Endometriosis, especially at the ovarian site has been shown to have a detrimental impact on ovarian physiology. Indeed, sonographic and histologic data tend to support the

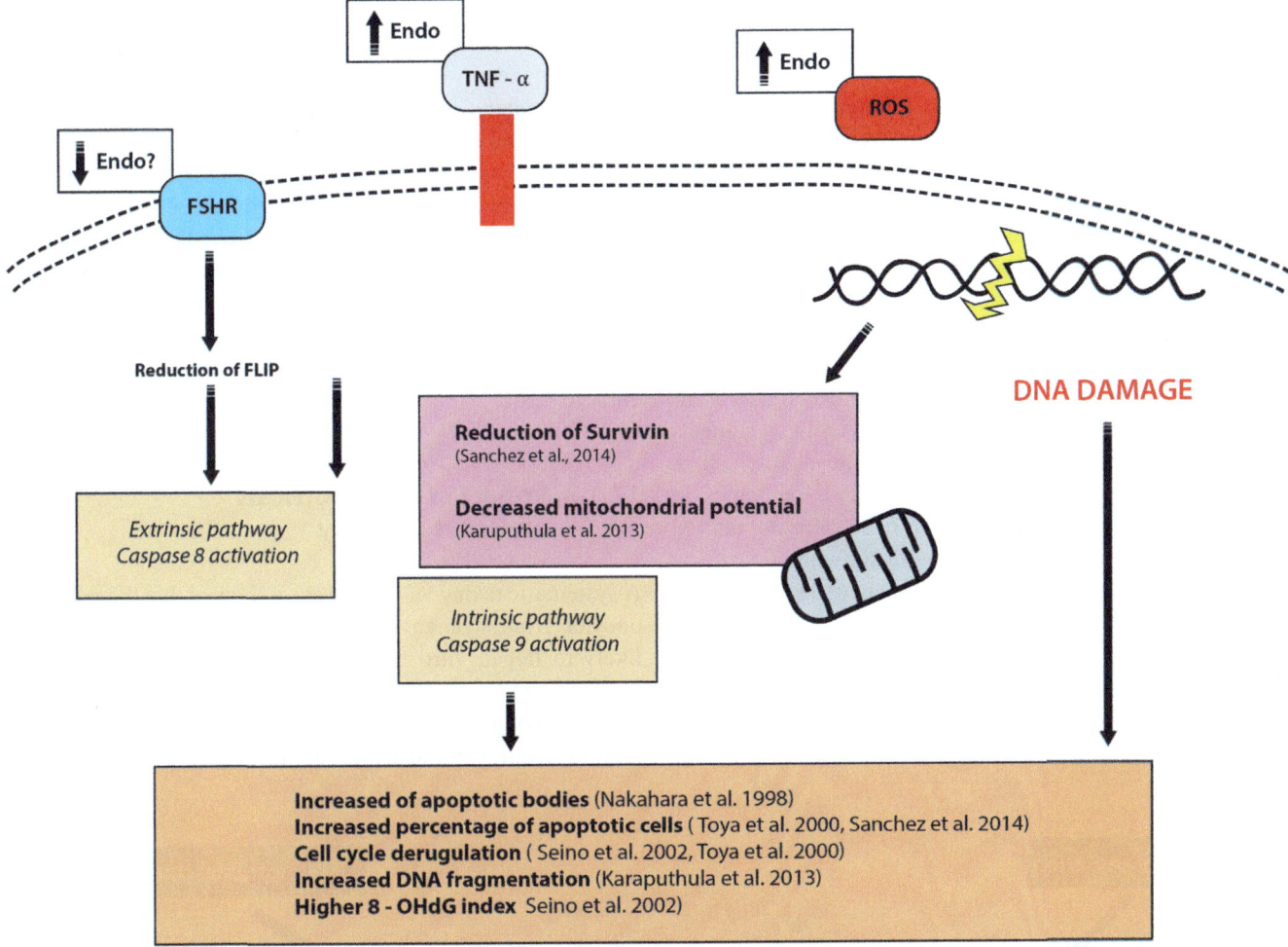

Fig. 17.9 Damage of endometriosis on tissues

idea that ovarian follicles of patients with endometriosis are decreased in number and more atretic. Moreover, the local intrafollicular environment of patients affected is characterized by alterations of the granulosa cell compartment including reduced P450 aromatase expression and increased intracellular reactive oxygen species generation [24].

Assessment of oocyte morphology is obligatory for the evaluation of oocyte quality and it has been known that quality of the oocyte has an impact on the fertilization outcomes [43].

Oocyte quality is determined by its morphological, cellular, and molecular evaluations [44].

Advances in reproductive medicine have made clear that one of the most important factors determining the outcome of embryo development is oocyte quality [45].

Many prognostic factors based on morphological characteristics of the oocyte have been devised that may allow prediction of oocyte quality, fertilization rates, and embryo development.

However, currently available techniques are not very reliable in predicting which metaphase II (MII) oocyte will lead

to an embryo which will implant and result in a clinical pregnancy [46] (Fig. 17.9).

One way indirectly to assess oocyte quality is to analyze markers in cumulus cells (CCs). During follicular development, the granulosa cells differ in the mural population, limiting the follicular antrum and in the CC population, which surrounds the oocyte. Mural cells are responsible for estrogen production and rupture of the follicle, whereas CCs are intimately associated with oocyte development. CCs are regulated, in part, by factors derived from the oocyte, while contributing to oocyte maturation and development potential.

In this context, some studies have suggested that the analysis of gene expression in CCs can be used as an indirect predictor of oocyte quality and outcomes of assisted reproduction technologies, with possible clinical applications [23].

Traditionally, poor oocyte quality has been held responsible for poor ART outcome in women with endometriosis.

Barnhart et al. observed lower number of oocytes retrieved and lower fertilization rates in oocytes recovered from women with endometriosis as compared to controls of tubal factor infertility but other authors have reported conflicting results [9].

Other researches have found no difference in folliculogenesis or the number of oocytes retrieved in patients with endometriosis, as compared to other etiologies such as tubal factor infertility [47, 48].

Adverse influence on the oocyte is therefore a likely central aspect in endometriosis-related infertility. This concept is strengthened by a study reporting significant improvement in the pregnancy rate in patients with endometriosis who received donated oocytes compared with their own oocytes. Conversely, the pregnancy rates were lower in subjects without endometriosis who received donor oocytes from subjects with endometriosis [49–51].

Moreover, a recent meta-analysis on IVF outcomes in endometriosis indicates that live birth rates were not altered in patients with minimal/mild endometriosis, whereas patients with moderate and severe endometriosis patients had poorer outcomes including lower retrieved oocytes, implantation rates, and birth rates [52].

When retrieved oocyte number is considered as ovarian response to controlled ovarian stimulation (COS) and as a success parameter, data in the literature are more conflicting.

The acquisition of oocyte competence is known to depend on adequate cytoplasmic and nuclear maturation, the latter being dependent on the presence of a normal spindle. The meiotic spindle of human oocytes in metaphase II, a temporary and dynamic structure composed of microtubules, is associated with the oocyte cortex and its subcortical microfilaments network and is essential to ensure the fidelity of chromosome segregation during meiosis. The meiotic spindle, however, is extremely sensitive to the action of various factors such as oxidative stress, which can promote meiotic abnormalities and chromosome instability, increase apoptosis and impair the development of the preimplantation embryo [23].

17.1.5 Impact of Endometriosis on Oocyte Quality

A systematic review of the literature showed that the retrieved oocytes from women affected by endometriosis are more likely to fail in vitro maturation and to show altered morphology and lower cytoplasmic mitochondrial content compared to women with other causes of infertility (Fig. 17.10). Results from meta-analyses addressing IVF outcomes in

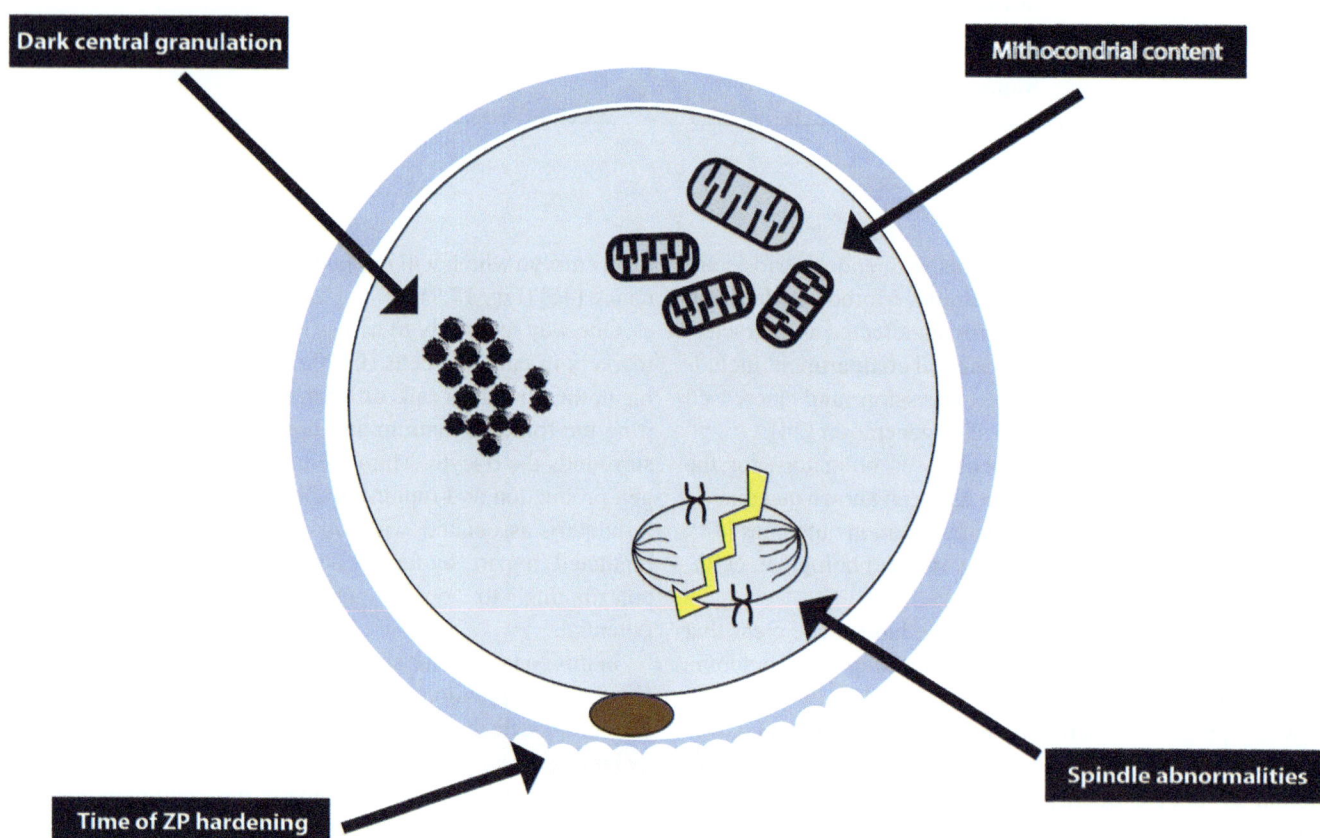

Fig. 17.10 Damage of endometriosis disease on oocyte quality

women affected would indicate that a reduction in the number of mature oocytes retrieved is associated with endometriosis while a reduction in fertilization rates is more likely to be associated with minimal/mild rather than with moderate/severe disease [24].

Women with endometriosis ovulate fewer oocytes than healthy women and those oocytes ovulated by women with endometriosis are both sometimes compromised, so that endometriosis negatively impacts embryo development [25].

Xu et al. examined the ultrastructure of oocytes from patients with minimal or mild endometriosis and control females undergoing IVF treatment by transmission electron microscopy (TEM) to investigate the physiological significance of oocyte quality for patients with minimal or mild endometriosis. The TEM results revealed that the oocytes from women with minimal or mild endometriosis exhibited abnormal mitochondrial structure and decreased mitochondria mass. Quantitative real-time PCR analysis revealed that the mitochondrial DNA copy number was significantly reduced in the oocytes from women with minimal or mild endometriosis compared with those of the control subjects. Their results suggested the decreased oocyte quality because of impaired mitochondrial structure and functions, probably an important factor affecting the fertility of patients with endometriosis [53].

A recent study has shown that women with endometriosis exhibit an increase in apoptosis of the cumulus cells surrounding the oocyte and apoptosis in ovarian cells is a good indicator of poor oocyte quality [54].

Death of cumulus cells probably leads to reduced oocyte quality and maturation attributable to the loss of the essential support that the cumulus cells give to the oocyte [55].

Aberrant nuclear and cytoplasmic events in embryos from women with endometriosis are six times more likely compared with women without endometriosis [56] (Fig. 17.11).

These events include cytoplasmic fragmentation, darkened cytoplasm, reduced cell numbers, and increased frequency of arrested embryos, leading to significantly fewer transferable blastocysts. Additionally, the quality of embryos that develop from patients with endometriosis has been shown to be reduced [57].

Treatment with a gonadotropin-releasing hormone agonist that temporarily causes regression of the endometriotic lesions and cessation of reproductive cyclicity helps to improve embryo quality in these patients [58].

Embryo quality and embryo implantation are also of particular concern in women with endometriosis. In a normal embryo, there are proteins called L-selectin that normally coat the trophoblast on the surface of the blastocyst. This protein is involved in binding of the embryo to the endometrium. Low levels of the enzyme involved in the synthesis of the endometrial ligand for L-selectin have been observed and is a possible etiology of decreased embryo receptivity in patients with endometriosis [59–61].

In addition, endometriosis-free patients who have oocytes donated from women with a known history of moderate to severe endometriosis have decreased implantation rates and reduced embryo quality. This decrease in implantation rate and embryo quality is in comparison with women with moderate to severe endometriosis that receive oocytes from endometriosis-free women [62].

The hormonal milieu was altered in the follicular fluid of patients with endometriosis, such as a decreased estradiol concentration [63].

A dysregulated intrafollicular hormone milieu, as well as an abnormal intrafollicular cytokine profile, might therefore be a cause of reduced fertility in endometriosis.

This suggestion is in line with studies from oocyte donation programs. Implantation rates were reduced with oocytes from women with endometriosis transferred to women without endometriosis, whereas embryos from healthy donors, transferred to women with endometriosis, did not affect implantation rates [29, 64].

Abnormal folliculogenesis, elevated oxidative stress (OS), altered immune function, changes in the hormonal milieu, or decreased endometrial receptivity may also contribute to reduced fertility [65].

OS can be considered as a process consisting in three distinct stages, with an increased production of reactive species occurring in the first stage, mobilization of antioxidant occurring in the second, and oxidative damage to the major targets (lipids, proteins, and nucleic acids) occurring in the third [66, 67].

The presence of OS markers in the follicular fluid of infertile women with endometriosis, submitted to in IVF, has been recently demonstrated (Table 17.1) [68, 69].

Donabela et al. demonstrated that infertile women with moderate and severe endometriosis showed increased expression of the superoxide dismutase 1 (SOD1) gene in cumulus cells, compared to women with minimal/mild endometriosis and controls. This evidence opens a new perspective for understanding the pathogenesis of endometriosis-related infertility, confirming that OS is involved in the worsening of oocyte quality in these women. These findings also suggest that analysis of expression of SOD1 gene in CCs might be used as a biomarker of ICSI success in women with infertility related to advanced stages of endometriosis [70].

Singh et al. evaluated the OS and trace elements in the oocytes environment in endometriosis and impact on IVF outcome. They aspirated FF at the time of oocyte retrieval from endometriosis ($n = 200$) and tubal infertility ($n = 140$) and it was analyzed. In endometriosis group, they showed an increased concentration of reactive oxygen species (ROS), nitric oxide (NO), lipid peroxidation (LPO), iron, lead, cadmium and reduced levels of total antioxidant capacity (TAC), superoxide dismutase (SOD), catalase, glutathione peroxidase

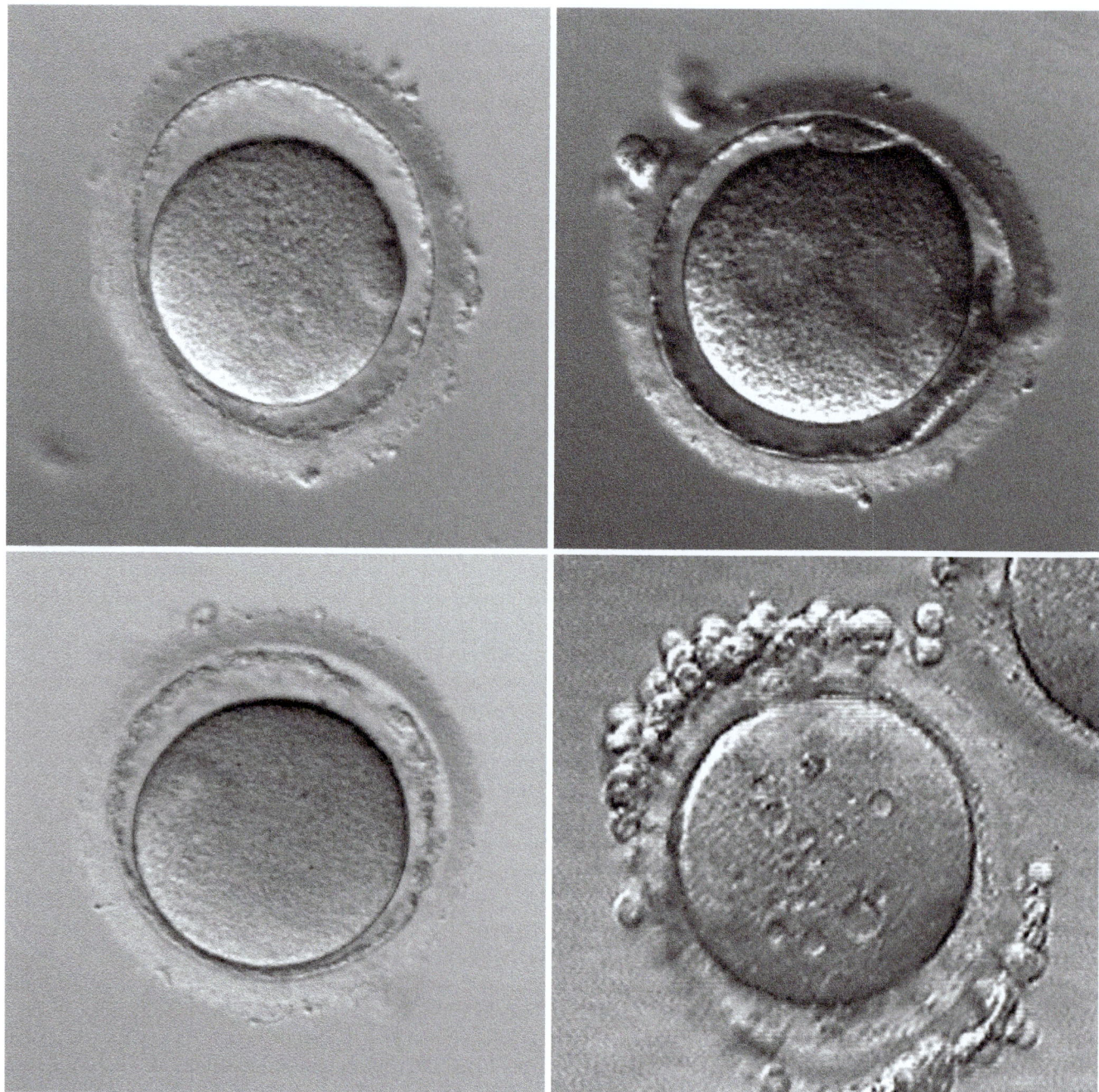

Fig. 17.11 Damage of endometriosis disease on oocyte quality (image under the microscope)

(GPx), glutathione reductase (GR), vitamins A, C, E, copper, zinc and selenium, compared to tubal infertility. Increased ROS and NO in endometriosis and tubal infertility are associated with poor oocytes and embryo quality. Increased levels of ROS, NO, LPO, cadmium, and lead were observed in women who did not become pregnant, compared to women who did. Intrafollicular zinc levels were higher in women with endometriosis who subsequently became pregnant following IVF.

The deleterious effect of intrafollicular ROS/NO on oocytes and embryo quality and IVF pregnancy prompted authors to ascertain the ROS threshold level, beyond which it appears to be toxic, and is associated with the formation of poor quality oocytes. Further, follicular levels of lead and cadmium showed a negative association with IVF pregnancy outcome, thereby highlighting the toxicity risk of environmental pollutants [71].

An imbalance between reactive oxygen species (ROS) production and antioxidant activity causes cellular damage and dysfunction and may affect folliculogenesis. Altered folliculogenesis in patients with endometriosis may contribute

Table 17.1 Change in OS concentration in oocytes after retrieval in patients with endometriosis

Endometriosis group
> ROS
> NO
> LPO
> Fe
> LEAD
> Cadmio
< TAC
< SOD
< Catalase
< Glutathione peroxidase
< GR
< Vit. A, C, E
< Cu, Zn, Se

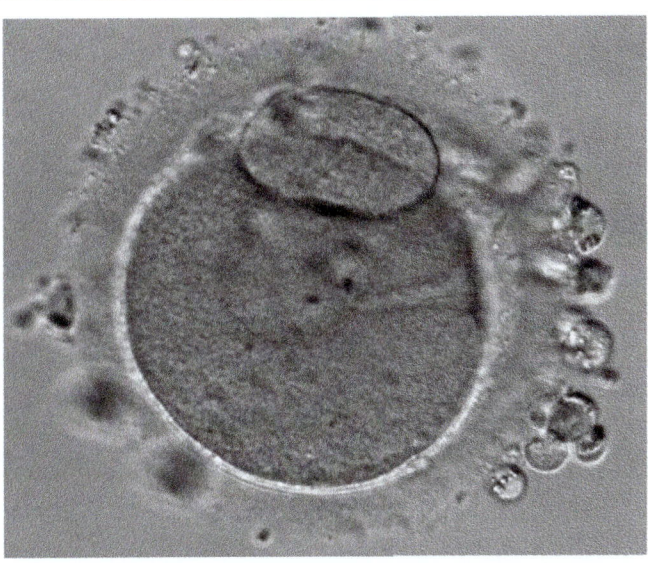

Fig. 17.12 Morphological alterations in oocyte pronucleus of endometriosis (A)

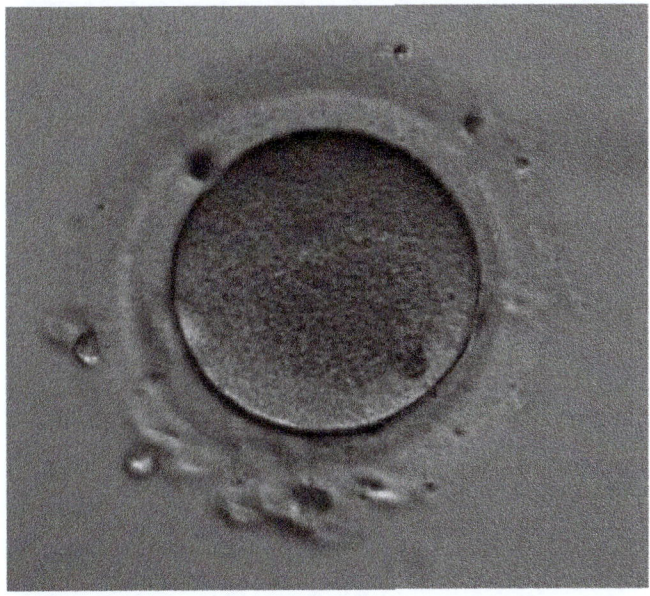

Fig. 17.13 Morphological alterations in oocyte pronucleus of patients with endometriosis (B)

to ovulatory dysfunction, poor oocyte quality, reduced fertilization, low-grade embryos, and reduced implantation [57].

Changes in the kinetics of granulosa cell cycle may also impair follicular growth and oocyte maturation in patients with endometriosis [72].

Thiols are organic sulfur derivatives, contributing to the infertility associated with endometriosis, since extracellular supply of thiols is critical for maintaining the redox state of the extracellular space or microenvironment [73].

Thus, endometriosis is associated with inflammatory changes in the intrafollicular microenvironment.

In addition, the levels of inflammatory cytokines, such as interleukin 6 (IL6), IL1b, and tumor necrosis factor alpha (TNFa), are increased in the ovarian follicular fluid (OFF) of patients with endometriosis [74].

Da Broi et al. detected a deleterious effect of FF taken from infertile women with mild endometriosis on the spindle and chromosome distribution of bovine oocytes matured in vitro, indicating the presence of harmful factors against oocyte quality in the FF of women with the disease and questioning the role of OS in the worsening of gamete quality [75].

Da Broi et al. also demonstrated both systemic and follicular oxidative stress in infertile patients with endometriosis. They demonstrate the presence of oxidative DNA damage, represented by higher 8OHdG concentrations in the follicular microenvironment of these patients, possibly related to compromised oocyte quality and associated with the pathogenesis of endometriosis-related infertility. These findings also suggest that some of the OS markers studied in serum and FF are predictive of clinical pregnancy and live birth after ICSI [76].

Baumann et al. demonstrated that endometriosis is linked with altered patterns of ovarian gene expression and demonstrated that a prominent epigenetic pathway, associated with oocyte quality and potential correct ovarian development, is severely disrupted in primate females with induced endometriosis [77].

Kasapoglu et al. showed dimorphisms significantly higher in oocytes retrieved from endometriosis group: dark cytoplasm; dark, large or thin zona pellucida; and flat or fragmented polar body ($p < 0.05$ for all) (Figs. 17.11, 17.12, and 17.13). When morphological parameters for oocytes of patients with endometriosis are evaluated, the oocyte defects have increased significantly in patients with endometriosis. Thus, the abnormal oocyte morphology is more common in patients with endometriosis than those with male factor infertility (Figs. 17.14, 17.15, 17.16, and 17.17).

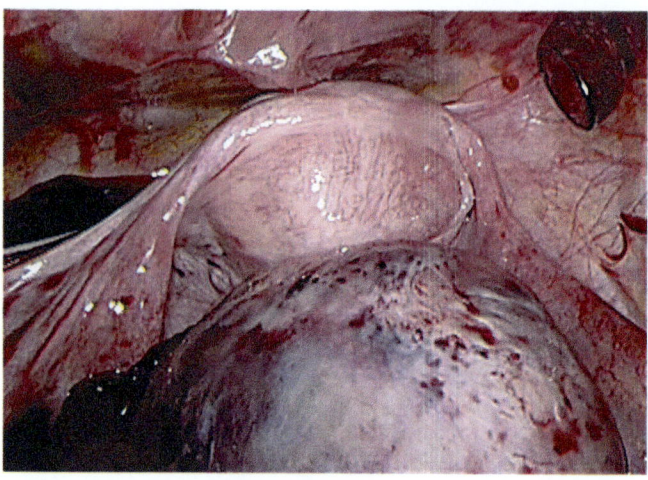

Fig. 17.14 Massive endometriotic ovarian cyst

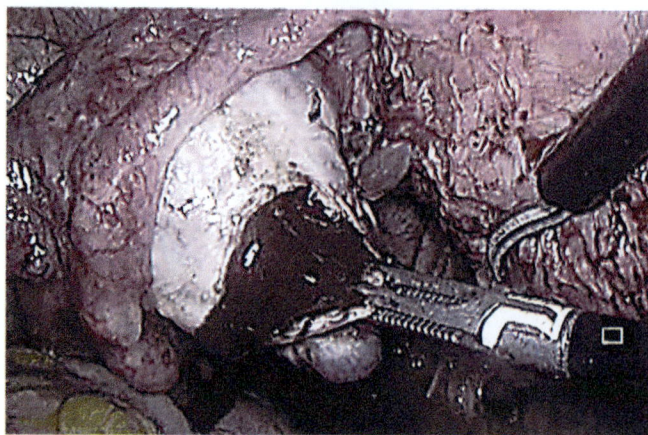

Fig. 17.17 Endoscopic image of chocolate cyst

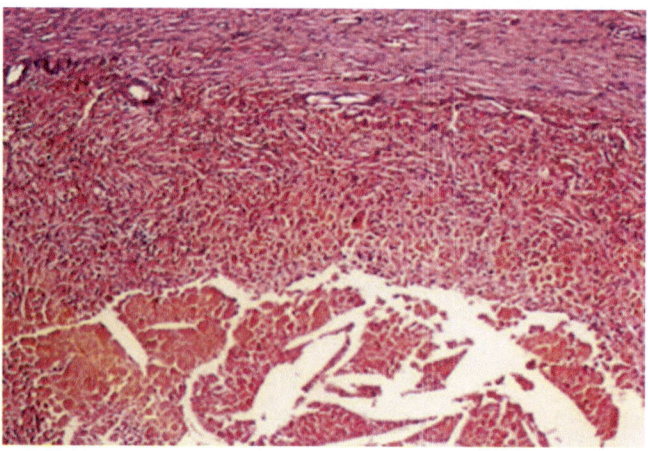

Fig. 17.15 The hemorrhagic event within an endometriotic cyst produces a slow re-adjustment of the blood with formation of a thick layer of siderotic macrophages and failure to reconstitute the endometrial mucosa. In these cases, the pathologist formulates a diagnosis of "endometriotic cyst" even without recognizing the endometrium

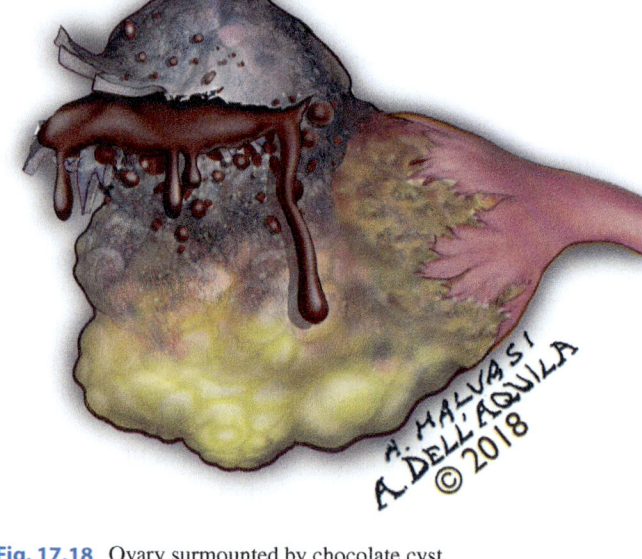

Fig. 17.18 Ovary surmounted by chocolate cyst

Thus, endometriosis may cause subfertility, and adversely affect outcomes of ART by its detrimental effects on oocyte morphology [78].

Santonastaso et al. analyzed and integrated different clinical chemistry parameters being specific of the metabolic profile, the inflammatory state, and the cell damage by H-Nuclear Magnetic Resonance (NMR) spectroscopy approach and biochemistry analysis, respectively, in follicular fluids of women with different stages endometriosis (I-II and III-IV) unrolled to IVF cycle (Figs. 17.18 and 17.19).

Their analysis evidenced that in the follicular fluids of the patients with endometriosis the levels of phospholipids, lactate, insulin, PTX3, CXCL8, CXCL10, CCL11, and VEGF were higher, whereas those of some fatty acids, lysine, choline, glucose, aspartate, alanine, leucine, valine, proline, phosphocholine, total LDH as well as its LDH-3 isoform were lower in comparison to control group. The levels of

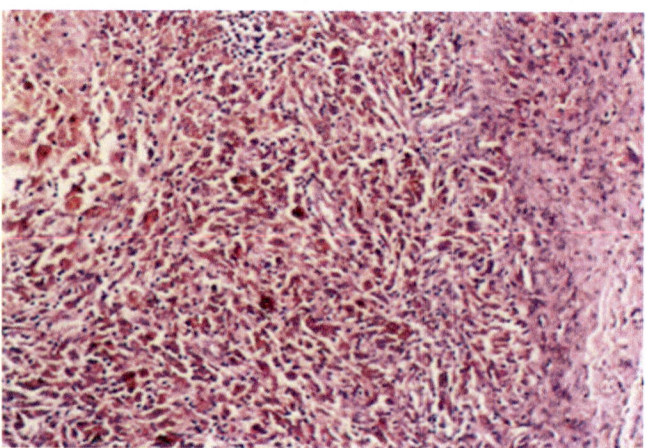

Fig. 17.16 At higher magnification we can see the large quantity of brownish pigment inside the macrophages

Fig. 17.19 Above, the graphic reconstruction of the endometriosic ovarian cyst; in the center the representation of transvaginal ultrasound used to diagnose the ovarian cyst of endometriotic appearance; below, the ultrasound image of the endometriotic cyst

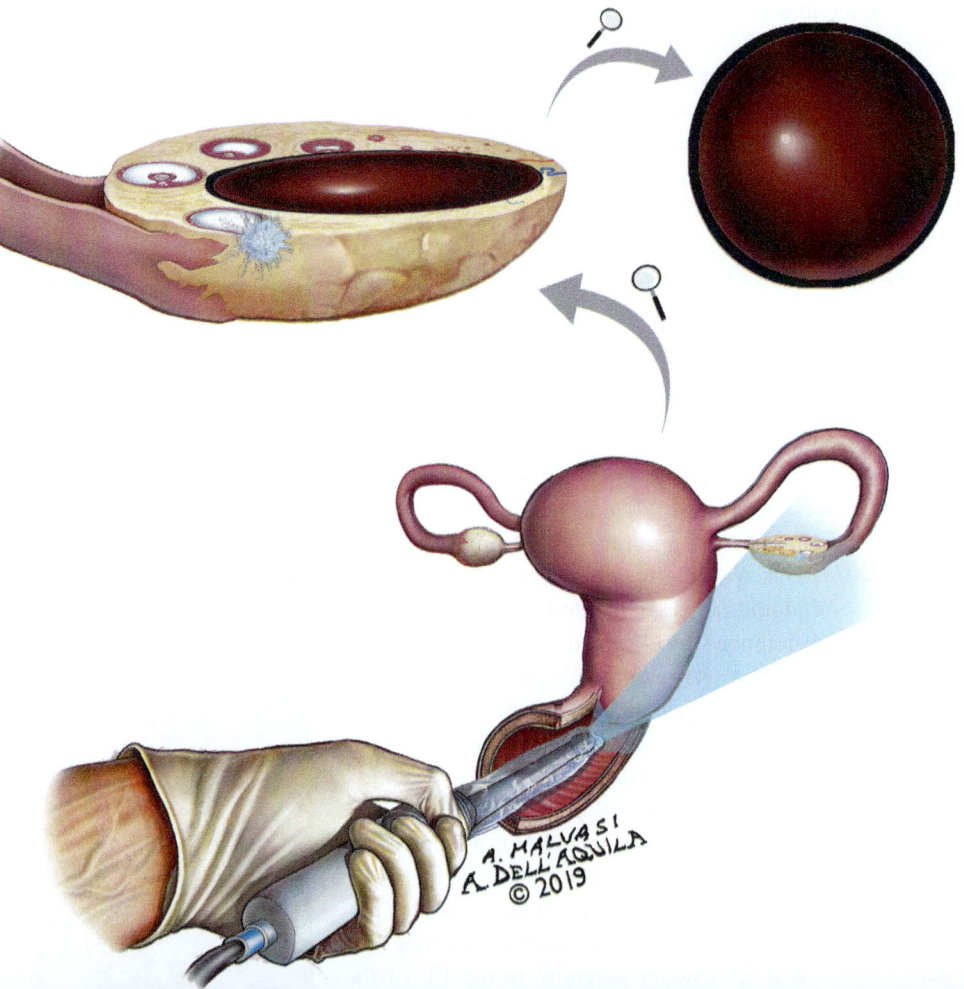

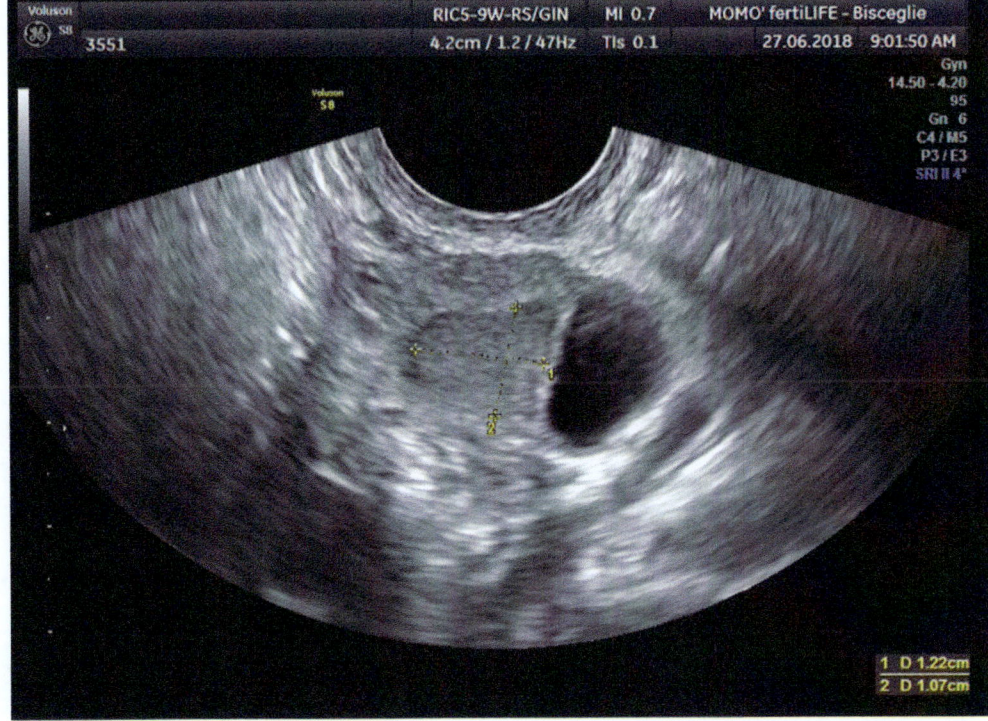

LDHB, PTX3, and insulin receptor were confirmed also by RT-PCR applied on cumulus cells surrounding oocytes retrieved from the patients. The reduced oocyte quality observed in patients with endometriosis can be certainly correlated to the different levels of these molecules [79].

Schebl et al. investigated morphological parameters of oocyte morphology in patients with endometriosis, describing oocyte morphology in patients undergoing intracytoplasmic sperm injection. Patients with endometriosis had a significantly lower rate of mature oocytes ($p < 0.03$) and morphologically normal oocytes ($p < 0.001$). In particular, brownish oocytes ($p < 0.009$; stage I-IV) and the presence of refractile bodies ($p < 0.001$; stage IV) were found to be increased. Endometriosis stage IV was associated with significantly worse-quality oocytes than stages I-III ($p < 0.01$). Fertilization was significantly reduced in conventional in vitro fertilization but not in intracytoplasmic sperm injection ($p < 0.03$). This was due to lower fertilization rates in stage III-IV endometriosis compared with stage I-II ($p < 0.04$). No difference was observed with respect to rates of implantation, clinical pregnancy, miscarriage, live birth, and malformation. Authors concluded that patients with endometriosis, in particular those with severe endometriosis, present lower-quality oocytes [80].

Nakagawa et al. measured the OS in the FF from a single follicle of patients with endometrioma (EM); we evaluated whether an EM might affect the environment of follicular growth. The FF was obtained during the first puncture of follicular aspiration and was evaluated. Authors showed that oxidative stress and antioxidant potential in the FF of the patients with unilateral EM showed values similar to those without an EM, and concluded that EMs do not affect the environment for follicle growth during ART treatment [81].

Nasiri et al. evaluated the levels of two OS markers including lipid peroxide (LPO) and total antioxidant capacity (TAC) in both serum and FF of women with endometriosis after puncture. They observed that women with endometriosis had significantly higher LPO and lower TAC levels in the serum and FF as compared with the control group. Therefore, authors noted that FF of women with endometriosis, regardless of disease stage, increases the proliferation power of endometrial cells in vitro, and presumed that inflammatory reactions-induced OS in ovary may be responsible for proliferation induction ability in FF obtained from women with endometriosis [82] (Figs. 17.20, 17.21, 17.22, 17.23, 17.24, 17.25, and 17.26).

Da Luz et al. compared the expression levels of PTGS2 in cumulus cells of infertile women, with and without endometriosis, undergoing ovarian stimulation for ICSI. A decreased expression of PTGS2 was found in cumulus cells of infertile women with endometriosis compared with controls, which might be related to reduced levels of COX-2 in the cumulus cells of women with the disease. Consequently, authors

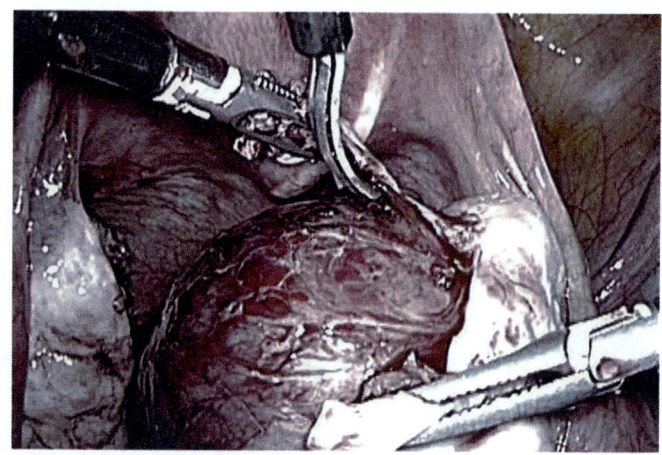

Fig. 17.20 Stripping technique for the removal of endometriotic cyst

Fig. 17.21 The causes of follicle loss during surgery for endometriosis involve injury to blood vessels and stroma and removal of healthy cortex. (1) Endometrioma. (2) Pseudocapsule of endometriosic ovarian cyst. (3) Healthy cortex containing significant number of follicles stripped with pseudocapsule. (4) Coagulation of vascular bed. (5) Blood vessels injuries. (6) Edema/inflammation

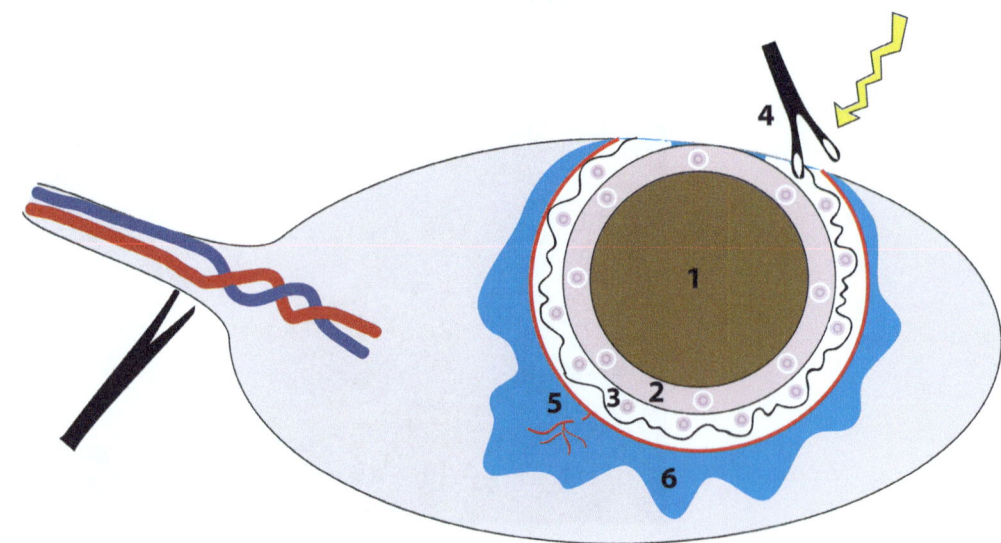

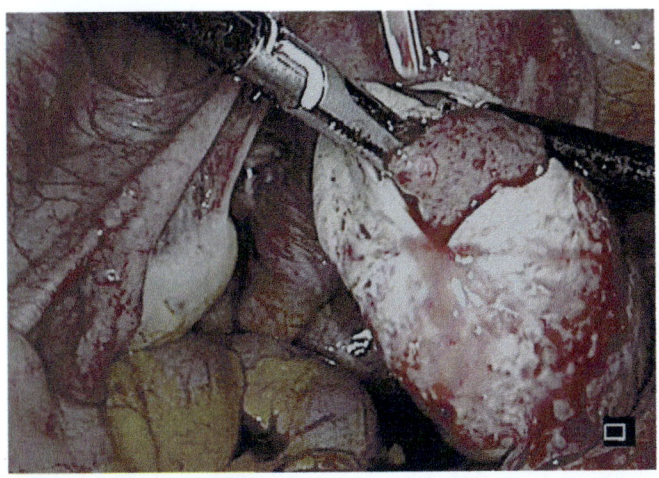

Fig. 17.22 Stripping technique for the removal of endometriotic cyst

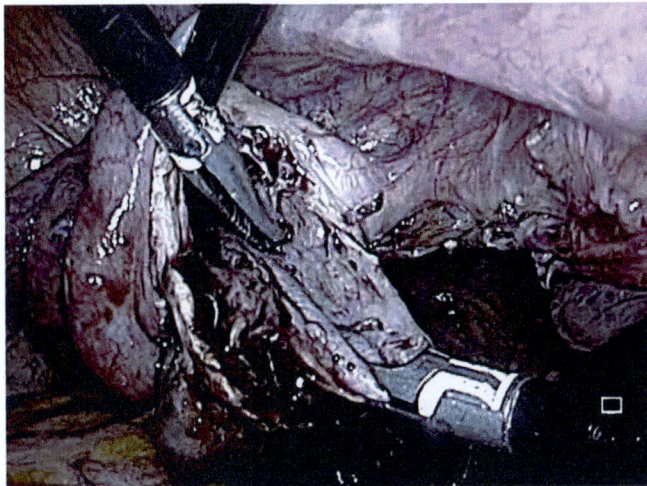

Fig. 17.23 Operative laparoscopy for endometriosis

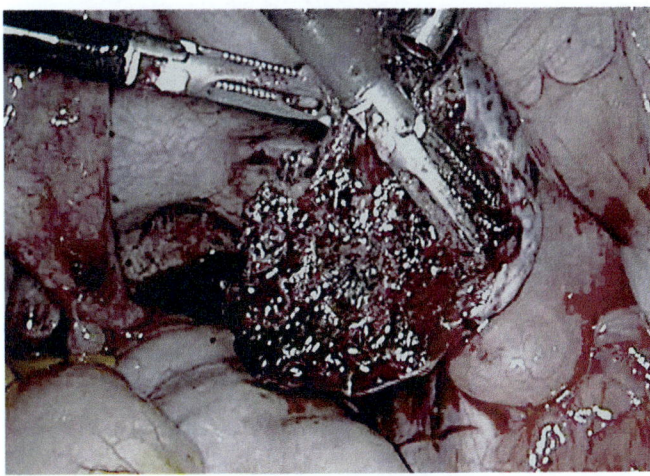

Fig. 17.24 Operative laparoscopy for endometriosis

hypothesized that lower transcript levels of PTGS2 in cumulus cells may be involved in the impairment of oocyte quality, suggesting a possible mechanism involved in disease-related infertility [83].

Pauli et al. analyzed and compared peripheral plasma (PP) and FF retinoid levels, retinol (ROL) including all-trans retinoic acid (ATRA), all essential for a number of reproductive processes, in women undergoing IVF. They investigated also the relationship between retinoid levels and embryo quality.

An analysis compared the retinoid levels with day 3 embryo grades between two groups of women, patients with endometriosis and control patients. Results demonstrated distinctive levels of retinoid metabolites and isomers in FF versus PP. There was a significantly larger percentage of high-quality grade I embryos derived from the largest versus smallest follicles. An increase in follicle size also correlated with a >50% increase in FF ROL and ATRA concentrations. Independent of follicle size, FF yielding grade I versus non-grade I embryos showed higher mean levels of ATRA but not ROL. In a nested case-control analysis, control participants had 50% higher mean levels of ATRA in their FF and PP than women with endometriosis. These findings strongly supported the proposition that ATRA should play a fundamental role in oocyte development and quality, and that reduced ATRA synthesis may contribute to decreased fecundity of participants with endometriosis [84].

Du et al. evaluated the effect of endometriosis on folliculogenesis and pregnancy, and to assess the involvement of inflammatory factors (IL1b, PGE2, PGF2a, and TGFb2) in follicular fluid. Authors aspirated FF in patients with endometriosis to measure the concentrations of inflammatory factors (IL1b, PGE2, PGF2α, and TGFβ2) and steroid hormones (E2, progesterone, FSH, and LH) within follicular fluid, as well as serum E2 and LH concentrations. The oocyte retrieval, rate of metaphase II oocyte, cleavage rate, effective embryo rate, and pregnancy rates of patients with endometriosis were all significantly lower than those of the control patients. In those with endometriosis, serum E2 concentrations were lower than those observed in controls. Aromatase levels in the granulosa cells of the endometriosis group were lower while concentrations of PGE2 in follicular fluid were higher than in the control group. Concentrations of PGE2, PGF2α, TGFβ2, and IL1b were significantly correlated with each other. The study conclusion was that the outcomes of ART, in relation to serum E2 concentration, were adversely affected by the presence of endometriosis [85] (Fig. 17.27).

Furthermore, severe ovarian damage and extensive follicle loss have been reported after cystectomy for endometriomas, resulting in a shorter reproductive life span or even immediate ovarian failure as reported in few cases [86–89].

The follicle loss during surgery for endometriosis has a negative impact of reproduction (Fig. 17.4).

Fig. 17.25 Adenomyotic nodule, small or large, which develops in deep adenomyosis in viscera (intestine, bladder) equipped with muscular tunic. The release of cytokines with stimulatory activity in the endometriotic focus causes reactive hyperplasia in the smooth muscle cells of the host organ. These fibers have an irregular pattern and do not respect the normal functional dynamics of the organ causing dyskinesias. Macroscopically, the hypertrophic lesion has a neoplastic-like character and causes extensive resections of the organ. Histologically, Peripherical endometrial stroma may be poor or absent, causing uncertainties about the invasive character of the glands

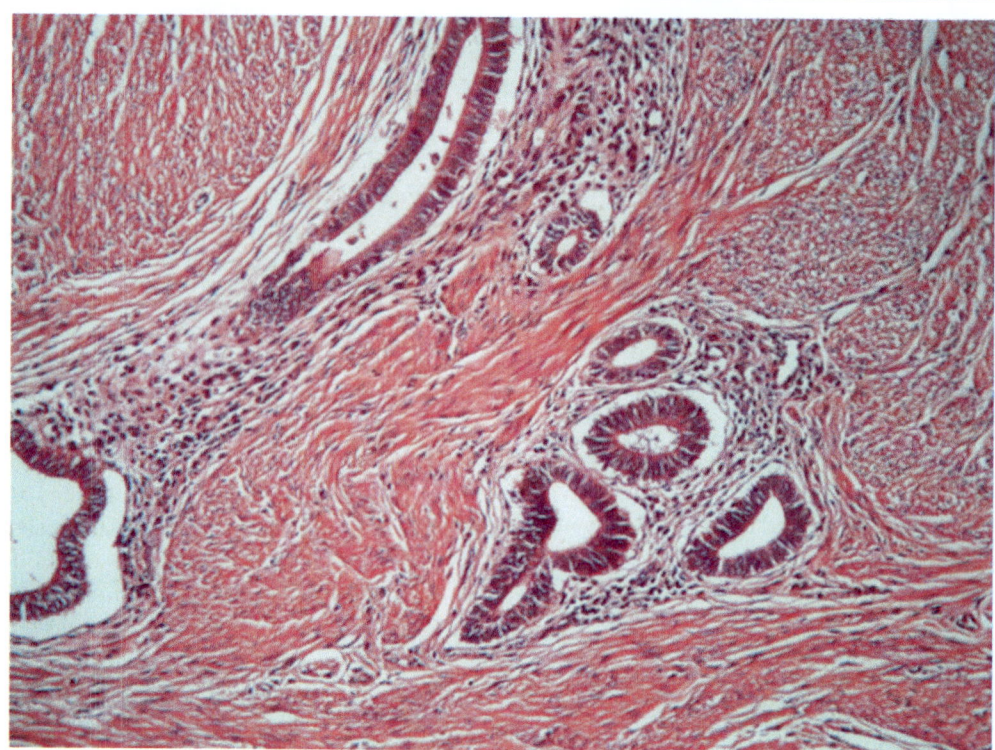

Fig. 17.26 The hemosiderin is not the only pigment present in endometriotic outbreaks. In the stroma of this outbreak, a light brown pigment is observed, vitreous with the characteristics of the ceroid pigment, linked to the deposition of complex fats coming from the erythrocyte wall

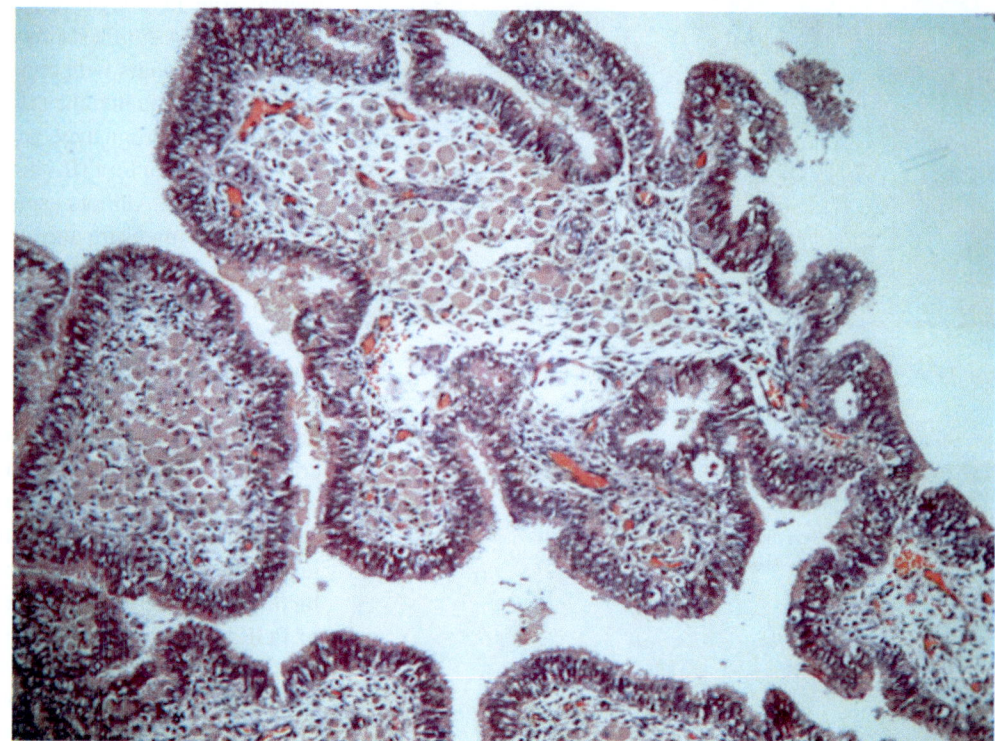

The amount of healthy tissue inadvertently lost during surgery is larger with excision of bilateral endometriomas and is also related to electrosurgical coagulation and the local inflammation associated with the procedure [90].

The endometrioma cyst wall contains different amounts of follicles, which are lost during surgery. The number of follicles in histological sections obtained from the cyst wall is related to patient's age: the younger the patient, the larger the number of follicles present in the endometrioma wall [91].

Young women also have a higher recurrence rate of their endometriomas (30–50%) that often leads to repeated ovarian surgery which further compromises ovarian reserve [92].

Fig. 17.27 An endometrioma exerting pressure on ovarian follicles on the day of oocyte aspiration

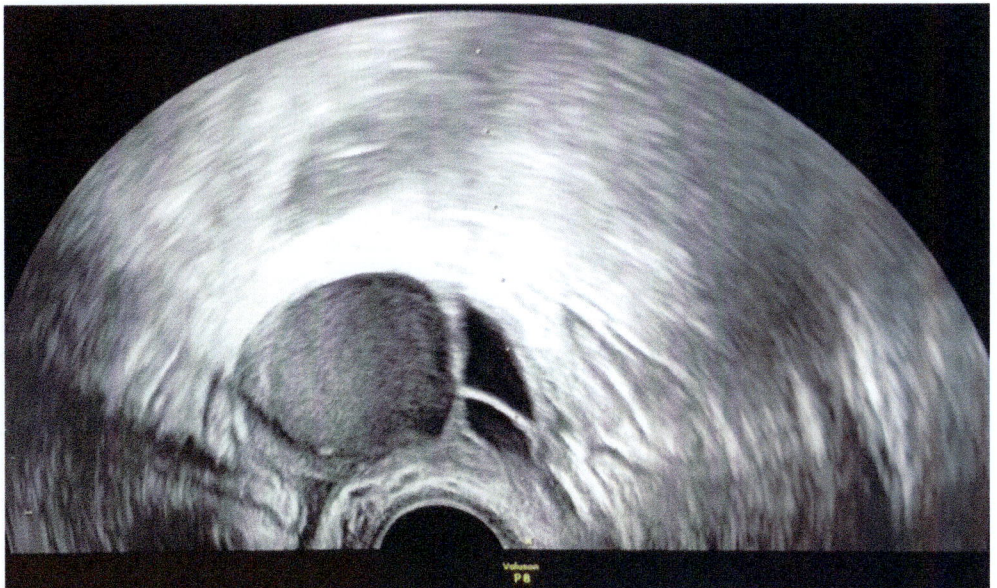

Lastly, extensive adhesiolysis even without direct surgery to the ovaries has been associated with a significant decline in ovarian reserve. This may derive from injury to ovarian vascular bed, resulting in reduced ovarian blood supply post-surgery [93].

17.2 Transvaginal Ultrasound-Guided Oocyte Retrieval in Patients with Endometriosis

The development of transvaginal ultrasound-guided oocyte retrieval transformed IVF in the 1980s. It became possible to retrieve oocytes from the ovaries using outpatient, minimally invasive approaches, utilizing IV sedation or even just local anesthetics [94]. Previously, laparoscopy was necessary with its increased cost and need for general anesthesia. Whether oocyte retrieval is being performed laparoscopically or trans-vaginally, the ovary needs to be held in place in order for the follicle to be punctured and aspirated. Several consequences of advanced stages of endometriosis include scarring of the ovary and adnexa within the cul-de-sac or obscuring by bowel or omental adhesions [95, 96]. Paradoxically during transvaginal oocyte retrieval, adhesion formation may actually immobilize the ovaries facilitating the aspiration of the follicles.

Endometriosis and associated endometriomas are common in patients coming for oocyte retrieval as part of the IVF process [97]. The development of large endometriomas is unusual outside the ovary, and the pathogenesis behind their development inside the ovary is unknown; however, different hypotheses do exist. It has been shown, while the formation of superficial cysts of superficial ovarian endometriosis is similar to extra-ovarian site endometriosis, the development of large endometriomas may be the result of secondary involvement of functional (follicular or luteal) ovarian cysts by the endometriotic process. Additionally, the ovary has several unique physiologic processes, such as high concentrations of ovarian steroids and growth factors which may impact the initiation, maintenance, and growth of endometrial implants; as well as, the regular follicular rupture at time of ovulation, also known as ovulation dehiscence, causes metaplasia of the ovarian mesothelium, or stigma, potentially allowing for the progressive invagination of the ovarian cortex and the invasion of follicles or corpora lutea from endometriotic cells [98, 99]. To note, the chance of correspondence between follicular dehiscence and an endometrial implant may be higher in natural cycles due to the concomitance of molecules involved in both endometriosis-associated inflammation and ovulation dehiscence. Furthermore, such correspondence can also occur during IUI but not during IVF cycles, when the stigma is controlled by physicians [100, 101]. These two unique features of the ovary in combination may play a role in the development of large ovarian endometriomas. Different clinical types of suspected endometriomas have been observed and classifications have been developed based on size, cyst contents, ease of capsule removal, adhesions of the cyst to surrounding structures, and location of superficial endometrial implants relative to the cyst [102, 103]; see Table 17.2.

At times, the surgical approach in these cases depends on the size and location of the endometrioma (Fig. 17.5). Ordinarily, follicles will be aspirated sequentially, moving from one to the next emptying the follicular contents. The larger problem faced during transvaginal oocyte retrieval in patients with endometriosis is the presence of endometriomas in the needle path from the vagina toward the target follicle [104]. Generally, the goal is to avoid the endometrioma and "go around it" if possible (Fig. 17.28).

Table 17.2 Classification of clinical types of suspected endometriomas [102]

TYPE I Primary endometrioma (or true endometrioma, like that found on peritoneal surfaces). Is called also "pure" endometriomas are characterized as small superficial cysts containing dark "chocolate" fluid. Typically, they firmly adhere to the tissue on the surface of the ovary making them difficult to remove surgically. Histological analysis reveals only endometrial glands and stroma

TYPE II Secondary endometrioma (or follicular or luteal ovarian cysts). They have been involved or invaded by cortical endometriotic implants or by primary endometriosis

TYPE IIa	*TYPE IIb*	*TYPE IIc*
– Usually large, with a capsule that is easily separated from the ovarian tissue – Follicular or luteal in origin – Endometrial implants (if present) do not penetrate the cyst wall – Histological analysis: walls are found to be clear of any endometrial tissue	– Have features of functional cysts but show deep involvement with surface endometriosis – Cyst lining is easily separated from the ovarian capsule and stroma, except where the ovarian capsule has adhered to the cyst wall adjacent to the area of endometriosis – Histological findings: endometriosis implants in the cyst wall	– Similar to Type IIb, functional cysts with extensive surface endometrial implants – PLUS deep penetration of endometriosis into the cyst wall, spreading to at least one area of the ovarian capsule – Histological findings: endometriotic extension into the wall of the ovarian cyst strong correlation with clinical findings of the presence of dense adhesions

There are difference between *TYPE IIa* and other *TYPE IIb* and *c*; but the difference between *TYPE IIb* and *TYPE IIc* is slight and depend on the degree of endometrial invasion into the cyst wall and progressive difficulty in removing the cysts capsule

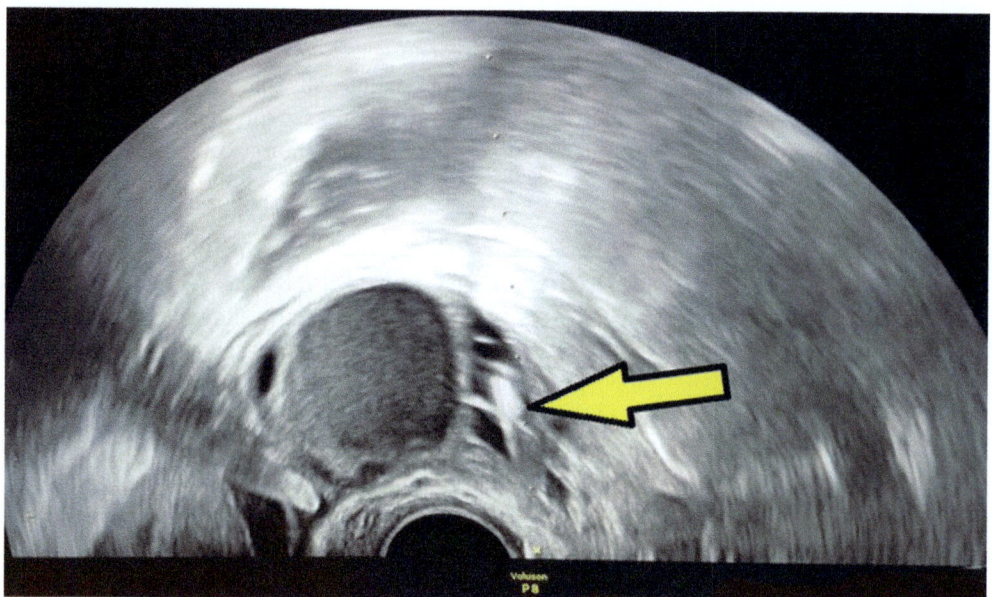

Fig. 17.28 Oocyte aspiration needle tip in follicle adjunct to ovarian endometrioma. (Image courtesy of Prof. Daniel Seidman, Tel Aviv, Israel)

The reason for this approach is because spillage of the endometrioma fluid can be toxic to the oocytes, the endometrium, and the peritoneal cavity [105]. Occasionally, it is hard to avoid the endometriomas and several methods exist to combat this inconvenience. (1) The vaginal ultrasound technique may be used to traverse the cyst with the aspirating needle without aspirating the cyst itself. This is usually successful and avoids the issues mentioned above; or (2) if the endometrioma is so large as to prevent a clear path to the normal follicle, it may be drained into a separate aspiration tube and the aspiration needle thoroughly rinsed prior to using it to aspirate a normal follicle.

IVF is an outstanding treatment option with excellent success rates for couples suffering from infertility caused by endometriosis [106]. Treatment for endometriosis via laparoscopy following previous IVF failures has been shown to increase odds of conceiving naturally and/or via IVF [107]. With a little planning and attention to detail, transvaginal ultrasound-guided oocyte retrieval can be carried out safely and efficiently in women with all stages of endometriosis.

References

1. Hirsch M, Begum MR, Paniz É, Barker C, Davis CJ, Duffy J. Diagnosis and management of endometriosis: a systematic review of international and national guidelines. BJOG. 2018;125(5):556–64.
2. Cho YJ, Lee SH, Park JW, Han M, Park MJ, Han SJ. Dysfunctional signaling underlying endometriosis: current state of knowledge. J Mol Endocrinol. 2018;60(3):R97–R113.

3. Patel BG, Lenk EE, Lebovic DI, Shu Y, Yu J, Taylor RN. Pathogenesis of endometriosis: interaction between endocrine and inflammatory pathways. Best Pract Res Clin Obstet Gynaecol. 2018;50:50–60. https://doi.org/10.1016/j.bpobgyn.2018.01.006. pii: S1521-6934(18)30023-3.

4. Clemenza S, Sorbi F, Noci I, Capezzuoli T, Turrini I, Carriero C, Buffi N, Fambrini M, Petraglia F. From pathogenesis to clinical practice: emerging medical treatments for endometriosis. Best Pract Res Clin Obstet Gynaecol. 2018;51:92–101. https://doi.org/10.1016/j.bpobgyn.2018.01.021. pii: S1521-6934(18)30039-7.

5. Greene AD, Lang SA, Kendziorski JA, Sroga-Rios JM, Herzog TJ, Burns KA. Endometriosis: where are we and where are we going? Reproduction. 2016;152(3):R63–78. https://doi.org/10.1530/REP-16-0052.

6. Donnez J, Donnez O, Orellana R, Binda MM, Dolmans MM. Endometriosis and infertility. Panminerva Med. 2016;58(2):143–50.

7. Matalliotakis M, Zervou MI, Matalliotaki C, Rahmioglu N, Koumantakis G, Kalogiannidis I, Prapas I, Zondervan K, Spandidos DA, Matalliotakis I, Goulielmos GN. The role of gene polymorphisms in endometriosis. Mol Med Rep. 2017;16(5):5881–6.

8. Hughes EG, Fedorkow DM, Collins JA. A quantitative overview of controlled trials in endometriosis-associated infertility. Fertil Steril. 1993;59(5):963–70.

9. Barnhart K, Dunsmoor-Su R, Coutifaris C. Effect of endometriosis on in vitro fertilization. Fertil Steril. 2002;77:1148–55.

10. Giudice LC, Kao LC. Endometriosis. Lancet. 2004;364(9447):1789–99.

11. Opoien HK, Fedorcsak P, Omland AK, Abyholm T, Bjercke S, Ertzeid G, Oldereid N, Mellembakken JR, Tanbo T. In vitro fertilization is a successful treatment in endometriosis-associated infertility. Fertil Steril. 2012;97:912–8.

12. Lin XN, Wei ML, Tong XM, Xu WH, Zhou F, Huang QX, Wen GF, Zhang SY. Outcome of in vitro fertilization in endometriosis-associated infertility: a 5-year database cohort study. Chin Med J (Engl). 2012;125:2688–93.

13. Dong X, Liao X, Wang R, Zhang H. The impact of endometriosis on IVF/ICSI outcomes. Int J Clin Exp Pathol. 2013;6(9):1911–8.

14. Barbosa MA, Teixeira DM, Navarro PA, Ferriani RA, Nastri CO, Martins WP. Impact of endometriosis and its staging on assisted reproduction outcome: systematic review and meta-analysis. Ultrasound Obstet Gynecol. 2014;44(3):261–78.

15. Tanbo T, Fedorcsak P. Endometriosis-associated infertility: aspects of pathophysiological mechanisms and treatment options. Acta Obstet Gynecol Scand. 2017;96(6):659–67.

16. Jeung I, Cheon K, Kim MR. Decreased cytotoxicity of peripheral and peritoneal natural killer cell in endometriosis. Biomed Res Int. 2016;2016:2916070.

17. D'Hooghe TM, Debrock S, Hill JA, Meuleman C. Endometriosis and subfertility: is the relationship resolved? Semin Reprod Med. 2003;21(2):243–54.

18. Khan KN, Kitajima M, Hiraki K, Fujishita A, Sekine I, Ishimaru T, Masuzaki H. Immunopathogenesis of pelvic endometriosis: role of hepatocyte growth factor, macrophages and ovarian steroids. Am J Reprod Immunol. 2008;60(5):383–404.

19. Oosterlynck DJ, Cornillie FJ, Waer M, Vandeputte M, Koninckx PR. Women with endometriosis show a defect in natural killer activity resulting in a decreased cytotoxicity to autologous endometrium. Fertil Steril. 1991;56(1):45–51.

20. Oosterlynck DJ, Meuleman C, Waer M, Vandeputte M, Koninckx PR. The natural killer activity of peritoneal fluid lymphocytes is decreased in women with endometriosis. Fertil Steril. 1992;58(2):290–5.

21. Bulletti C, Coccia ME, Battistoni S, Borini A. Endometriosis and infertility. J Assist Reprod Genet. 2010;27(8):441–7.

22. Garrido N, Navarro J, Remohí J, Simón C, Pellicer A. Follicular hormonal environment and embryo quality in women with endometriosis. Hum Reprod Update. 2000;6(1):67–74.

23. Da Broi MG, Navarro PA. Oxidative stress and oocyte quality: ethiopathogenic mechanisms of minimal/mild endometriosis-related infertility. Cell Tissue Res. 2016;364(1):1–7.

24. Sanchez AM, Vanni VS, Bartiromo L, Papaleo E, Zilberberg E, Candiani M, Orvieto R, Viganò P. Is the oocyte quality affected by endometriosis? A review of the literature. J Ovarian Res. 2017;10(1):43.

25. Stilley JA, Birt JA, Sharpe-Timms KL. Cellular and molecular basis for endometriosis-associated infertility. Cell Tissue Res. 2012;349(3):849–62.

26. Miller JE, Ahn SH, Monsanto SP, Khalaj K, Koti M, Tayade C. Implications of immune dysfunction on endometriosis associated infertility. Oncotarget. 2017;8(4):7138–47.

27. Prasad S, Tiwari M, Pandey AN, Shrivastav TG, Chaube SK. Impact of stress on oocyte quality and reproductive outcome. J Biomed Sci. 2016;23:36.

28. Missmer SA, Chavarro JE, Malspeis S, Bertone-Johnson ER, Hornstein MD, Spiegelman D, Barbieri RL, Willett WC, Hankinson SE. A prospective study of dietary fat consumption and endometriosis risk. Hum Reprod. 2010;25(6):1528–35.

29. Hauzman EE, Garcia-Velasco JA, Pellicer A. Oocyte donation and endometriosis: what are the lessons? Semin Reprod Med. 2013;31(2):173–7.

30. Afshar Y, Hastings J, Roqueiro D, Jeong JW, Giudice LC, Fazleabas AT. Changes in eutopic endometrial gene expression during the progression of experimental endometriosis in the baboon, Papio anubis. Biol Reprod. 2013;88(2):44.

31. Bulun SE, Monsivais D, Kakinuma T, Furukawa Y, Bernardi L, Pavone ME, Dyson M. Molecular biology of endometriosis: from aromatase to genomic abnormalities. Semin Reprod Med. 2015;33(3):220–4.

32. Bulun SE. Endometriosis. N Engl J Med. 2009;360(3):268–79.

33. Pavone ME, Dyson M, Reirstad S, Pearson E, Ishikawa H, Cheng YH, Bulun SE. Endometriosis expresses a molecular pattern consistent with decreased retinoid uptake, metabolism and action. Hum Reprod. 2011;26(8):2157–64.

34. Chen GY, Nuñez G. Sterile inflammation: sensing and reacting to damage. Nat Rev Immunol. 2010;10(12):826–37.

35. Haney AF, Muscato JJ, Weinberg JB. Peritoneal fluid cell populations in infertility patients. Fertil Steril. 1981;35(6):696–8.

36. Beste MT, Pfäffle-Doyle N, Prentice EA, Morris SN, Lauffenburger DA, Isaacson KB, Griffith LG. Molecular network analysis of endometriosis reveals a role for c-Jun-regulated macrophage activation. Sci Transl Med. 2014;6(222):222ra16.

37. Osborn BH, Haney AF, Misukonis MA, Weinberg JB. Inducible nitric oxide synthase expression by peritoneal macrophages in endometriosis-associated infertility. Fertil Steril. 2002;77(1):46–51.

38. Goud AP, Goud PT, Diamond MP, Gonik B, Abu-Soud HM. Activation of the cGMP signaling pathway is essential in delaying oocyte aging in diabetes mellitus. Biochemistry. 2006;45(38):11366–78.

39. Somigliana E, Viganò P, Gaffuri B, Candiani M, Busacca M, Di Blasio AM, Vignali M. Modulation of NK cell lytic function by endometrial secretory factors: potential role in endometriosis. Am J Reprod Immunol. 1996;36(5):295–300.

40. Kokcu A. Possible effects of endometriosis-related immune events on reproductive function. Arch Gynecol Obstet. 2013;287(6):1225–33.

41. Heitmann RJ, Tobler KJ, Gillette L, Tercero J, Burney RO. Dexamethasone attenuates the embryotoxic effect of endometriotic peritoneal fluid in a murine model. J Assist Reprod Genet. 2015;32(9):1317–23.

42. Riccio LDGC, Santulli P, Marcellin L, Abrão MS, Batteux F, Chapron C. Immunology of endometriosis. Best Pract Res Clin Obstet Gynaecol. 2018;50:39–49. https://doi.org/10.1016/j.bpobgyn.2018.01.010. pii: S1521-6934(18)30028-2.

43. Harris SE, Faddy M, Levett S, et al. Analysis of donor heterogeneity as a factor affecting the clinical outcome of oocyte donation. Hum Fertil (Camb). 2002;5:193–8.

44. Wang Q, Sun QY. Evaluation of oocyte quality: morphological, cellular and molecular predictors. Reprod Fertil Dev. 2007;19:1–12.

45. Cohen Y, Malcov M, Schwartz T, Mey-Raz N, Carmon A, Cohen T, et al. Spindle imaging: a new marker for optimal timing of ICSI? Hum Reprod. 2004;19:649–54.

46. De Santis L, Cino I, Rabellotti E, Calzi F, Persico P, Borini A, et al. Polar body morphology and spindle imaging as predictors of oocyte quality. Reprod Biomed Online. 2005;11:36–42.

47. Dmowski WP, Rana N, Michalowska J, Friberg J, Papierniak C, el-Roeiy A. The effect of endometriosis, its stage and activity, and of autoantibodies on in vitro fertilisation and embryo transfer success rates. Fertil Steril. 1995;63:555–62.

48. Bergendal A, Naffah S, Nagy C, Bergqvist A, Sjöblom P, Hillensjö T. Outcome of IVF in patients with endometriosis in comparison with tubal factor infertility. J Assist Reprod Genet. 1998;15:530–4.

49. Simón C, Gutiérrez A, Vidal A, de los Santos MJ, Tarín JJ, Remohí J, Pellicer A. Outcome of patients with endometriosis in assisted reproduction: results from in-vitro fertilization and oocyte donation. Hum Reprod. 1994;9(4):725–9.

50. Garrido N, Navarro J, Remohí J, Simón C, Pellicer A. Follicular hormonal environment and embryo quality in women with endometriosis. Hum Reprod Update. 2000;6(1):67–74.

51. Garrido N, Navarro J, García-Velasco J, Remoh J, Pellice A, Simón C. The endometrium versus embryonic quality in endometriosis-related infertility. Hum Reprod Update. 2002;8(1):95–103.

52. Hamdan M, Omar SZ, Dunselman G, Cheong Y. Influence of endometriosis on assisted reproductive technology outcomes: a systematic review and meta-analysis. Obstet Gynecol. 2015;125:79–88.

53. Xu B, Guo N, Zhang XM, Shi W, Tong XH, Iqbal F, Liu YS. Oocyte quality is decreased in women with minimal or mild endometriosis. Sci Rep. 2015;5:10779.

54. Díaz-Fontdevila M, Pommer R, Smith R. Cumulus cell apoptosis changes with exposure to spermatozoa and pathologies involved in infertility. Fertil Steril. 2009;91(5 Suppl):2061–8.

55. Wu R, Van der Hoek KH, Ryan NK, Norman RJ, Robker RL. Macrophage contributions to ovarian function. Hum Reprod Update. 2004;10(2):119–33.

56. Brizek CL, Schlaff S, Pellegrini VA, Frank JB, Worrilow KC. Increased incidence of aberrant morphological phenotypes in human embryogenesis—an association with endometriosis. J Assist Reprod Genet. 1995;12(2):106–12.

57. Garrido N, Pellicer A, Remohí J, Simón C. Uterine and ovarian function in endometriosis. Semin Reprod Med. 2003;21(2):183–92.

58. Kimura F, Takahashi K, Takebayashi K, Fujiwara M, Kita N, Noda Y, Harada N, et al. Fertil Steril. 2007;87(6):1468.e9–12.

59. Burney RO, Talbi S, Hamilton AE, et al. Gene expression analysis of endometrium reveals progesterone resistance and candidate susceptibility genes in women with endometriosis. Endocrinology. 2007;48:3814–26.

60. Kao LC, Germeyer A, Tulac S, et al. Expression profiling of endometrium from women with endometriosis reveals candidate genes for disease-based implantation failure and infertility. Endocrinology. 2003;144:2870–81.

61. Kemmann E, Ghazi D, Corsan G, et al. Does ovulation stimulation improve fertility in women with minimal/mild endometriosis after laser laparoscopy? Int J Fertil Menopausal Stud. 1993;38:16–21.

62. Evans MB, Decherney AH. Fertility and endometriosis. Clin Obstet Gynecol. 2017;60(3):497–502.

63. Wunder DM, Mueller MD, Birkhäuser MH, Bersinger NA. Steroids and protein markers in the follicular fluid as indicators of oocyte quality in patients with and without endometriosis. J Assist Reprod Genet. 2005;22(6):257–64.

64. von Wolff M, Kollmann Z, Flück CE, Stute P, Marti U, Weiss B, et al. Gonadotrophin stimulation for in vitro fertilization significantly alters the hormone milieu in follicular fluid: a comparative study between natural cycle IVF and conventional IVF. Hum Reprod. 2014;29:1049–57.

65. Härkki P, Tiitinen A, Ylikorkala O. Endometriosis and assisted reproduction techniques. Ann N Y Acad Sci. 2010;1205:207–13.

66. Gupta S, Agarwal A, Krajcir N, Alvarez JG. Role of oxidative stress in endometriosis. Reprod Biomed Online. 2006;13(1):126–34.

67. Agarwal A, Said TM, Bedaiwy MA, Banerjee J, Alvarez JG. Oxidative stress in an assisted reproductive techniques setting. Fertil Steril. 2006;86(3):503–12.

68. Navarro PA, Liu L, Ferriani RA, Keefe DL. Arsenite induces aberrations in meiosis that can be prevented by coadministration of N-acetylcysteine in mice. Fertil Steril. 2006;85(Suppl 1):1187–94.

69. Prieto L, Quesada JF, Cambero O, et al. Analysis of follicular fluid and serum markers of oxidative stress in women with infertility related to endometriosis. Fertil Steril. 2012;98(1):126–30.

70. Donabela FC, Meola J, Padovan CC, de Paz CC, Navarro PA. Higher SOD1 gene expression in cumulus cells from infertile women with moderate and severe endometriosis. Reprod Sci. 2015;22(11):1452–60.

71. Singh AK, Chattopadhyay R, Chakravarty B, Chaudhury K. Markers of oxidative stress in follicular fluid of women with endometriosis and tubal infertility undergoing IVF. Reprod Toxicol. 2013;42:116–24.

72. Saito H, Seino T, Kaneko T, Nakahara K, Toya M, Kurachi H. Endometriosis and oocyte quality. Gynecol Obstet Invest. 2002;53(Suppl 1):46–51.

73. Turkyilmaz E, Yildirim M, Cendek BD, Baran P, Alisik M, Dalgaci F, Yavuz AF. Evaluation of oxidative stress markers and intra-extracellular antioxidant activities in patients with endometriosis. Eur J Obstet Gynecol Reprod Biol. 2016;199:164–8.

74. Wunder DM, Mueller MD, Birkhäuser MH, Bersinger NA. Increased ENA-78 in the follicular fluid of patients with endometriosis. Acta Obstet Gynecol Scand. 2006;85(3):336–42.

75. Da Broi MG, Malvezzi H, Paz CC, Ferriani RA, Navarro PA. Follicular fluid from infertile women with mild endometriosis may compromise the meiotic spindles of bovine metaphase II oocytes. Hum Reprod. 2014;29(2):315–23.

76. Da Broi MG, de Albuquerque FO, de Andrade AZ, Cardoso RL, Jordão Junior AA, Navarro PA. Increased concentration of 8-hydroxy-2′-deoxyguanosine in follicular fluid of infertile women with endometriosis. Cell Tissue Res. 2016;366(1):231–42.

77. Baumann C, Olson M, Wang K, Fazleabas A, De La Fuente R. Arginine methyltransferases mediate an epigenetic ovarian response to endometriosis. Reproduction. 2015;150(4):297–310.

78. Kasapoglu I, Kuspinar G, Saribal S, Turk P, Avcı B, Uncu G. Detrimental effects of endometriosis on oocyte morphology in intracytoplasmic sperm injection cycles: a retrospective cohort study. Gynecol Endocrinol. 2018;34(3):206–211.11.

79. Santonastaso M, Pucciarelli A, Costantini S, Caprio F, Sorice A, Capone F, Natella A, Iardino P, Colacurci N, Chiosi E. Metabolomic profiling and biochemical evaluation of the follicular fluid of endometriosis patients. Mol Biosyst. 2017;13(6):1213–22.

80. Shebl O, Sifferlinger I, Habelsberger A, Oppelt P, Mayer RB, Petek E, Ebner T. Oocyte competence in in vitro fertilization and intracytoplasmic sperm injection patients suffering from endometriosis and its possible association with subsequent treatment outcome: a matched case-control study. Acta Obstet Gynecol Scand. 2017;96(6):736–44.

81. Nakagawa K, Hisano M, Sugiyama R, Yamaguchi K. Measurement of oxidative stress in the follicular fluid of infertility patients with an endometrioma. Arch Gynecol Obstet. 2016;293(1):197–202.

82. Nasiri N, Moini A, Eftekhari-Yazdi P, Karimian L, Salman-Yazdi R, Arabipoor A. Oxidative stress statues in serum and follicular fluid of women with endometriosis. Cell J. 2017;18(4):582–7.

83. da Luz CM, da Broi MG, Donabela FC, Paro de Paz CC, Meola J, Navarro PA. PTGS2 down-regulation in cumulus cells of infertile women with endometriosis. Reprod Biomed Online. 2017;35(4):379–86.

84. Pauli SA, Session DR, Shang W, Easley K, Wieser F, Taylor RN, Pierzchalski K, Napoli JL, Kane MA, Sidell N. Analysis of follicular fluid retinoids in women undergoing in vitro fertilization: retinoic acid influences embryo quality and is reduced in women with endometriosis. Reprod Sci. 2013;20(9):1116–24.

85. Du YB, Gao MZ, Shi Y, Sun ZG, Wang J. Endocrine and inflammatory factors and endometriosis-associated infertility in assisted reproduction techniques. Arch Gynecol Obstet. 2013;287(1):123–30.

86. Hwu YM, Wu FS-Y, Li S-H, Sun F-J, Lin M-H, Lee RK-K. The impact of endometrioma and laparoscopic cystectomy on serum anti-Mullerian hormone levels. Reprod Biol Endocrinol. 2011;9:80.

87. Busacca M, Riparini J, Somigliana E, Oggioni G, Izzo S, Vignali M, et al. Postsurgical ovarian failure after laparoscopic excision of bilateral endometriomas. Am J Obstet Gynecol. 2006;195(2):421–5.

88. Coccia ME, Rizzello F, Mariani G, Bulletti C, Palagiano A, Scarselli G. Ovarian surgery for bilateral endometriomas influences age at menopause. Hum Reprod. 2011;26(11):3000–7.

89. Roman H, Tarta O, Pura I, Opris I, Bourdel N, Marpeau L, et al. Direct proportional relationship between endometrioma size and ovarian parenchyma inadvertently removed during cystectomy, and its implication on the management of enlarged endometriomas. Hum Reprod. 2010;25:1428–32.

90. Li CZ, Liu B, Wen ZQ, Sun Q. The impact of electrocoagulation on ovarian reserve after laparoscopic excision of ovarian cyst: a prospective clinical study of 191 patients. Fertil Steril. 2009;92:1428–35.

91. Romualdi D, Franco Zannoni G, Lanzone A, Selvaggi L, Tagliaferri V, Gaetano Vellone V, et al. Follicular loss in endoscopic surgery for ovarian endometriosis: quantitative and qualitative observations. Fertil Steril. 2011;96(2):374–8.

92. Tandoi I, Somigliana E, Riparini J, Ronzoni S, Vigano P, Candiani M. High rate of endometriosis recurrence in young women. J Pediatr Adolesc Gynecol. 2011;24(6):376–9.

93. Hirokawa W, Iwase A, Goto M, Takikawa S, Nagatomo Y, Nakahara T, et al. The post-operative decline in serum anti-Mullerian hormone correlates with the bilaterality and severity of endometriosis. Hum Reprod. 2011;26(4):904–10.

94. Tanbo T, Henriksen T, Magnus O, Abyholm T. Oocyte retrieval in an IVF program. A comparison of laparoscopic and transvaginal ultrasound-guided follicular puncture. Acta Obstet Gynecol Scand. 1988;67(3):243–6.

95. Ota Y, Andou M, Ota I. Laparoscopic surgery with urinary tract reconstruction and bowel endometriosis resection for deep infiltrating endometriosis. Asian J Endosc Surg. 2018;11(1):7–14.

96. King CR, Lum D. Techniques in minimally invasive surgery for advanced endometriosis. Curr Opin Obstet Gynecol. 2016;28(4):316–22.

97. Khine YM, Taniguchi F, Harada T. Clinical management of endometriosis-associated infertility. Reprod Med Biol. 2016;15(4):217–25.

98. Nezhat F, Nezhat C, Allan CJ, Metzger DA, Sears DL. Clinical and histologic classification of endometriomas: implications for a mechanism of pathogenesis. J Reprod Med. 1992;37(9):771–6.

99. Vigano P, Vanni VS, Corti L, Garavaglia E, Tandoi I, Pagliardini L, et al. Unravelling the ovarian endometrioma pathogenesis: "the long and winding road across the various theories.". J Endometr Pelvic Pain Disord. 2013;5:62–7.

100. Gerard N, Caillaud M, Martoriati A, Goudet G, Lalmanach AC. The interleukin-1 system and female reproduction. J Endocrinol. 2004;180:203–12.

101. Somigliana E, Vigano P, Benaglia L, Busnelli A, Vercellini P, Fedele L. Adhesion prevention in endometriosis: a neglected critical challenge. J Minim Invasive Gynecol. 2012;19:415–21.

102. Nezhat C, Nezhat F, Nezhat CH, Seidman DS. Classification of endometriosis: improving the classification of endometriotic ovarian cysts. Hum Reprod. 1994;9(12):2212–3.

103. Nezhat C, Nezhat F, Nezhat CH. Nezhat's video-assisted and robotic-assisted laparoscopy and hysteroscopy. 4th ed. New York: Cambridge University Press; 2013.

104. Benaglia L, Busnelli A, Biancardi R, Vegetti W, Reschini M, Vercellini P, Somigliana E. Oocyte retrieval difficulties in women with ovarian endometriomas. Reprod Biomed Online. 2018;37(1):77–84.

105. Somigliana E, Vigano P, Filippi F, Papaleo E, Benaglia L, Candiani M, et al. Fertility preservation in women with endometriosis: for all, for some, for none? Hum Reprod. 2015;20:1280–6.

106. Cecchino GN, Garcia-Velasco JA. Endometrioma, fertility, and assisted reproductive treatments: connecting the dots. Curr Opin Obstet Gynecol. 2018;30(4):223–8.

107. Littman E, Giudice L, Lathi R, Berker B, Milki A, Nezhat C. Role of laparoscopic treatment of endometriosis in patients with failed in vitro fertilization cycles. Fertil Steril. 2005;84(6):1574–8.

The Adhesion of the Blastocyst: A Question of Bonds

18

Leonardo Resta, Roberta Rossi, and Graziana Arborea

Contents

Almost 75% of pregnancy loss that occurs before the 20th week of gestation (when the vast majority of miscarriage takes place) is due to the failure of implantation of the embryo in the uterus.

The implantation takes place approximately 6 days after conception when the blastocyst has been formed by cell division of the original cells.

The blastocyst state of the embryo is a microscopic sphere ($d = 250$ μ) and is composed of about 64 cells which are divided into the outer layer of the trophoblast, which will generate both the placenta and the other tissues necessary for the foetus during its inter-uterine life, and an inner mass of cells from which all the cells of the human body will develop (Figs. 18.1 and 18.2). The mechanisms through which implantation is governed and controlled are not yet perfectly understood, though it is evident that during these phases what is crucial are the strong relationships which develop between the specialized cells of the trophoblast and the cells of the endometrium taken together as epithelium, stroma and blood vessels (Fig. 18.3).

Three distinct phases can be identified in blastocyst implantation:

1. *Adhesion of the blastocyst to the endometrium*
2. *Invasion of endometrial mucosa by the trophoblast and embedding*

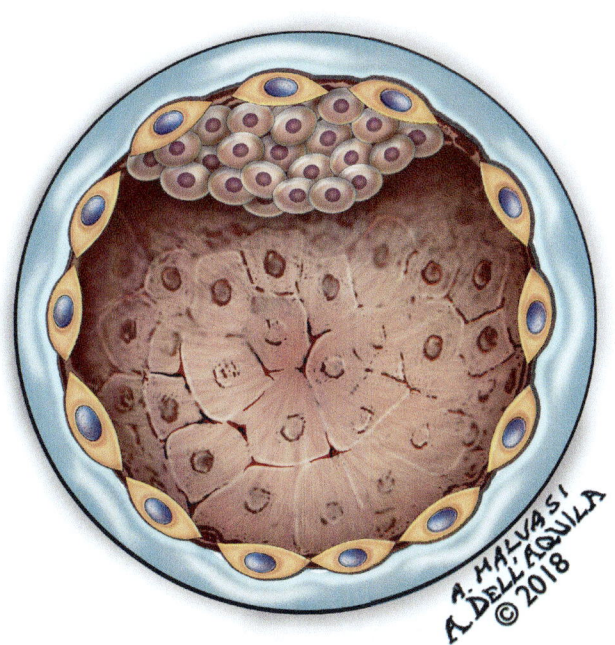

Fig. 18.1 Schematic representation of blastocyst

3. *Maintenance of the implantation through a complex operation consisting of invasion, transformation of the matrix and the vascular structures, overcoming of immunitary defences and auto-limiting of the invasive activity.*

The first phase of adhesion would seem to be the simplest; however, it is premised by a series of exceptionally delicate mother–embryo interactions which can compromise the final result.

In humans, the endometrium shows maximum receptivity for embryo implantation during the mid-secretory phase,

L. Resta (✉) · R. Rossi
Dipartimento dell'Emergenza e dei Trapianti d'Organo (DETO), Università degli Studi di Bari "Aldo Moro", Bari, Italy
e-mail: leonardo.resta@uniba.it; roberta.rossi@uniba.it

G. Arborea
U.O. Anatomia e Istocitopatologia Ospedale "Sacro Cuore di Gesù", Gallipoli, Italy

there being a precise "window of implantation" which corresponds to the 21st day of a hypothetical regular menstrual cycle of 28 days. The window is when there is the maximum

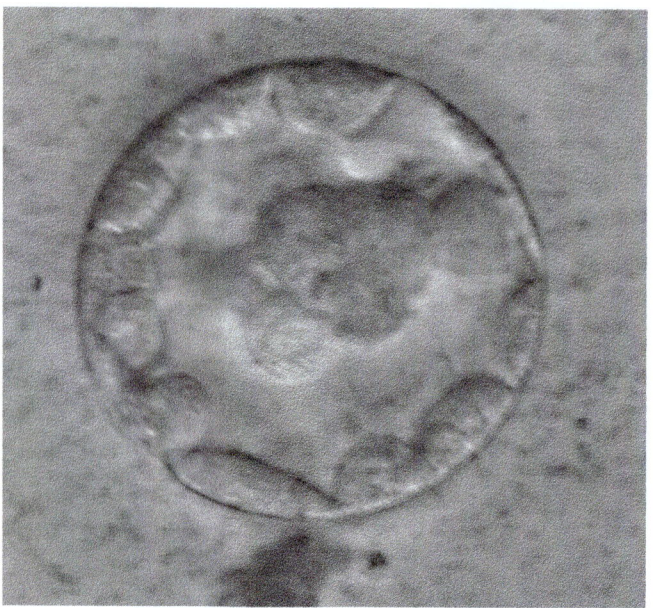

Fig. 18.2 Image of blastocyst under a microscope

level of glandular secretion, interstitial edema and optimal blood flow. These conditions of course do not explain how the adhesion of the blastocyst to the endometrium becomes stable.

In 2003, Genbacev et al. [1] discovered the protein L-selectin functioned as a type of "Velcro" allowing the outer layer trophoblast cells to adhere to the walls of the uterus, thus it is possibly one of the most important ways of mediating early stage embryo–endometrium interaction.

The outer layer of the blastocyst expresses L-selectin and the uterus expresses high quantities of glycoproteins with oligosaccharide domains which interact at a molecular level with the protein so creating "sticky" conditions between them. The blastocyst moves along the uterus sticking and unsticking to it so slowing its progress until finally it sticks to one point and there begins the embedding process. This phase is crucial for embryo development (Figs. 18.4, 18.5, 18.6, and 18.7a, b).

The body's immune response to cell damage makes use of the process of leukocyte extravasation which needs the leukocytes to attach themselves to the vessel walls under conditions of shear stress, as is the case in the need for the blastocyst to attach itself to the uterus. These similar activities have led several scientists to propose similar mecha-

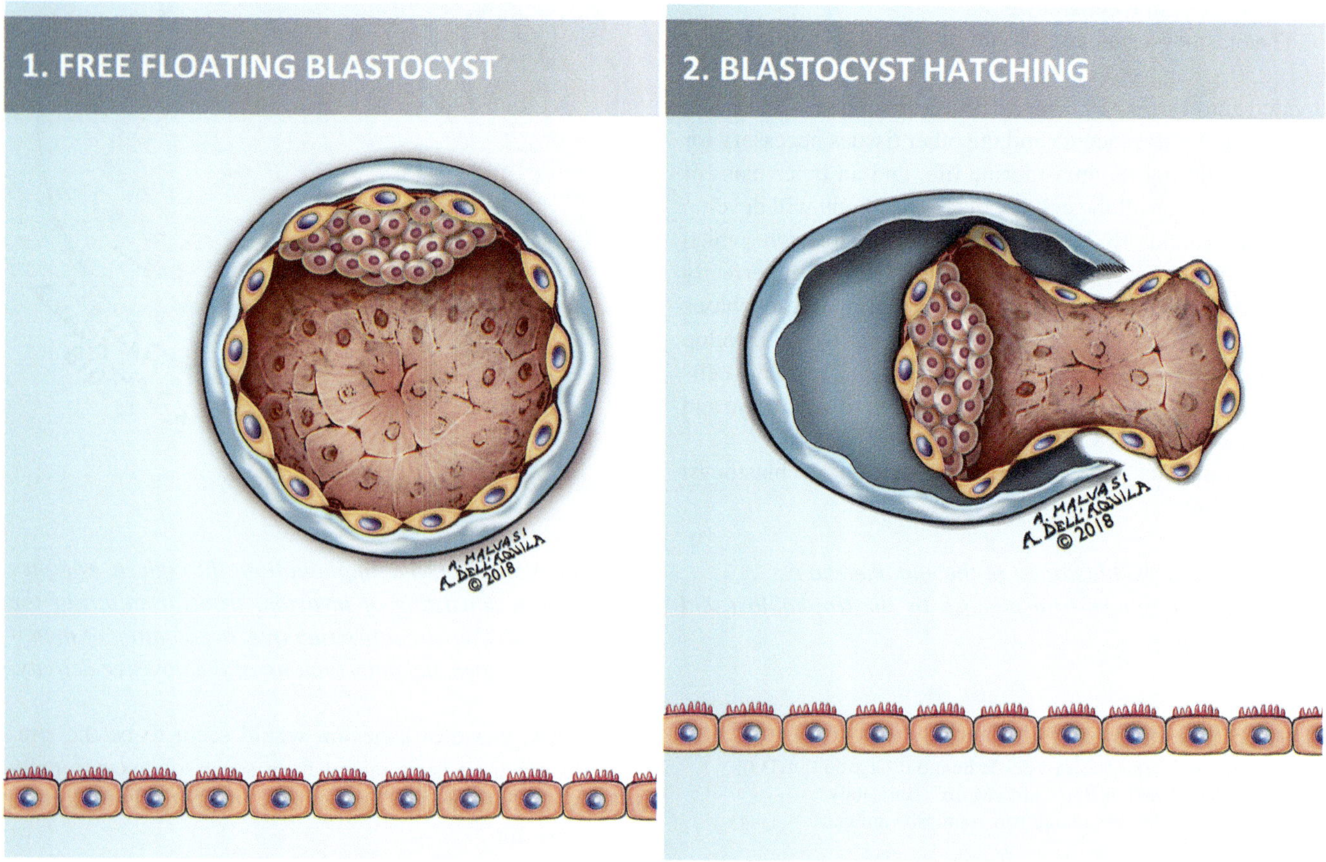

1. FREE FLOATING BLASTOCYST

2. BLASTOCYST HATCHING

Fig. 18.3 In (1–6) succession the nesting of the blastocyst in the endometrium

3. BLASTOCYST APPOSITION

4. BLASTOCYST ADHESION

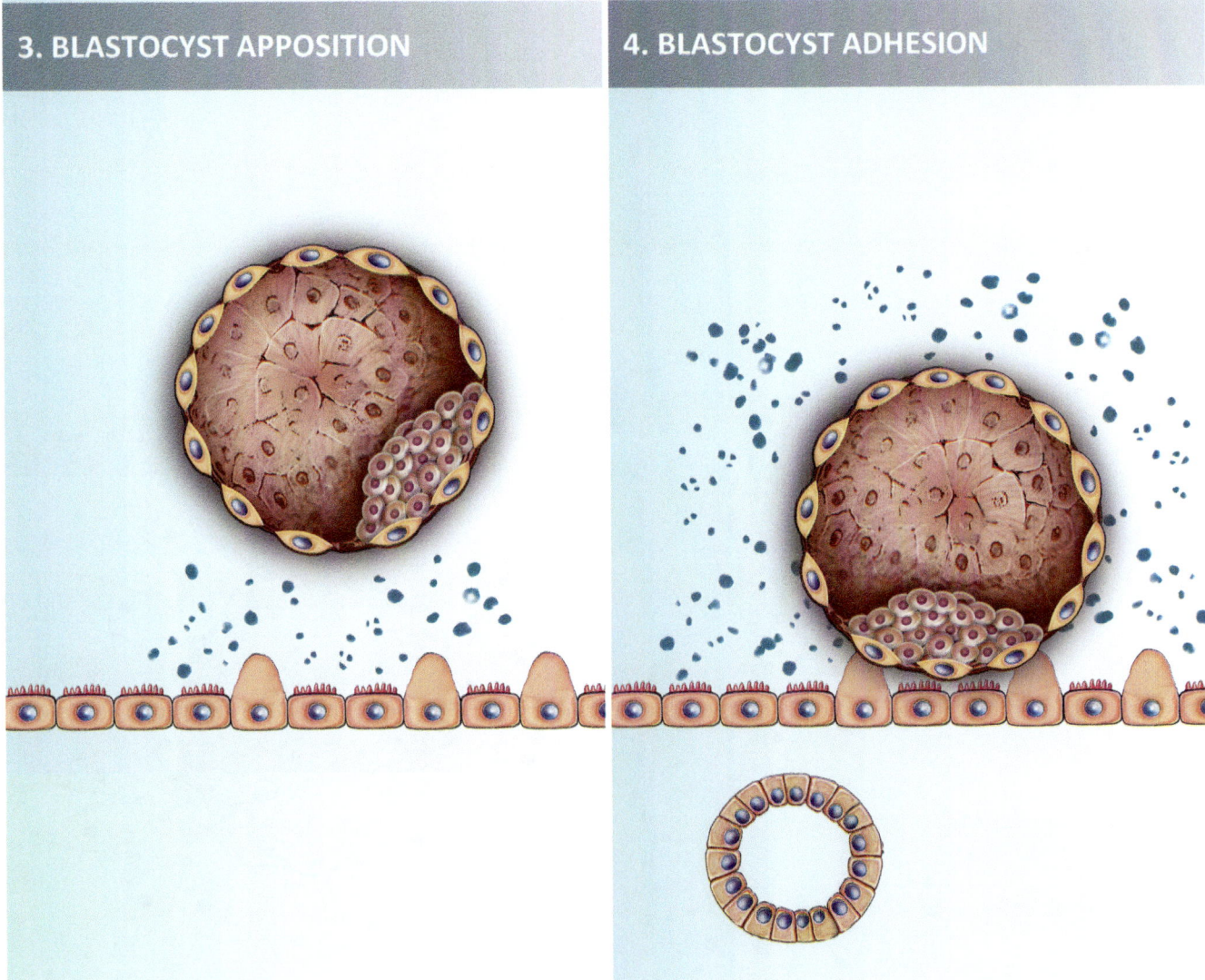

Fig. 18.3 (continued)

5. BLASTOCYST INVASION   ## 6. IMPLANTATION COMPLETE

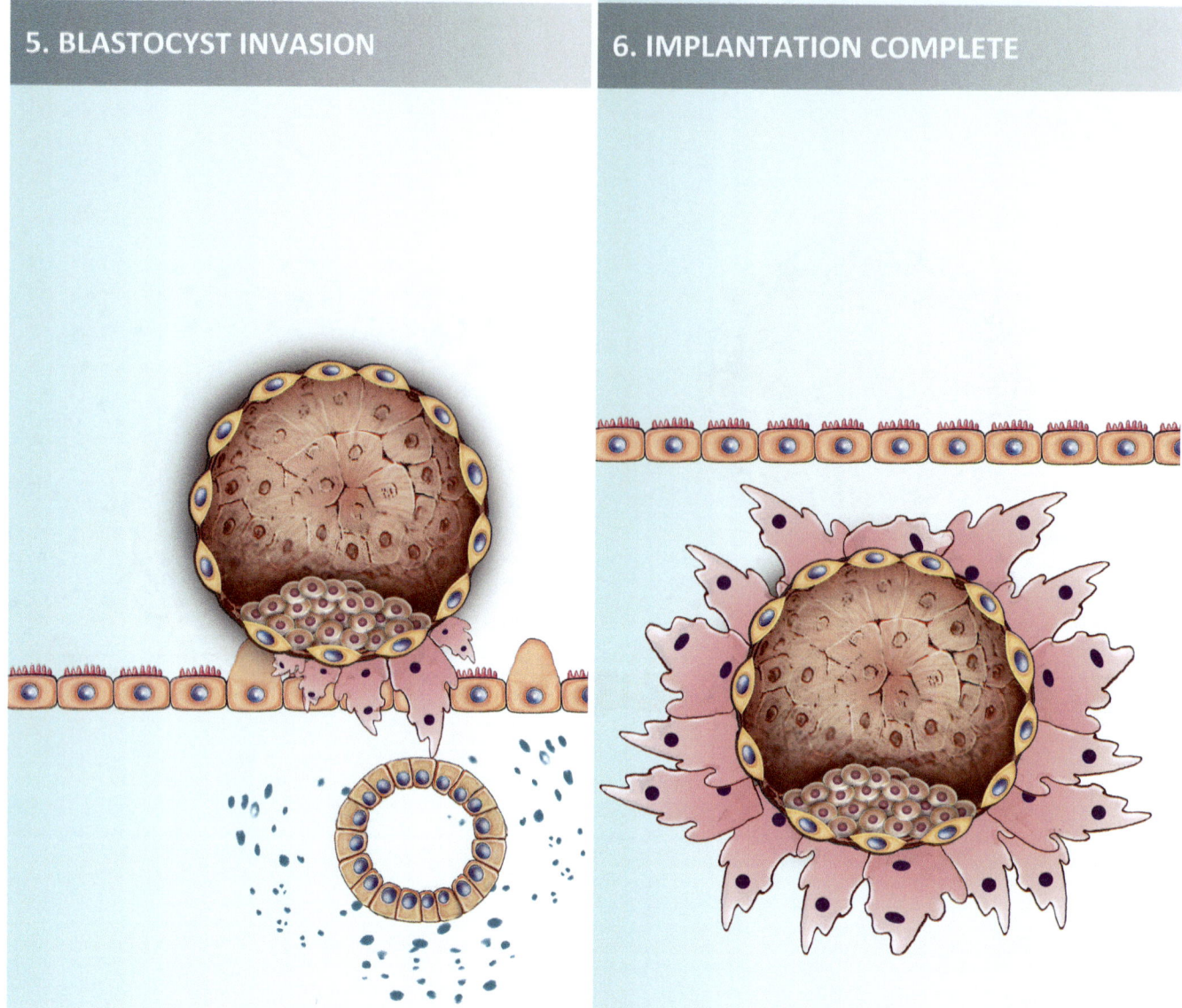

Fig. 18.3 (continued)

nisms for the two events. They affirm that the molecular basis for embryo implantation must be similar to that of the transmigration process of the leukocytes through the endothelial cells of the blood vessels, which initially functions by blocking the movement of the leukocytes in the blood by molecular "stickiness" using the selectin and other proteins expressed by the leukocytes and the carbohydrate ligands on the endothelium [2].

Selectins are a C-type lectin (glycoproteins which bind to sugar molecules and require calcium for the binding) which are expressed on the surface of leukocytes, platelets and activated endothelial cells.

They are part of the linking mechanism of rolling adhesion of leukocytes and platelets onto vessel endothelium and

are important for the homing of the lymphocytes to secondary lymphoid organs and for the recruiting of leukocytes to inflammation sites [3] (Fig. 18.8).

There are three types of selectins:

- **L-selectin** (Fig. 18.9) expressed by all leukocytes except T-lymphocytes.
- **E-selectin** (Fig. 18.10) expressed by endothelial cells activated by cytokines from transcriptional stimulation.
- **P-selectin** (Fig. 18.11) expressed by platelets and activated endothelial cells where it is stored in α-granules and Weibel–Palade bodies, respectively, as pre-formed transmembrane proteins and is translocated to the plasma membrane when stimulated.

Fig. 18.4 The fifth day of the blastocyst and the particular of the blastocyst's relationship with the endometrium

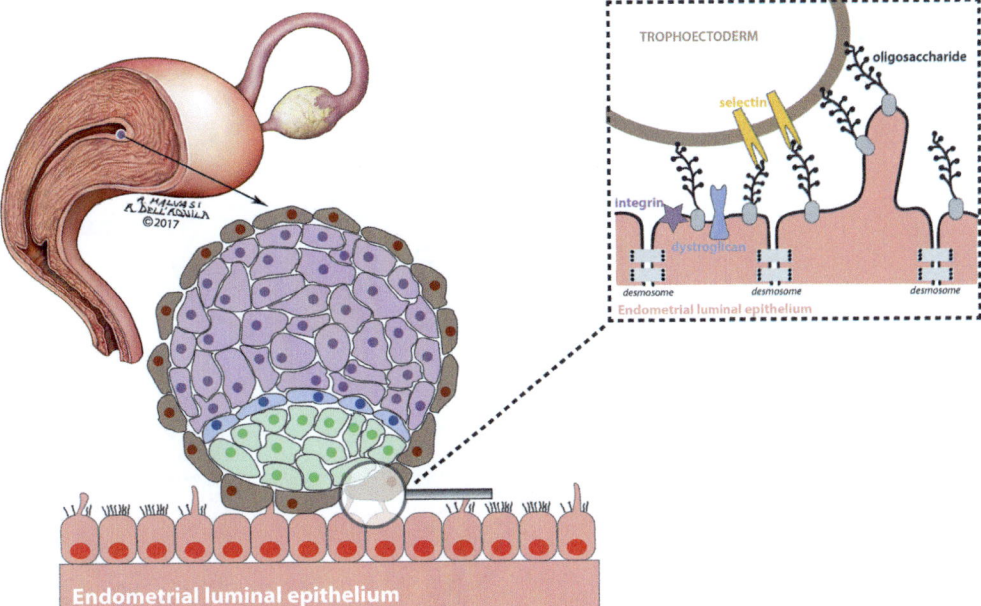

Fig. 18.5 The sixth day of the blastocyst

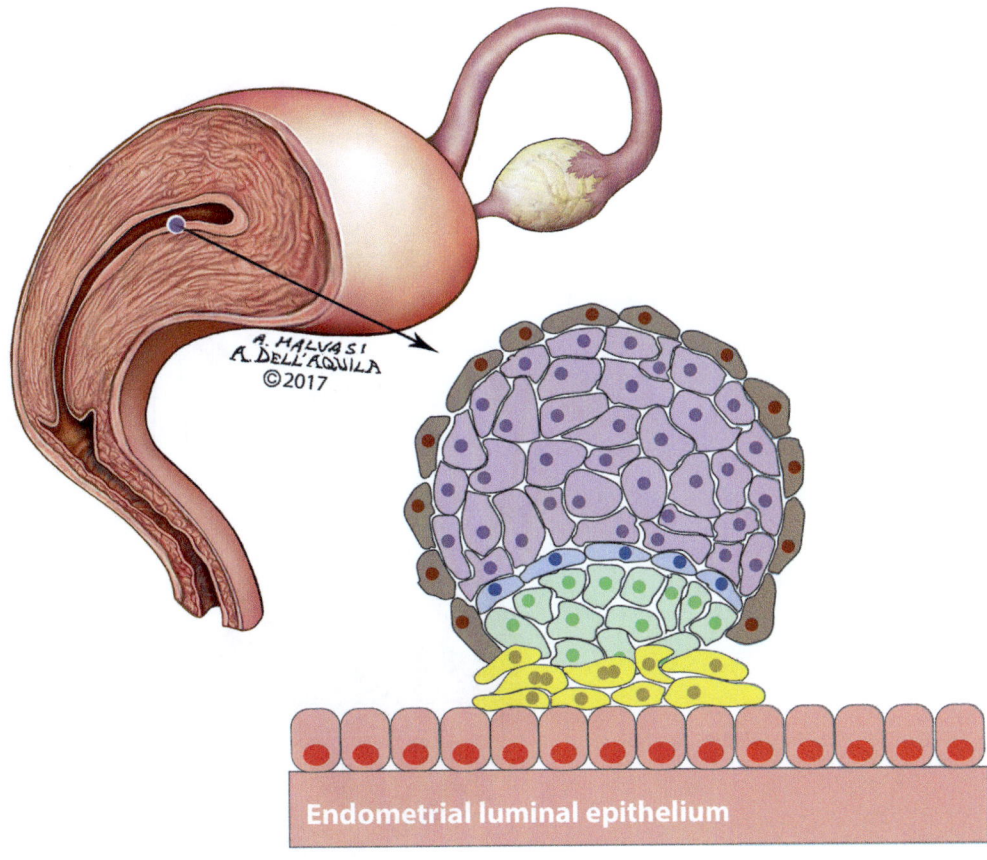

It is capable of heterophilic binding and interacts with glycoproteins and glycolipids which contain structures with α2-3-linked sialic acid and α1-3-linked fucose in their terminal branches.

Selectin-mediated cellular adhesion is determined by the recognition of carbohydrates by calcium-dependent lectin.

In general, L-selectin ligands are found on endothelial cells while E- and P-selectin ligands are found on leukocytes.

C-type lectins are carbohydrate-binding proteins characterized by a "carbohydrate recognition domain" (CRD). They are extended rigid molecules and contain an N-terminal CRD domain, which links to the carbohydrate components

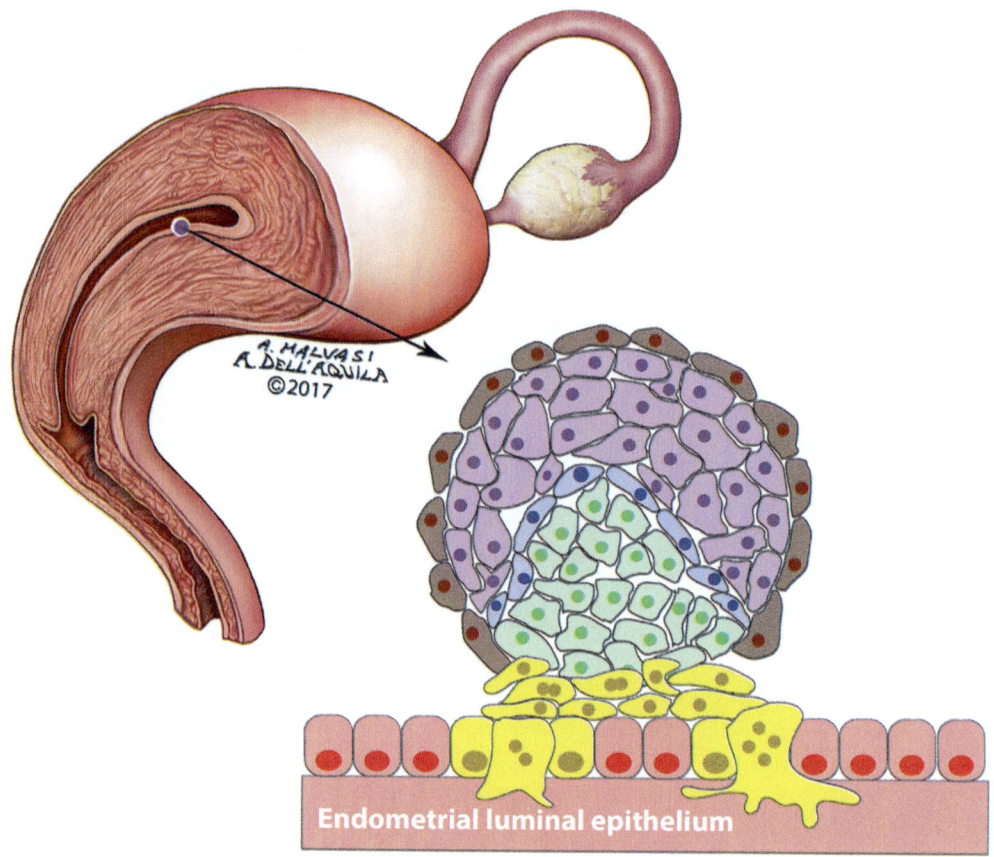

Endometrial luminal epithelium

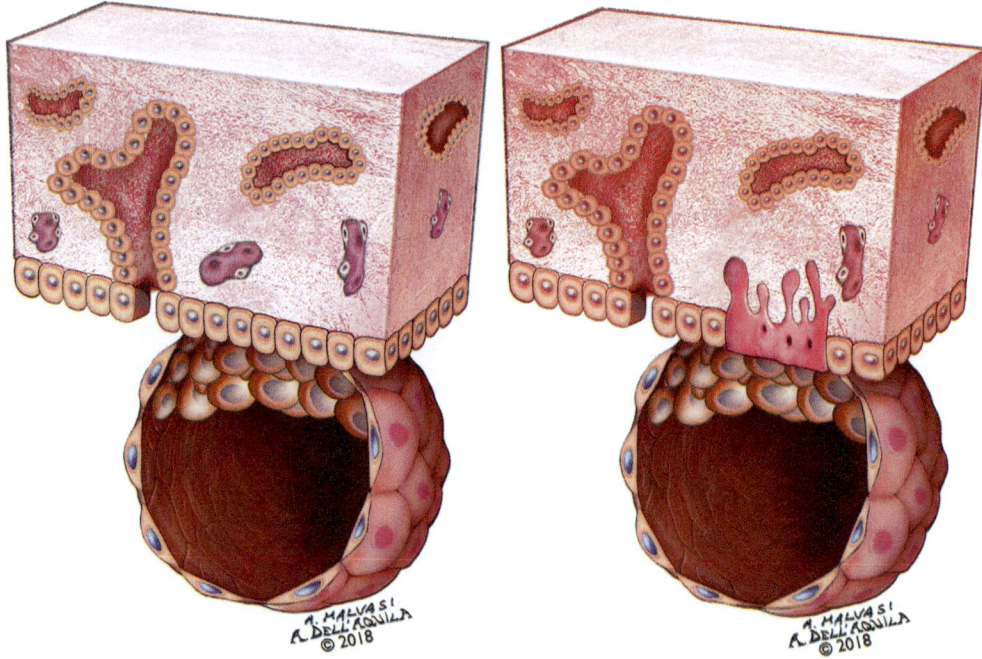

of other molecules, an epidermal growth factor (EGF)-like domain and a variable number of short consensus repeat (SCR) units. The difference in size between the three selectins is a factor of the number of SCRs in each type (2, 6, and 6 or 9 for L-, E-, and P-selectin, respectively).

The transmembrane and intracytoplasmatic domains are non-consistent between the three types, showing that they interact with different intracellular proteins.

During the inflammatory response, the adhesion of the leukocytes to the endothelial cells is controlled by the bind-

Fig. 18.8 Selectin activity in chronic inflammation

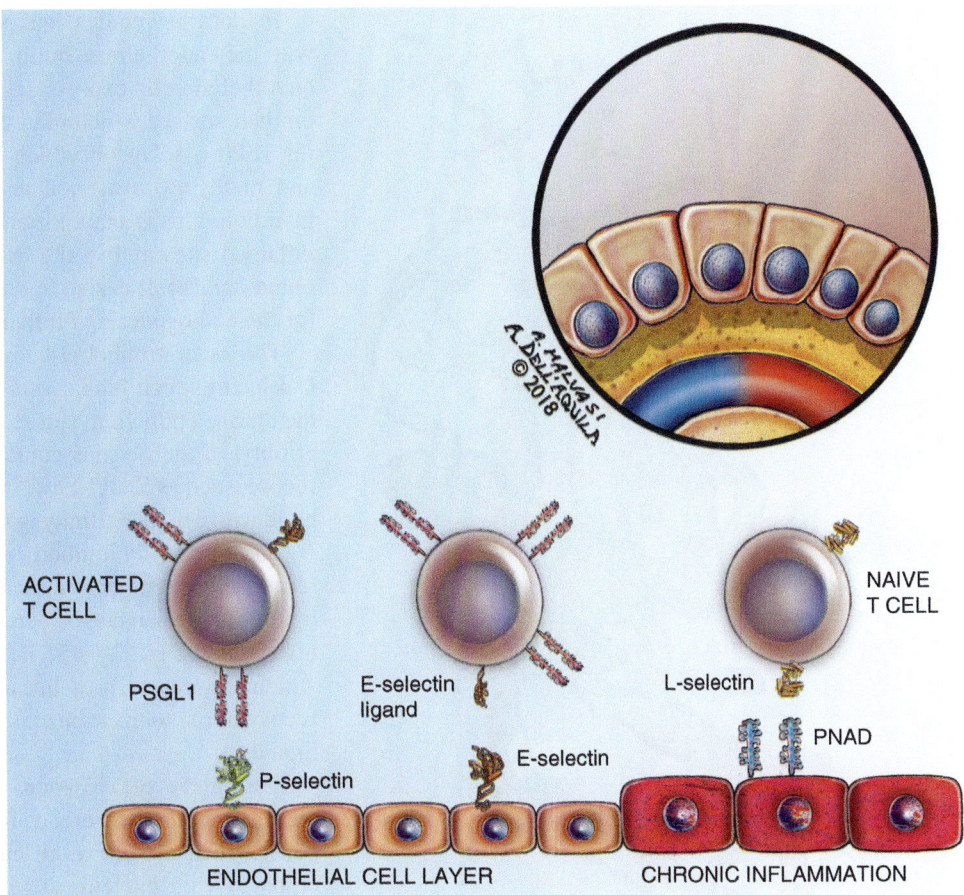

Fig. 18.9 L-selectin

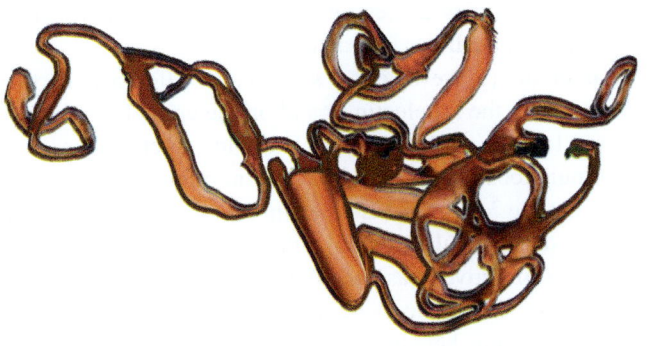

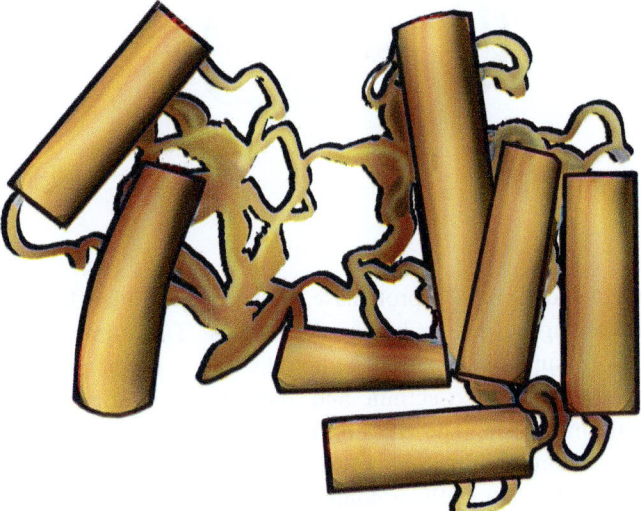

Fig. 18.10 E-selectin

ing of the inner vessel wall selectins to their complementary carbohydrates on the leukocytes. All known ligands are transmembrane glycoproteins which present oligosaccharidic structures to the selectins. The formation of transitory bonds between selectins and their ligands determine the first steps in the adhesion cascade. All three types of selectin can recognize glycoproteins and/or glycolipids which contain the tetrasaccharide Sialyl-Lewis x, which is found in all the circulating myeloid cells and is composed of sialic acid, galactose, fucose and *N*-acetylgalactosamine. It is still not

clear how the selectins are able to carry out specific interactions with their ligands, seeing that they use the same molecule for carbohydrate recognition.

L-selectin is constitutively expressed in the microvilli of leukocytes. Its surface levels are regulated by scission,

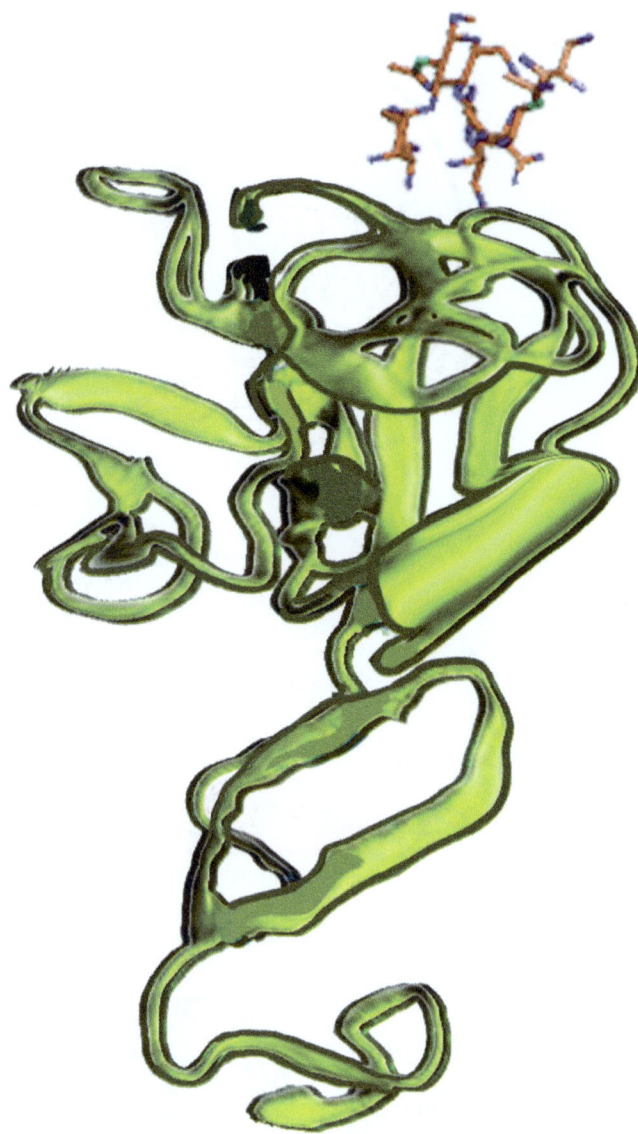

Fig. 18.11 P-selectin

mediated by metalloproteinase, of the extracellular domain following activation by the leukocytes. The intracellular cytoplasmic tail binds to calmodulin and to the actin cytoskeleton using α-actinin and the protein family ezrin/radixin/moesin. The equilibrium between these competing cytoplasmic interactions can influence the proteolytic scission of the extracellular domain.

The extracellular domain of L-selectin binds both to the glycoprotein PSGL-1 on the myeloid cells or on the activated T-lymphocytes and to the glycoproteins that are found on the specialized endothelial cells within the venules of the peripheral lymphoid tissue.

In normal venules leukocytes flow without interaction with the endothelium, but in the vessels in an inflamed area, endothelial cells express selectins and ligands for integrins on their surface which bind the circulating leukocytes, causing rolling adhesion which transforms into tight adhesion and finally extravasation and transmigration to the site of infection. This is an important process both in autodefence of inflamed sites and in the homing of lymphocytes (to lymphoid organs). It is also important as the process responsible for the pathogenesis of inflammatory disorders.

The outer trophoblast layer of the blastocyst expresses L-selectin which binds with the oligosaccharides present on the uterine epithelium surface. Generally it bonds, with a low affinity, to the glycans containing α2,3 sialic acid and α1,3 fucose, such as Sialyl-Lewis x (sLe x), while it is also able to bond with a higher affinity to sulfated and fucosylated ligands.

The MECA-79 antibody recognizes the high affinity sulfation dependent determinant, 6-sulfo-sLex, on L-selectin ligands [4] which can be detected on the surface of the endometrial cells. HECA-452 is, instead, an anti-sLex antibody which requires the presence of both α2,3 sialylation and α1,3 fucosylation to recognize the epitope of the low affinity ligand.

During the development period of the mouse embryo, there is a marked difference in the expression of surface antigens, which are above all carbohydrates. Treatment of the embryos with haptenic sugars, with biosynthetic inhibitors of glycosyltransferase or with glycosidases has induced development arrest in certain stages, suggesting that the carbohydrate antigens are essential, probably owing to their involvement in cellular interaction.

Lai et al. [5] revealed a significant difference in the expression of the L-selectin ligand on the epithelium during the proliferative, early-secretory and mid-secretory phases.

Immunolocalization studies on normal endometrium show that the MECA-79 L-selectin ligand is overexpressed from the day of ovulation until 6 days after and reduced during the proliferative phase and the anovulatory cycles. Other studies have shown the overexpression of HECA-452 when the endometrium becomes receptive during the "implantation window". Quantitatively, MECA-79 expression is always higher than that of HECA-452.

In our experience the expression of MECA-79 and HECA-452 concerns only the surface and glandular epithelium, with higher concentration in the uppermost part of the cell (Figs. 18.12, 18.13, 18.14a, b, and 18.15a, b). There is evidently an accumulation of signal in the glandular secretion and correspondingly there is a reduction in infertile women, especially those affected by endometritis. The reduction is more marked for the HECA-452 antibody (Figs. 18.16 and 18.17a, b).

Fig. 18.12 Typical histological pattern of the endometrium at 21° day of the menstrual cycle, corresponding to the most probably "implantation window" for the blastocyst. The glands contain a large amount of secretion; the stroma is edematous and hyperaemic

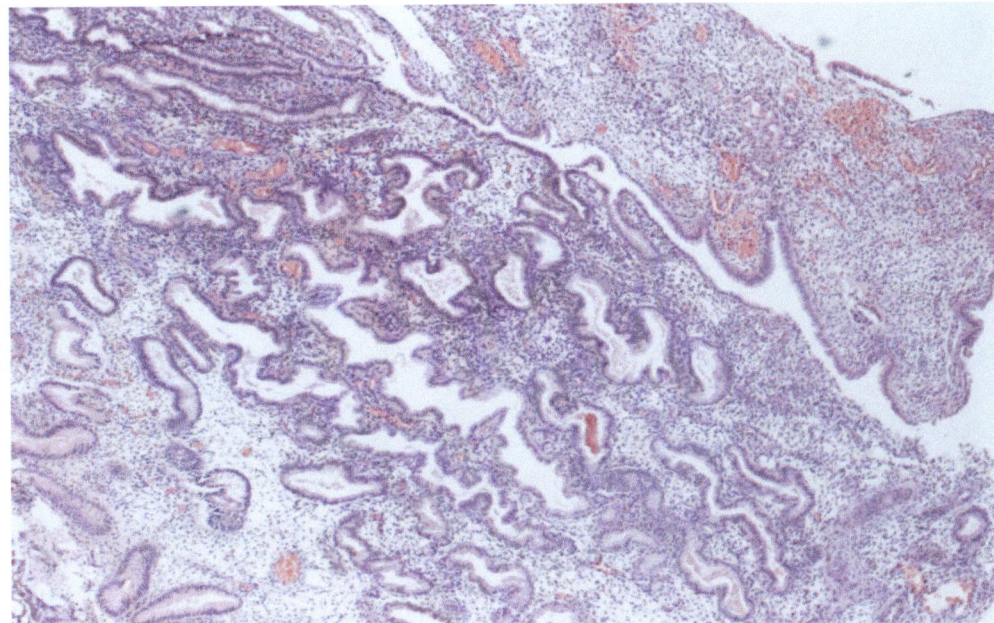

Fig. 18.13 Same case of the previous figure. The MECA-79 antibody is negative in the stroma, while it is expressed in the glandular secretion and in the luminal margin of the epithelial cells

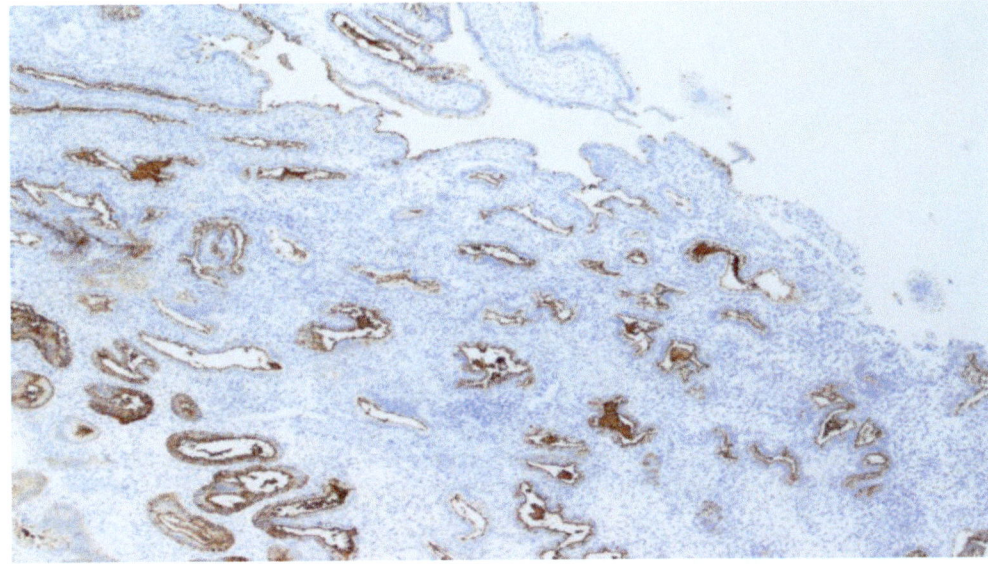

Research into the different levels of immunohistochemical expression of the two ligands in fertile and infertile women is on-going and several studies have been carried out on infertility due to endometriosis or PCOS or other unknown causes. In these patients, emphasis has been put on the reduction in expression of MECA-79 and an increase in that of HECA-452 [6]. However, a more careful analysis of the published tables shows that the expression of HECA-452 in the infertile group compared to the control group varies at the limit of significance and the expression in the lumen of the gland is the same.

Other studies have analysed the expression of these ligands in women who underwent hormonal stimulation (Figs. 18.18 and 18.19) with either a positive or negative outcome for the implanting of the blastocysts [7]. Measurements of ligand levels carried out at the gland apex and cytoplasm and at the surface show minimum variation between the two groups. This variation is then amplified by mathematical artifice (HSCORE) to show a significant difference in favour of

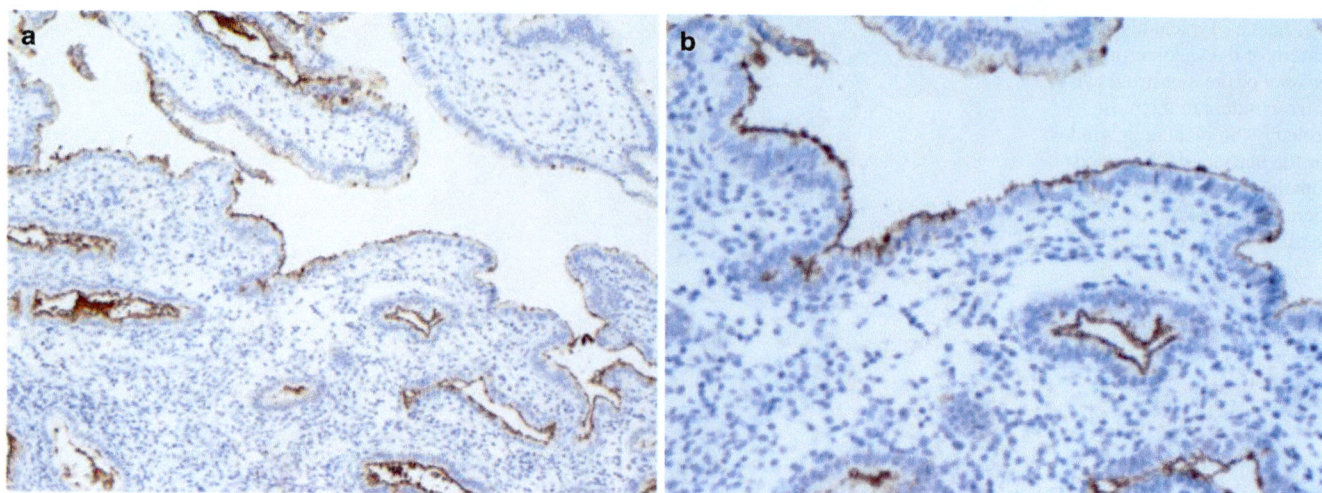

Fig. 18.14 (**a**) The immunohistochemical expression of MECA-79 is strong and linear at the free border of the superficial epithelium and in luminal border of the gland epithelium. (**b**) The positivity is of cupular morphology in several of the superficial cells

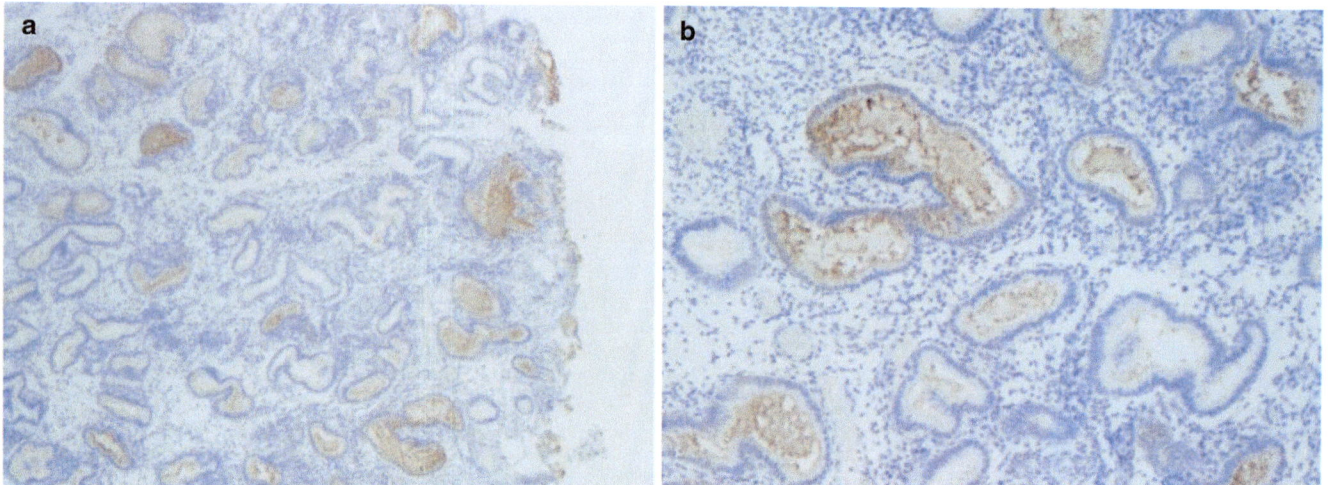

Fig. 18.15 (**a**) The HECA-452 antibody expresses a less intense positivity only in the epithelial cells. (**b**) At higher magnification, the expression is more intense in the luminal secretion than in the epithelial border

fertile women, especially if the comparison is made based on the quality parameters of the embryo. In our experience, stimulated patients with a failed implantation show high values of MECA-79 expression and almost inexistent levels of HECA-452.

Our previous studies [8, 9] have clearly shown the correlation between aspecific chronic endometritis and sterility. Such correlation can be associated with the production of cytokines which interfere with those expressed by the trophoblast, or with the asynchrony of the maturation of the endometrium often present in endometritis, that is with the modifications of the stroma which accompany many cases of endometrial inflammation [9].

Our experience also shows no significant differences in the expression of MECA-79 between fertile and unfertile women suffering endometritis, though with an absolute value in favour of the healthy control group (6.85 vs. 6.41), while there is a significant reduction in the expression of HECA-452 (5.00 vs. 3.41). It is likely that the variation can be associated with the factors which mediate the inflammation. And considering as the same type of ligands interact with inflammatory cells and endothelium cells in the leukocyte margination and adhesion process [10], it is also possible to hypothesize that the ligands can interact with the selectins of the trophoblast so interfering in the implantation process.

Fig. 18.16 Endometrium in secretive phase (21° day) in patient with chronic endometritis. The inflammatory cells are present in some glandular lumen and in the stroma. The glandular maturation is abnormal: few glandular secretion and absence of the initial glandular convolution

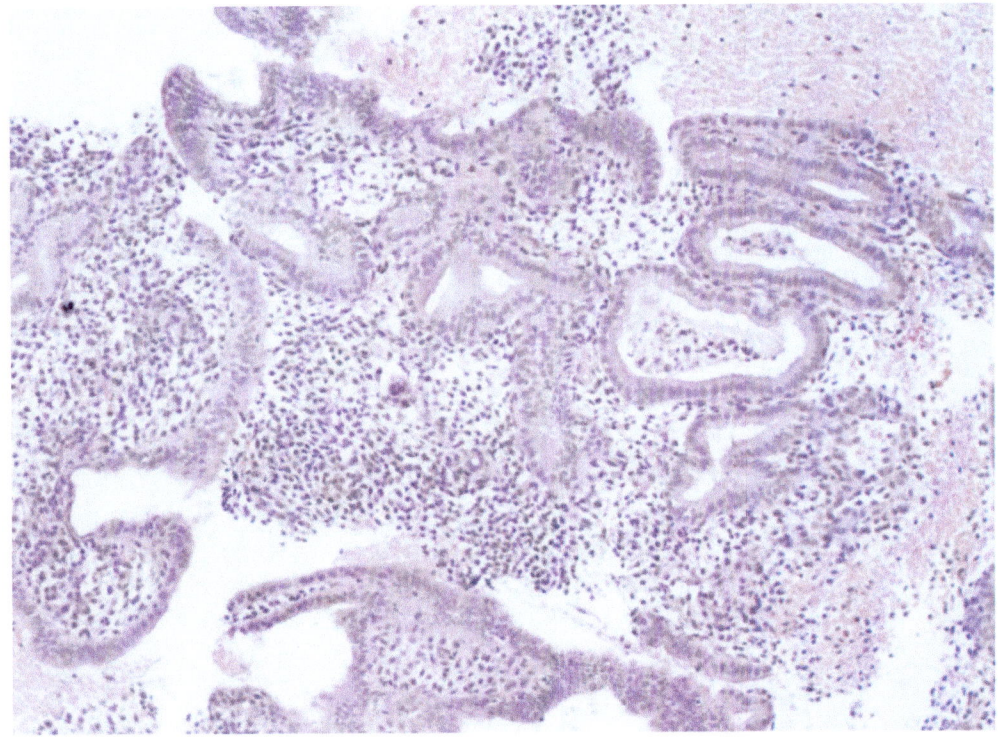

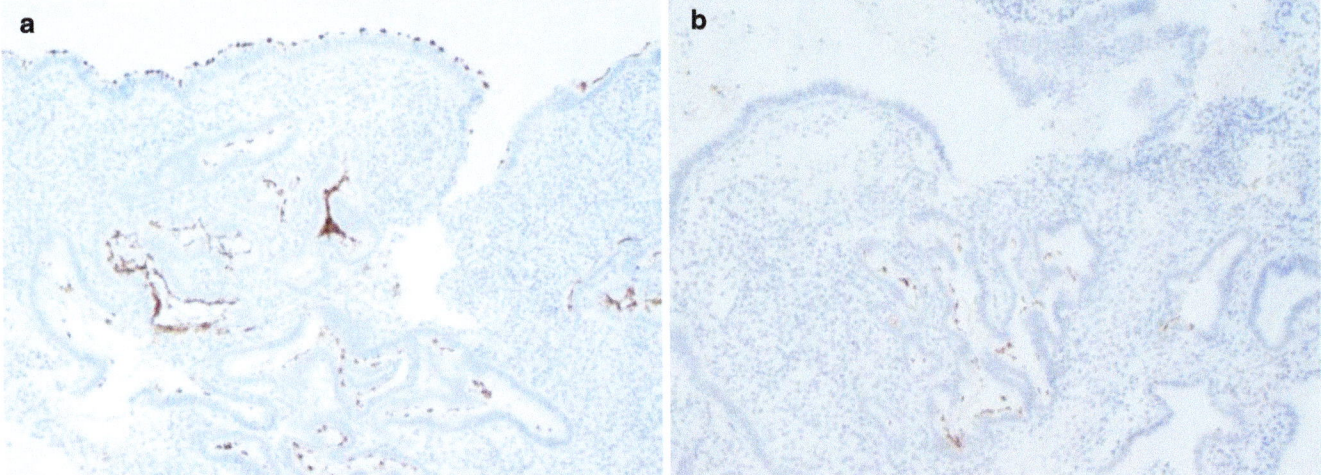

Fig. 18.17 Same case of the previous figure. (**a**) The expression of MECA-79 in the superficial and glandular epithelium is not different with respect to the endometrium of fertile women. (**b**) The expression of HECA-452 is reduced

The actual effects of these variations on the adhesion process is still to be established though it would be logical to assume that a reduction in ligands, including those of low affinity, would lead to a reduction in the ability of the blastocyst to attach itself to the uterine wall. It is in fact known that the establishment of multiple consecutive bonds between the blastocyst and endometrium is indispensible for the progressive slowing of the rolling movement of the blastocyst along the uterine wall until its final stopping.

Ultrastructural investigation with immunogold (Fig. 18.20) confirmed the transmembrane surface distribution of the L-selectin ligand MECA-79 [11]. The correlation between ligand expression and the presence of pinopodes, as shown by scanning electron microscope, could explain the cupular morphology of the endometrial surface, as seen in immunohistochemistry.

Recently [12], by methodical one-step quantitative RT-PCR, five types of L-selectin ligand peptide compo-

Fig. 18.18 Endometrium of a patient submitted to hormonal therapy in view of an intervention of medical fertilization. The glands are dilated by a large amount of secretion. However, with respect to a normal subject, the glands are dysmetric, and focally distorted, and the stroma is more compact. In some glands, the secretion is dense and hypereosinophilic

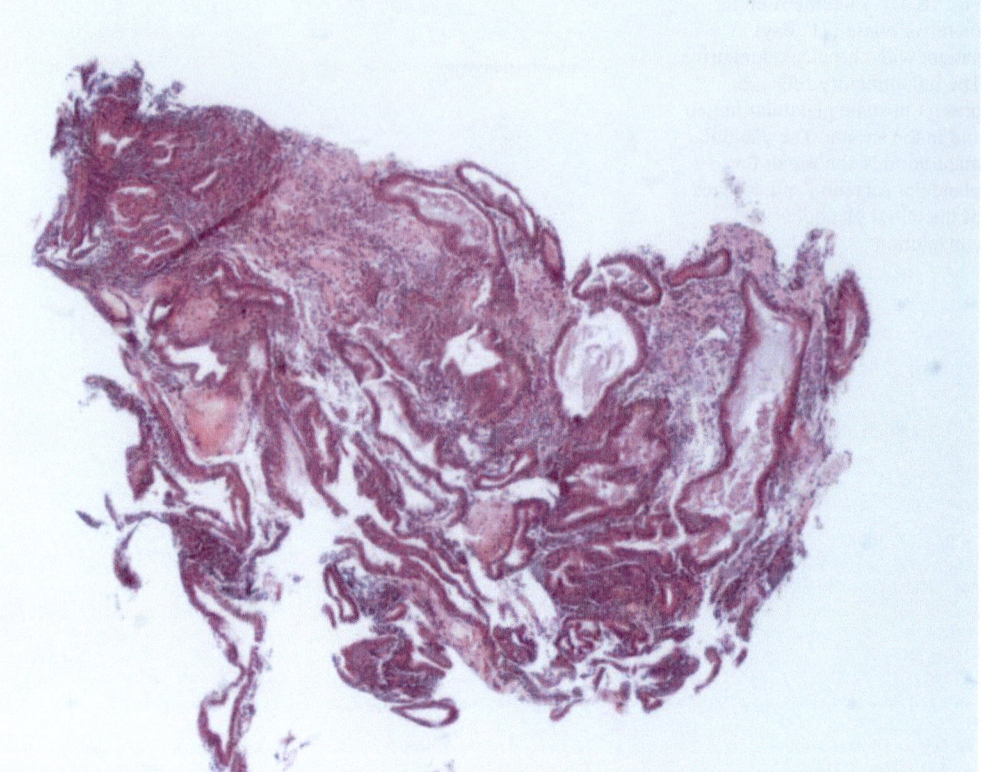

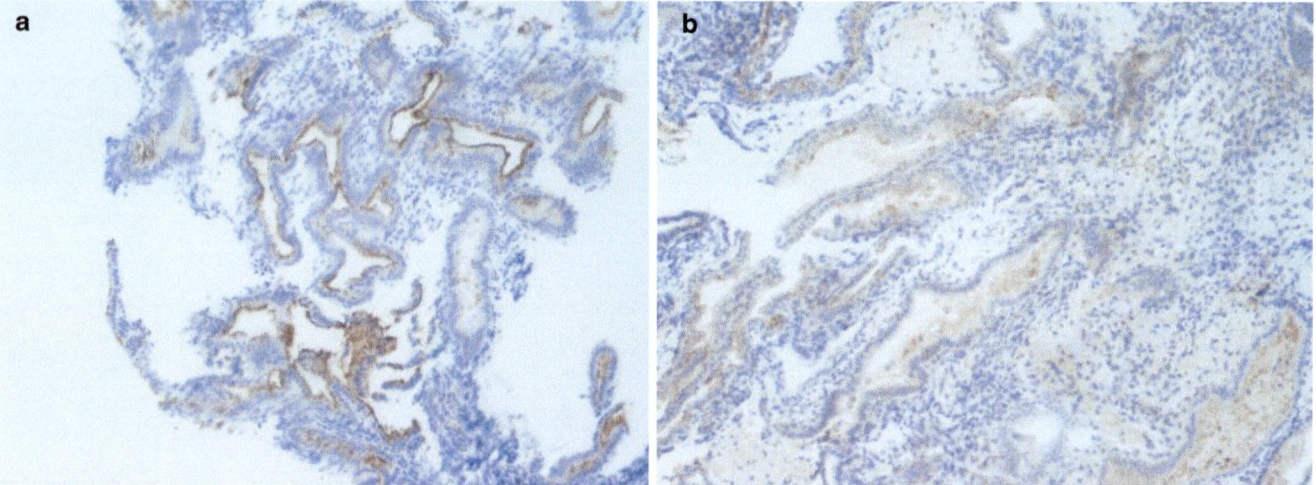

Fig. 18.19 Same case of the previous figure. (**a**) The expression of MECA-79 is normally continuous in the apex of the superficial and glandular cells. (**b**) HECA-452 offers a week signal in the glandular secretion

nents were detected in the endometrium: podocalyxin, endomucin, nepmucin, GlyCAM-1 and CD34. All have a mucin-like structure with sulphate-linked glycans (recognized by the MECA-79 antibody). Endomucin, nepmucin and CD34 are highly present in the proliferative phase, but only endomucin shows a significant increase in the secretory phase. The genes CHST2 and CHST4 involved in the induction of the formation of the epitopes of the L-selectin ligands (sulfotransferase) do not show any significant differences in the various phases of the menstrual cycle. At the same time, in the same endometrium samples the expression of oestrogen receptors alpha remains constant during the cycle, while the expression of progesterone receptors gradually decreases from the proliferative phase to the late secretory phase. The authors note that very probably the expression of many ligands begins in the proliferative phase, while in the early-secretory phase there is the translational modification with the oligosaccharides, perhaps in association with the cycling levels of serum oestrogens, but all is not yet clear. The translational modi-

Fig. 18.20 The electron microscopy identifies the presence of MECA-79 (**a**) and HECA-79 (**b**) antibodies in the microvilli present at the border of superficial and glandular epithelial cells and in the intervillous space, by the immunogold technique (arrows)

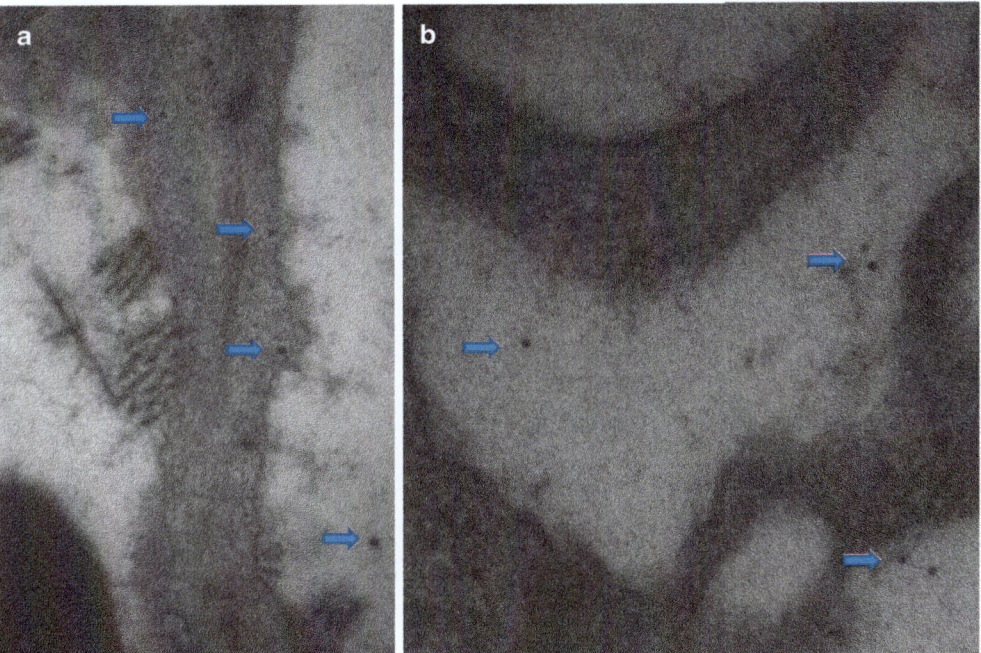

fication makes the ligand recognizable to the MEGA 79 antibody and, more importantly, more attractive to the trophoblast selectin.

Endomucin is a transmembrane L27.5 kD polypeptide with many glycosylation sites which is found in the endothelium of many organs such as heart, lungs and kidneys. Many lymphatic organs overexpress this protein in the postcapillary high endothelium venules (HEV), where it carries out an important role in the downregulation of the adhesion of immunocompetent cells [13, 14]. In this regard, the expression of MECA-79 in the HEV of the reactive lymphocytic infiltrate of melanomas [15] and other solid tumours recall the observations already made on the interactions between blastocyst implanting and infertility due to endometritis.

References

1. Genbacev OD, Prakobphol A, Foulk RA, Krtolica AR, Ilic D, Singer MS, Yang ZQ, Kiessling LL, Rosen SD, Fisher SJ. Trophoblast L-selectin-mediated adhesion at the maternal-fetal Interface. Science. 2003;299:405–8.
2. Zak I, Lewandowska E, Gnyp W. Selectin glycoprotein ligands. Acta Biochim Pol. 2000;4:393–412.
3. Uchimura K, Rosen SD. Sulfated L-selectin ligands as a therapeutic target in chronic inflammation. Trends Immunol. 2006;27:559–65.
4. Pablos J, Santiago B, Tsay D, Singer M, Palao G, Galindo M, Rosen SDA. HEV-restricted sulfotransferase is expressed in rheumatoid arthritis synovium and is induced by lymhotoxin-alpha/beta and TNF-alpha in cultured endothelial cells. BMC Immunol. 2005;7(6):6.
5. Lai TH, Shih IM, Vlahos N, Ho CL, Wallach E, Zhao Y. Differential expression of L-selectin ligand in the endometrium during the menstrual cycle. Fertil Steril. 2005;83(Suppl 1):1297–302.
6. Margarit L, Gonzalez D, Lewis PD, Hopkins L, Davies C, Conlan RS, Joels L, White JO. L-selectin ligands in human endometrium: comparison of fertile and infertile subjects. Hum Reprod. 2009;24:2767–77.
7. Shamonki M, Kligman I, Shamonki JM, Schattman G, Hyjek E, Spandorfer SD, Zanonic N, Rosenwaks Z. Immunohistochemical expression of endometrial L-selectin ligand is higher in donor egg recipients with embryonic implantation. Fertil Steril. 2006;86:1365–75.
8. Cicinelli E, De Ziegler D, Nicoletti R, Colafiglio G, Saliani N, Resta L, Rizzi D, De Vito D. Chronic endometritis: correlation among hysteoscopic, histologic, and bacteriologic findings in a prospective trial with 2190 consecutive office hysteroscopies. Fertil Steril. 2008;89:677–84.
9. Resta L, Palumbo M, Rossi R, Piscitelli D, Fiore MG, Cicinelli E. Histology of micro polyps in chronic endometritis. Histopathology. 2012;60:670–4.
10. Bevilacqua MP. Endothelial-leukocyte adhesion molecules. Annu Rev Immunol. 1993;11:767–804.
11. Nejatbakhsh R, Kabir-Salmani M, Dimitriadis E, Hosseini A, Taheripanah R, Sadeghi Y, Akimoto Y, Iwashita M. Subcellular localizzation of L-selectin ligand in the endometrium implies a novel function for pinopodes in endometrial receptivity. Reprod Biol Endocrinol. 2012;15(10):46.
12. Lai T-H, Chang F-W, Lin J-J, Ling Q-D. Gene expression of human endometrial L-selectin ligand in relation to the phases of the natural menstrual cycle. Sci Rep. 2018;8:1443.
13. Zahr A, Alcaide P, Yang J, Jones A, Gregory M, dela Paz NG, Patel-Hett S, Nevers T, Koirala A, Luscinskas FW, Saint-Geniez M, Ksander B, D'Amore PA, Argüeso P. Endomucin prevents leukocyte-endothelial cell adhesion and has a critical role under resting and inflammatory conditions. Nat Commun. 2016;2(7):10363.
14. Park-Windhol C, Ng YS, Yang J, Primo V, Saint-Geniez M, D'Amore PA. Endomucin inhibits VEGF-induced endothelial cell migration, growth, and morphogenesis by modulating VEGFR2 signaling. Sci Rep. 2017;7(7):17138.
15. Avram C, Sànchez-Sendra B, Martìn JM, Terràdez L, Ramos D, Monteagudo D. The density and type of MECA-79-positive high endothelial venules correlate with lymphocytic infiltration and tumour regression in primary cutaneous melanoma. Histopathology. 2013;63:852–61.

Complications in Oocyte Retrieval

19

Michail Pargianas, Styliani Salta, Stelis Fiorentzis,
Lamprini G. Kalampoki, Renata Beck, Damiano Vizziello,
and Ioannis Kosmas

Contents

M. Pargianas
Department of Obstetrics and Gynecology, Medical School,
University of Ioannina, Ioannina, Greece

S. Salta
Cancer Biology and Therapeutics, Centre de Recherche Saint-Antoine, Institut Nationalde la Santé et de la Recherche Médicale, (INSERM) U938 and Institut Universitaire de Cancérologie, Faculté de Médecine, Sorbonne Université, Paris, France

Service d'Hématologie Biologique Hôpital Tenon, Hôpitaux, Assistance Publique Hôpitaux de Paris (AP-HP), Universitaires Est Parisien, Paris, France

S. Fiorentzis
Agios Nikolaos Crete, Crete, Greece

L. G. Kalampoki
Department of Obstetrics and Gynecology, Chatzikosta General Hospital, Ioannina, Epirus, Greece

R. Beck
Department of Anesthesia, Santa Maria Hospital, GVM Care and Research, Bari, Italy

D. Vizziello
I.R.C.C.S. Policlinico San Donato, Department of Urology, University of Milano, Milano, Italy
e-mail: Damiano.vizziello@grupposandonato.it

I. Kosmas (✉)
Department of Obstetrics and Gynecology, Ioannina State General Hospital G. Chatzikosta, Ioannina, Greece

© Springer Nature Switzerland AG 2020
A. Malvasi, D. Baldini (eds.), *Pick Up and Oocyte Management*, https://doi.org/10.1007/978-3-030-28741-2_19

19.1   Introduction

The most important step for the in vitro fertilization (IVF) process is oocyte retrieval. Under ultrasound guidance, a needle is inserted through the vagina and directed to the ovary and the follicles. Subsequently, the follicular fluid together with the oocyte is aspirated. Although it is a very precise technique, complications may occur. Although these complications are rare, they could be serious and life threatening. In this chapter, we present the complications after oocyte retrieval for IVF as they are reported in case reports and studies with small series of cycles. All studies conclude that these events are associated with pelvic inflammatory disease or endometriosis that may coexist with infertility.

19.2   Incidence of IVF Complications as Reported Through the Years

In a retrospective report, Tureck et al. in 1993 [1] included 674 patients that underwent oocyte retrieval in the same unit, covering a period of 3 years. All surgeons had extensive experience with OPU. About 1.5% (10) of patients required hospitalization, nine for intravenous antibiotics, and one for broad ligament hematoma observation. Two patients had significant vaginal arterial bleeding after the procedure. Most of the hospitalized patients had a history of extensive pelvic adhesions with or without a history of salpingitis. Authors conclude that a history of previous pelvic inflammatory disease and/or adnexal adhesions is a risk factor for perioperative morbidity. In a narrative review, El-Shawarby et al. in 2004 [2] described the OPU complications presented at that time in literature. Eventually, he formed a table of general recommendations, to increase safety during oocyte retrieval. These include a detailed preoperative evaluation, the construction of a risk assessment list for complications during OPU, and the establishment of a clinical risk management group at each unit to evaluate and solve eventual problems. In addition, he advises to avoid multiple penetrations of the ovary and vaginal wall, in order to prevent intraperitoneal bleeding and pelvic infection. He emphasizes the need for clinical guidelines and the importance of training for junior doctors on oocyte retrieval. He suggests that clinical research is needed to optimize this procedure while the use of color Doppler might be beneficial.

Ludwig et al. in 2006 [3] reported the perioperative and postoperative complications after 1058 OPUs. There were no complications from general anesthesia. Vaginal bleeding was evident in 2.8% of the participants (29 patients). For 28 of them, the bleeding was stopped by compression for more than 1 min and for the remaining one patient tamponade was required for more than 2 h without the need for suturing. The majority of patients (41.6%) experienced mild pain 2 h after oocyte retrieval, 16.9% presented with medium pain, 2.7% with severe pain, and 0.4% with very severe pain. Most importantly, the mean pain score was dependent on the number of oocytes retrieved. Regarding the persistence of pain, 2–3 days after oocyte retrieval, 7.6% of the patients reported medium pain, 1.5% severe pain, and 0.2% very severe pain. Only 25.6% of them suffered from mild pain on the day of embryo transfer. Overall, only 98 patients were hospitalized for ovarian hyperstimulation, complications from oocyte retrieval, pain and complications during early pregnancy. Only one patient was hospitalized for injury to the ureter. Authors conclude that oocyte retrieval is a procedure that is well tolerated with a minority of women developing severe pain.

Bodri et al. in 2008 [4] evaluated the complications of 4052 IVF cycles, of which 1238 were downregulated with agonist and 2814 with antagonist. Fourteen patients developed intra-abdominal bleeding, two presented with severe pain, and one had an ovarian torsion. Among oocyte retrievals, almost half of them (1917) have been for egg donation. For patients who received GnRH antagonists, oocytes final maturation was triggered either by hCG or GnRH agonist, in order to prevent ovarian hyperstimulation. Nevertheless, 22 oocyte donors developed early onset moderate/severe OHSS. One patient had to undergo ascites puncture by culdocentesis. Surprisingly more patients developed ovarian hyperstimulation in the GnRH antagonist/hCG protocol that in the GnRH agonist/hCG one although this did not reach statistical significance. In the oocyte donation group, 11 patients developed intra-abdominal bleeding. Of these, six required observation only, four needed laparoscopy for cauterization, and one required laparotomy due to ovarian torsion resulting in acute abdomen. Most of them had a large number of oocytes retrieved, except for two patients hospitalized for observation that had a small amount of oocytes collected. In the IVF group, two women developed intra-abdominal bleeding, eight presented with an early onset moderate/severe ovarian hyperstimulation, and seven with late onset moderate/severe OHSS.

In a very large series of 7098 IVF cycles, Aragona et al. in 2011 [5], monitored the complications of transvaginal oocyte retrieval. Four patients developed severe peritoneal bleeding and required surgical intervention while two patients developed pelvic abscesses. Intraperitoneal bleeding was developed immediately, in 2 h and 12 h, respectively, for these four patients. Three patients underwent laparoscopic hemostasis and one had a laparotomy. Three patients had an embryo transfer while the laparotomy patient received no embryo. Regarding the two patients who developed pelvic abscesses, this was evident at 7 and 10 days after embryo transfer and oocyte retrieval, respectively. The first patient had a left oophorectomy while for the second patient, right ovarian abscess drainage was performed.

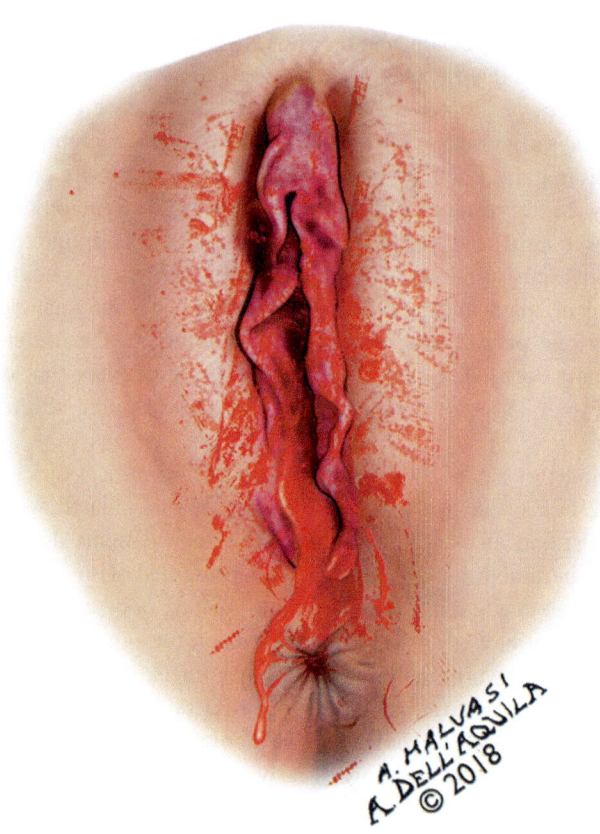

Fig. 19.1 Vaginal bleeding

In a retrospective study, Siristatidis et al. in 2013 [6], presented the complications arising from 542 oocyte retrievals in a 7-year period. Most of them (18.08%) had minor vaginal bleeding (controlled by <2 min pressure). Mild vaginal bleeding (Fig. 19.1) was evident in 5.9% (32 cases), similarly controlled by <2 min pressure. Twelve patients developed mild OHSS and only five were involved in severe ovarian hyperstimulation. No injuries of other internal organs have been reported although in one case, the suspicion of iliac artery trauma existed. One cervical pregnancy occurred that was followed by hysterectomy. Two cases of peritoneal bleeding have been documented, both involving women at prophylactic dose of LMWH. Two patients developed bronchospasm during general anesthesia. In all cases, appropriate measures have been taken.

19.3 Complications Developed in the Uterus, Ovaries, and Fallopian Tubes

19.3.1 Tubo-Ovarian Abscess in General

19.3.1.1 Overview

In a case series of 7098 patients that underwent transvaginal oocyte retrieval, only two cases of pelvic abscess have been reported. Abscesses have been developed despite antibiotic prophylaxis. These abscesses have not been developed early and did not involve the tubo-ovarian complex entirely, but developed alone, one in the left ovary and the other at the right ovary [5]. The authors suggest that it might be beneficial to perform vaginal culture for infections and antibiotic prophylaxis before the oocyte retrieval. Only if patient is found negative for vaginal infections, then it is allowed to proceed to the OPU.

19.3.1.2 Risks of Developing Tubo-Ovarian Abscess

In another retrospective study covering four consecutive years, Villette et al. [7] tried to associate tubo-ovarian abscess with the likelihood of endometriosis and oocyte retrieval. Only three out of ten women that hospitalized for ovarian abscess, presented with factors, the oocyte retrieval and the endometrioma. This complication developed in different time after OPU (16, 57 and 102 days later). The other seven patients had tubo-ovarian abscesses without undergoing oocyte retrieval, previously. Authors do not associate ART with tubo-ovarian abscess but rather these constitute sporadic occurrences in women with endometriosis (Figs. 19.2 and 19.3).

19.3.2 Tubo-Ovarian Abscess from Specific Microorganisms Actinomycosis

19.3.2.1 Tubo-Ovarian Abscesses from Actinomycosis urogenitalis

Van Hoecke et al. in 2013 [8] reported a tubo-ovarian abscess in a 40-year-old woman with Crohn's disease and previously right hemi-colectomy. The responsible microorganism was Actinomyces urogenitalis. Patient presented 14 days after OPU with infection signs and antibiotics have been administered (amoxicillin–clavulanic acid (two doses, 2 g each) and doxycycline (two doses, 100 mg each)). She was discharged but pelvic inflammatory disease continued. Patient was admitted again after 2 days and underwent laparoscopic exploration that ended in laparotomy and right adnexal abscess drainage. Authors found a large right adnexal multiocular collection with abscess formation and bacteremia, while after the pelvic exploration, amoxicillin–clavulanic acid for four doses (1 g each one), was administered. Eventually she was discharged 8 days after surgery.

19.3.2.2 Actinomycosis israelii Pelvic Abscess

In another case report, infection with Actinomyces israelii, presented as pelvic abscess. In a 31-year-old woman, with no previous pregnancies and male factor as a cause for infertility, pelvic infection developed 6 days after oocyte retrieval. She was presented with pelvic pain, nausea, vomiting, uri-

Fig. 19.2 Ovaric and tubal abscess

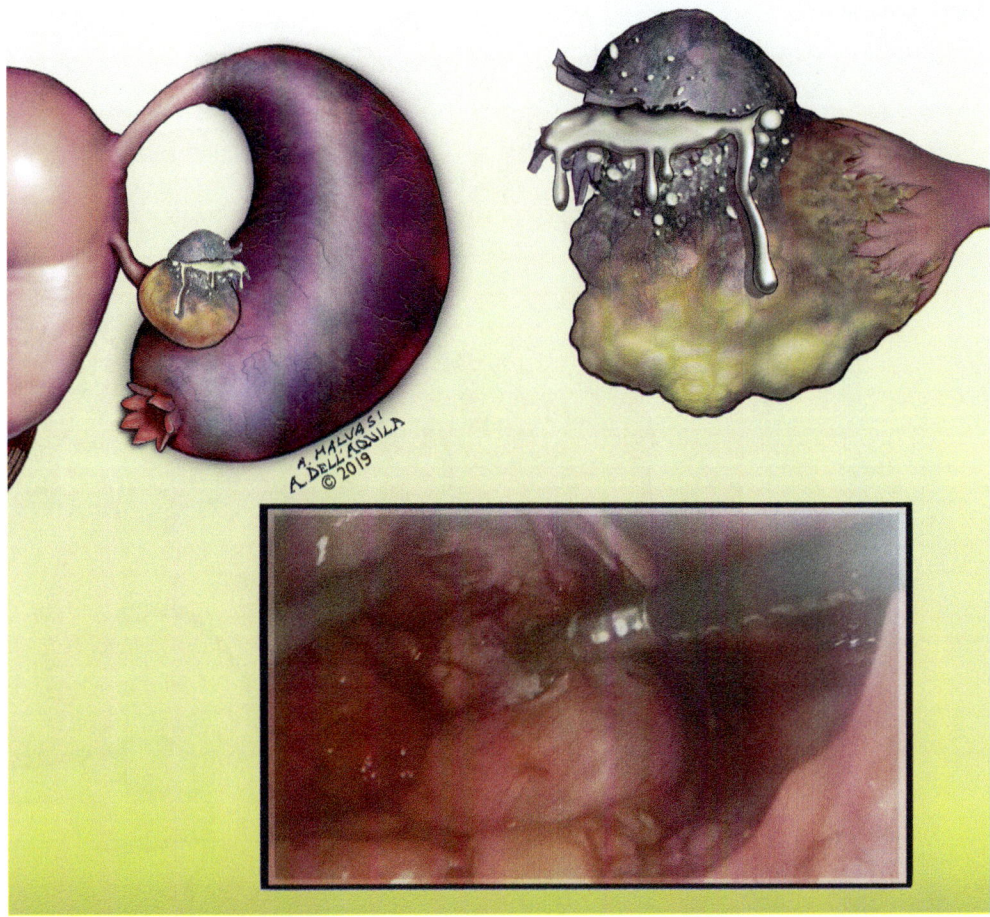

nary urgency, anorexia, and fever. A diagnosis of urinary tract infection was set up before 2 days and nitrofurantoin, (100 mg daily for 3 days) was administered. On pelvic ultrasound and computed tomography, large bilateral loculated pelvic abscesses have been diagnosed and (IV) vancomycin, gentamicin, and clindamycin were administered for 7 days. At that time, a CT-guided drainage was performed with a pig-tailed drain to be left in situ. This is where the diagnosis of Actinomyces israelii was set. Same antibiotic regimen continued for the next 4 days. Patient was discharged on ninth day, and continued oral amoxicillin/clavulanate potassium and metronidazole for 14 days [9].

19.3.2.3 Ureaplasma Parvum Peritonitis

Bébéar et al. in 2014 [10], reported an infection, 72 h after oocyte retrieval for male factor infertility. Patient presented with severe pelvic pain and fever, indicating an abdominal infection. She had (IV) cefoxitin 2 mg during oocyte pickup. By TVS, pelvic fluid collection reported in the pouch of Douglas and a perriapendiceal collection. An exploratory laparoscopy was performed and a retro-uterine collection of pus was found. Abscess was drained and on bacteriology, Ureaplasma parvum was reported while blood cultures at the

time of admission have been negative. Neither her husband nor she has been infected from U parvum during OPU. As a treatment, she received ticarcillin, clavulanic acid, and ciprofloxacin. This regimen was changed to (o) ciprofloxacin, 2 days after she established apyrexia. This treatment continued for 21 days. No pregnancy was stated.

19.3.2.4 Pelvic Tuberculosis

Annamraju et al. in 2008 [11], reported pelvic tuberculosis reactivation in a 40-year-old, nulliparous woman with three previous unsuccessful IVF attempts. Last attempt was 9 months before symptoms development. She developed a biloculated cystic mass in the left iliac fossa. By ultrasound, it was found, that it was ovarian in origin, thin walled, avascular, and uniform. A laparotomy revealed a large left retroperitoneal mass, between the descending colon, sigmoid colon, and uterus while the fimbrial end, including the left ovary, was encapsulated in the mass. Operators left this ovary intact while dissected the mass and cleaned the discharge. The examination of the mass, by pathology, suggested tuberculosis. Patient had (IV) cefuroxime and metronidazole for 48 h and for the next 14 days continued on oral medications. Patient advised that before any IVF attempts, a hysteroscopic

Fig. 19.3 Ovaric and tubal
abscess peritonitis

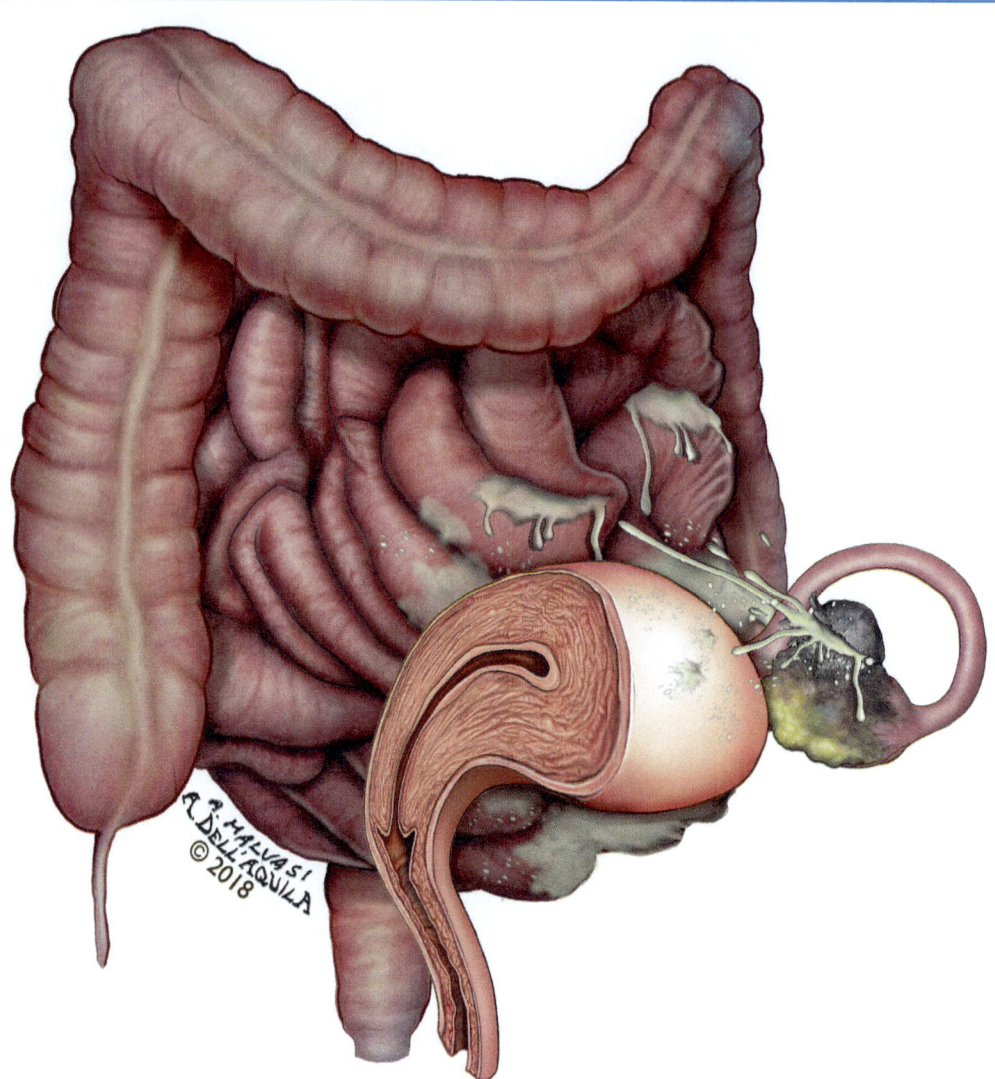

evaluation of the uterus and a laparoscopic evaluation of the peritoneal cavity (or hysterosalpingogram), is needed. In addition, an endometrial biopsy has to be performed to rule out active tuberculosis lesions.

19.4 Complication During Pregnancy

19.4.1 Early Pregnancy Complicated Tubo-ovarian Abscess

Matsunaga et al. in 2003 [12], reported a tubo-ovarian abscess during pregnancy after oocyte retrieval. Patient delivered at 22 weeks of pregnancy and a left salpingo oophorectomy was performed afterwards. Varras et al. in 2003 presented a case of tubo-ovarian abscess in a 38-year-old patient with primary infertility and bilateral hydrosalpinx aspiration, at

the time of TVOR. The authors consider that the possible cause of this infection was PID reactivation of latent pelvic infection [13]. Patient previously had PID. They also conclude that tubo-ovarian abscess has to be taken into diagnosis of peritonitis after OPU. Fertility preservation should be opted for with uterus and ovary preservation. Laparoscopic drainage was the choice for operating a left ovarian abscess with diffuse pus, which developed 3 weeks after oocyte retrieval. This patient was 26 years old and underwent ART for male factor infertility [14]. She was presented with mild abdominal pain and fever that remained even after antibiotic treatment. After laparoscopic drainage and whole pelvis irrigation, three microorganisms have been found (Escherichia coli, bacteroides and peptostreptococcus species). Patient was discharged 5 days after the surgery. She was pregnant at 5 weeks of gestation, during surgery, but miscarried at 8 weeks. No recurrence took place.

19.4.2 Pregnancy at Second Trimester Complicated Tubo-ovarian Abscess

Den Boon et al. in 1999 [15] described the rupture of a bilateral ovarian abscess, at the end of second trimester and the acute abdomen development. Patient had two IVF cycles in the past for male infertility. She had a previous pregnancy delivered at the 28 weeks of gestation with cesarean section (after IVF). From her medical history, patient had a laparotomy for an ovarian endometrioma. During the second IVF procedure, operators detected an endometrioma that was not punctured, in the left ovary. Antibiotic prophylaxis was administered the day before, during, and after the OPU. A diamniotic dichorionic pregnancy was the result of this IVF. At 25 weeks of gestation, she was admitted to the hospital with symptoms of labor. Tocolysis was performed and cervical effacement and dilatation was evident. The days of admission, she developed an infection, acute abdomen, rebound tenderness, and guarding. An emergency laparotomy was performed. Pus in the pouch of Douglas originating from the right ovary has been found. Both ovaries had small abscesses that drained with multiple incisions. A drain was placed in the pouch of Douglas. Antibiotics have been administered. Peritoneal cultures revealed Staphylococcus aureus and mixed anaerobic bacteria. At 26 weeks of gestation, she went into labor delivering two boys. Pulmonary edema and peritonitis was developed. On the fifth postpartum day, a second laparotomy was performed but no pus was found. She was discharged after 3 weeks from her delivery. One of the infants died 9 weeks postpartum.

19.4.3 Term Delivery Complicated Tubo-ovarian Abscess

Kim et al. in 2013 [16] reported a tubo-ovarian abscess after oocyte retrieval. This infertility treatment, ended to a pregnancy. A 33-year-old patient, with 4 years of infertility, presented with a history of a left tubal pregnancy, bilateral tubal obstruction, and a 4.5-cm endometrioma on the right ovary. Tubal factor was considered the reason for infertility treatment. Before ovarian stimulation, she had a course of ciprofloxacin 250 mg for 5 days because of vaginitis due to Ureaplasma urealyticum and Mycoplasma hominis. During OPU, no puncture of endometrioma took place. After the procedure, patient became pregnant and at 7 weeks of pregnancy, presented with right lower abdominal pain and growth of an endometrioma mass. At that time, conservative management and observation was decided. At 14 weeks gestation, patient presented with lower abdominal pain mimicking appendicitis. After ultrasonography and MRI, a pelvic abscess was found, that arise from the right adnexa, adherent to the posterior wall of the uterus, right pelvic sidewall, and sigmoid colon. On laparoscopic examination, it was found that the abscess was encapsulated within the ovary and there was no pus within the pelvis. Pus drainage was performed and a drain was placed in the pouch of Douglas. Cefotiam (IV) (1 g every 12 h) and metronidazole (500 mg every 8 h) was administered for treatment. The drain was retained for 2 days, while patient was discharged after 10 days. Her pregnancy continued at 8 months while no recurrence was observed.

19.4.4 Late in Pregnancy Complicated Tubo-ovarian Abscess

Younis et al. in 1997 [17] reported three cases of pelvic abscess that developed on ovarian endometriosis. The first one was a 34year-old woman with 12 years of primary infertility. The second one was a 36-year-old with 10 years primary infertility and the last one was 29 years old with 4.5 years of infertility. Both the first and the second had a stage IV endometriosis and the last one had diffuse pelvic endometriosis with bilateral endometrioma. These have been considered the reason for infertility. The first case received laparoscopic adhesiolysis, bilateral tubolasty, and right endometriosis cystectomy. The last two had laparoscopy with the second one to receive bilateral endometriosis cystectomy. All three patients received GnRH agonist downregulation. In the first case, a 4-cm endometrioma was aspirated while in the other two cases, aspiration was not performed. All three patients received prophylactic antibiotics (IV cefazolin). The first patient, 40 days after oocyte retrieval, admitted to the hospital with signs of abdominal infection and a left ovarian multicystic mass. Laparotomy was performed and chocolate-like material was expelled from the cyst. Patient received broad spectrum antibiotics and discharged. Eight weeks later, she developed pelvic peritonitis. In TVS, bilateral complex adnexal masses compatible with bilateral tubo-ovarian abscesses have been revealed. IV antibiotics have been administered again but sonographic findings remained the same. Three weeks later, she had bilateral salpingo-oophorectomy with spillage of pus coming from both ovaries. She recovered uneventfully. The second patient developed high temperature, 24 days after oocyte retrieval. She had no signs from the ovaries, and admitted to the internal medicine department to be treated for Q fever. She was discharged and after 4 weeks, was admitted with high temperature, low abdominal pain, and bilateral tender adnexal masses. On transvaginal ultrasound, bilateral adnexal multicystic complex masses have been observed and the diagnosis was set up for tubo-ovarian abscesses. Patient received intravenous antibiotics and a laparotomy with bilateral salpingo-oophorectomy was performed. In addition, the second patient, recovered uneventfully. The third patient, 22 days after OPU, developed low abdominal pain, bilateral tender adnexal masses, and high temperature. These masses were also complex and compatible with tubo-ovarian abscess. She received IV antibiotics and clinical improvement was evident, although fever remained up to 38 C. On the sixth day of admission, IV treatment was changed and fever and WBC fell to normal levels. Patient was discharged home, after 15 days of intravenous antibiotics, and continued on oral antibiotics. She became pregnant, with an intrauterine viable fetus and at 14 weeks pregnancy, a viable pregnancy was observed. Patient delivered at term.

19.4.5 Pyometra Development and Hysterectomy

A 43-year-old woman, with three previous IVF attempts and no pregnancy, underwent the last oocyte retrieval. Four weeks after OPU, she presented with fever and chills and left lower quadrant tenderness. Laboratory studies showed an ever-increasing infection while CT and MRI revealed a large heterogeneous myomatosus uterus with several fibroids. Patient was administered vancomycin, aztreonam, metronidazole, and ciprofloxacin but her condition did not resolve. After that diagnostic laparoscopic and hysteroscopy was performed to evaluate focal points of infection. On laparoscopy, an old pelvic inflammatory disease with bilateral hydrosalpinges and perihepatic adhesions was seen. On the contrary, hysteroscopy revealed pyometra. Endometrial cultures were taken and revealed vancomycin-resistant enterococci. Linezolid added to the treatment scheme and vancomycin was taken out. Patient discharged on linezolid and metronidazole. Two weeks later patient readmitted with signs of infection and the CT scan showed resistant pyometra. Severe infection and signs of shock have been developed while fever remained at high levels. For that reason, total abdominal hysterectomy was performed and her condition was substantially improved. Patient discharged after 5 days. No other postoperative problems have been reported [18].

19.5 Endometriosis-Endometrioma Associated Complications

19.5.1 Endometrioma Abscess

19.5.1.1 General
In a retrospective study, Benaglia et al. in 2008 [19], poses the question whether ovarian endometrioma abscesses are a

true risk after oocyte retrieval, or a rare event. They included patients with 1, 2, 3, or more ovarian endometriomas that underwent ovarian hyperstimulation and OPU, from 2004 to 2006. Diameters ranged from <20 mm to >30 mm with the majority of them to be at the first group. All women were covered with ceftriaxone 1 g for 4 days, starting at oocyte retrieval. Overall, 214 cycles have been examined for pelvic pain, fever, antibiotic use, and hospitalization. There was no difference between the three groups, on the duration of stimulation and pregnancy rates was at 43%. Only three cases had an IVF-correlated complication. Two of them presented with moderate ovarian hyperstimulation and one had unexplained fever starting 7 days after OPU. Patient recovered in 2 days. None of the women developed endometriotic abscess either when endometriomas punctured accidentally or not (Figs. 19.4 and 19.5). Authors conclude that endometriotic pelvic abscesses after oocyte retrieval are very low. Although in this study, the diagnosis of endometriomas has been done only by ultrasound and not by histology, care has been taken to exclude other functional ovarian cysts.

19.5.2 Endometrioma and Pregnancy Outcome

In another study [20], 24 patients with an ovarian endometrioma that aspirated at the time of OPU, completed 29 cycles. These patients have been compared retrospectively with 84 patients (147 cycles) for all main IVF parameters. No adverse outcomes have been reported following endometrioma aspiration and a similar total number of embryos have been obtained. There was no difference in clinical pregnancies, between the two groups. It appears that endometriosis does not adversely affect pregnancy rates and ovarian endometriomas after IVF, have a minimal impact on pregnancy rates.

19.5.3 Endometriosis-Pelvic Infection

Moini et al. in 2005 [21], answered the question, whether endometriosis raises the risk of pelvic inflammatory disease (Fig. 19.5), after OPU. In his retrospective study, out of 5958 cycles, ten patients developed pelvic inflammatory disease. Diagnosis of PID was set up on certain criteria, and usually was evident 4–7 days after oocyte retrieval. Eight out of the ten women that diagnosed with PID, had endometriosis. It was found after clinical symptoms for endometriosis and diagnostic laparoscopy. One of them had an endometrioma, and the others had stage II, III, IV endometriosis. The non-endometriosis patients had bilateral tubal obstruction and a history of PID. After

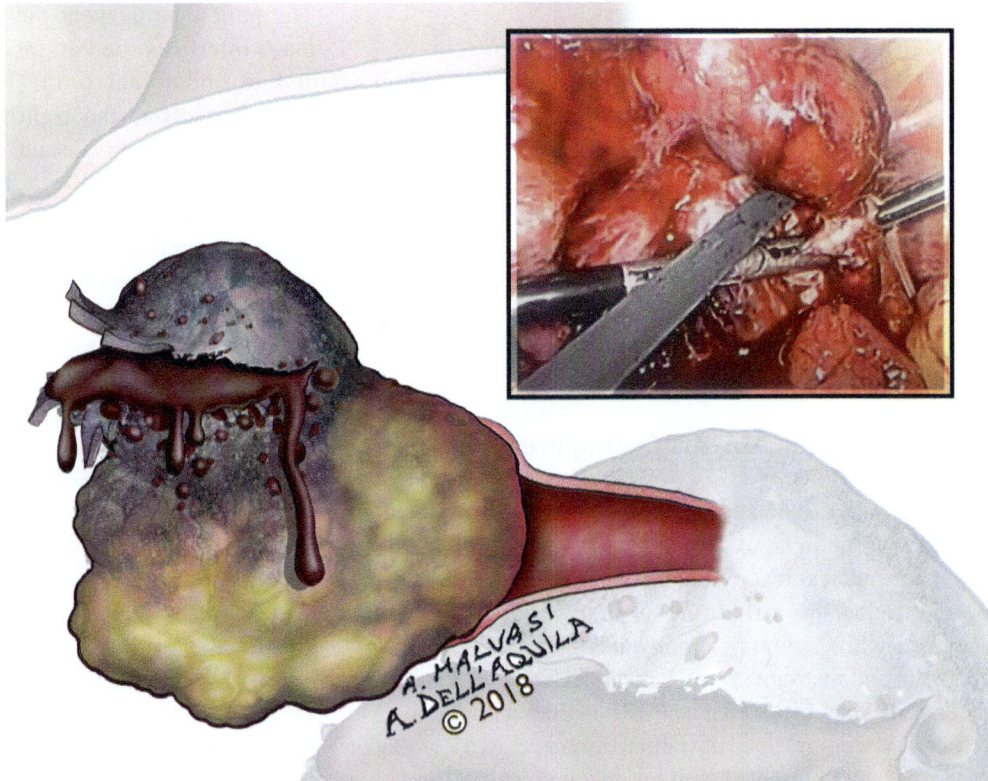

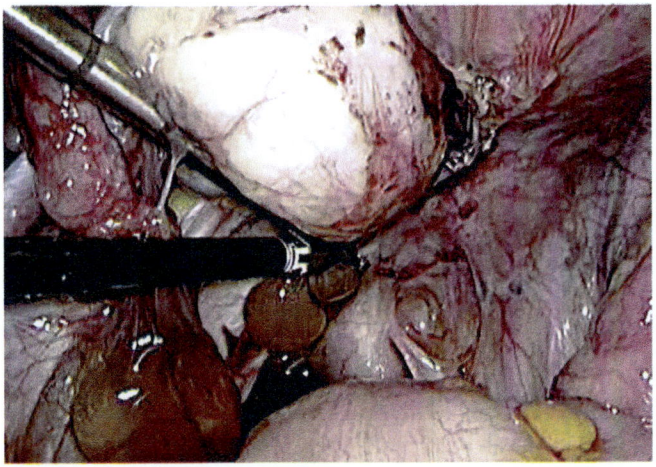

Fig. 19.5 Chocolate cysts in patient with PID

the diagnosis of pelvic inflammatory disease, five of them treated conservatively with antibiotics, while the other three needed surgical intervention. Two of the patients had laparoscopic drainage of abscess; one of them had a transvaginal drainage of abscess, while the other two needed laparotomy. All patients recovered well. Authors conclude that inoculation of vaginal bacteria and anaerobe microorganisms after oocyte retrieval can cause pelvic inflammatory disease. On the contrary, no pelvic infection has been reported in the literature, after laparoscopic or abdominal oocyte retrieval.

19.5.4 Bilateral Ovarian Abscess

Kelada et al. in 2007 [22], reported on a 35-year-old woman, with no previous pregnancies and a bilateral ovarian abscess formation. Patient presented with left iliac fossa pain and diarrhea, 16 days after oocyte retrieval. Also she presented with vaginal bleeding. Ovarian hyperstimulation syndrome was evident and at first, clexane 20 mg/day administered. On further evaluation with transvaginal ultrasonography, bilateral ovarian masses have been seen. Although, infection was not evident, at the later stage, she developed fever (over 38 °C). Patient administered cefuroxime and metronidazole for 48 h but infection continued. Even after a replacement to clindamycin and gentamicin, there is no improvement on infection signs while abdominal guardening and generalized tenderness was developed. Consumption coagulopathy was evident while her condition has been deteriorating. Laparotomy has been performed and the abscess capsule was excised, from each ovary. Pus drained and the culture showed staphylococci. Peritoneal cavity was washed out from pus while two drains where left in the site. As a treatment, clindamycin and gentamicin were continued postoperatively while the patient was discharged on the fourth day. Authors did not mention further complications but they conclude that if antibiotics response in 72 h is minimal, then exploratory laparoscopy or laparotomy should take place.

19.5.5 Right Ovarian Abscess

In one of the earliest reports for endometrioma abscess after oocyte retrieval, it was documented the development of a right ovarian endometrioma that aspirated during OPU [23]. Patient after OPU had an embryo transfer. Two weeks after oocyte retrieval, she developed signs of peritonitis and an immediate laparoscopy revealed a ruptured right ovarian abscess. The patient had laparoscopic drainage and IV antibiotics. Fortunately she achieved a single ongoing pregnancy, at the time of the publication.

19.5.6 Ovarian Abscess During Pregnancy

Sharpe et al. in 2006 [24] described an ovarian abscess in a 35-year-old nulliparous woman with long-term infertility. From her medical history, she had endometriosis and a right ovarian endometrioma. During OPU, this endometrioma was aspirated while antibiotic prophylaxis was administered (IV cefazolin and metronidazole). Patient became pregnant with a dichorionic diamniotic pregnancy. Thirteen weeks after oocyte retrieval, she complained of vaginal discharge. At 17 weeks of pregnancy, she presented with an ongoing vaginal discharge and low-grade fever, nausea, vomiting, and malaise. Vaginal and blood cultures, chest X-rays and ultrasound have been performed. Except the twin pregnancy, no other findings have been found to indicate the infection origin. Patient improved transiently on azithromycin but vaginal discharge increased. On 18th week, after a repeat ultrasound, a mild enlargement in the right ovarian mass was observed. Metronidazole was administered but with no effect. After 30 weeks of pregnancy, discharge was increasing while by ultrasound and MRI, a right ovarian abscess was revealed. A vaginal fistula was evident clinically while cefotaxime and metronidazole was started. On first instance, S. viridans was recognized. Despite clinical improvement, a cesarean section was performed at 31 weeks of pregnancy and two healthy twins have been delivered. In abscess fluid, S. viridans, Escherichia Coli, Bacteroides, and Peptostreptococcus species, have been identified. At that time, it was preferred not to drain. A percutaneous drain was inserted, 23 days later. Patient discharged 10 days postpartum while parenteral antibiotic therapy was continued for 4.5 weeks. Antibiotics sustained for another 4 weeks, orally. Authors agree that delayed diagnosis and therapy was made, due to variable symptoms. The continuation of pregnancy did not allow for surgical intervention before 32 weeks.

19.5.7 Gigantic Ovarian Abscess

Hameed et al. in 2010 [25], reported a rare case of De Novo gigantic ovarian abscess within an endometrioma.

The patient, a 47-year-old nulliparous woman, with primary infertility, had an increase in temperature (38.5 °C) and in abdominal girth. The abdominal extension was more evident in the right side and the whole abdomen was tender. On a CT scan, a large ovarian mass, ascites, and obstruction of the left ureter were evident. Patient started on antibiotics and a midline laparotomy incision, was performed. A large cystic mass in the right adnexa was identified, after aspiration of 6 L of pus. Ovarian cyst was drained and 5 L of pus aspirated. Inside the cavity wall there was necrotic tissue. Many fibroids existed on the large uterus. For this reason, a subtotal hysterectomy with right oophorectomy was performed. As a next step, a left oophorectomy with adjunct endometriotic cysts was performed. Patient remained in intensive care and transfused six units of blood. On pus cultures, Bacteroides fragilis was developed, and treated with tazocin. She remained on antibiotics for 10 days and discharged on the 14th postoperative day. On histology, marked inflammation was on the right ovarian cyst wall with glandular foci, indicating endometriosis. In addition, the left ovary had an endometriotic cyst. Authors conclude that patient's primary infertility was due to undiagnosed endometriosis. An infection, ascending from the vaginal canal, was spread to the endometrioma. Pus leakage from the abscess created peritonitis and transformed ovarian abscess to an acute gynecological emergency.

19.6 Hydrosalpinx and Its Management

19.6.1 Starting Recommendation

Tubal disease and hydrosalpinx are important factors for reduced pregnancy rates after in vitro fertilization. Hydrosalpinges, when found by ultrasound (Figs. 19.6 and 19.7), need laparoscopic salpingectomy because clinical pregnancy and ongoing pregnancy rates are increased [26]. Even if laparoscopic occlusion of the fallopian tube is performed then there is significant increase in the clinical pregnancy rates [27]. Both methods are of equal importance, in terms of ongoing pregnancy. Ultrasound-guided aspiration of hydrosalpinges (Fig. 19.8) and its effect on pregnancy rates remains to be elucidated.

19.6.2 Hydrosalpinx Aspiration

In a case report, Hinckley and Milki in 2003 [28] reported two patients that had hydrosalpinges aspiration at the time of oocyte retrieval and rapid accumulation of hydrometra before embryo transfer. The first patient had bilateral distal tubal occlusion and prominent hydrosalpinx on the left

Fig. 19.6 Ultrasonography of hydrosalpinx

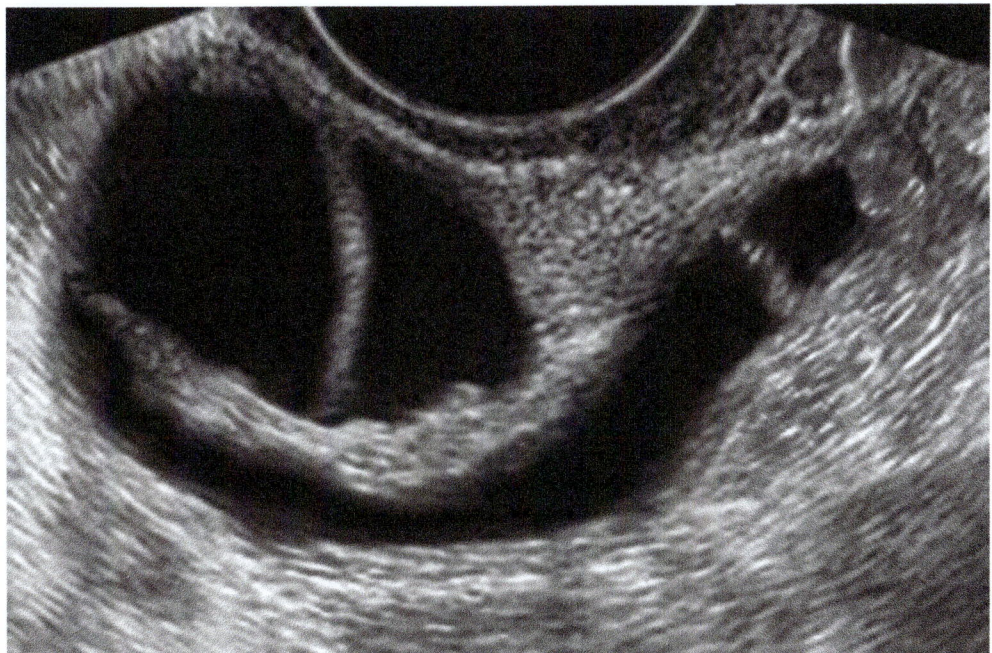

Fig. 19.7 Schematic rappresentation of hydrosalpinx

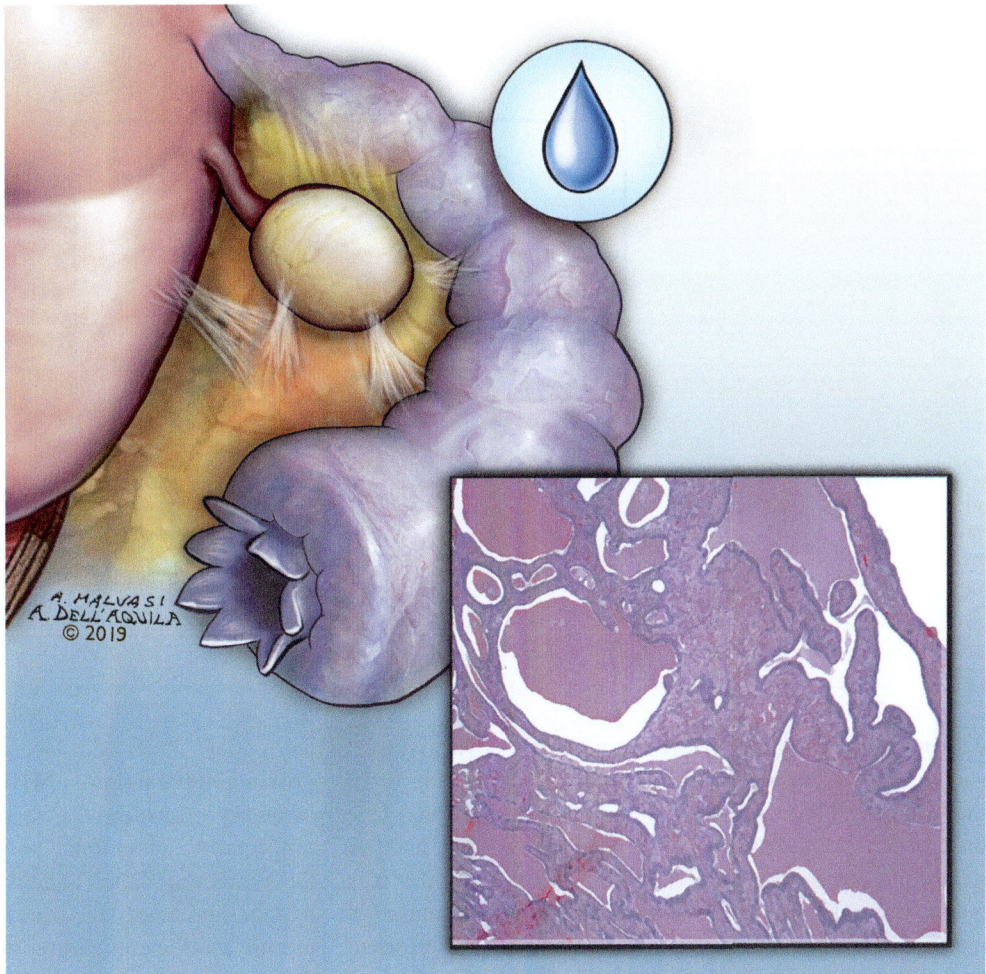

Fig. 19.8 Transvaginal aspiration of hydrosalpinx

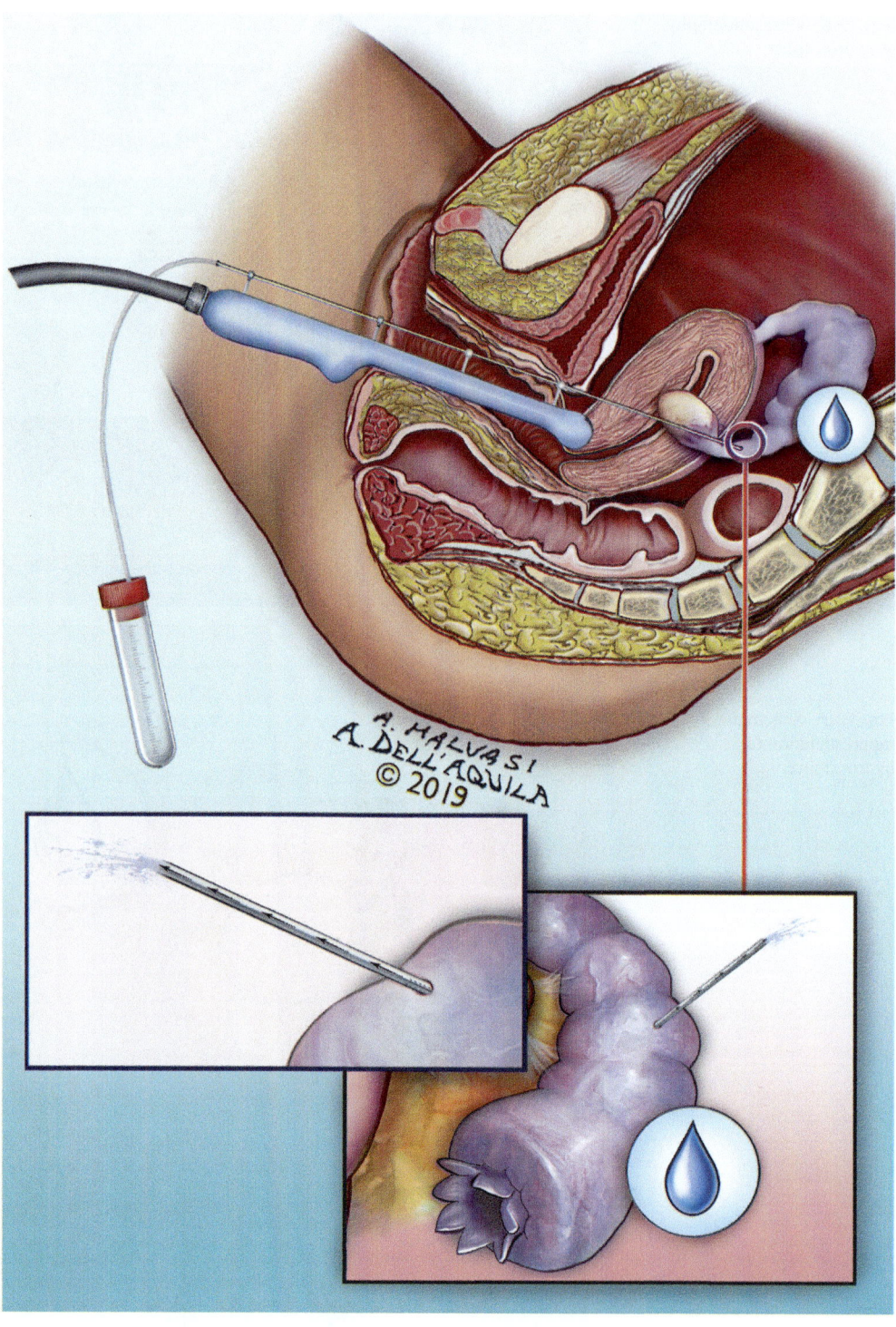

with no visualization of hydrometra. After oocyte retrieval and aspiration, an ultrasound was performed on day three that suggested fluid accumulation inside the uterus. This fluid was aspirated and partially accumulated 1 h later. A second aspiration was performed and embryo transfer was postponed until day five. At this day, fluid accumulation in the uterus was increased, aspirated again but returned to the same size 2 h later. Embryo transfer was postponed

and patient underwent laparoscopic salpingectomy and left proximal tubal ligation. No hydrometra was seen at the time of embryo transfer. The second patient had a previous salpingectomy for ectopic pregnancy and a hydrosalpinx of the remaining tube. Patient underwent controlled ovarian hyperstimulation, and at day 3 just before embryo transfer, uterine fluid accumulation was suspected. Hydrometra was 5 mm, hydrosalpinx was refilled to 1.9 cm. Embryo transfer was postponed until day five, and aspiration was performed. Fluid disappearance was evident with ultrasound. Embryo transfer was canceled and blastocyst cryopreservation was performed. Patient underwent proximal tubal ligation and after that frozen/thaw, embryo transfer was performed with no hydrometra to be seen at the time of embryo transfer.

19.6.3 Hydrosalpinx Aspiration and Pregnancy Rates

In a randomized controlled trial, Hammadieh et al. in 2008 [29], examined the effect of ultrasound-guided hydrosalpinx aspiration on pregnancy rates. The control group consisted of patients with hydrosalpinges, which received no intervention. Aspiration was performed on the day of the oocyte retrieval. There is significant difference in biochemical pregnancy rates favoring the aspiration group. As a next step, authors examined the time of fluid re-accumulation. They scanned 2–3 days after the aspiration and 14 days later. About 38% of the patients that had fluid accumulation at 14 days got pregnant while 39% of the patient that did not get fluid re-accumulation became pregnant. Authors conclude that fluid re-accumulation after aspiration does not impair pregnancy rates. Most importantly, after microbiological cultures only one patient found positive to Escherichia coli. Improvement in the clinical pregnancy and implantation rates, in the aspiration group, did not reach statistical significance. No ectopic pregnancy was reported in this study.

19.6.4 Hydrosalpinx Aspiration/Pregnancy Rates Trials

Sharara in 2009 [30], in a letter to the journal of Human Reproduction, poses certain questions that need to be taken into account in the design of clinical trials for ultrasound-guided hydrosalpinx aspiration. All patients have to have hysterosalpingography or a prior laparoscopy for diagnosis of hydrosalpinx. Endometrial fluid collection should be noted and hydrosalpinx fluid accumulation to be recorded. The time needed for fluid re-accumulation should be associated with pregnancy rates. Bilateral hydrosalpinx need to be compared to unilateral hydrosalpinx, in terms of pregnancy rates.

19.6.5 Hydrosalpinx Aspiration and Mouse Embryo Assay

Chen et al. in 2012 [31] presented a case report of ultrasound-guided hydrosalpinx aspiration combined with the mouse embryo assay of hydrosalpinx fluid for selection

of appropriate treatment. Left hydrosalpinx was recognized at the seventh day of ovarian stimulation that increased in size. On the day of hCG administration, endometrial fluid collection of 15 mm was organized. At oocyte retrieval, hydrosalpinx aspiration was performed transvaginally, until it completely collapsed. Microbiological cultures of the fluid were performed and bacterial infection was not found. After that, the mouse embryo assay was performed with hydrosalpinx fluid. Two days after oocyte retrieval, an ultrasound examination, indicated that the endometrial fluid was reduced to 5 mm. A decision was taken, to perform a day three embryo transfer. Seven days later, no endometrial fluid collection or hydrosalpinx, was noted. A singleton pregnancy was established and delivered at 39 weeks of gestation.

19.6.6 Hydrosalpinx Aspiration vs. Laparoscopic Salpingectomy

In a randomized controlled trial that compared hydrosalpinx fluid aspiration versus laparoscopic salpingectomy, no significant difference was found in clinical and ongoing pregnancy rates. Laparoscopic salpingectomy performed at least 2 months before oocyte retrieval while hydrosalpinx aspiration performed at the time of OPU. Fluid re-accumulation was examined on the day of embryo transfer and 2 weeks after, by ultrasound. In the ultrasound, aspiration group three patients had re-accumulation of hydrosalpinx fluid and uterine collection on the day of embryo transfer and did not become pregnant. At the same group, eight other patients had fluid re-accumulation. Obviously, rapid accumulation of hydrosalpinx after aspiration decreases pregnancy rates [32].

19.6.7 Unilateral Hydrosalpinx Fluid Aspiration

In a case report of ultrasound-guided aspiration of unilateral hydrosalpinx, at the time of oocyte retrieval, a patient became pregnant in the same cycle. She had a left hydrosalpinx with blocked right tube that was found 6 years before IVF. She received hydrosalpinx drainage, immediately after oocyte retrieval. Hydrosalpinx fluid was sterile. Patient became pregnant and she had an uneventful antenatal period [33].

19.6.8 Long-Term vs. Short-Term Diagnosis for Hydrosalpinx Fluid Aspiration

Zhou et al. in 2016 [34] have retrospectively tested, whether hydrosalpinx aspiration during oocyte retrieval had a positive effect on embryo implantation and clinical pregnancy rates. In this study, unilateral or bilateral hydrosalpinges have been included, after diagnosed by hysterosalpingography and ultrasound. Four groups have been assigned and further partitioned. The first group included hydrosalpinx diagnosis before IVF while the second group had diagnosis during treatment. Both these two groups received ultrasound-guided hydrosalpinx aspiration immediately after oocyte retrieval. The third group included hydrosalpinges that received no treatment, while the fourth group included women with no hydrosalpinges and received no treatment. This group served as control. All patients received the same downregulation protocol and the same criteria for diagnosing hydrosalpinx either by hysterosalpingography or ultrasound. Study results show that embryo implantation and clinical pregnancy rates are lower in the group of hydrosalpinx diagnosed before IVF and received treatment and the group with hydrosalpinges that received no treatment when compared with the other two groups. There is no difference in these two factors between control group and the second group. Abortion rate was higher in the first and the third group. Ongoing pregnancy rates have been significantly lower in the third group compared with the fourth group. It is not clear why there was significant difference in pregnancy rates between the two groups (A and B) that received hydrosalpinx aspiration immediately after oocyte retrieval. Authors conclude that ultrasound-guided aspiration during controlled ovarian hyperstimulation improves the clinical outcome of IVF, only for hydrosalpinx diagnosed during COH.

19.7 Ureteric Injury

19.7.1 Ureteral Stricture

Fugita and Kavoussi in 2001 [35] reported a ureteral stricture after oocyte retrieval. A 41-year-old woman with a history of laparoscopic myomectomy and five oocyte retrievals underwent IVF. After the last OPU, she experienced dysuria and left-sided flank pain. After 2 weeks, she came to the hospital. On renal ultrasound, it was revealed left ureterohydronephrosis. A nephrostomy tube was placed and retrograde pyelography revealed hydronephrosis and a left distal ureteral obstruction. A CT scan confirmed this obstruction at a level between the vagina and the left ovary. A laparoscopic approach was used to reimplant the left ureter. Laparoscopy was a choice to minimize pain and length of hospitalization. Patient was discharged 2 days after the operation. No complications arose after 6 months of observation when examined by either ultrasound, IV pyelography, or diuretic renography.

19.7.2 Ureteral Obstruction

Miller et al. in 2002 [36] reported an acute ureteral obstruction after oocyte retrieval. A 34-year-old woman with pri-

mary unexplained infertility, and a history of diagnostic laparoscopy and hysteroscopy, underwent OPU. After 7 h, from OPU, she presented with right lower quadrant tenderness and guarding. On transvaginal ultrasound, a small amount of fluid was revealed in the pelvis. On renal ultrasound, a mild right hydronephrosis with debris on the right collection system was evident. Patient was administered (IV) amoxicillin and sulbactam. On a CT scan, the next day, a right hydronephrosis and mild hydroureter was revealed, down to the right adnexa. A ureteral stent was inserted through cystoscopy. Patient had an embryo transfer but did not become pregnant. The stent was removed 3 weeks after, in an office cystoscopy. No complications were reported 6 weeks after stent removal.

19.7.3 Uro-retroperitoneum

Fiori et al. in 2006 [37] reported a different complication of ureteric injury after OPU, the development of uro-retroperitoneum. A 33-year-old woman, with two previous pregnancies that were delivered by cesarean section, presented with uro-retroperitoneum. This complication developed in the first 2 days after OPU. She has no medical history of endometriosis or renal pathology. Two hours after oocyte retrieval, patient presented with severe abdominal pain, dysuria and fluid in the pouch of Douglas. She was hospitalized with IV paracetamol but in the next day she developed fever, nausea, urinary urgency, and bladder tenesmus with abdominal guarding in the right iliac fossa. She started ofloxacin and metronidazole (IV). On the next day an MRI revealed a right lateral uterine collection in the broad ligament and dilation of the right urinary tract collection system. An abdominal CT showed a leakage of the medium through a pelvic-ureter lesion, near the right vesicoureteral junction. A right ureteral stent was inserted through cystoscopy. Patient discharged after 6 days, and the ureteral stent was removed 10 weeks later.

19.7.4 Ureteric Injury and OHSS

Grynberg et al. in 2011 [38] reported a ureteric injury in a 26-year-old woman with ovulatory infertility due to PCOs. This patient, after oocyte retrieval developed mild OHSS. One day after retrieval, she was admitted with pelvic pain (diffuse tenderness with localized hypogastric guarding) and cervical motion tenderness. Minor intra-abdominal fluid was evident due to OHSS, after transabdominal and transvaginal ultrasound. Patient was hospitalized and (IV) paracetamol was administered. Improvement of symptoms was noted and at the second day an embryo transfer was performed. Eight hours later, pelvic pain with radiation to the right lumbar region and polyuria was developed. The clinical picture resembled ureteric injury. On renal sonogram and subsequent uro-computed tomography, a mild right dilatation of pyelocalyceal cavities and proximal ureter was observed, with leakage of contrast medium through a right pelvic-ureter lesion. A cystoscopy and a right ureteral stent was placed. Patient was discharged 24 h later. In 3 weeks, the ureteral stent was removed. At 6 weeks, an IV pyelogram revealed a normal right urinary tract. Patient delivered at 38 weeks gestation (Fig. 19.9).

19.7.5 Hematuria

Papler et al. in 2015 [39] reported a case of delayed massive hematuria (Fig. 19.10) on a 28-year-old woman with 2 years of primary infertility. From her medical history, she has a resection of uterine septum, electrocoagulation of peritoneal endometriosis lesions, and resection of endometriosis nodes on both sacrouterine ligaments, 4 months before IVF. One day after OPU, she presented with bilateral adnexal tenderness and a drop at Hb levels. On ultrasound, a hematoma in the left side of the pouch of Douglas was presented. With cystoscopy (Fig. 19.10), left ureter active bleeding was observed and hemostasis was achieved using monopolar coagulation with wire electrode. A double J-stent was inserted at that time while gentamycin (IV) was administered along with transfusion of concentrated erythrocytes and fresh frozen plasma. On the next day, Hb levels return to normal and blood clots have been disappeared. She received a second cystoscopy at 7 days and the urine catheter was removed. She was discharged the same day. Six weeks later, operators removed the double J-stent.

19.7.6 Early Ureteric Injury

Vilos et al. in 2015 [40] reported an early ureteric injury after OPU, on a 37-year-old patient, gravida 1, with three past IVF trials and a miscarriage. From medical history she had high BMI (42 kg/m^2) and was a carrier of factor V Leiden mutation. Twelve hours after OPU, she noted a watery vaginal discharge. After an immediate CT scan, a right ureteric injury was noted, 1 cm from vesicoureteral junction. A ureteral stent was placed, by cystoscopy, for the next 3 weeks. No fertilization was achieved in this cycle and the patient asked for a second cycle. A diagnostic laparoscopy and hysteroscopy were performed. In laparoscopy, endometriosis type II was found, mainly in the left side of the pelvis. Extensive adhesions have been noted while endometriotic scarring pulled both ovaries toward the pelvic brim. Authors used laser to excise all adhesions and endometriotic implants. Bilateral ureteric stents had been inserted, 1 week before starting the next cycle. During OPU, these stents had been clearly visualized on ultrasound. They remained in position until 48 h post-retrieval. On this IVF cycle, patient became pregnant but miscarried at 8 weeks of gestation.

Catanzarite et al. in 2015 [41] reported a ureteral trauma after OPU. Bleeding from the left ureter was revealed after cystoscopy, laparoscopy, and retrograde pyelography. A left ureteral stent was inserted through cystoscopy and ureteral trauma was managed successfully.

Choudhary et al. in 2017 [42] reported a case of ureteric injury, on a 28-year-old woman, with primary infertility due to male factor. After OPU and still in anesthesia, operator noticed a 4 × 3 cm collection, above the right ovary and minimal fluid collection in the anterior pouch. Abdominal ultrasonography revealed no abdominal fluid. On patient catheterization, frank hematuria was noted while in accompanied cystoscopy, injury of the right ureter was noticed. Continuous trickling of blood from the right ureteric orifice was evident and a ureteric stent was positioned at the same time. Secondary measures included continuous bladder irrigation and intravenous antibiotics. Hematuria was diminished over the next 2 days and the patient discharged after 3 days. This OPU complication did not recur, when patient tested with ultrasound, after 7 days from the discharge and after 6 weeks. After 6 weeks, the stent was removed.

19.8 Uterovaginal and Vesicovaginal Fistulas

Coroleu et al. in 1997 [43] presented a case of a ureteral lesion after oocyte retrieval. A 33-year-old patient, with male factor infertility, and 7 years of infertility had an OPU. After 5 days, patient developed a severe abdominal pain located in the right iliac fossa, dysuria and vesical tenesmus while later, pain spread to right lumbar fossa. On ultrasonography, she had mild OHSS while renal ultrasound revealed pyelocalyceal hydronephrosis of the right kidney with proximal ureter dilation. Also, an irregular enlargement of the right posterolateral wall of the urinary wall was noted.

A diagnostic cystoscopy revealed an edematous area showed neo-formation of tissue occupying all the right hemitrigone. Vesical integrity has been tested and found no need for drainage. In 24 h, all symptoms have ceased and minimal pyelocalyceal dilatation was noted. Unfortunately, loss of vaginal fluid (urine) was reported and transurethral and IV methylene blue was instilled. Ureterovaginal fistula secondary to ureteral lesions was noted. A surgical reimplantation of right ureter was performed by laparotomy. Patient was discharged 12 days after the operation while she was pregnant with a dizygotic twin and delivered at 38 weeks by cesarean section.

Fig. 19.9 Renal injury from needle pickup, this is rare, but in cases of ectopic kidney it can be a really possible complication

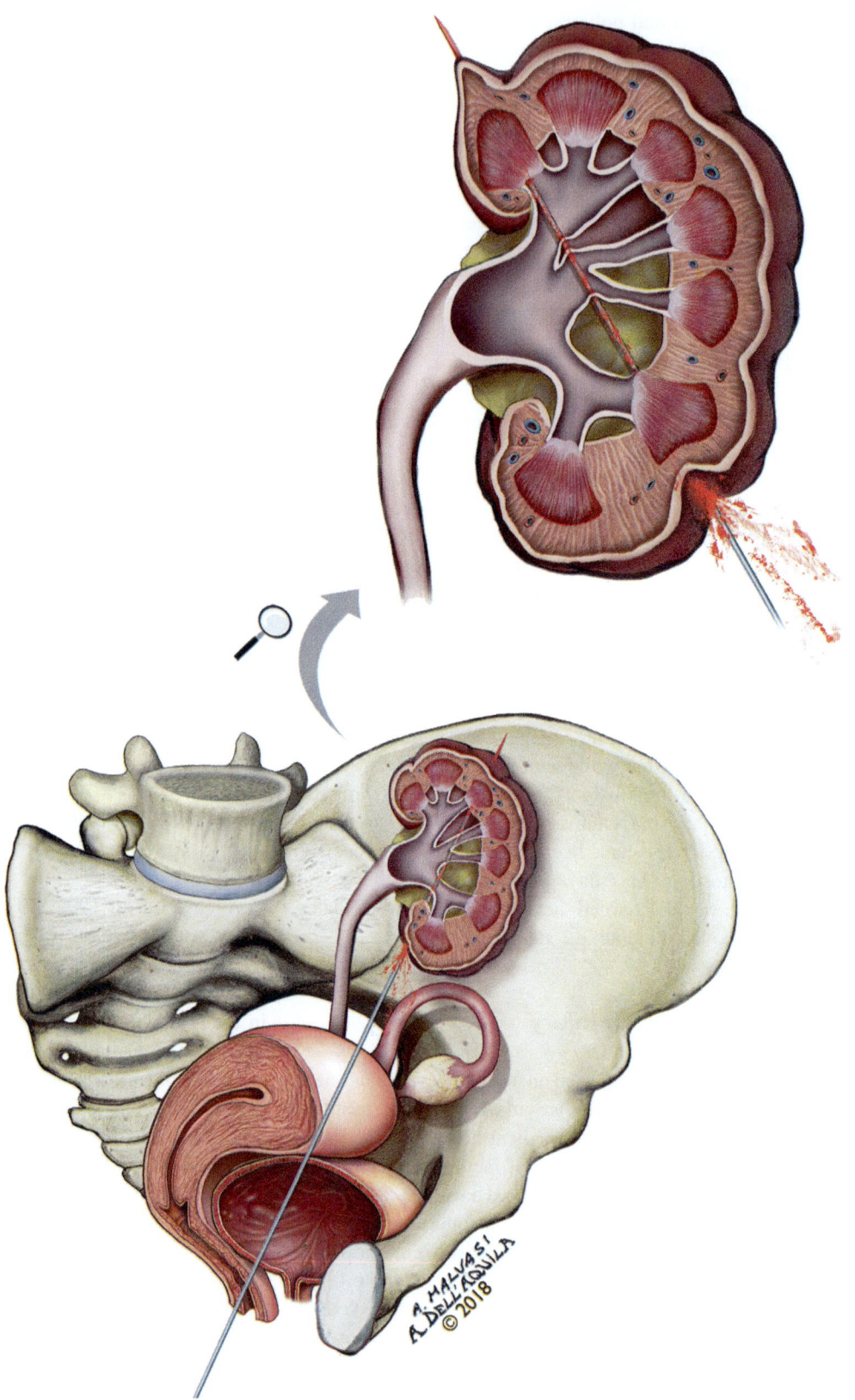

Fig. 19.10 Hematuria after oocyte retrieval by needle pickup

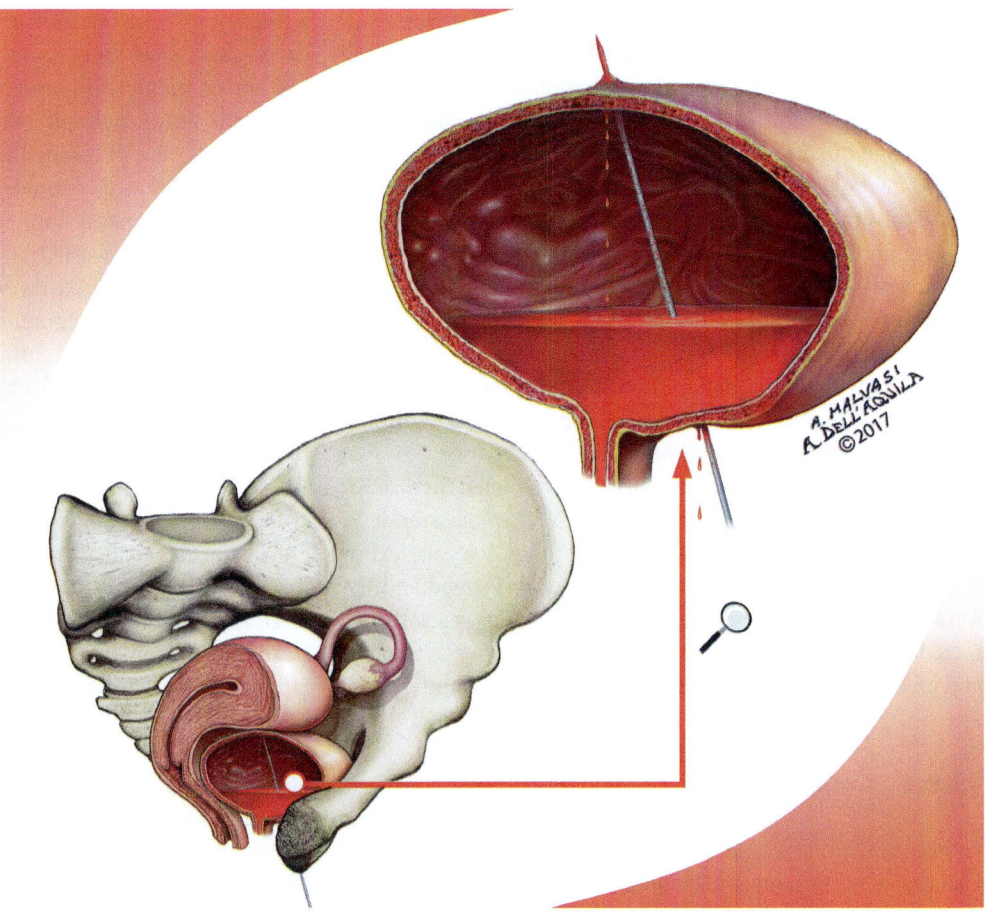

Mongiu et al. in 2009 [44] reported the formation of ureterovaginal fistula, 7 days after oocyte retrieval. A 33-year-old g0p0 with a history of two previous IVF cycles had third oocyte retrieval. After 2 days, she presented with right lower quadrant abdominal pain and fever. WBC was raised to 24.2 K/µL and she received IV antibiotics. No symptoms from the ureter or the bladder, was evident at that time. She had a blastocyst transfer and discharged with antibiotic coverage for another 7 days. After 2 days, she had urinary leakage from her vagina that continued till 21 days after oocyte retrieval. No other symptoms accompanied this leakage. Moderate right renal hydronephrosis was revealed with renal ultrasound. Efflux was observed from the left ureteral orifice with flexible cystoscopy. A tampon was placed to the vagina and bladder was distended with a methylene blue, but no leakage was observed. Under cystoscopic observation and a cone-tipped catheter, methylene blue was instilled to the left and the right ureter. No leakage to the vagina was observed from the left ureter but this was evident from the right ureter confirming a right ureterovaginal fistula. A different approach was used to close this fistula, secondary. Under ultrasound guidance, a percutaneous nephrostomy tube was placed to the dilated right kidney, because fluoroscopic guidance to the ureters was not possible due to the early pregnancy. In 2 days,

vaginal drainage has completely resolved. Unfortunately, on first trimester screening, embryo was found with trisomy 21 and pregnancy was terminated at 15 weeks gestation, on patient's decision. After that, in 2 weeks' time, on contrast instillation from the right nephrostomy tube, no evidence of leakage or fistula was evident. A small defect like ureteral diverticulum was evident. The nephrostomy tube was closed and removed 1 week later. No recurrence took place.

Al-Shaikh et al. in 2012 [45] reported a vesicovaginal fistula after OPU, for male factor infertility. Patient had a fresh embryo transfer while in parallel had watery vaginal discharge. On examination, the bladder was filled with methylene blue and leakage was noted from the vaginal apex at lateral fornix on the left side. Patient declined voiding cystogram and only a 14-Foleys catheter was inserted for full bladder drainage. Catheter remained in position for the next 3 weeks, and no leakage was observed at all. Even with methylene blue dye, no leakage was evident. After that, Foleys catheter was removed. At 17 weeks of pregnancy, patient had a magnetic resonance imaging, for confirmation of bladder integrity. No leakage was observed till the end of the pregnancy.

A case report of an acute uterovaginal fistula was presented in a 33-year-old patient with primary anovulatory infertility and class II obesity [46]. She had a difficult OPU, especially at the left ovary. Immediately after oocyte retrieval, she developed pain that was controlled with analgetics. On her way home, she developed lower abdominal pain, emesis, and leakage of vaginal fluid. She developed abdominal tenderness and infection signs. On urinalysis, she had hematuria. Ovaries were seen with TVS, as usual ovaries after OPU. A freeze-all embryo cycle was planned. A CT scan revealed nothing about the leakage. Even on vaginal examination, no fistula was identified but fluid was pooling in the vagina. On creatinine measurements of the fluid it was found that it was urine. On a CT urogram of the abdomen/pelvis with IV contrast, a small fistula extending from the distal left ureter to the vagina was observed. Bladder cystoscopy revealed no injury, while left retrograde pyelogram revealed contrast extravasation from the distal ureter without associated hydroureteronephrosis. She was inserted with a left double J ureteral stent with Foley catheter to be removed after 2 weeks. After 4 weeks, a left retrograde pyelogram was performed and the stent was removed because uterovaginal fistula was self-corrected. Eight weeks later, patient had a day 5 embryo transfer and an ongoing pregnancy till publication of this study.

19.8.1 Conclusion

Ureteric injury is a rare complication after oocyte retrieval. Usually it is presented with abdominal pain to the side of the injury. Fistula formation is very rare (only two cases reported till now) and becomes evident in about 7 days after OPU. Physician should be aware of this rare complication. Extensive investigations are needed to define the level of the injury. Abdominal or vaginal scans are not sufficient for an early diagnosis. Correction of the injury can be done, with pregnancy continuation, so an embryo transfer is allowed. At the moment, there is no universal method of treatment, but rather inserting a stent in the site of the injury or inserting a nephrostomy tube, diverting the urine flow, and leaving the ureter to heal. In case of a small (<1 cm) vesicovaginal fistula that is diagnosed within 7 days after OPU, conservative management might be sufficient to resolve the situation. Conservative management includes at least 4 weeks of constant bladder drainage because this time interval is correlated with success. For large vesicovaginal fistulas, conservative management offers lower closure rates (12–18%). IVF specialists should know that for this rare complication, early intervention with Foley catheter drainage can cure the condition without long-term morbidity.

19.9 Pseudoaneurysm

A pseudoaneurysm has been developed after transmyometrial and transabdominal oocyte retrieval for the right and left ovaries, respectively. Both procedures have been under ultrasound guidance. The patient, a 34-year-old woman, had a history of four miscarriages. She had received curettages twice and had two spontaneous expulsions. No other history of pelvic inflammation or pelvic surgery has been reported. After ovarian stimulation protocol with GnRH antagonists, she developed more than 53 follicles. The right ovary was located behind the middle uterine settlement and was firmly fixed while the left ovary was beneath left lower abdominal wall. For the transmyometrial puncture, the needle was guided through the right posterior portion of the lower uterine segment to access the right ovary. After this the transabdominal follicular aspiration was performed. The next day, the patient experienced slight bleeding while 6 days later, intermittent vaginal bleeding was evident, and in the seventh day with massive vaginal bleeding. Bleeding was a major symptom. Transvaginal and transabdominal color Doppler ultrasound revealed a pseudoaneurysm. During a CT scan, a vascular lesion of 2.5 cm was seen in the lower uterine segment. Three-dimensional CT angiography showed a ruptured pseudoaneurysm, starting from the peripheral branch of the right uterine artery. Uterine preservation was needed and transcatheter arterial embolization was performed. The pseudoaneurysm and the feeding artery have been embolized. This secured hemostasis and hemodynamic stability. The overall amount of blood loss from the pseudoaneurysm rupture was about 1000–1500 mL. An MRI evaluated the pelvic condition and the position of the ovaries. Patient was discharged 3 days after embolization without any other symptoms. Although arterial embolization is an option for uterine artery pseudoaneurysms, there are concerns about future fertility. Uterine ischemia may influence endometrial receptivity. From the other side, transmyometrial oocyte retrieval should be avoided and early recognition of pseudoaneurysms is mandatory for uterus preserving management.

A very late pseudoaneurysm of the left ovary was presented by Pappin and Plant in 2006 [47]. Patient had an OPU, 6 years earlier. She presented at 12 weeks gestation as a complete miscarriage. Conservative management was decided and after 10 days, on transvaginal ultrasound with color Doppler, a left ovarian cyst with pulsating flow was observed. A diagnosis of 4.5-cm pseudoaneurysm was suspected and an MRI angiogram was performed. This structure originated from anterior branches of the left internal iliac artery. After the diagnosis, patient understood the pulsating cessation of the pseudoaneurysm. Selective embolization was performed and conservative management of miscarriage was continued due to the risk of aneurysm rupture during ERPC. Pseudoaneurysm flow was ceased and she was discharged with advice to avoid pregnancy for a year. After 13 months, with the use of MRI I angiogram, this structure remained occluded.

Another case of pseudoaneurysm reported from Bozdag et al. in 2007 [48]. A 22-year-old woman with primary infertility of 6 years, had oocyte retrieval and an embryo transfer,

Fig. 19.11 Hemaperitoneum from rupture of an ovarian vessel

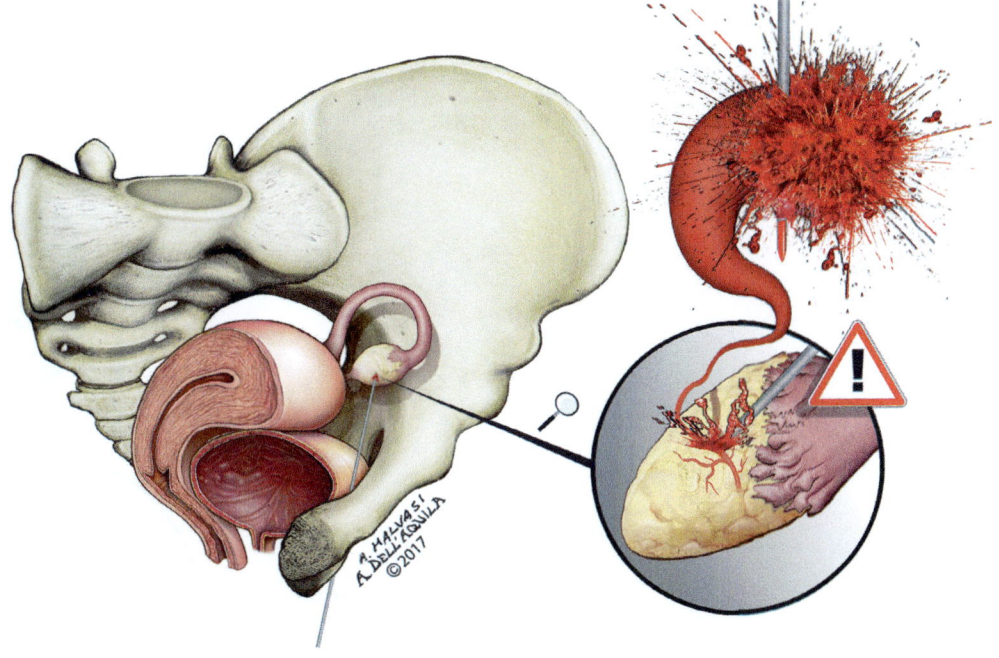

3 days after. She became pregnant and at 29 weeks of gestation and at a planned visit, a unilocular anechoic mass was found in the left upper side of the uterus. Doppler examination for the diagnosis of pseudoaneurysm was set and angiographic MRI revealed this pseudoaneurysm originated from the left internal iliac artery. Patient delivered at 32 weeks gestation due to preterm labor. At this time, a change of the pseudoaneurysm was noted. Eventually this structure was visualized in the left inferior pudendal artery and successfully embolized. The patient was examined at 6 weeks after the procedure with no other changes.

19.9.1 Pseudoaneurysm and Massive Hematuria

Jayakrishnan et al. in 2011 [49] reported massive hematuria in a 34-year-old patient with 8 years of primary infertility and severe endometriosis. She had an embryo transfer 2 days after retrieval. Seven days after oocyte retrieval, patient presented with severe dysuria and frank hematuria. In the next day, she developed severe pain in the abdomen with tachycardia, hypotension, and urinary retention. Patient presented with a hemoglobin fall from 12.8 to 6 g/dL while in parallel she received four units of packed RBCs. She had an emergency cystoscopy and pseudoaneurysm was found in the right ureteric orifice. Pseudoaneurysm cauterization was performed while after that, no other episodes of hematuria was recorded. Hemoglobin rose to 10.5 g/dL. Patient was discharged 3 days after cystoscopy with oral antibiotics. No pregnancy was achieved.

19.10 Hemoperitoneum

Zhen et al. in 2010 [50] investigated the factors that contribute to hemoperitoneum after oocyte retrieval (Figs. 19.11 and 19.12).

In a retrospective study of 10,251 oocyte retrievals, only 22 patients had intraperitoneal bleeding. Only five of them had severe bleeding and underwent laparoscopy or laparotomy. The other patients were managed conservatively. There is significant difference in the number of oocytes retrieved between mild and severe bleeding. Paradoxically mild intraperitoneal bleeding is associated with more oocytes retrieved than the severe one. Also patients with lower body mass index (BMI) have been significantly more susceptible for severe bleeding. Mild bleeding is associated with younger patients and more than 15 oocytes retrieved while 6 of the 17 patients that have been managed conservatively had previous surgical history, either ovarian cystectomy or salpingectomy.

Chatrian et al. in 2012 [51] reported a case report of a 33-year-old woman with male factor infertility undergoing oocyte retrieval. Three hours after oocyte retrieval, developed abdominal pain and hemoglobin was 9.9 g/L but dropped to 9.0 g/L after 6 h. Ultrasound revealed massive hemoperitoneum. Patient had an emergency laparoscopy, 7 h after OPU and at that time, hemoglobin was 7.7 g/L. Active bleeding was recognized from the site of left ovarian puncture. Hemostasis achieved with the use of human fibrinogen and thrombin sponge while in parallel a transfusion of three units of packed red cells were administered. Patient was discharged after 2 days but no embryo transfer took place and all embryos have been cryopreserved.

Fig. 19.12 Hemaperitoneum from rupture of an omental vessel

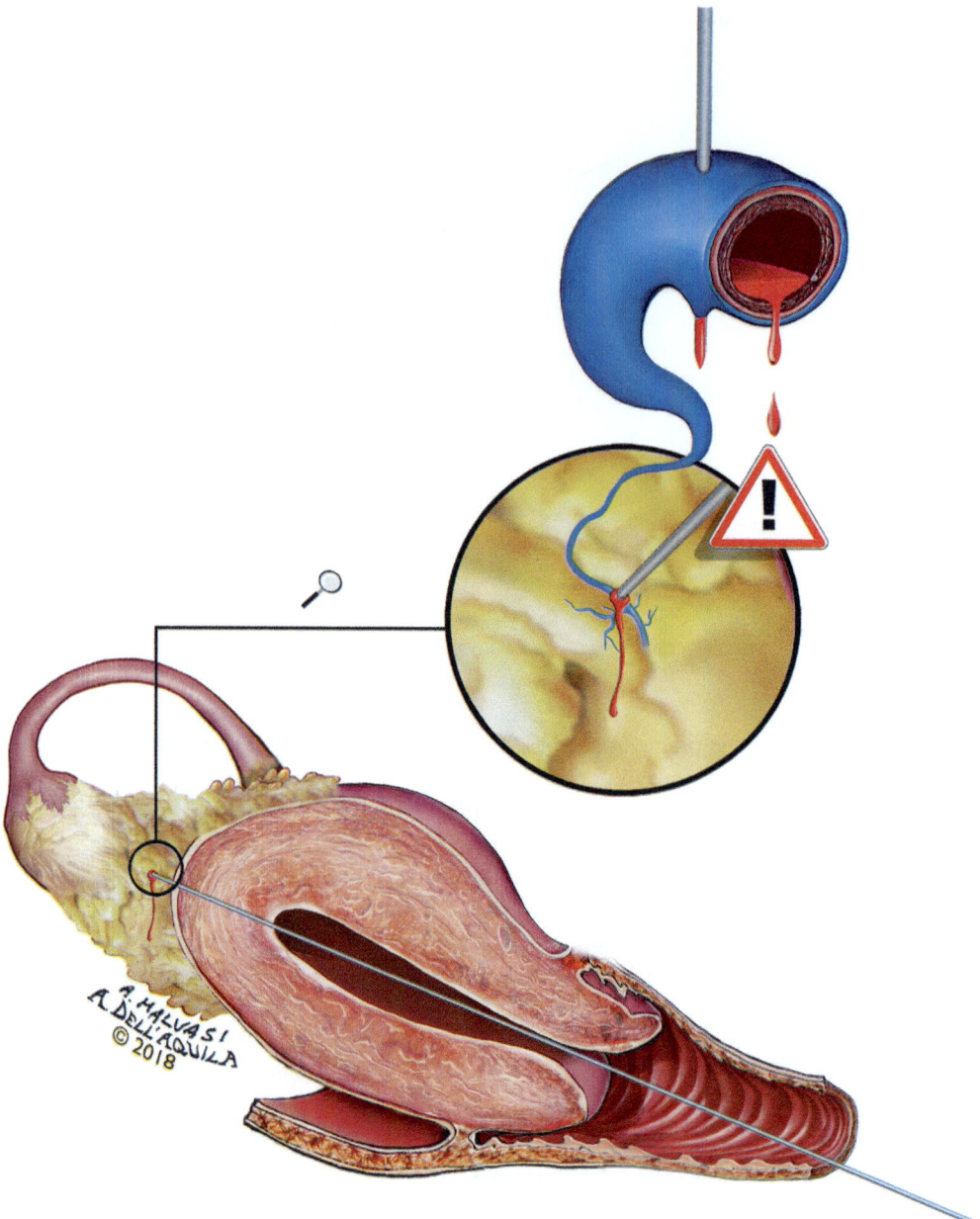

Nouri et al. in 2014 [52] performed a retrospective analysis of hemoperitoneum cases after oocyte retrieval. He examined 28,416 patients where 34 of them had hemoperitoneum. Hemoglobin drop was between 4.5 and 9 g/L (median 6.7 g/L). Some factors that may have contributed to hemoperitoneum were: prolongation of the activated partial thromboplastin time, a combination of the previous factor and decreased factors XI and XII, mild factor VIII deficiency, and IV diclofenac before oocyte retrieval. No consistent risk factor has been recognized from this study while from other studies leanness of the patients (BMI around 20 kg/m^2) and polycystic ovarian syndrome was

evident. Median time of surgical intervention after oocyte retrieval was 10 h (range 1–5 h) while laparoscopy or laparotomy was the main method of treatment, while angiographic embolization of the right and left uterine arteries was performed in one woman. In all except three cases, the bleeding ovary was preserved. One patient had ovarian wedge resection. It is important to mention, that patients, which preserved their ovaries, had significantly shorter time intervals between oocyte retrieval and onset of symptoms. Patients were discharged after 2–10 days (median time of hospitalization 5 days). He concludes that these cases should be better reported.

19.11 Periumbilical Hematoma (Cullens Sign)

Bentov et al. in 2005 [53] presented two cases that developed periumbilical hematoma (Cullens sign) after oocyte retrieval. The first case was a 34-year-old patient with a total of seven IVF cycles due to polycystic selected ovary syndrome, an ectopic pregnancy, and a full-term pregnancy. Patient underwent cryopreservation due to the high number of oocytes retrieved and the possible ovarian hyperstimulation. The days after the procedure, patient presented with urinary tract infection, while and nontender bluish discoloration around umbilicus was noticed. No signs of peritonitis was evident while all clotting tests are normal. She received cefuroxime and metronidazole while skin discoloration disappeared after 2 weeks. The second case report was a 32-year-old woman with primary infertility due to male factor, and a medical history of a laparoscopic ovarian detorsion a year ago. At the end of oocyte retrieval, no active bleeding and no hemoperitoneum were present. A week after oocyte retrieval patient presented with abdominal pain and a periumbilical hematoma with a dark red-blue color. All hematological and clotting factors where in normal range. On the second day, she developed abdominal tenderness and laparoscopy revealed a bilateral ovarian torsion similar to the previous year. Detorsion was performed and patient was discharged on the next day. In general, Gullens sign is associated with hemorrhagic pancreatitis and retroperitoneal hematoma. Other pathological situations that is associated with, is ruptured amoebic liver abscess, malignant liver diseases, intra-abdominal non-Hodgin lymphoma, and ruptured ectopic pregnancy. In this case, authors conclude that hemoperitoneum may spread to the peritoneal folds to the retroperitoneum and from this space may spread to the periumbilical region via the falciform ligament.

19.12 Vertebral Osteomyelitis

Almog et al. in 2000 [54] presented the first case of a vertebral osteomyelitis after IVF treatment. The patient, a 41-year-old woman with unexplained infertility had four previous failed attempts. After the oocyte pickup she had a day two embryo transfer. Nine days after oocyte retrieval she was presented with low back pain, high temperature, and signs of mild infection. She had amoxicillin plus clavulanic acid and fever dropped for a few days. Low back pain insisted radiating symmetrically to both posterior thighs and was unrelieved by the rest. Temperature rose again with signs also of mild infection. Seven days after admission, a spinal MRI did not reveal anything specific. In the next 2 days spiking fevers

have been continuously evident in the evenings. Repeat MRI on the 16th day of hospitalization disclosed an inflammatory process (Fig. 19.13) involving L5, disk L5-S1, and foramen L5-S1. Antibiotic treatment was instituted on the fifth day of hospitalization but was discontinued after 10 days. The days after, a CT-guided needle aspiration of the infected foci was performed but no microorganism was found. On another, temperature rise, blood cultures have been obtained and revealed, Escherichia Coli. This infection was treated with ciprofloxacin for 6 weeks. Patient recovered without any other recurrence of the infection.

Another case of infectious spondylitis has been reported after ultrasound-guided oocyte retrieval, 14 weeks after OPU [55]. Patient had an embryo transfer on day three. The patient, a 31-year-old woman, developed lower back pain for the last 3 weeks and on a lumbar spine magnetic resonance imaging (MRI), high signal intensity of the second and third lumbar vertebrae has been seen. Infectious spondylitis was the first diagnosis, and a spinal biopsy was performed. The spinal biopsy results showed Staphylococcus aureus and IV cefazolin was the antibiotic of choice. In parallel, amniotic fluid cultures showed no infection with an infant in good development. Transthoracic echocardiogram showed that no vegetations have been developed in the mitral or aortic valves. Repeat blood culture on day 9 indicated elimination of Staphylococcus aureus. Pelvic and lower back pain has been improved on day 12. Cefazolin treatment was continued for 6 weeks and patient remained in the hospital for 44 days. She delivered a female at 38 weeks with no other recurrence of the infection.

Some of the routes of vertebral osteomyelitis after oocyte retrieval include the direct inoculation of vaginal organisms, trauma to the loop of the large bowel, and reactivation of previous pelvic infection. The most likely explanation for pelvic infection is the direct implantation of vaginal organisms, followed by reactivated pelvic infection. Large bowel trauma is less likely to take place and has to be accompanied by abdominal or pelvic infection. Trauma to the bone causes the pain, infects the area with microorganisms, and causes inflammation. Vaginal preparation for the procedure is mandatory.

19.13 General Conditions That Predispose to Complications

19.13.1 Hematological Conditions and Its Effect on Hemorrhage After OPU

19.13.1.1 Factor XI Deficiency

In a case report, Battaglia et al. in 2000 [56] described a hemoperitoneum in a 34-year-old woman who underwent

Fig. 19.13 Rare complication, vertebral osteomyelitis after puncture of the needle to pick

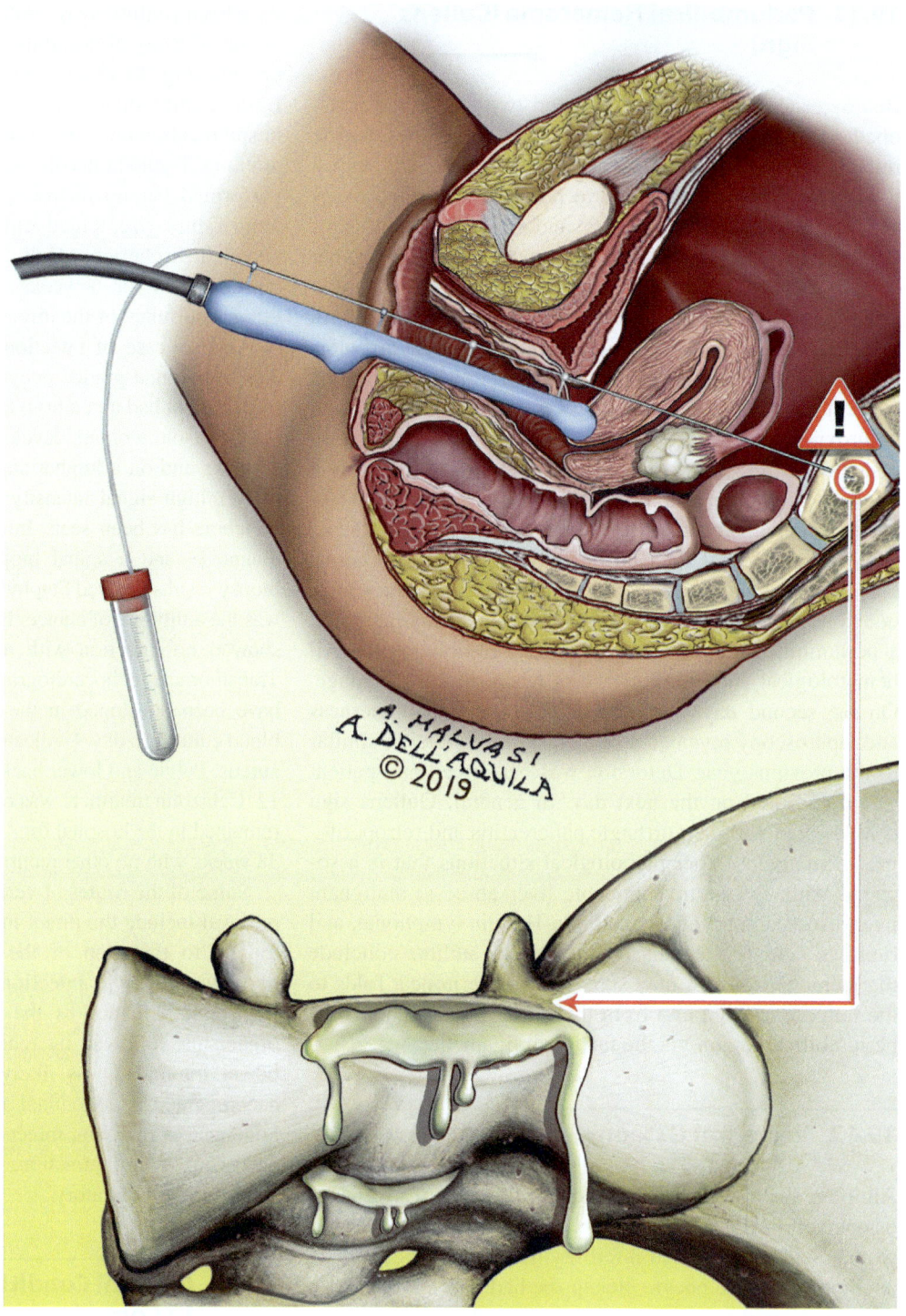

in vitro fertilization for primary infertility of male origin. The patient's bleeding history consisted of easy bruising and two episodes of menorrhagia. As per protocol, 35 h after hCG administration, the transvaginal oocyte retrieval was performed uneventfully, according to standard procedures, followed by a pelvic ultrasound to exclude blood leakage. Three hours later, while the patient was waiting in the observation ward, she suffered from a lipothymic episode. An ulterior drop of the hemoglobin and the appearance of an abdomen rebound, promptly suggested hemorrhage which was confirmed by both transvaginal and transabdominal ultrasonography. An exploratory laparotomy was performed that revealed blood leakage from both ovaries without evidence of iatrogenic damage. Pelvic blood drainage and accurate hemostasis successfully controlled the hemorrhage and the patient was discharged from the hospital 10 days later. A retrospective analysis of the patient's frozen plasma showed a mild prolongation of the activated partial thrombloplastin time (aPTT) (ratio 1.31; normal range 0.82–1.24) that led to a further exploration of the intrinsic pathway coagulation factors and the discovery of Factor XI deficiency (39%; normal range 60–150%).

Although severe hemorrhagic complications after transvaginal oocyte retrieval are rare, they can be life threatening. A thorough family and personal bleeding history as well as global coagulation tests are sufficient to guide the physician toward a more targeted research of a hemostatic disorder. Clinicians should be vigilant about a prolonged aPTT that should always be investigated especially if the patient is about to undergo an invasive procedure. FXI deficiency is not associated with spontaneous bleeding, and therefore, it could remain silent and unrecognized for years. Furthermore, there is no correlation between FXI level and bleeding risk making patient's management complicated [57]. A specialist's approach along with an individual care plan is recommended to prevent bleeding complications.

19.13.1.2 Other Coagulation Factors Deficiencies

In an observational retrospective study, Fatum et al. in 2008 [58] reviewed 1800 patients who underwent oocyte retrieval from 2002 until 2008 and identified eight with a bleeding disorder. For half of them the need for assisted reproduction was of male origin, three had unexplained infertility, and for one patient the cause was mechanical. In two patients, the disorder was already known and the rest was diagnosed in the course of routine preoperative blood tests. Three patients had factor VII deficiency, other three had factor XI deficiency, one had von Willebrand type B2 disease, and one had immune thrombocytopenia (ITP). All patients with factor deficiencies received plasma before the ovum pickup, while the patient with von Willebrand disease had factor VIII infusion and to the patient with ITP were given steroids and intravenous immunoglobulin. None of them experienced bleeding complications and no relation was found between bleeding disorder and IVF outcome. Currently, there is no strong evidence to support the predictive value of preoperative indiscriminate coagulation screening [59]. Assessment of bleeding risk in view of an invasive procedure is based on thorough personal and family bleeding history which will then guide the need for subsequent laboratory tests [60]. If the bleeding history is positive or there is evidence from physical examination, a comprehensive assessment which includes prothrombin Time (PT), aPTT, fibrinogen level, and von Willebrand screen is done. A specialist's opinion is recommended to evaluate the bleeding risk in relation to the severity of coagulopathy (Figs. 19.14 and 19.15) in order to avoid unnecessary blood products or coagulation factors infusion.

19.13.1.3 Thrombocythemia

El-Shawarby et al. in 2004 [61] reported a case of a 37-year-old woman with essential thrombocythemia (ET) who developed an extensive hemoperitoneum after transvaginal ultrasound-guided oocyte retrieval. She underwent medically assisted reproduction for primary infertility of male origin. Her platelet count at the time was 1372 × 109/L and was treated with clopidogrel and low dose aspirin to reduce the risk of thrombosis. No cytoreductive therapy was administered by patient's choice but she was on prophylactic dalteparin injections throughout the ovarian stimulation, which was discontinued on the day of the procedure. Screening coagulation tests were performed preoperatively with no evidence of abnormality. The transvaginal ovum pickup was performed successfully according to the institute's protocol with no complications. Twenty eight hours later, the patient presented lower abdominal pain that quickly ended in hypovolemic shock and a hemoglobin level of 5 g/dL. A prompt resuscitation was followed by an urgent exploratory laparotomy which revealed active bleeding from the right ovary and a massive hemoperitoneum of approximately 3 L of blood. A right salpingoophorectomy had to be carried out to achieve hemostasis. The patient received several units of blood products during and after surgery and was finally discharged 9 days later.

Essential thrombocythemia is not uncommon among women of reproductive age. One of the main concerns for this indolent myeloproliferative disorder is the occurrence of vascular events, both thrombosis and bleeding. The main objective of therapy is to minimize the risk for these events taking into account the patient's age, platelet count, and personal history of thrombosis or major bleeding. Any concomitant cardiovascular risk factors such as hypertension, diabetes, or dyslipidemia should be evaluated for the therapeutic decision and adequately treated. Therapy is essentially focused on antiplatelet agents with or without cytoreductive therapy. However, if PLT count is >1000 109/L and/or the patient has a history of bleeding, the possibility of an acquired von Willebrand syndrome should be considered and investigated [62]. If this is confirmed, the use of antiplatelet agents is contraindicated because the patient is at high risk of bleeding. A careful evaluation from a hematologist is recommended before undertaking any invasive procedure to balance the hemorrhagic and thrombotic risk.

In general, no predisposing factors have been associated with hemoperitoneum during oocyte retrieval. Only when woman have a BMI around 20 kg/m² and have polycystic ovary syndrome may be more susceptible for hemoperitoneum. The reason for that is the increased number of oocytes retrieved or the fragility of the ovarian tissue as it is observed in ovarian lacerations. In case of abnormalities detection in the coagulation system, transfusion of fresh frozen plasma, concentrated preparations of the deficient

Fig. 19.14 Rare complication, thrombotic event of the retinal artery

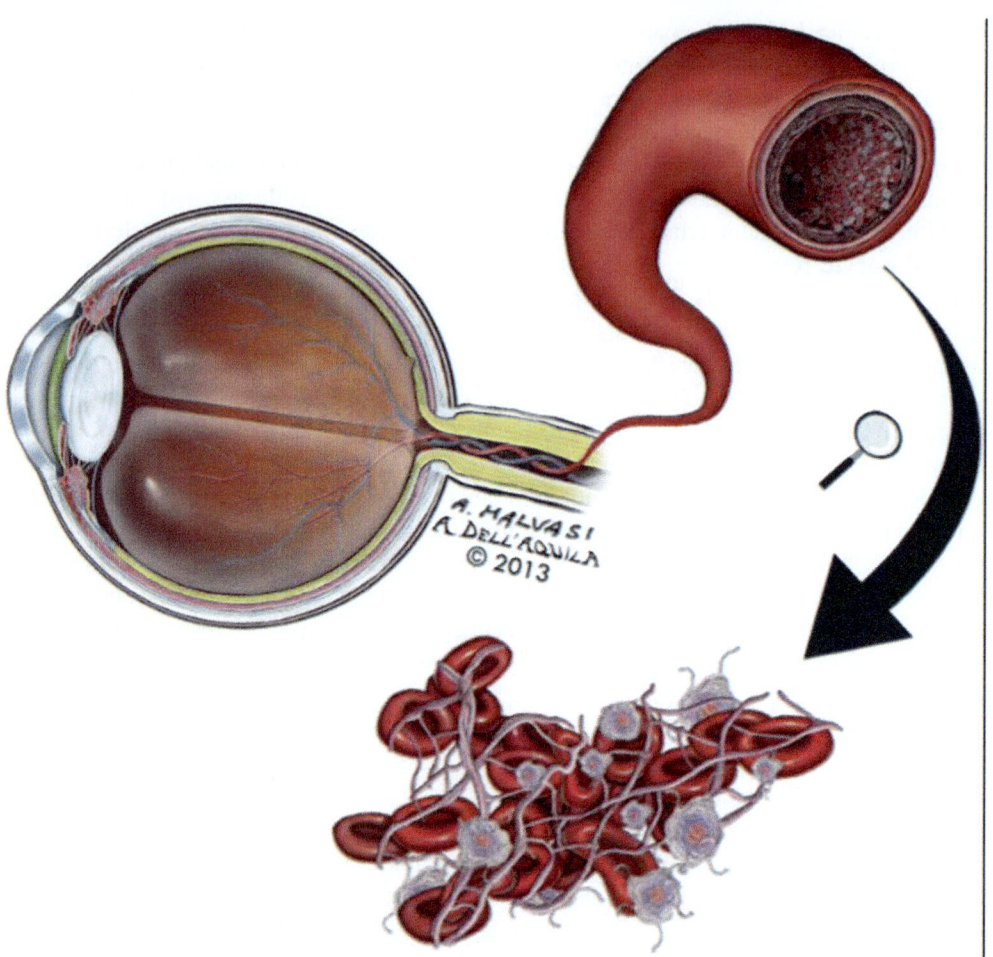

clotting factor. Intravenous immunoglobulins (IVIG) and steroids are recommended. The use of color Doppler during oocyte retrieval is not found as capable to predict peritoneal bleeding.

19.14 Complications After Special Oocyte Retrievals

19.14.1 In Vitro Maturation

Seyhan et al. in 2013 [63] reported the complications of transvaginal ultrasound follicular aspiration for in vitro maturation. For IVM, 19 gauge single lumen needles are used. There are specific differences between IVM and IVF cycles and their management. In IVM, hCG is administered when the leading follicle reaches 10–12 mm while in IVF, the follicle has to reach 17–18 mm before oocyte maturation. Antibiotics have been administered in both protocols. There was no significant difference in the complications reported. Most of the patients (97.3% in the IVM group and 94.1% in the IVF group) experienced no complication.

Ovarian and vaginal bleeding, endometrioma perforation, and severe postoperative pain are the common incidents between the two groups. Fever was experienced only in the IVM group while an ovarian abscess developed only in the IVF group. More patients with severe postoperative pain existed in the IVF group but this did not reach statistical significance. Obviously, a significantly higher number of polycystic ovaries' patients were in the IVM group, and significantly more time was needed for an IVM oocyte retrieval (22 versus 15 min). Authors conclude that higher complication rates after IVM oocyte pickup was not observed comparing with IVF.

19.14.2 Transabdominal Oocyte Retrieval

In a retrospective study, Barton et al. in 2011 [64], examined the transabdominal (Fig. 19.16) and the transvaginal oocyte aspiration approach. They included also in the study, cases of mixed abdominal/vaginal follicular aspiration. There is no

Fig. 19.15 Rare complication, thrombotic event of the cerebral vessel

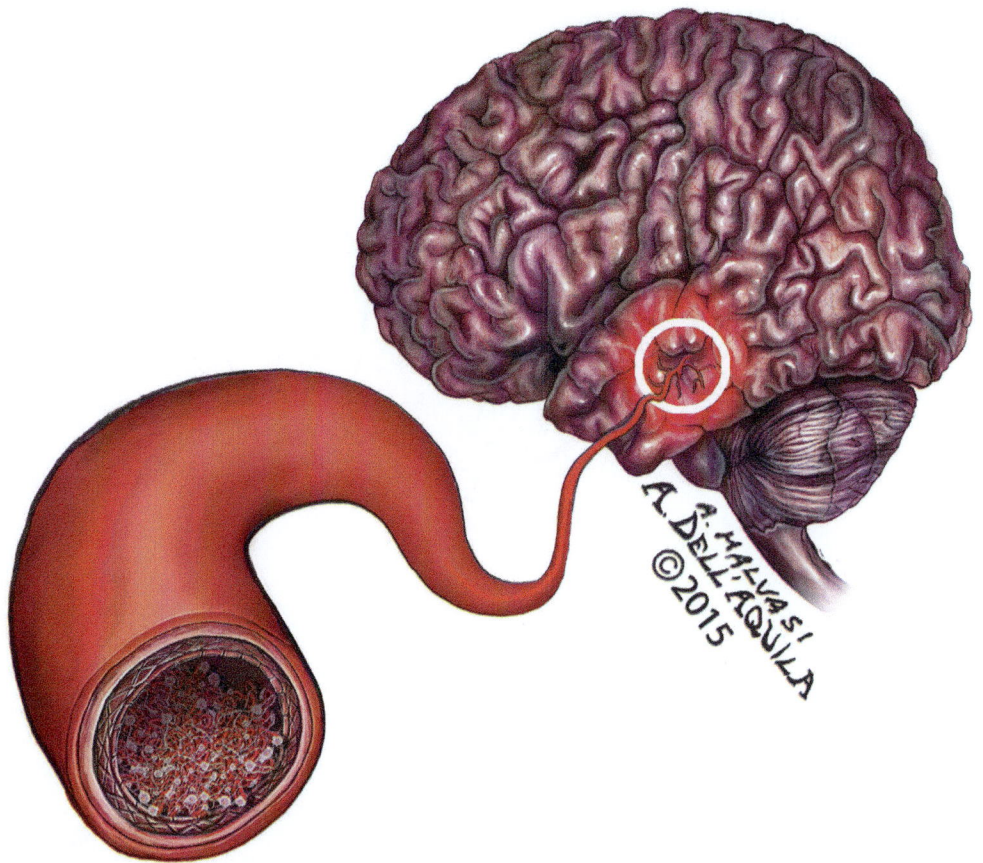

difference in all parameters of stimulated cycles in the two groups, except the transabdominal approach had less number of total oocytes retrieved but similar clinical and ongoing pregnancy rates. No serious intraoperative complications were observed but two postoperative infections have been noted in the transabdominal group and one mixed case of transabdominal/transvaginal retrieval had bleeding in the vaginal puncture site. Antibiotics have been administered to the patients that developed infection and complete symptom resolution has been observed.

Roman-Rodriguez et al. in 2015 [65] retrospectively compared the transabdominal and transvaginal ultrasound-guided follicular aspiration and eventually developed a risk score for the transabdominal approach. Three groups have been formed, one with entirely the transvaginal approach, the second with the transabdominal one, and the third group that started transvaginally for the first ovary and continued transabdominally for the second inaccessible one. No difference in pregnancy rates were observed while no complications took place. The final risk score included the BMI, the history of pelvic surgery, and whether ovaries are difficult to be seen on ultrasound. This model can serve as a useful screening tool for women that are for increased risk of transabdominal oocyte retrieval.

19.15 Methods to Improve Safety During Oocyte Retrieval

19.15.1 Prevention of Infection with Vaginal Disinfection

Many studies reported on the use of povidone iodine and saline douching, alone or in combination, for prevention of pelvic infection after oocyte retrieval. All studies agree that there are no significant differences in the fertilization rates, embryo morphology, and other embryological parameters. The same does not apply for the clinical pregnancy rates between the two groups as examined by van Os HC et al. in 1992 [66]. In this study, significantly higher pregnancy rates have been observed in the normal saline group. In addition, in the study by Hannoun et al. in 2008 [67], an increased rate of chemical pregnancies has been observed in the povidone iodine group, so they suggest thorough cleaning with saline irrigation before oocyte retrieval. When comparing the use of saline alone or with a combination of povidone and subsequent saline douching, no significant difference was observed in all embryo parameters, including clinical and ongoing pregnancy rates [68]. In this study, four patients from the saline douching group had an

Fig. 19.16 Oocytes retrieval by transabdominal

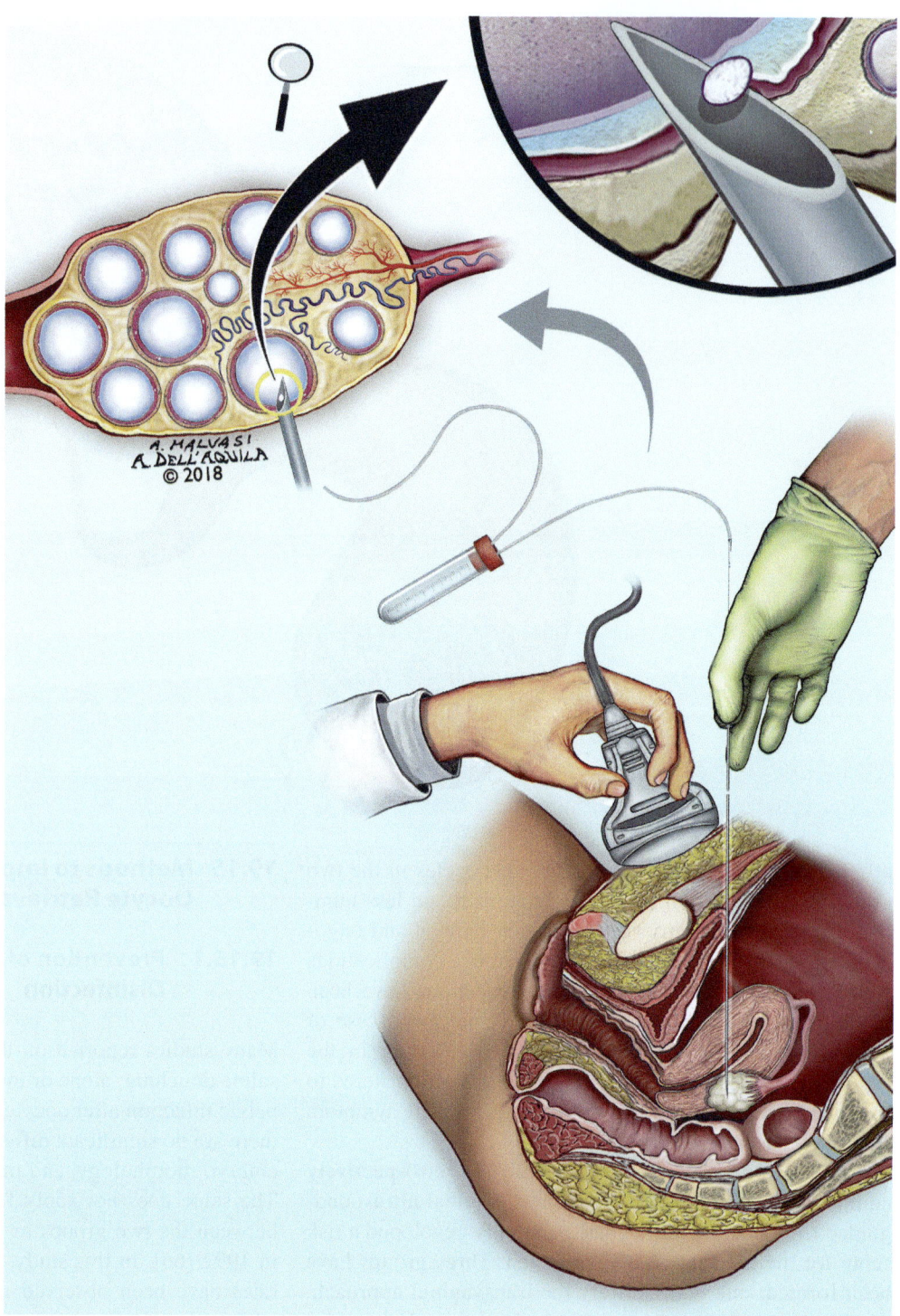

incidence OPU-associated pelvic inflammation. Tsai et al. in 2005 [69], compared the use of aqueous povidone iodine followed by saline or the use of saline alone, specifically to the patients with endometriomas. No significant difference was found in fertilization parameters and pregnancy rates. On the contrary, two patients in the saline only group developed a right and a left tubo-ovarian abscess, respectively. For the first patient, a right salpingoophorectomy was per- formed while for the second one, ovarian preservation was achieved through abscess drainage. Both cultures revealed E. Coli.

Summarizing evidence, vaginal disinfection with normal saline achieves better pregnancy rates than povidone iodine but with incidences of pelvic infection and ovarian abscesses. An effective solution is to clean the vagina with povidone iodine and subsequently rinse with normal saline [68].

Fig. 19.17 The use of the Doppler decreases the risk of perforation of blood vessels during the oocyte retrieval

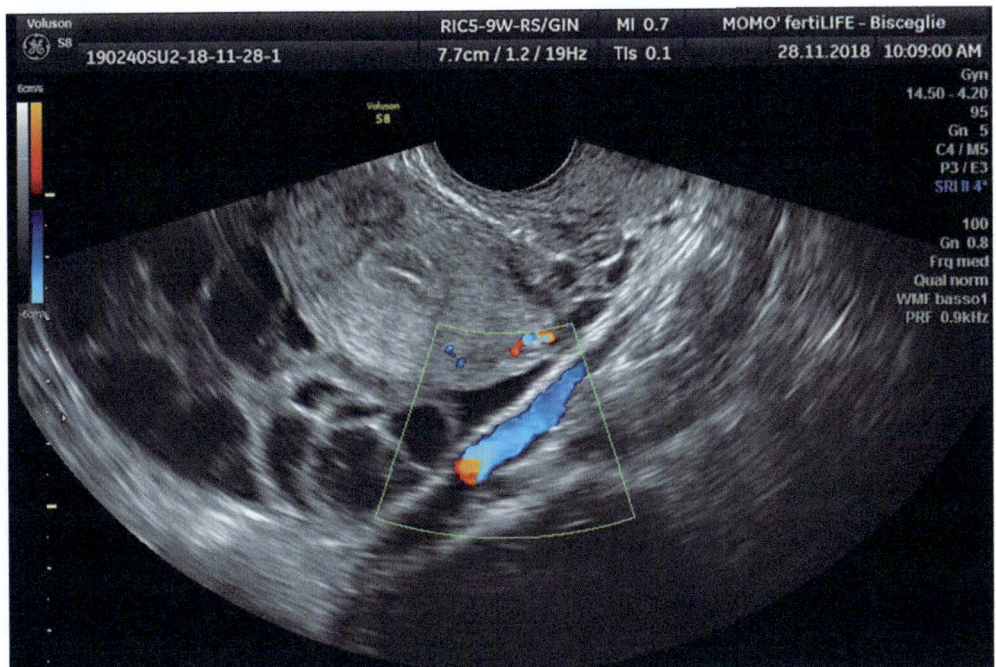

19.15.2   Transvaginal Ultrasound-Guided Oocyte Retrieval Plus Doppler

Transvaginal ultrasound-guided oocyte retrieval with the use of Doppler and the appropriate ultrasound-guided simulation training techniques has been proposed as a method to increase safety (Fig. 19.17) and avoid bleeding by Porter in 2008 [70]. Rísquez et al. in 2010 [71], evaluated the use of Doppler ultrasound during oocyte pickup, to predict moderate peritoneal bleeding. Authors measured the fluid pockets to predict hemoperitoneum. Pockets measured less than 2 cm have been considered as mild hemoperitoneum while if at least one pocket with maximum diameter 2–4 cm existed, then moderate hemoperitoneum was defined. If one pocket measured more than 5 cm then bleeding was considered. Unfortunately, a large percentage (45%) of patients with bleeding was not predicted. The incidence of vaginal bleeding was 1% with the use of Doppler ultrasound, while the expected incidence is 2.8%. Authors raise certain questions about the validity of this method to minimize hemoperitoneum. The visualization of vascularized ovarian areas during OPU mandates the clinician take a decision whether to risk hemorrhage in order to harvest an extra number of oocytes.

19.15.3   Ethanol Sclerotherapy

19.15.3.1   Ethanol Sclerotherapy in Endometriotic Cysts

Ethanol sclerotherapy might be used also for recurrent endometriotic cyst before ovarian stimulation. In order to avoid unwanted consequences of ovarian poor response after ovarian surgery, ethanol sclerotherapy is a good alternative [72]. This technique includes a needle insertion into the endometrioma, through vagina. The cyst content is aspirated and sent for pathological review. Pure sterile ethanol at an amount of 80% of the aspirated volume is instilled to the cyst. Care is taken to avoid over distention, cyst rupture, and pelvic leakage. Ethanol remains in the cyst for 10 min and afterwards it is entirely aspirated. Significantly, higher number of oocytes retrieved was observed in the sclerotherapy group. As a second result of this technique, a significant number of ongoing pregnancies were observed in the ethanol sclerotherapy group compared with the control group. The same applied for the cumulative pregnancy rates (after three cycles). Authors conclude that except efficiency, this technique is safe because no ovarian abscesses were seen.

19.15.3.2   Ethanol Sclerotherapy Design of Studies

In a letter to the editor for the previous study, Kumbak and Sahin in 2010 [73], point some methodology flows of the study and propose a different control group. Secondly, they define that the benefits and the mechanism of ethanol sclerotherapy and recurrent endometrioma are not clear. They conclude that it is not the cyst, but the endometriosis that affects pregnancy rates.

19.15.3.3   Ethanol Sclerotherapy in Hydrosalpinx

Song et al. in 2017 [74] tested whether ultrasound sclerotherapy treatment before ovarian hyperstimulation offered the same pregnancy rates with hydrosalpinx aspiration and laparoscopic bilateral salpingectomy, before an IVF cycle. About 265 cycles were included to the ultrasound sclerotherapy pretreatment group, while 109 cycles had hydrosalpinx aspiration under ultrasound guidance on the day of oocyte retrieval. The third group included 108 cycles and bilateral salpingectomy was performed before IVF treatment. Hydrosalpinx sclerotherapy treatment and the bilateral salpingectomy methods performed equally in terms of embryo implantation, biochemical, and clinical pregnancy rates. The ultrasound-guided aspiration of hydrosalpinx had lower pregnancy and higher abortion rates than the other two groups. Authors conclude that ultrasound sclerotherapy has a position in the surgical management of hydrosalpinges. Benefits of this method include the avoidance of risks from bilateral salpingectomy, like reduced ovarian responsiveness and increased risk from severe pelvic adhesions.

19.15.4 SIPS Technique

Shah and Walmer in 2010 [75] tried to evaluate the pelvic anatomy with a technique called saline intraperitoneal sonogram. They included ten women with unexplained infertility and normal hysterosalpingogram while five of them had known adhesive disease. The technique involved two steps. First of all they performed a sonohysterogram with saline and observed for a pocket of fluid in the peritoneal cavity. Secondly, they directed at 17-g oocyte retrieval needle into the pocket of peritoneal fluid and infused of 600 mL of normal saline. At this step, they evaluated with 3D and 4D ultrasound the pelvic anatomy. More saline was infused (up to 1500 mL) in case tubes and ovaries did not float easily. At the end of the procedure, saline was aspirated from the peritoneal cavity and antibiotics have been administered. Then they evaluated the images and considered as normal if the uterus, fallopian tubes and ovaries where completely surrounded from saline and no abnormal pathology was observed. In case the structures were not completely surrounded by saline, then the images were considered nondiagnostic. From the other side, if these images have been suspicious for pelvic adhesions or hydrosalpinges, then they were considered abnormal. Diagnostic laparoscopy was offered for patients that included in the last two groups. The average time for this procedure was 45 min. Eventually, with this technique, all patients finished the procedure. Eight of them requested sedation and pain management and one developed signs of abdominal infection. This patient was admitted and treated with IV antibiotics. For patients with known risk factors for adhesions, SIPS technique was very accurate finding pelvic adhesions, evidence of prior peritonitis (Fitz-Hugh-Curtis adhesions), and peritoneal adhesions involving 75% the peritoneal cavity after myomectomy. Of the five subjects without risk factors for intraperitoneal disease, four had studies that were judged to be normal and one had findings with unilateral hydrosalpinx and bilateral pelvic adhesions not seen in a previous hysterosalpingogram. This technique is considered feasible and cost-effective for patients that would like to avoid laparoscopy while in parallel evaluating the intraperitoneal cavity for pathology that affects fertility treatment (Fig. 19.18).

19.16 Anesthesia for Assisted Reproductive Techniques

In vitro fertilization (IVF) and embryo transfer in the last two decades became popular for the treatment of infertility. For stimulation of maturation of plenty of follicles, hormone therapy is used. Under ultrasound, the preovulatory oocytes are aspirated through transvaginal approach. After microscopic control combine with semen, and formed embryos are transferred into uterine cavity.

19.16.1 Planning the Anesthetic Approach

The preanesthetic evaluation is similar to that for other preoperative patients, with a focus on assessment of the airway, lower back, and coexisting patient's medical conditions. Challenges and complications related to anesthesia are more common in obese patients, which include difficulty with monitoring, positioning, airway management, and neuraxial techniques [54]. In patients with specific medical issues, such as predicted difficult airway or (rarely) malignant hyperthermia susceptibility, there are additional reasons to avoid general anesthesia. Therefore, anesthesiology consultation is recommended.

19.16.2 IVF Procedures Can Be Conducted with Local Infiltration, Neuraxial, or in General Anesthesia

1. Local infiltration of posterolateral vaginal fornix, in combination with small doses of sedatives and narcotics, can be used successfully. This technique doesn't give complete immobilization to the patient, and this can be negative side of local anesthesia.
2. Complication during infiltration of local anesthetics: intravascular injection is most often heralded by agitation, visual disturbance, tinnitus, and convulsions and may lead to loss of consciousness. If any of these symptoms is noted, the injection should be stopped and immediate attention is given to airway.

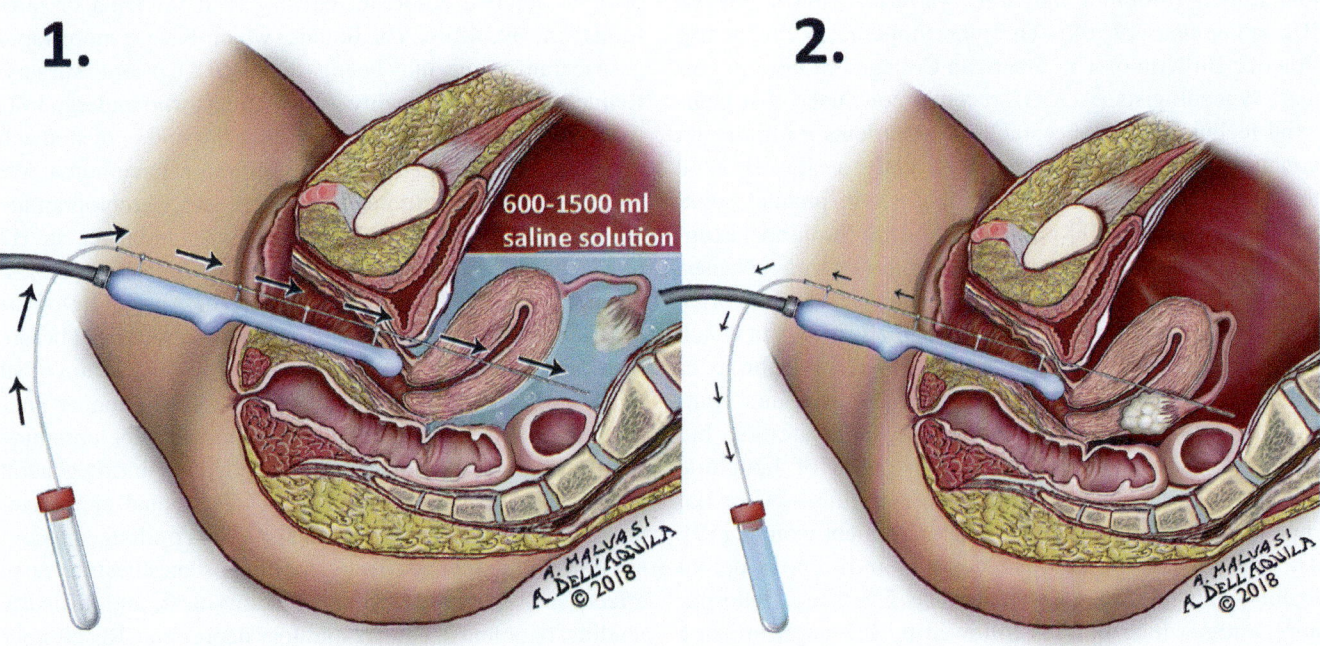

Fig. 19.18 The first two time of SIPS technique

19.16.3 Spinal Anesthesia

Spinal anesthesia can provide an excellent operating condition for IVF. The needles presently in use, as Withacre or Sprotte, decrease the incidence of postdural puncture headache (PDPH) to 1% [76, 77]. Furthermore, use of low dose of local anesthetic in combination with narcotics as fentanyl or sufetanil can produce neuraxial blockade that decrease pain with preserved leg mobility [5, 11].

19.16.4 Complication During Regional Anesthesia

Regional anesthesia is an extremely safe technic, but like all surgical procedures, rarely, cardiovascular, neurologic, infective, or hematologic complications may occur. This may take place also in total spinal anesthesia [9]. (a) Hypotension is one of the cardiovascular complications of neuraxial technique. The most frequently applied definition is systolic arterial blood pressure less than 100 mmHg from baseline or if patient becomes symptomatic. Dense neuraxial blockade at the high sensory level, for example fourth thoracic dermatome, includes sympathetic block and vasodilation that often results in hypotension. The hypotension can be prevented with low doses of local anesthetics in combination with intravenous fluid pre- or co-loading with crystalloids and ephedrine prophylaxis. (b) Bradycardia and cardiac arrest are the most feared complications and have

higher incidence in neuraxial than in general anesthesia. The blockade of the preganglionic cardio accelerator fibers originating between vertebra T1 and T4 may progress in heart block or asystole. First-line therapy in this case is atropine; ephedrine is used when hypotension is associated with bradycardia or in unresponsive case to atropine. (c) Postdural puncture headache (PDPH) is a common complication after inadvertent puncture of the dura matter. The risk factors included sex, young age, pregnancy, vaginal delivery, low body mass index, and being non-smoker. The PDPH is a postdural headache that worsens with sitting or standing and improves with lying down. Conservative therapies such as bed rest, hydration, and caffeine are commonly used treatments, and the blood epidural patch in the patients with unsuccessful conservative therapy [76]. (d) Infective complications can occur if the meticulous aseptic technique during neuraxial block procedures in operating room has not been followed. The infection concerns the central nervous system such as arachnoiditis, meningitis, and abscess following spinal anesthesia. The source of infection is contamination by the hands or nasopharynx of the operating anesthesiologist. Using of sterile overalls, gloves, surgical cup, and face mask should be of procedural routine. (e) Hematoma is a rare and well-recognized complication in patients who have received regional anesthesia. The literature suggest that routine platelet count can predict anesthesia-related complications in patient with disorders associated with coagulopathy, or in patient in therapy with low molecular weight heparin, other factor Xa inhibitors, direct thrombin inhibitor, warfarin, aspirin, GPIIb/IIIa antagonists [9, 64]. Thrombocytopenia in Pregnancy, Practice Bulletin of The American College of Obstetricians and Gynecologists (ACOG), recently concluded that neuraxial techniques are acceptable in parturients with platelet counts greater than 80,000 mm^3. Recently, a safe neuraxial technique was suggested in patients whose platelet count was more than 56,000 mm^3 with normal thromboelastography value [10, 19, 56]. (f) Nausea and vomiting—Nausea is a common complaint during cesarean delivery. It is often related to hypotension from the sympathetic block, in which case restoring the blood pressure (with phenylephrine or ephedrine) should alleviate the nausea. Nausea and vomiting is common after spinal morphine administration, but unlikely following neuraxial administration of lipophilic opioids (e.g., fentanyl, sufentanil). (g) Pruritus—Neuraxial opioids lead to pruritus in 60–100% of patient women [19]. This may resolve with small doses of intravenous opioid agonist–antagonists (e.g., nalbuphine 2.5–5 mg, butorphanol 1 mg, which may be followed by 0.2 mg/h infusion (14)), or antagonists (e.g., naloxone 40–100 mcg IV boluses, which may be followed by 0.25–1 mcg/kg/h infusion) [19]. (h) Total spinal anesthesia can happen when local anesthetic interferes with the normal neuronal function in the cervical spinal cord and brain stem. The onset is usually rapid and severe hypotension bradycardia, and respiratory arrest can occur. Management of total spinal anesthesia is mainly supportive: fluid administration, inotrope or vasopressors drugs to raise blood pressure, and atropine to treat bradycardia. Respiratory insufficiency may need tracheal intubation and mechanical ventilation [9].

19.17 General Anesthesia Can Be Used for Oocyte Retrieval

Usually, the induction is made with benzodiazepine, narcotics, and propofol. General anesthesia may preserve spontaneous ventilation or may require mechanical ventilation through an endotracheal tube or a laryngeal mask airway [9]. General anesthesia-associated patients' morbidities include airway-related complications (e.g., aspiration of stomach contents, failed intubation). The consequences of airway problems may be severe, but the incidence is low, if the device for difficult airway management is present.

19.17.1 Patient Preparation

Preoperative fasting—We agree with the American College of Obstetricians and Gynecologists (ACOG) and the American Society of Anesthesiologists (ASA) recommendation that patients abstain from solid food for at least 6 h

prior to elective cesarean delivery (8 h for fried or fatty foods) [4, 39, 48]. Clear liquids, which have a more rapid gastric transit time, may be ingested until 2 h prior to surgery. Reduction of gastric acidity—For patients who undergo IVF, we administer medications that reduce the acidity of stomach contents as prophylaxis against aspiration pneumonia. We administer sodium citrate, 30 mL PO, and metoclopramide 10 mg IV, slowly. If time permits, we administer an H2 blocker (e.g., ranitidine 50 mg IV) 40–60 min prior to anesthesia as well. The American Society of Anesthesiologists Practice Guidelines for Obstetric Anesthesia state that before surgical procedures (i.e., cesarean delivery, postpartum tubal ligation) clinicians should consider administration of nonparticulate antacids, H2 antagonists, and/or metoclopramide for aspiration prophylaxis [48]. Complication during general anesthesia, accomplished either by inhalational or intravenous agents, is frequently associated with a prolonged recovery time and an increased incidence of postanesthesia adverse effects such as nausea, vomiting, drowsiness, and difficulty voiding, hypotension and respiratory depression. Respiratory depression was defined as apnea, hypopnea, oxyhemoglobin desaturations, or episodes of severe pain despite moderate to profound sedation. Weingarten et al. [78] found in their study that 23.7% cases of 11,970 patients had respiratory depression in postoperative period after sedating analgesics. A higher rate of respiratory depression was observed among patients who underwent general anesthesia (312 per 1000 cases; 95% CI, 301–323) than neuraxial anesthesia (144 per 1000 cases; 95% CI, 135–153) ($P < 0.001$) [79]. Induction of general anesthesia tends to transiently reduce patients' blood pressure. Hypotension should be treated with fluid and vasopressor administration, aiming for blood pressure near or at baseline. Patients who required flumazenil postoperatively had received a higher dosage of benzodiazepines and utilized more postoperative health care resources. More conservative perioperative use of benzodiazepines may improve postoperative recovery and use of health care resources [41]. Other adverse systemic effects of general anesthesia that may have a potential detrimental effect on reproductive outcome include transient elevations of serum prolactin levels and suppression of progesterone production by the corpus luteum.

Standard I. Major conduction anesthesia (lumbar or caudal subarachnoid or bilateral lumbar sympathetic block) shall be initiated and maintained only in locations with appropriate resuscitation equipment and drugs immediately available to manage procedurally related problems (e.g., hypotension, respiratory depression, convulsion, myocardial depression)

Resuscitation Equipment: (a) It must be present with sources of oxygen and suction, (b) equipment to maintain an airway and perform endotracheal intubation, (c) possibility to provide positive pressure ventilation, and (d) drugs and equipment for cardiopulmonary resuscitation shall be immediately available.

Standard II. Major conduction anesthesia should not be administered until the patient has been examined.

Standard III. An intravenous infusion shall be established before initiation and maintained throughout the duration of major conduction block.

Standard IV. The patient oxygenation, ventilation, and circulation shell be monitored continually.

Standard V. The anesthetist should be always present.

Standard VI. All patients recovering from major conduction anesthesia shall receive appropriate postanesthesia care.

References

1. Tureck RW, García CR, Blasco L, Mastroianni L. Perioperative complications arising after transvaginal oocyte retrieval. Obstet Gynecol. 1993;81:590–3. http://www.ncbi.nlm.nih.gov/pubmed/8459973.

2. El-Shawarby S, Margara R, Trew G, Lavery S. A review of complications following transvaginal oocyte retrieval for in-vitro fertilization. Hum Fertil (Camb). 2004;7:127–33. https://doi.org/10.1080/14647270410001699081.

3. Ludwig AK, Glawatz M, Griesinger G, Diedrich K, Ludwig M. Perioperative and post-operative complications of transvaginal ultrasound-guided oocyte retrieval: prospective study of >1000 oocyte retrievals. Hum Reprod. 2006;21:3235–40. https://doi.org/10.1093/humrep/del278.

4. Bodri D, Guillén JJ, Polo A, Trullenque M, Esteve C, Coll O. Complications related to ovarian stimulation and oocyte retrieval in 4052 oocyte donor cycles. Reprod Biomed Online. 2008;17:237–43. http://www.ncbi.nlm.nih.gov/pubmed/18681998.

5. Aragona C, Mohamed MA, Espinola MSB, Linari A, Pecorini F, Micara G, Sbracia M. Clinical complications after transvaginal oocyte retrieval in 7,098 IVF cycles. Fertil Steril. 2011;95:293–4. https://doi.org/10.1016/j.fertnstert.2010.07.1054.

6. Siristatidis C, Chrelias C, Alexiou A, Kassanos D. Clinical complications after transvaginal oocyte retrieval: a retrospective analysis. J Obstet Gynaecol. 2013;33:64–6. https://doi.org/10.3109/01443615.2012.721818.

7. Villette C, Bourret A, Santulli P, Gayet V, Chapron C, de Ziegler D. Risks of tubo-ovarian abscess in cases of endometrioma and assisted reproductive technologies are both under- and overreported. Fertil Steril. 2016;106:410–5. https://doi.org/10.1016/j.fertnstert.2016.04.014.

8. Van Hoecke F, Beuckelaers E, Lissens P, Boudewijns M. Actinomyces urogenitalis bacteremia and tubo-ovarian abscess after an in vitro fertilization (IVF) procedure. J Clin Microbiol. 2013;51:4252–4. https://doi.org/10.1128/JCM.02142-13.

9. Asemota OA, Girda E, Dueñas O, Neal-Perry G, Pollack SE. Actinomycosis pelvic abscess after in vitro fertilization. Fertil Steril. 2013;100:408–11. https://doi.org/10.1016/j.fertnstert.2013.04.018.

10. Bébéar C, Grouthier V, Hocké C, Jimenez C, Papaxanthos A, Creux H. Ureaplasma parvum peritonitis after oocyte retrieval for in vitro fertilization. Eur J Obstet Gynecol Reprod Biol. 2014;172:138–9. https://doi.org/10.1016/j.ejogrb.2013.10.025.

11. Annamraju H, Ganapathy R, Webb B. Pelvic tuberculosis reactivated by in vitro fertilization egg collection? Fertil Steril. 2008;90:2003.e1–3. https://doi.org/10.1016/j.fertnstert.2008.02.147.

12. Matsunaga Y, Fukushima K, Nozaki M, Nakanami N, Kawano Y, Shigematsu T, Satoh S, Nakano H. A case of pregnancy complicated by the development of a tubo-ovarian abscess following in vitro fertilization and embryo transfer. Am J Perinatol. 2003;20:277–82. https://doi.org/10.1055/s-2003-42772.

13. Varras M, Polyzos D, Tsikini A, Antypa E, Apessou D, Tsouroulas M. Ruptured tubo-ovarian abscess as a complication of IVF treatment: clinical, ultrasonographic and histopathologic findings. A case report. Clin Exp Obstet Gynecol. 2003;30:164–8. http://www.ncbi.nlm.nih.gov/pubmed/12854869.

14. Pabuccu EG, Taskin S, Atabekoglu C, Sonmezer M. Early pregnancy loss following laparoscopic management of ovarian abscess secondary to oocyte retrieval. Int J Fertil Steril. 2014;8:341–6. http://www.ncbi.nlm.nih.gov/pubmed/25379164.

15. den Boon J, Kimmel CE, Nagel HT, van Roosmalen J. Pelvic abscess in the second half of pregnancy after oocyte retrieval for in-vitro fertilization: case report. Hum Reprod. 1999;14:2402–3. http://www.ncbi.nlm.nih.gov/pubmed/10469720.

16. Kim JW, Lee WS, Yoon TK, Han JE. Term delivery following tuboovarian abscess after in vitro fertilization and embryo transfer. Am J Obstet Gynecol. 2013;208:e3–6. https://doi.org/10.1016/j.ajog.2013.01.040.

17. Younis JS, Ezra Y, Laufer N, Ohel G. Late manifestation of pelvic abscess following oocyte retrieval, for in vitro fertilization, in patients with severe endometriosis and ovarian endometriomata. J Assist Reprod Genet. 1997;14:343–6. http://www.ncbi.nlm.nih.gov/pubmed/9226514.

18. Nikkhah-Abyaneh Z, Khulpateea N, Aslam MF. Pyometra after ovum retrieval for in vitro fertilization resulting in hysterectomy. Fertil Steril. 2010;93:268.e1–2. https://doi.org/10.1016/j.fertnstert.2009.08.023.

19. Benaglia L, Somigliana E, Iemmello R, Colpi E, Nicolosi AE, Ragni G. Endometrioma and oocyte retrieval-induced pelvic abscess: a clinical concern or an exceptional complication? Fertil Steril. 2008;89:1263–6. https://doi.org/10.1016/j.fertnstert.2007.05.038.

20. Isaacs JD, Hines RS, Sopelak VM, Cowan BD. Ovarian endometriomas do not adversely affect pregnancy success following treatment with in vitro fertilization. J Assist Reprod Genet. 1997;14:551–3. http://www.ncbi.nlm.nih.gov/pubmed/9447452.

21. Moini A, Riazi K, Amid V, Ashrafi M, Tehraninejad E, Madani T, Owj M. Endometriosis may contribute to oocyte retrieval-induced pelvic inflammatory disease: report of eight cases. J Assist Reprod Genet. 2005;22:307–9. https://doi.org/10.1007/s10815-005-6003-2.

22. Kelada E, Ghani R. Bilateral ovarian abscesses following transvaginal oocyte retrieval for IVF: a case report and review of literature. J Assist Reprod Genet. 2007;24:143–5. https://doi.org/10.1007/s10815-006-9090-9.

23. Padilla SL. Ovarian abscess following puncture of an endometrioma during ultrasound-guided oocyte retrieval. Hum Reprod. 1993;8:1282–3. http://www.ncbi.nlm.nih.gov/pubmed/8408527.

24. Sharpe K, Karovitch AJ, Claman P, Suh KN. Transvaginal oocyte retrieval for in vitro fertilization complicated by ovarian abscess during pregnancy. Fertil Steril. 2006;86:219.e11–3. https://doi.org/10.1016/j.fertnstert.2005.12.045.

25. Hameed A, Mehta V, Sinha P. A rare case of de novo gigantic ovarian abscess within an endometrioma. Yale J Biol Med. 2010;83:73–5. http://www.ncbi.nlm.nih.gov/pubmed/20589187.

26. Johnson NP, Mak W, Sowter MC. Surgical treatment for tubal disease in women due to undergo in vitro fertilisation. Cochrane Database Syst Rev. 2004;CD002125. https://doi.org/10.1002/14651858.CD002125.pub2.

27. Johnson N, van Voorst S, Sowter MC, Strandell A, Mol BWJ. Surgical treatment for tubal disease in women due to undergo in vitro fertilisation. Cochrane Database Syst Rev. 2010;CD002125. https://doi.org/10.1002/14651858.CD002125.pub3.

28. Hinckley MD, Milki AA. Rapid reaccumulation of hydrometra after drainage at embryo transfer in patients with hydrosalpinx.

Fertil Steril. 2003;80:1268–71. http://www.ncbi.nlm.nih.gov/pubmed/14607587.

29. Hammadieh N, Coomarasamy A, Ola B, Papaioannou S, Afnan M, Sharif K. Ultrasound-guided hydrosalpinx aspiration during oocyte collection improves pregnancy outcome in IVF: a randomized controlled trial. Hum Reprod. 2008;23:1113–7. https://doi.org/10.1093/humrep/den071.

30. Sharara FI. Ultrasound-guided hydrosalpinx aspiration during oocyte collection improves outcome in IVF. Hum Reprod. 2009;24:756. https://doi.org/10.1093/humrep/den448; author reply 756–7.

31. Chen C-D, Chao K-H, Wu M-Y, Chen S-U, Ho H-N, Yang Y-S. Ultrasound-guided hydrosalpinx aspiration during oocyte retrieval and a mouse embryo assay of hydrosalpinx fluid in a woman with hydrosalpinx and hydrometra during in vitro fertilization treatment. Taiwan J Obstet Gynecol. 2012;51:106–8. https://doi.org/10.1016/j.tjog.2012.01.021.

32. Fouda UM, Sayed AM, Abdelmoty HI, Elsetohy KA. Ultrasound guided aspiration of hydrosalpinx fluid versus salpingectomy in the management of patients with ultrasound visible hydrosalpinx undergoing IVF-ET: a randomized controlled trial. BMC Womens Health. 2015;15:21. https://doi.org/10.1186/s12905-015-0177-2.

33. Okohue JE, Ikimalo JI. IVF pregnancy and delivery following ultrasound scan guided aspiration of a left hydrosalpinx—a case report. Niger Postgrad Med J. 2015;22:123–5. http://www.ncbi.nlm.nih.gov/pubmed/26259161.

34. Zhou Y, Jiang H, Zhang W-X, Ni F, Wang X-M, Song X-M. Ultrasound-guided aspiration of hydrosalpinx occurring during controlled ovarian hyperstimulation could improve clinical outcome of in vitro fertilization-embryo transfer. J Obstet Gynaecol Res. 2016;42:960–5. https://doi.org/10.1111/jog.13013.

35. Fugita OE, Kavoussi L. Laparoscopic ureteral reimplantation for ureteral lesion secondary to transvaginal ultrasonography for oocyte retrieval. Urology. 2001;58:281. http://www.ncbi.nlm.nih.gov/pubmed/11489721.

36. Miller PB, Price T, Nichols JE, Hill L. Acute ureteral obstruction following transvaginal oocyte retrieval for IVF. Hum Reprod. 2002;17:137–8. http://www.ncbi.nlm.nih.gov/pubmed/11756377.

37. Fiori O, Cornet D, Darai E, Antoine JM, Bazot M. Uro-retroperitoneum after ultrasound-guided transvaginal follicle puncture in an oocyte donor: a case report. Hum Reprod. 2006;21:2969–71. https://doi.org/10.1093/humrep/del252.

38. Grynberg M, Berwanger AL, Toledano M, Frydman R, Deffieux X, Fanchin R. Ureteral injury after transvaginal ultrasound-guided oocyte retrieval: a complication of in vitro fertilization-embryo transfer that may lurk undetected in women presenting with severe ovarian hyperstimulation syndrome. Fertil Steril. 2011;96:869–71. https://doi.org/10.1016/j.fertnstert.2011.07.1094.

39. Burnik Papler T, Vrtačnik Bokal E, Šalamun V, Galič D, Smrkolj T, Jančar N. Ureteral injury with delayed massive hematuria after transvaginal ultrasound-guided oocyte retrieval. Case Rep Obstet Gynecol. 2015;2015:760805. https://doi.org/10.1155/2015/760805.

40. Vilos AG, Feyles V, Vilos GA, Oraif A, Abdul-Jabbar H, Power N. Ureteric injury during transvaginal ultrasound guided oocyte retrieval. J Obstet Gynaecol Can. 2015;37:52–5. http://www.ncbi.nlm.nih.gov/pubmed/25764037.

41. Catanzarite T, Bernardi LA, Confino E, Kenton K. Ureteral trauma during transvaginal ultrasound-guided oocyte retrieval: a case report. Female Pelvic Med Reconstr Surg. 2015;21:e44–5. https://doi.org/10.1097/SPV.0000000000000176.

42. Choudhary RA, Bhise NM, Mehendale AV, Ganla KN. Ureteric injury during transvaginal oocyte retrieval (TVOR) and review of literature. J Hum Reprod Sci. 2017;10:61–4. https://doi.org/10.4103/jhrs.JHRS_124_16.

43. Coroleu B, Lopez Mourelle F, Hereter L, Veiga A, Calderón G, Martinez F, Carreras O, Barri PN. Ureteral lesion secondary to vag-

inal ultrasound follicular puncture for oocyte recovery in in-vitro fertilization. Hum Reprod. 1997;12:948–50. http://www.ncbi.nlm.nih.gov/pubmed/9194645.

44. Mongiu AK, Helfand BT, Kielb SJ. Ureterovaginal fistula formation after oocyte retrieval. Urology. 2009;73:444.e1–3. https://doi.org/10.1016/j.urology.2008.02.042.

45. Al-Shaikh GK, Abotalib ZM. Vesicovaginal fistula formation after oocyte retrieval. Taiwan J Obstet Gynecol. 2013;52:597–8. https://doi.org/10.1016/j.tjog.2013.10.028.

46. Spencer ES, Hoff HS, Steiner AZ, Coward RM. Immediate ureterovaginal fistula following oocyte retrieval: a case and systematic review of the literature. Urol Ann. 2017;9:125–30. https://doi.org/10.4103/UA.UA_122_16.

47. Pappin C, Plant G. A pelvic pseudoaneurysm (a rare complication of oocyte retrieval for IVF) treated by arterial embolization. Hum Fertil (Camb). 2006;9:153–5. https://doi.org/10.1080/14647270600595952.

48. Bozdag G, Basaran A, Cil B, Esinler I, Yarali H. An oocyte pick-up procedure complicated with pseudoaneurysm of the internal iliac artery. Fertil Steril. 2008;90:2004.e11–3. https://doi.org/10.1016/j.fertnstert.2008.02.010.

49. Jayakrishnan K, Raman VK, Vijayalakshmi VK, Baheti S, Nambiar D. Massive hematuria with hemodynamic instability—complication of oocyte retrieval. Fertil Steril. 2011;96:e22–4. https://doi.org/10.1016/j.fertnstert.2011.04.046.

50. Zhen X, Qiao J, Ma C, Fan Y, Liu P. Intraperitoneal bleeding following transvaginal oocyte retrieval. Int J Gynaecol Obstet. 2010;108:31–4. https://doi.org/10.1016/j.ijgo.2009.08.015.

51. Chatrian A, Vidal C, Equy V, Hoffmann P, Sergent F. Hemoperitoneum presenting with the use of a topical hemostatic agent in oocyte retrieval: a case report. J Med Case Rep. 2012;6:395. https://doi.org/10.1186/1752-1947-6-395.

52. Nouri K, Walch K, Promberger R, Kurz C, Tempfer CB, Ott J. Severe haematoperitoneum caused by ovarian bleeding after transvaginal oocyte retrieval: a retrospective analysis and systematic literature review. Reprod Biomed Online. 2014;29:699–707. https://doi.org/10.1016/j.rbmo.2014.08.008.

53. Bentov Y, Levitas E, Silberstein T, Potashnik G. Cullen's sign following ultrasound-guided transvaginal oocyte retrieval. Fertil Steril. 2006;85:227. https://doi.org/10.1016/j.fertnstert.2005.06.054.

54. Almog B, Rimon E, Yovel I, Bar-Am A, Amit A, Azem F. Vertebral osteomyelitis: a rare complication of transvaginal ultrasound-guided oocyte retrieval. Fertil Steril. 2000;73:1250–2. http://www.ncbi.nlm.nih.gov/pubmed/10856494.

55. Kim HH, Yun NR, Kim D-M, Kim SA. Successful delivery following Staphylococcus aureus bacteremia after in vitro fertilization and embryo transfer. Chonnam Med J. 2015;51:47–9. https://doi.org/10.4068/cmj.2015.51.1.47.

56. Battaglia C, Regnani G, Giulini S, Madgar L, Genazzani AD, Volpe A. Severe intraabdominal bleeding after transvaginal oocyte retrieval for IVF-ET and coagulation factor XI deficiency: a case report. J Assist Reprod Genet. 2001;18:178–81. http://www.ncbi.nlm.nih.gov/pubmed/11411435.

57. Davies J, Kadir R. The management of factor XI deficiency in pregnancy. Semin Thromb Hemost. 2016;42:732–40. https://doi.org/10.1055/s-0036-1587685.

58. Fatum M, Ozcan C, Simon A, Lewin A, Laufer N. The safety of ultrasound-guided oocyte pick-up in IVF patients with haemostatic disorders. Eur J Obstet Gynecol Reprod Biol. 2008;137:259–61. https://doi.org/10.1016/j.ejogrb.2007.01.010.

59. Chee YL, Crawford JC, Watson HG, Greaves M. Guidelines on the assessment of bleeding risk prior to surgery or invasive procedures. British Committee for Standards in Haematology. Br J Haematol. 2008;140:496–504. https://doi.org/10.1111/j.1365-2141.2007.06968.x.

60. Borges NM, Thachil J. The relevance of the coagulation screen before surgery. Br J Hosp Med (Lond). 2017;78:566–70. https://doi.org/10.12968/hmed.2017.78.10.566.

61. El-Shawarby SA, Margara RA, Trew GH, Laffan MA, Lavery SA. Thrombocythemia and hemoperitoneum after transvaginal oocyte retrieval for in vitro fertilization. Fertil Steril. 2004;82:735–7. https://doi.org/10.1016/j.fertnstert.2004.01.044.

62. Rumi E, Cazzola M. How I treat essential thrombocythemia. Blood. 2016;128:2403–14. https://doi.org/10.1182/blood-2016-05-643346.

63. Seyhan A, Ata B, Son W-Y, Dahan MH, Tan SL. Comparison of complication rates and pain scores after transvaginal ultrasound-guided oocyte pickup procedures for in vitro maturation and in vitro fertilization cycles. Fertil Steril. 2014;101:705–9. https://doi.org/10.1016/j.fertnstert.2013.12.011.

64. Barton SE, Politch JA, Benson CB, Ginsburg ES, Gargiulo AR. Transabdominal follicular aspiration for oocyte retrieval in patients with ovaries inaccessible by transvaginal ultrasound. Fertil Steril. 2011;95:1773–6. https://doi.org/10.1016/j.fertnstert.2011.01.006.

65. Roman-Rodriguez CF, Weissbrot E, Hsu C-D, Wong A, Siefert C, Sung L. Comparing transabdominal and transvaginal ultrasound-guided follicular aspiration: a risk assessment formula. Taiwan J Obstet Gynecol. 2015;54:693–9. https://doi.org/10.1016/j.tjog.2015.02.004.

66. van Os HC, Roozenburg BJ, Janssen-Caspers HA, Leerentveld RA, Scholtes MC, Zeilmaker GH, Alberda AT. Vaginal disinfection with povidon iodine and the outcome of in-vitro fertilization. Hum Reprod. 1992;7:349–50. http://www.ncbi.nlm.nih.gov/pubmed/1587940.

67. Hannoun A, Awwad J, Zreik T, Ghaziri G, Abu-Musa A. Effect of betadine vaginal preparation during oocyte aspiration in in vitro fertilization cycles on pregnancy outcome. Gynecol Obstet Investig. 2008;66:274–8. https://doi.org/10.1159/000156378.

68. Funabiki M, Taguchi S, Hayashi T, Tada Y, Kitaya K, Iwaki Y, Karita M, Nakamura Y. Vaginal preparation with povidone iodine disinfection and saline douching as a safe and effective method in prevention of oocyte pickup-associated pelvic inflammation without spoiling the reproductive outcome: evidence from a large cohort study. Clin Exp Obstet Gynecol. 2014;41:689–90. http://www.ncbi.nlm.nih.gov/pubmed/25551964.

69. Tsai Y-C, Lin MYS, Chen S-H, Chung M-T, Loo T-C, Huang K-F, Lin L-Y. Vaginal disinfection with povidone iodine immediately before oocyte retrieval is effective in preventing pelvic abscess

formation without compromising the outcome of IVF-ET. J Assist Reprod Genet. 2005;22:173–5. http://www.ncbi.nlm.nih.gov/pubmed/16021862.

70. Porter MB. Ultrasound in assisted reproductive technology. Semin Reprod Med. 2008;26:266–76. https://doi.org/10.1055/s-2008-1076145.

71. Rísquez F, Confino E. Can Doppler ultrasound-guided oocyte retrieval improve IVF safety? Reprod Biomed Online. 2010;21:444–5. https://doi.org/10.1016/j.rbmo.2010.04.035.

72. Yazbeck C, Madelenat P, Ayel JP, Jacquesson L, Bontoux LM, Solal P, Hazout A. Ethanol sclerotherapy: a treatment option for ovarian endometriomas before ovarian stimulation. Reprod Biomed Online. 2009;19:121–5. http://www.ncbi.nlm.nih.gov/pubmed/19573300.

73. Kumbak B, Sahin L. Ethanol sclerotherapy for ovarian endometriomas before ovarian stimulation. Reprod Biomed Online. 2010;20:163. https://doi.org/10.1016/j.rbmo.2009.10.003; author reply 164.

74. Song X-M, Jiang H, Zhang W-X, Zhou Y, Ni F, Wang X-M. Ultrasound sclerotherapy pretreatment could obtain a similar effect to surgical intervention on improving the outcomes of in vitro fertilization for patients with hydrosalpinx. J Obstet Gynaecol Res. 2017;43:122–7. https://doi.org/10.1111/jog.13152.

75. Shah AA, Walmer DK. A feasibility study to evaluate pelvic peritoneal anatomy with a saline intraperitoneal sonogram (SIPS). Fertil Steril. 2010;94:2766–8. https://doi.org/10.1016/j.fertnstert.2010.04.066.

76. American College of Obstetricians and Gynecologists' Committee on Practice Bulletins—Obstetrics. Practice bulletin no. 166: thrombocytopenia in pregnancy. Obstet Gynecol. 2016;128:e43–53. https://doi.org/10.1097/AOG.0000000000001641.

77. Practice guidelines for obstetric anesthesia: an updated report by the American Society of Anesthesiologists Task Force on Obstetric Anesthesia and the Society for Obstetric Anesthesia and Perinatology. Anesthesiology. 2016;124:270–300. https://doi.org/10.1097/ALN.0000000000000935.

78. Weingarten TN, Jacob AK, Njathi CW, Wilson GA, Sprung J. Multimodal analgesic protocol and postanesthesia respiratory depression during phase I recovery after total joint arthroplasty. Reg Anesth Pain Med. 2015;40:330–6. https://doi.org/10.1097/AAP.0000000000000257.

79. Cahill DJ, Fox R, Wardle PG. Ureteral obstruction—a complication of oocyte retrieval. Fertil Steril. 1994;61:787–8. http://www.ncbi.nlm.nih.gov/pubmed/8150128.

Oocytes Freezing in Patient with Cancer

Fabrizio Signore, Raffaella Votino, Evangelos Sakkas,
Domenico Baldini, Simona Zaami, and Antonio Malvasi

Contents

Ovarian tissue cryopreservation was first performed more than 20 years ago. The first live birth after ovarian tissue transplantation after cryopreservation was reported in 2004 [1] followed by a second one the following year [2]. Today, with more than 120 live births and a 30% success rate, this technique is no longer considered experimental. However, the evolution of oocyte and embryo vitrification techniques has limited the ovarian cryopreservation to a selected number of patients. The

F. Signore (✉) · R. Votino · E. Sakkas
Department of Obstetrics, Gynaecology and Reproductive
Medicine, Misericordia Hospital, Grosseto, Italy
e-mail: fabrizio.signore@uslsudest.toscana.it;
raffaella.votino@uslsudest.toscana.it;
evangelos.sakkas@uslsudest.toscana.it

D. Baldini
Center of Medically Assisted Procreation, MOMO' fertiLIFE,
Bisceglie, Italy

S. Zaami
Department of Anatomical, Histological, Forensic and Orthopaedic
Sciences, Sapienza University of Rome, Rome, Italy

A. Malvasi
Department of Obstetrics and Gynecology, GVM Care
and Research Santa Maria Hospital, Bari, Italy

Laboratory of Human Physiology, Phystech BioMed School,
Faculty of Biological and Medical Physics, Moscow Institute
of Physics and Technology (State University), Dolgoprudny,
Russia

ASRM (American Society for Reproductive Medicine) recognizes the cryopreservation of oocytes and embryos as only valid methods for the preservation of fertility.

Premature ovarian failure (POF) can occur in woman spontaneously or due to iatrogenic causes. Chemotherapy and radiotherapy have significantly increased life expectancy in cancer patients but at the same time they can become deleterious for the ovarian function and reserve.

Chemotherapy treatments (Fig. 20.1) are divided into three categories of gonadotoxicity risk: low, medium, and high risk.

The *low-risk* group includes:
- methotrexate
- 5-fluorouracil
- vincristine
- bleomycin
- actinomycin D
- mercaptopurine

The *medium-risk* group includes:
- doxorubicin
- cisplatin
- carboplatin

The *high-risk* group includes:
- cyclophosphamide

© Springer Nature Switzerland AG 2020
A. Malvasi, D. Baldini (eds.), *Pick Up and Oocyte Management*, https://doi.org/10.1007/978-3-030-28741-2_20

- chlorambucil
- nitrogen mustard
- dacarbazine
- ifosfamide
- thiotepa
- melphalan
- busulfan
- procarbazine (Fig. 20.1)

Cyclophosphamide is the agent which causes the greatest damage to oocytes and granulosa cells. The ovarian damage depends on patient's age and on the type of treatment administered.

As far as radiotherapy is concerned it has been stated that a dose of 5–20 Gy administered to the ovary is sufficient to completely impair gonadal function, whatever the age of the patient [3, 4].

Patients who undergo bone marrow transplantation associated to total body irradiation and/or intensive chemotherapy, the percentage of POF after the treatment is nearly 100% [5–7].

Three options can be proposed to preserve fertility before radiotherapy or chemotherapy: oocyte cryopreservation, embryo cryopreservation, and ovarian tissue cryopreservation. The vitrification of oocytes (in metaphase II) is the ideal technique in pubertal and adult age for the preservation of fertility

Fig. 20.1 Categories of chemotherapy associated to gonadotoxicity risk

Degree of risk	Treatment protocol
High risk More than 80% of woman develop amenorrhea post-treatment	• CAF x 6 cycles in women ages 40 and older (cyclophosphamide,doxorubicin, 5-FU) • CEF x 6 cycles in women ages 40 and older (cyclophosphamide, epirubicin, 5-FU) • CMF x6 cycles in wome ages 40 older (cyclophosphamide,methotrexate,5-fluorouracil)
Intermediate risk Approximately 30-70% of woman develop amenorrhea post-treatment	• CMF x6 cycles in wome ages 30-39 (cyclophosphamide,methotrexate,5-fluorouracil) • CAF x 6 cycles in women ages 30-39 (cyclophosphamide,doxorubicin, 5-FU) • CEF x 6 cycles in women ages 30-39 (cyclophosphamide, epirubicin, 5-FU) • AC x 4 in women ages 40 and older (doxorubicin, cyclophosphamide
Low risk Approximately 20% of woman develop amenorrhea post-treatment	• AC x 4 in women ages 30-39 (doxorubicin, cyclophosphamide) • CAF x 6 cycles in women under 30 (cyclophosphamide,doxorubicin, 5-FU) • CEF x 6 cycles in women under 30 (cyclophosphamide, epirubicin, 5-FU) • CMF x6 cycles in women under 30 (cyclophosphamide,methotrexate,5-fluorouracil)
Very low/ no risk No effects	• MF (methotrexate, 5-FU)
Unknown risk There has been limited research on this treatment	• Trastuzamab(Herceptin) • Paclitaxel • Docetaxel

in cases of benign diseases such as autoimmune diseases or in cases of neoplasia. Moreover, it is the only method that guarantees that no malignant cell is reintroduced when the oocytes will be used again. The embryo cryopreservation would be a better option because of the known oocyte loss at thawing but it requires the presence of a partner or donor sperm. Studies show a survival rate of mature oocytes after thawing of 90% and a 50% pregnancy rate. However, we must consider that in order to have a live birth, it is necessary to have at least 20 vitrified oocytes [5]. In both cases, the patient must be in pubertal age and the start of the chemotherapy has to be postponed for 2 weeks, the time interval needed to stimulate the ovaries and collect mature oocytes. In prepubertal patients or in patients with oncological diseases in which the beginning of chemotherapy cannot be delayed, ovarian tissue cryopreservation represents the only possibility of preserving fertility.

The indications for cryopreservation of ovarian tissue in case of malignant and nonmalignant diseases are summarized here below (Table 20.1) [8]. In gynecological neoplasia, proposing an ovarian cryopreservation should be taken into consideration before realizing a fertility preservation surgery and spare the uterus given the restriction in surrogacy. The indication for ovarian cryopreservation can be also considered in patients, especially children, who undergo a unilateral oophorectomy for nonmalignant diseases. Jadoul et al. in 2017 analyzed all ovarian cryopreservation cases realized in their institution between 1997 and 2013; in 545 cases, 17% were done for benign diseases as shown in Table 20.2 [9]. The indications of cryopreservation must be discussed in a multidisciplinary team after taking into consideration the type of treatment administered to the patient after the surgery and its gonadotoxic risk.

However, in some types of neoplasia such as leukemia and lymphoma, ovarian tissue autotransplantation should be avoided due to the high possibility of reintroducing malignant cells. Rosendahl et al. demonstrated that there was suspicion of malignant cell infiltration in 7% of cases of ovarian tissue autotransplantation [10]. Dolmans et al. have evidenced the prevalence of minimal residual disease (MRD) in cryopreserved ovarian tissue in patients with chronic myeloid leukemia and lymphoblastic leukemia; these percentages are 33% and 70%, respectively [9]. In vitro maturation (IVM) and isolated follicle transplantation from ovarian tissue could be a promising option for these cases [12, 13]. However, primordial follicles do not grow properly in culture and the current studies are trying to identify the ideal culture system (Table 20.3).

20.1 The Surgical Technique

In cases in which it is not possible to postpone the chemotherapy or in prepubertal age, ovarian tissue cryopreservation is the only possibility of fertility preservation.

Table 20.1 Indications for cryopreservation of ovarian tissue in case of malignant and nonmalignant diseases (adopted from Donnez et al. [1])

(A)	**Malignant**
(a)	***Extrapelvic diseases***
	Bone cancer (osteosarcoma and Ewing sarcoma)
	Breast cancer
	Melanoma
	Neuroblastoma
	Bowel malignancy
(b)	***Pelvic diseases***
	Non gynecologic malignancy
	Pelvic sarcoma
	Rhabdomyosarcoma
	Sacral tumors
	Rectosigmoid tumors
	Gynecologic malignancy
	Early cervical carcinoma
	Early vaginal carcinoma
	Early vulvar carcinoma
	Selected cases of ovarian carcinoma (stage IA)
	Borderline ovarian tumors
(c)	***Systemic diseases***
	Hodgkin disease
	Non-Hodgkin lymphoma
	Leukemia
	Medulloblastoma
(B)	**Nonmalignant**
	(a) Uni/bilateral oophorectomy
	Benign ovarian tumors
	Severe and recurrent endometriosis
	BRCA1 or BRCA2 mutation carriers

Table 20.2 Causes of ovarian cryopreservation [6]

	N(%) patients	*N(%)* deaths	*N(%)* autografts
Hematological pathology	191(35)	15(8)	11
Lymphoma	127(23)	6(5)	
Leukemia	50(9)	9(18)	
Benign	14(3)	0	
Breast cancer	94(17)	5(5)	
Sarcoma	51(9)	17(33)	
Gynecological malignancy	33(6)	4(12)	
Neurological malignancy	26(5)	7(27)	
Gastrointestinal malignancy	16(3)	5(31)	
Systemic disease	11(2)	0	
Benign and borderline ovarian pathology	95(17)	0	
Generic diseases	19(3)	0	
Other	9(2)	1(11)	

There are three different techniques to realize the ovarian cryopreservation:

1. Large ovarian biopsies and orthotopic or heterotopic graft
2. Follicular isolation and IVM followed by transplantation (not yet realized in humans)

Table 20.3 Series of 60 live births after trasplantation of frozen-thawed ovarian cortex [18]

	Cryopreservation procedure	No of transplanted women desiring pregnancy	No of live birth = ongoing pregnancies
Donnez, Dolmans	SF	19	8 (+1)
Meirow et al.	SF	NA	6
Demeestere et al.	SF	NA	3
Andersen's et al.	SF	25	8
Silber et al.	SF	6	4
Piver et al., Roux et al.	SF	NA	3 (+1)
Pellicer et al.	SF	33	6ª (+3)
Revel et al.	SF	NA	2
Dittrich et al.	SF	20	6
Revelli et al.	SF	NA	1
Callejo et al.	SF	NA	1
Stem, Gook and Rozen	SF	14	3ª
Kawamura, Suzuka et al.	VF	NA	2
Burmeister, Kovacs, et al.	SF	2	1
Rodriguez-Wallberg, Hovatta et al.	SF	NA	1
Tanbo et al.	SF	2	2
Agarwal et al.	SF	NA	1
Makolkin et al., Kalugina et al.	SF	NA	2

SF slow freezing, *VF* vitrification
ªTwins

3. Removal of the entire ovary in order to preserve the vascularization and reduce the follicular loss due to ischemia [5]

The first technique is the most frequently used. The ovarian biopsies are taken by laparoscopic or laparotomic surgery depending on the surgical team and patient's age. The operation is done under general anesthesia. The following four laparoscopic puncture sites, including the umbilicus, are used:

- 10 mm umbilical.
- 5 mm right.
- 10 mm medial (allowing the use of 5-mm instruments) and 5 mm left lower quadrant, just above the pubic hairline.
- Lateral incisions are made next to the deep epigastric vessels. A cannula is placed in the cervix for appropriate uterine mobilization.

Then, multiple biopsies (Fig. 20.2) of one or both ovaries are performed. In prepubertal patients, it is preferred to remove the entire ovary or half of it (Fig. 20.3). Bipolar coagulation is avoided as far as possible in order to reduce the follicular damage.

The size of biopsies is in general 1.5–2 cm × 5 mm. The number of follicles found in the ovarian cortex depends on the patient's age: 350 and 400 follicles/mm³ in patients aged <10 years; 70–80/mm³ in patients between 10 and 15 years; 30–35/mm³ in patients between 15 and 34 years [10, 11]. The removed biopsies or ovary are then immediately handed over to a second team that is present in the operating room

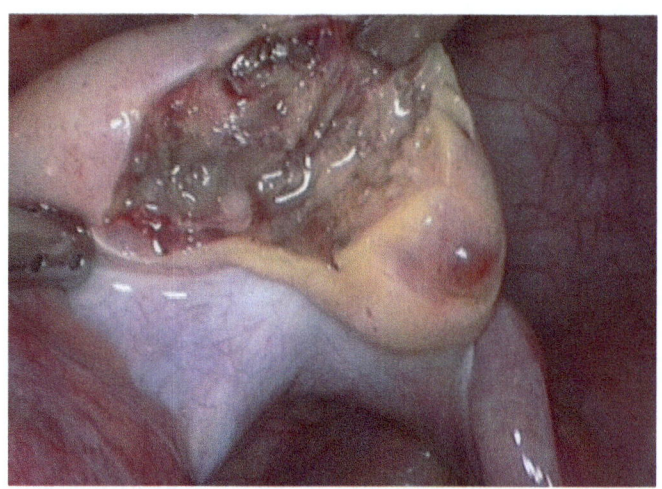

Fig. 20.2 Laparoscopic surgery: biopsy of ovarian cortical tissue for cryopreservation

and that includes a microsurgeon and biologist. A part of one of the biopsies is directly sent to anatomopathology in order to detect the presence of any malignant cell. The surgery can be realized in day hospital. After surgery, patients can undergo their programmed treatment immediately.

20.2 Transplantation

The transplantation can be realized when the patient has finished the treatment and is considered disease-free according to the oncologist and radiotherapist. The ovarian cortex can be implanted into the pelvic site (orthotopic site) or in another site in the body as the abdominal wall (heterotopic site). There are a few reports about the heterotopic autotransplantation of cryopreserved human ovarian tissue [14, 15]. Studies have reported heterotopic transplantation in rectus and pectoralis muscle. However, more is known on orthotopic transplantation.

The transplantation is performed with a laparoscopic surgery. At the time of transplantation, the ovarian fragments are placed on the ovaries by using stitches, glue, or intercede (Figs. 20.4 and 20.5). During transplantation, the cortex of

the ovary is cut in order to create a window with a new vascularization. If the ovaries were removed in first place, the ovarian fragments are placed in a peritoneal window created at the ovarian fossa or at the large ligament. Orthotopic transplantation has a 95% recovery rate of ovarian endocrine activity and 40% restoration of fertility [15, 16].

20.3 Results

When primordial follicles are present in the reimplanted ovarian tissue in orthotopic reimplantation, the ovarian function is almost always restored. Generally, the ovarian function begins about 4 months (between 31/2 and 61/2 months) after the transplantation [17, 18]. The reduction of FSH starts about 3 months after surgery and gains its normal baseline levels after 5 months. The peak of estradiol (E2) concomitant with decline of FSH is more later, between 51/2 and 61/2 months after the surgery. The peak of E2 depends on the follicular reserve and on the patient's age at the time of the cryopreservation [19, 20]. Meirow et al. demonstrated that the decline of FSH depends on the detrimental effect of previous chemotherapy on the vascularization [2]. According to Donnez et al., the decline of FSH depends also on the existent blood vessels in grafts tissue. The restauration of ovarian activity is lower in patients who had received chemotherapy before the cryopreservation and depends on the type of chemotherapy.

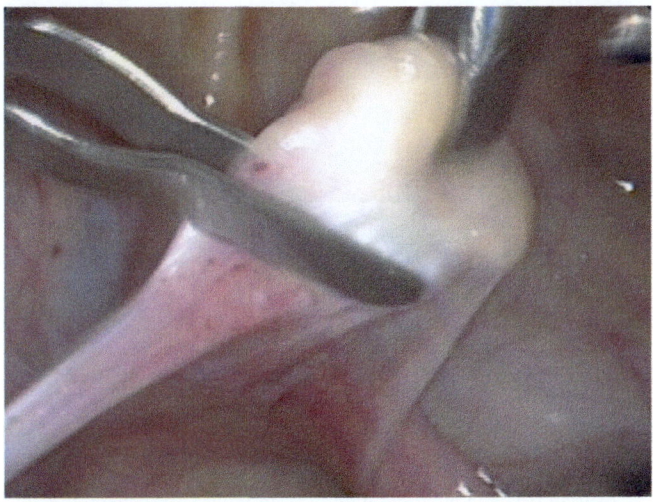

Fig. 20.3 Laparoscopic surgery: unilateral oophorectomy for ovarian cryopreservation

Fig. 20.4 (**a**) Remaining ovary. (**b**) The cortex of the remaining ovary is removed. (**c**) Ovarian cortical pieces were grafted with stitches. (**d**) Pieces are covered with interceed. (Images kindly offered by St Luc Hospital in Bruxelles)

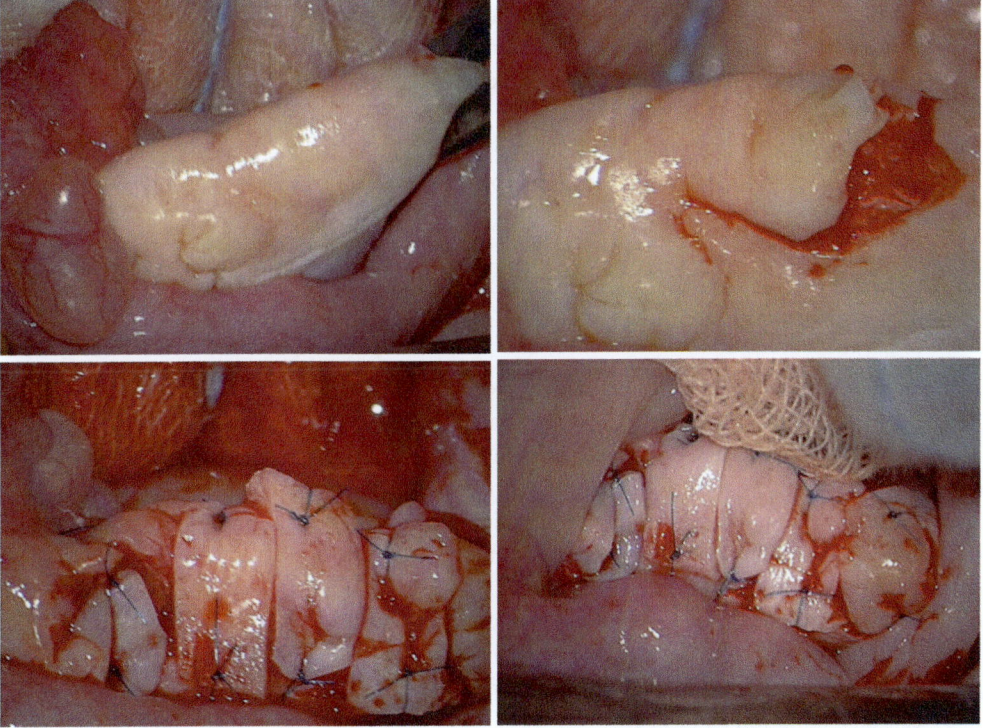

Fig. 20.5 Decortication of ovarian cortex (**a**); fixation of interceed (**b**); small ovarian biopsies are placed on the ovary (**c**); the interceed cover the ovarian fragments and is fixed (**d**). Large strips 8–10 mm × 5 mm and small cubes 2 mm × 2 mm. (Images kindly offered by St Luc Hospital in Bruxelles)

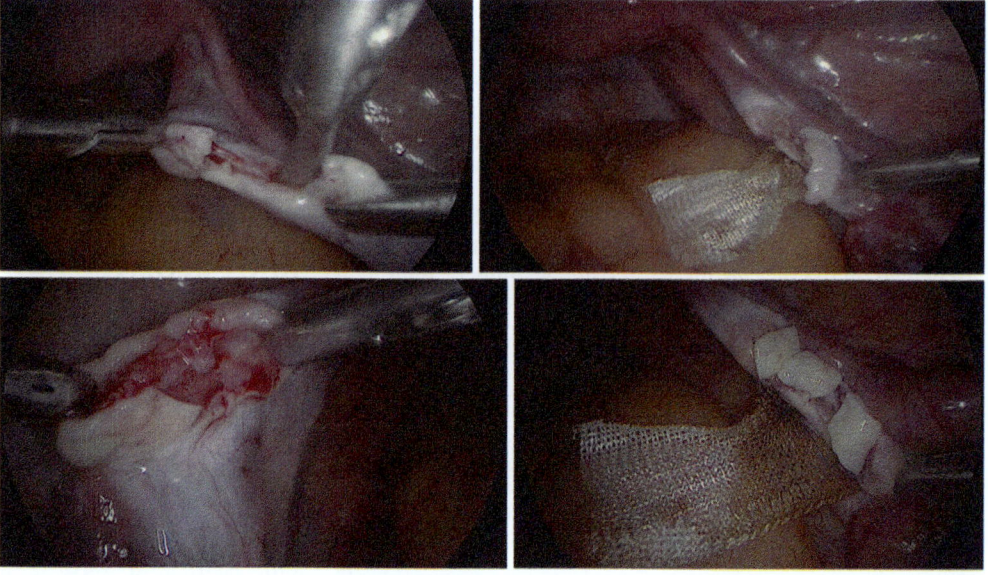

The ovarian activity is maintained for an average of 5 years but in the patients who received the chemotherapy before cryopreservation the ovarian activity lasts 1–2 years.

Spontaneous pregnancies have been reported after orthotopic and heterotopic transplantation. However, in many cases, the patients will have to follow an in vitro fertilization (IVF) treatment. In these patients, there is a higher rate of empty follicles (29–35%) [2, 21–23]; this rate is higher than in the general population undergoing IVF. Different factors can determine the higher empty follicles such as the delay of revascularization after the graft.

According to Donnez and Demesteere, the orthotopic transplantation should be preferred to the heterotopic because it provides the optimal environment for follicular development in terms of pressure, temperature, and paracrine factors. It should be emphasized that ovarian tissue transplantation can be repeated in order to prolong the ovarian activity for more than 10 years [24–30].

20.4 Conclusion

Approximately, one-third of young women exposed to chemotherapy develop ovarian failure. The ovarian tissue cryopreservation is an invasive and experimental procedure compared to the embryo and oocyte cryopreservation. However, it represents the only solution in patients who have to undergo a gonadotoxic chemotherapy immediately or in cancer patients of prepubertal age. In some neoplasia such as the lymphoma, the transmission of malignant cells exists but it should be proposed in these patients when there are no other possibilities. More research is expected on the isolated oocytes transplantation and IVM.

References

1. Donnez J, Dolmans MM, Demylle D, Jadoul P, Pirard C, Squifflet J, Martinez-Madrid B, Van Langendonckt A. Livebirth after orthotopic transplantation of cryopreserved ovarian tissue. Lancet. 2004;364:1405–10. Erratum in Lancet 2004;364:2020.
2. Meirow D, Levron J, Eldar-Geva T, Hardan I, Fridman E, Zalel Y, Schiff E, Dor J. Pregnancy after transplantation of cryopreserved ovarian tissue in a patient with ovarian failure after chemotherapy. N Engl J Med. 2005;353:318–21.
3. Wallace WH, Thomson AB, Saran F, et al. Predicting age of ovarian failure after radiation to a field that includes the ovaries. Int J Radiat Oncol Biol Phys. 2005;62:738–44.
4. Wallace WH, Thomson AB, Kelsey TW. The radiosensitivity of the human oocyte. Hum Reprod. 2003;18(1):117–21.
5. Cobo A, Garcia-Velasco JA, Coello A, Domingo J, Pellicer A, Remohi J. Oocyte vitrification as an efficient option for elective fertility preservation. Fertil Steril. 2016;105:755–64.
6. Doyle JO, Richter KS, Lim J, Stillman RJ, Graham JR, Tucker MJ. Successful elective and medically indicated oocyte vitrification and warming for autologous in vitro fertilization, with predicted birth probabilities for fertility preservation according to number of cryopreserved oocytes and age at retrieval. Fertil Steril. 2016;105(2):459–66. Epub 2015 Nov 18.
7. Chang CC, Elliott TA, Wright G, Shapiro DB, Toledo AA, Nagy ZP. Prospective controlled study to evaluate laboratory and clinical outcomes of oocyte vitrification obtained in in vitro fertilization patients aged 30 to 39 years. Fertil Steril. 2013;99(7):1891–7.
8. Donnez J, Dolmans MM. Cryopreservation and transplantation of ovarian tissue. Clin Obstet Gynecol. 2010;53(4):787–96.
9. Jadoul P, Guilmain A, Squifflet J, Luyckx M, Votino R, Wyns C, Domans MM. Efficacy of ovarian tissue cryopreservation for fertility preservation: lessons learned from 545 cases. Hum Reprod. 2017;32(5):1046–54.
10. Rosendahl M, Greve T, Andersen CY. The safety of transplanting cryopreserved ovarian tissue in cancer patients: a review of the literature. J Assist Reprod Genet. 2013;30(1):11–24. https://doi.org/10.1007/s10815-012-9912-x.
11. Dolmans MM, Marinescu C, Saussoy P, Van Langendonckt A, Amorim C, Donnez J. Reimplantation of cryopreserved ovarian tissue from patients with acute lymphoblastic leukemia is not safe. Blood. 2010;116:2908–14.

12. Luyckx V, Dolmans MM, Vanacker J, Legat C, Fortuno Moya C, Donnez J, Amorim CA. A new step toward the artificial ovary: survival and proliferation of isolated murine follicles after autologous transplantation in a fibrin scaffold. Fertil Steril. 2014;101:1149–56.
13. Chiti MC, Dolmans MM, Lucci CM, Paulini F, Donnez J, Amorim CA. Further insights into the impact of mouse follicle stage on graft outcome in an artificial ovary environment. Mol Hum Reprod. 2017;23(6):381–92.
14. Oktay K, Buyuk E, Veeck L, et al. Embryo development after heterotopic transplantation of cryopreserved ovarian tissue. Lancet. 2004;363:837–40.
15. Kim SS, Lee WS, Chung MK, et al. Long-term ovarian function and fertility after heterotopic autotransplantation of cryobanked human ovarian tissue: 8-year experience in cancer patients. Fertil Steril. 2009;91:2349–54.
16. Donnez J, Manavella DD, Dolmans MM. Techniques for ovarian tissue transplantation and results. Minerva Ginecol. 2018;70(4):424–31. https://doi.org/10.23736/S0026-4784.18.04228-4.
17. Donnez J, Dolmans MM, Pellicer A, Diaz-Garcia C, Sanchez Serrano M, Schmidt KT, Ernst E, Leuyckx V, Andersen CY. Restoration of ovarian activity and pregnancy after transplantation of cryopreserved ovarian tissue: a review of 60 cases of reimplantation. Fertil Steril. 2013;99:1503–13.
18. Donnez J, Dolmans MM. Ovarian tissue freezing: current status. Curr Opin Obstet Gynecol. 2015;27:22–30.
19. Poirot C, Vacher-Lavenue MV, Helardot P, Guilbert J, Brugieres L, Jouannet P. Human ovarian tissue cryopreservation: indications and feasibility. Hum Reprod. 2002;17(6):1447–52.
20. Poirot CJ, Martelli H, Genestie C, Golmard JL, Valteau-Couanet D, Helardot P, Pacquement H, Sauvat F, Tabone MD, Philippe-Chomette P, Esperou H, Baruchel A, Brugieres L. Feasibility of ovarian tissue cryopreservation for prepubertal females with cancer. Pediatr Blood Cancer. 2007;49(1):74–8.
21. Dolmans MM, Donnez J, Camboni A, Demylle D, Amorim C, Van Langendonckt A, et al. IVF outcome in patients with orthotopically transplanted ovarian tissue. Hum Reprod. 2009;24:2778–87.
22. Andersen CY, Rosendahl M, Byskov AG, Loft A, Ottosen C, Dueholm M, et al. Two successful pregnancies following autotransplantation of frozen/thawed ovarian tissue. Hum Reprod. 2008;23:2266–72.
23. Bedaiwy MA, El-Nashar SA, El Saman AM, Evers JL, Sandadi S, Desai N, Falcone T. Reproductive outcome after transplantation of ovarian tissue: a systematic review. Hum Reprod. 2008;23(12):2709–17.
24. Donnez J, Dolmans MM. Ovarian cortex transplantation: 60 reported live births brings the success and worldwide expansion of the technique towards routine clinical practice. J Assist Reprod Genet. 2015;32:1167–70.
25. Lutchman Singh K, Davies M, Chatterjee R. Fertility in female cancer survivors: pathophysiology, preservation and role of ovarian reserve testing. Hum Reprod Update. 2005;11(1):69–89.
26. Desolle L, Darai E, Cornet D, Rouzier R, Coutant C, Mandelbaum J, Antoine JM. Determinants of pregnancy rate in the donor oocyte model: a multivariate analysis of 450 frozen-thawed embryo transfers. Hum Reprod. 2009;24(12):3082–9.
27. Donnez J, Dolmans MM. Fertility preservation in women. N Engl J Med. 2017;377(17):1657–65.
28. Winkler-Crepaz K, Ayuandari S, Ziehr SC, Hofer S, Wildt L. Fertility preservation in cancer survivors. Minerva Endocrinol. 2015;40(2):105–18.
29. Dittrich R, Maltaris T, Hoffmann I, Oppelt PG, Beckmann MW, Mueller A. Fertility preservation in cancer patients. Minerva Ginecol. 2010;62(1):63–80.
30. Chuai Y, Xu X, Wang A. Preservation of fertility in females treated for cancer. Int J Biol Sci. 2012;8(7):1005–12.

Eggs Retrieval. Adverse Events, Complications, and Malpractice: A Medicolegal Perspective

21

Simona Zaami, Michael Stark, Antonio Malvasi, and Enrico Marinelli

Contents

21.1 Standard and Substandard Care Concepts

Ovum pickup (OPU) or egg retrieval, also known as follicular or follicle puncture, is instrumental in carrying out in vitro fertilization (IVF) procedures.

S. Zaami (✉) · E. Marinelli
Department of Anatomical, Histological, Forensic and Orthopedic Sciences, Sapienza University of Rome, Rome, Italy
e-mail: simona.zaami@uniroma1.it; enrico.marinelli@uniroma1.it

M. Stark
The New European Surgical Academy, Berlin, Germany

Charitè University Hospital, Berlin, Germany

ELSAN Group Hospitals, Paris, France
e-mail: mstark@nesacademy.org

A. Malvasi
Department of Obstetrics and Gynecology, GVM Care and Research Santa Maria Hospital, Bari, Italy

Laboratory of Human Physiology, Phystech BioMed School, Faculty of Biological and Medical Physics, Moscow Institute of Physics and Technology (State University), Dolgoprudny, Russia

It is a surgical process aimed at harvesting oocytes from the ovarian follicles. The intervention in itself is swiftly performed, usually under anesthesia (sedation). By virtue of ovum-retrieval being an invasive kind of practice, it is consequently prone to bringing about adverse events, throughout the various stages of the procedure, from hormonal stimulation to management of retrieved oocytes, in addition to possible mishaps occurring in the pickup phase.

Guidelines have been devised as a means to facilitate clinical practice and to provide, beforehand, a set of standards of conduct to be adopted as guiding principles in health care practice. Over time, guidelines have, de facto, taken up ever greater legal significance, since they have been applied as parameters of judgment in almost all nations, even across different legal and judicial systems, for the purpose of formulating assessments as to the suitability and soundness of health care choices made by professionals.

It is therefore safe to say that the main assessment criteria applicable to evaluate the clinical and legal tenability of any given medical procedure, including MAP and egg retrieval, is the compliance with relevant sets of guidelines pertaining to a given medical specialty [1].

In some instances, however, there may not be specific guidelines for a certain field of medicine, or those available may not be universally acknowledged. In such cases, the judiciary has often shown a tendency to rely on good practices, which are typically based on scientific literature and research findings of recognized merit. Those standards constitute the cornerstone, from a legal perspective, needed to outline the standards of care. Any health care choice that fails to meet those standards, which prove unwarranted by either available guidelines or best practices, is likely to be deemed unorthodox, inappropriate, liable to be punishable in a court of law, especially if a connection is proven with adverse outcomes following such actions (the so-called substandard of care, i.e., a breach of standards of care). In that respect, it is worth pointing out that the very definition of complication, however, widely used, may often prove unsatisfactory and hazy, in order to properly identify an area of non-liability, unlike the notion of malpractice, clearly associated with punishable events.

The medical concept of complication stands for any damaging event arising during treatment which may result in an unfavorable deviation with respect to the expected clinical path, whatever the cause may be.

Such definition, widely accepted in medicine, does not satisfy fundamental law requirements, as often observed in medicolegal disputes (Fig. 21.1).

In fact, legal approaches which came about in the field of medical malpractice both in Anglo-Saxon countries (common law) and in those of Roman tradition (civil law) do not consider nullifying the fact that clinical statistics foresee a particular adverse event as a complication. In legal proceeding terms, the concept of complication is much more restrictive than that provided in medicine.

In fact, the complication that does not involve responsibility is only the so-called unpredictable or unavoidable event. In particular, unpredictability or inevitability of complications excludes liability if the expected favorable outcome is not feasible in practice, not just on the basis of the statistical data. In Italy, this principle has been repeatedly stated in court decisions and has been recently confirmed by the Italian Supreme Court [2].

The logic behind this approach is: in treatments of choice (i.e., treatments performed not in emergency-urgency conditions) a favorable outcome should follow the treatment on the basis of the principle of clinical-statistical regularity. The latter is closely related to the doctrine of res ipsa loquitur, which is applied in most European countries and in the United States.

This doctrine, peculiar of the Anglo-Saxon jurisprudence, affects the burden of proof between the plaintiff and the defendant and consists in a rule of evidence that involves the presumption that the surgeon acted negligently for the very fact that the claimed damage occurred. In the commonly accepted interpretation, the presumptive liability, in order to be applied, must see to meet three conditions:

(a) The material means that determined the damage (i.e., instruments) were under the operator's direct control.
(b) The damage could have occurred only for the operator's negligence or mistake.
(c) The behavior of the damaged party has not contributed to the injury.

Experience demonstrates that this rule is applied by the courts in a less strict way than the original version, and in cases of uncertainty the judgment is usually in favor of the damaged parties.

Based on the actual features of the arising complication, physicians may avoid the debt of liability only if said developments could not be avoided in that specific case. In all other cases, it is likely that surgeons are held responsible.

Moreover, even in those cases of unavoidable complications, the physician's responsibility is considered as factual if complications were not treated according to the standard of care, which anyhow was inadequate. This evaluation, which should be made case by case, unavoidably calls for the consultation of experts that the courts rely on in the case of legal disputes that require specific technical knowledge. They should have expertise on both the methodology under discussion and the medical testimony, also

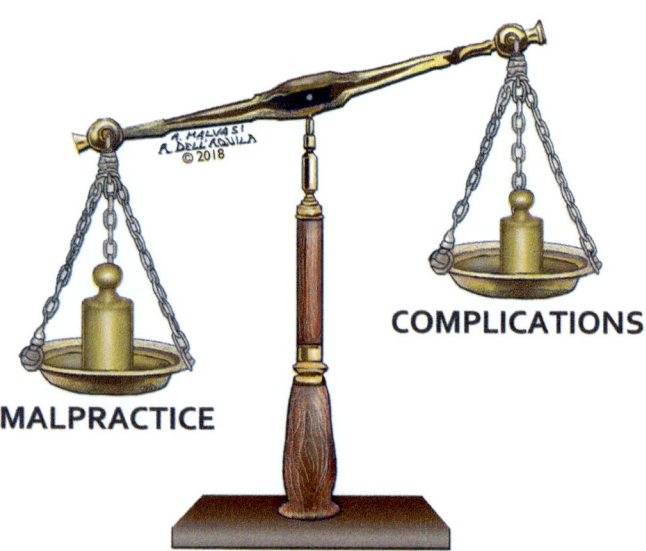

Fig. 21.1 The medical concept of complication stands for any damaging event arising during treatment which may result in an unfavorable deviation with respect to the expected clinical path, whatever the cause may be. Such definition, widely accepted in medicine, does not satisfy fundamental law requirements, as often observed in medicolegal disputes

in order to avoid any procedural error in the evaluation of the responsibilities that could lead to legally invalidate the assessing procedure.

A person can testify as a medical expert only after his/her credentials are established before the court. An attorney can assess the medical expert credentials by asking questions about their education, training, skills, and experience within a particular field. Once the required qualifications for an expert witness status have been established, a judge will qualify the witness as an expert. Most expert witnesses must be paid to testify on behalf of one of the parties. There may be more than one medical expert witness in a case [3]. Since it is difficult that only one professional has both technical-operational skills and expertise as expert fitness in medical litigations, the collective legal assessment is becoming a legal practice (a physician actually applying the method and a professional medical expert witness).

This practice is supported by some codes of medical ethics [4], and in Italy by a law enacted on article 15 of 8th March 2017 [5].

This awareness justifies the great interest on the issue of complications, both in terms of improving the individual performance of each operator and the ability to prevent and manage possible damages in order to avoid charges of malpractice or, at least, reduce the consequences.

21.2 The Issue of Informed Consent

Egg-retrieval procedures and IVF must be carried out in compliance with available guidelines, such as those laid out by the European Society of Human Reproduction and Embryology, and after gaining informed consent from patients made fully aware of the risks involved in the procedures.

As with any medical procedure, patients must provide informed consent to fertility treatments such as artificial insemination and in vitro fertilization (IVF).

Informed consent occurs when a patient understands the nature of the proposed treatment as well as the potential benefits and risks of the treatment and potential alternatives, and voluntarily chooses to proceed with the treatment.

Many fertility clinics have standardized forms for patients to complete as part of the informed consent process. Typically, the physician will have the informed consent discussion with patients simultaneously with the completion of the informed consent paperwork. However, it is unrealistic to expect a physician to understand the nuances of the unsettled field of parentage law.

The informed consent paperwork often goes beyond the concepts of procedures, benefits and risks, and delves into issues such as the establishment and relinquishment of parental rights [6].

Clinic consent forms have played an important role in litigation surrounding the use of cryopreserved genetic material following the divorce of the intended parents. Courts have taken different approaches toward evaluating the preferences expressed in the clinic consent forms.

The clinical consent forms at issue would typically be filled out by the intended parents before the creation of the embryos, at a time when the patients' interests are typically focused only on maximizing the chance of success of their upcoming IVF cycle.

Thoughtful deliberation is necessary to determine the ultimate disposition of their unused embryos at this stage of the process.

It should be highlighted that the definition of the main complications as part of the informed consent procedure is not in itself sufficient to ensure that gynecologists will not incur in charges in case any of these complications occur. In deciding whether the physician is free from any responsibility, the judge will consider only the inevitable or unforeseeable complications. However, timely and complete information avoids the charge of violating the patient's self-determination freedom that a poor information does not allow.

From a practical point of view, it is therefore necessary to consider the problem of what are the minimum requirements of the information to be given to patients. In theory, any form of information could be disputed for being inappropriate, most frequently due to its being somehow incomplete.

However, respecting some logical criteria (which could constitute a sort of checklist of the information to be given to the patient) the risks can be limited to a minimum.

The necessary information requirements, according to the patient's right-to-know should include:

- Usefulness, purpose, and method of execution of the procedure.
- If, and whenever feasible, there are alternative and equally efficient therapeutic procedures.
- Degree of tolerability of the procedure (in terms of pain, discomfort, time).
- Need to use drugs specifying their nature, route of administration, dosage, side effects, and possible interactions with any other medications that the patient is taking.
- Risks of the procedure with an indication of the statistically significant adverse events (ovarian hyperstimulation syndrome, hemoperitoneum, anesthetic adverse events, and long-term effects).
- Physician's skills in the execution of the procedure. In this context, it is still debated whether it is sufficient that physicians provide general statistical information on the frequency of adverse events or whether it is essential they make available also their own personal statistics. The latter information is preferable not only because it is more specific, but also because it is more transparent.

This aspect should not be underestimated because in many countries, especially in Italy, courts can punish physicians who have not fulfilled this obligation even when the procedure used has a favorable outcome, by imposing a compensation calculated on the basis of a fair, equitable method (discretionary), if the patient claims that the information provided was insufficient and the physician is not able to demonstrate that there was no lack of information [7].

21.3 Ovum PickUp Related Injuries: All Potential Claims

Ovum pickup associated complications may include damage to pelvic organs, hemorrhage, and infection (Fig. 21.2) [8].

Thorough information, as previously pointed out, entails that such potential developments should be explained to prospective donors. The provision of thorough information, however, is not necessarily enough to stave off lawsuits in case of adverse outcomes. It can be confidently asserted that almost all kinds of complications laid out in scientific literature may give rise to doctors being sued. The main kinds of recurring damages are outlined below, in terms of their assessed potential to lead to indemnity payments being awarded.

21.3.1 Candidate Selection. Obesity-Related Risks and Medicolegal Issues

Obesity is a growing problem in many parts of the world. It is generally defined using the body mass index (BMI) measurement in the units, kg/m^2.

Based on World Health Organization (WHO) standards, a BMI of 18.5–24.9 is considered normal, 25–29.9 overweight, and ≥30 as obese.

In obese patients, the egg retrieval technique is more challenging, difficult, and dangerous (Fig. 21.3) [9]. For this reason, many IVF centers have imposed various cutoffs for BMI and IVF egg retrievals under conscious sedation [10].

Some women with a BMI over 40 (morbid obesity) may not be able to proceed to egg retrieval and conscious sedation. At Fertility Centers of Illinois, any obese women with a BMI over 35 must obtain counseling regarding the increased risks to both the mom and baby, and provide authorization to proceed with IVF in light of the risks [11].

In addition, any woman whose BMI is between 40 and 50 may proceed with IVF and anesthesia, as long as they pass medical clearance and anesthesia clearance. A consultation with a Maternal Fetal Medicine specialist may also be required to discuss potential risks to mother and baby. In regards to the effect of obesity on oocyte retrieval: a review reflects that eight studies reported lower numbers and nine

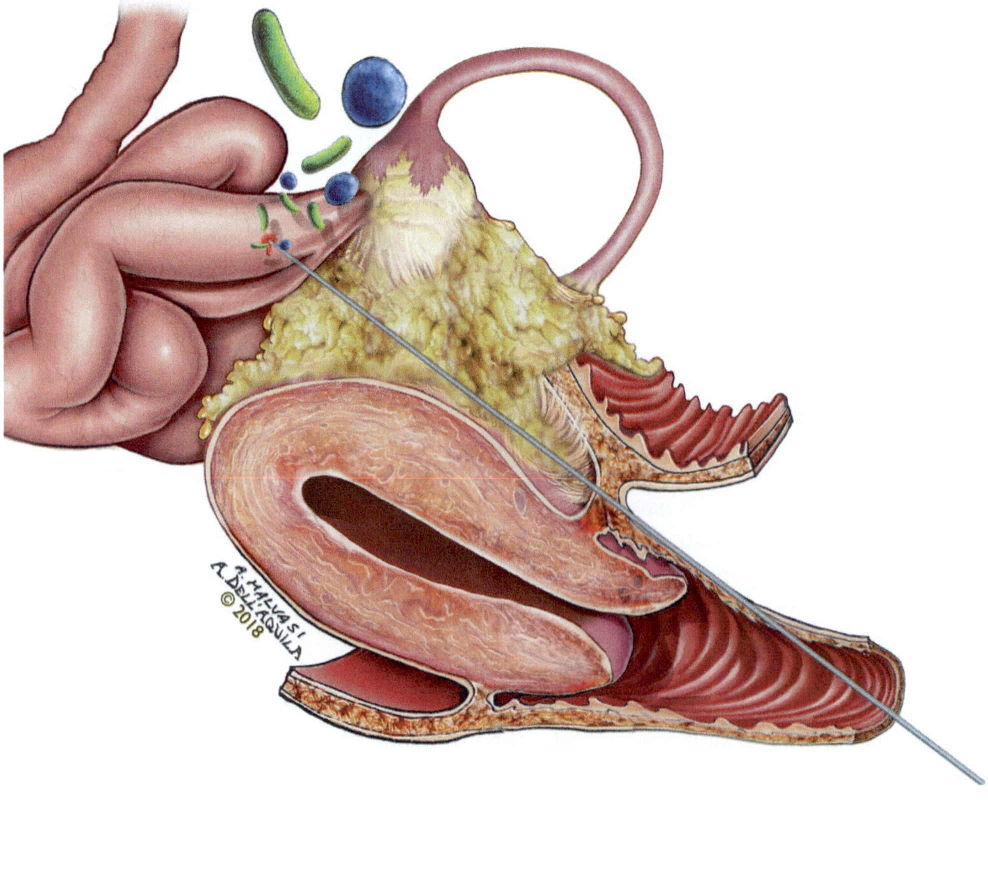

Fig. 21.2 Ovum pickup in patients with the uterine bowel adhesions and accidental intestinal perforation and subsequent peritoneal infection: a potential claim issue

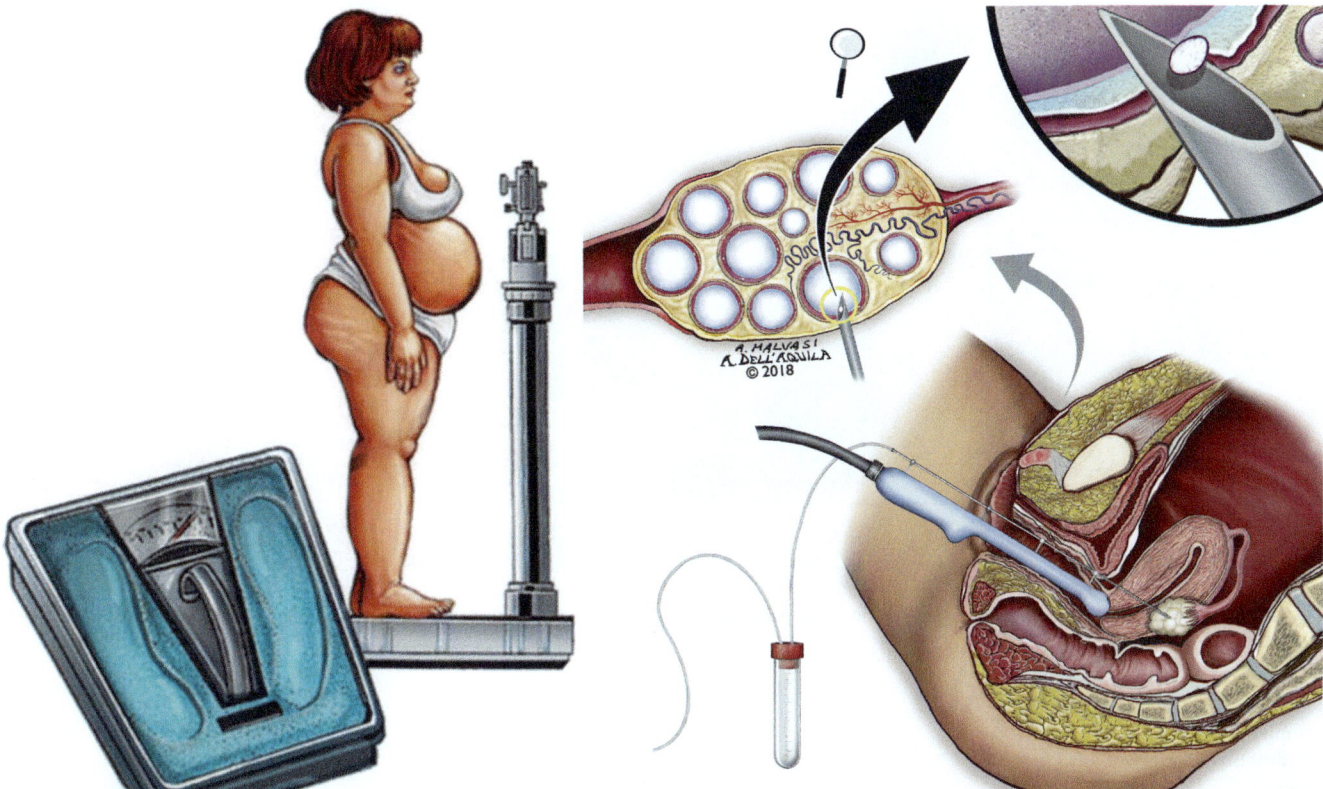

Fig. 21.3 In obese patients, the egg retrieval technique is more challenging, difficult, and dangerous

found no difference; oocyte quality or maturity: six studies found an adverse effect and one found no effect [12].

Women with polycystic ovarian syndrome (PCOS) and obesity were also reported to have smaller oocyte diameter at the time of retrieval [13].

Because of the heightened associated risks, patients with a BMI over 50 will not be permitted to proceed with fertility treatment [14].

Obesity can result in fewer mature follicles and a decreased chance for oocyte retrieval [15–17]. Any failure to abide by the disqualifying criteria (BMI > 50, for instance) would be bound to lead to malpractice claims against doctors.

21.3.2 Ovum PickUp and Anesthetic Complications

A retrospective study of 1.031 patients showed that OPU is a safe and well-tolerated procedure. In this study, there were no anesthetic complications in patients who underwent sedoanalgesia or local anesthesia [18].

Two studies in the literature reported complications due to anesthesia performed for OPU; one was conducted on a

series of 542 patients, and intensive care was needed for two patients due to bronchospasm, which occurred after general anesthesia [19, 20]. The harmful potential of these adverse events is relative because these are usually reversible events.

Additional complications may result from the administration of intravenous sedation or general anesthesia. These include asphyxia caused by airway obstruction, apnea, hypotension, and pulmonary aspiration of stomach contents (Fig. 21.4) [21]. Such developments result in high likelihood of generating legal claims, especially relative to the possibility of brain damage arising from them.

The second complication type, described in a not so recent case report, was cardiac conduction disorder, which occurred in a patient who received paracervical anesthesia with 400 mg mepivacaine [22]. This event turned out to be reversible. Aside from these cases, no other anesthesia-induced complications were found in the literature [23].

21.3.3 Hemorrhagic Complications

Limited vaginal bleeding is relatively common (8%) at the entrance site of the OPU needle; this can often be stopped by compression, although suturing is sometimes required [24].

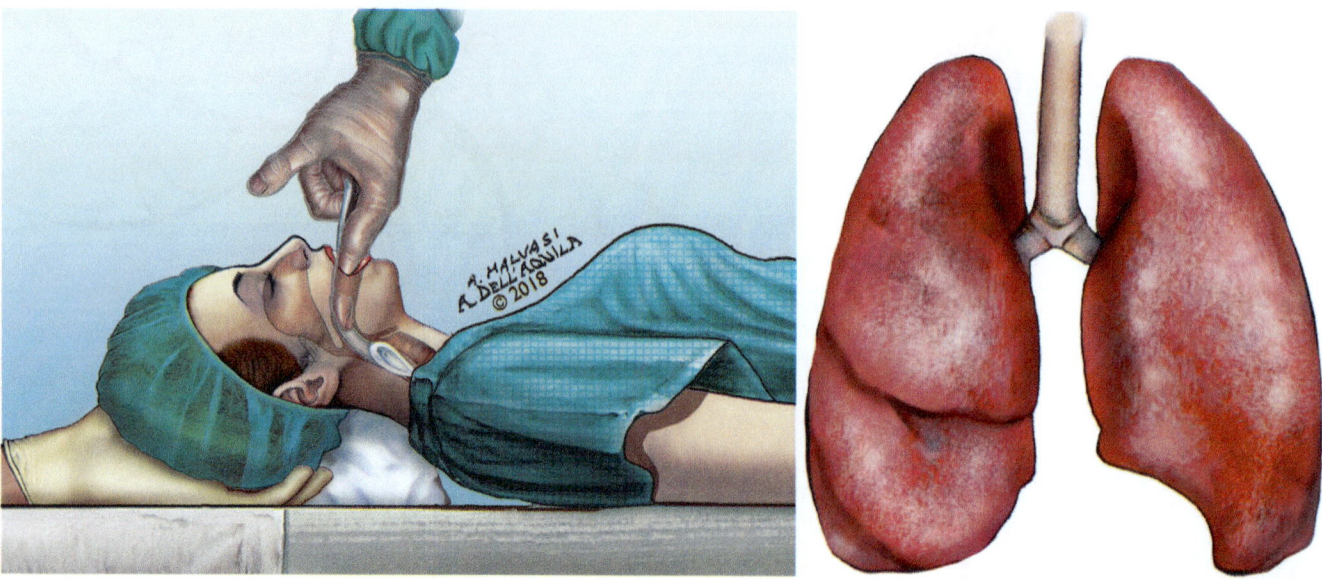

Fig. 21.4 Oocytes retrieval and general anesthetic complications: asphyxia caused by airway obstruction, apnea, ipotension, and pulmonary aspiration

Fig. 21.5 Hemorrhagic complication during oocyte retrieval on the artery of left ovary

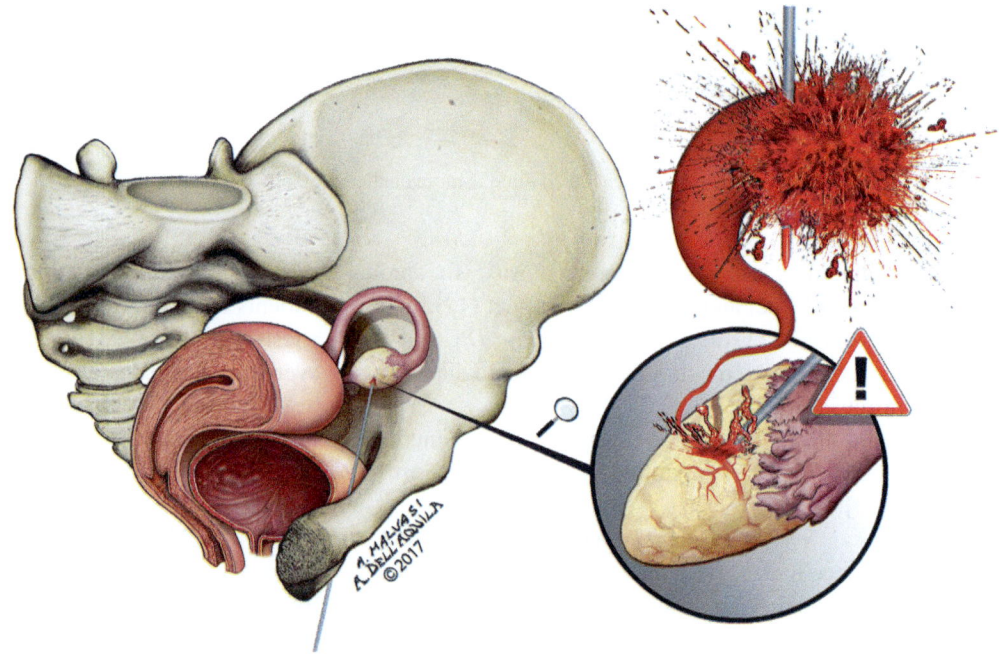

Acute hemorrhage from the ovary (Fig. 21.5), and bleeding or hematomas due to vascular damage in the uterus, ovary, and iliac vein are very rare (0.04–0.07%), but may require surgical intervention when they do occur [25].

Ovarian hemorrhage after transvaginal oocyte retrieval (TVOR) is a potentially catastrophic complication, even life-threatening, and has been observed to occur more often in lean patients with polycystic ovary syndrome [26]. Such a risk factor must be carefully assessed in women candidate to procedure. Luckily this is an event rarely detected in literature.

In the realm of such events, it is often difficult to draw the line between complication (i.e., unavoidable adverse event) and malpractice [27]. Courts of law have frequently shown a tendency to take into account the scope of consequences, thus opting for a principle of proportionality between risks and achievable benefits: the more severe the event turns out, the less excusable it is deemed, particularly when it occurs in healthy patients.

21.3.4 Ovarian Hyperstimulation Syndrome (OHSS) and Liability

HCG injections as a trigger for ovulation may give rise to the risk of ovarian hyperstimulation syndrome (OHSS), especially in patients suffering from polycystic ovary syndrome who may have been hyperstimulated during previous assisted reproduction cycles. Most cases involving patients who undergo egg retrieval are mild to moderate cases that resolve themselves within a few days.

In order to stave off these complications, patients should undergo a thorough female pelvic ultrasound exam to prevent fluid from accumulating in the pouch of Douglas. In that clinical field, the use of diagnostic ultrasonography could go a long way in warding off malpractice litigation, based on the allegedly untimely detection and treatment of OHSS; in that regard, ultrasonography should be combined with a thorough documentation process of all tests and monitoring activities implemented, as it is the case in other gynecological specialties [28].

Patient follow-up studies from Canada indicate that about one-third of women who undergo ovarian stimulation suffer "mild" OHSS. In a British study tracking 339 women, roughly 14% were hospitalized for OHSS after stimulation cycles yielded more than 20 eggs [29].

The results of a study by Kramer et al. seem to be in agreement with previous reports of the prevalence of OHSS following ovarian stimulation, now recognized as a common adverse effect [30].

Ovarian hyperstimulation entails a significant degree of risk, which seems to become worse with the number of cycles undergone. Provided that five or fewer successive stimulation cycles do not seem to impair ovarian response, the American Society of Reproductive Medicine (ASRM) [31] cautions that the number of adverse events after a given number of procedures is additive and, therefore, recommends a maximum limit of six cycles of oocyte donation [32].

Patients experiencing mild OHSS may complain of mild pain, bloated feeling, mild abdominal swelling, mild nausea, mild weight gain, and diarrhea [33].

Moderate OHSS presents symptoms similar to mild OHSS, but the swelling and bloating is worse, as are abdominal pain and vomit. There might be fluid build-up in the abdominal cavity causing discomfort. Severe OHSS carries even worse swelling and bloating in addition to abdominal pain and vomiting (Fig. 21.6).

Patients might experience shortness of breath and a reduction in the amount of urine output. Severe OHSS is typical in an IVF cycle with the intended mothers own eggs and the intended mother having a transfer of the embryos into herself after undergoing egg retrieval. The worst cases seem to be associated with pregnancy.

If hyperstimulation is mild to moderate, it can be managed at home on bed rest. The study of Kramer et al. shows that 11.6% of respondents had required paracentesis and/or hospitalization for OHSS [30].

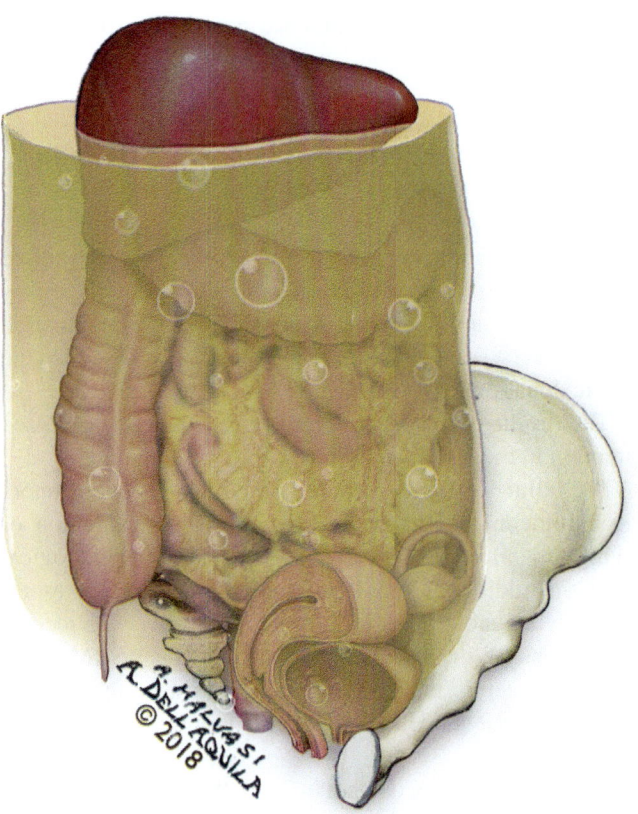

Fig. 21.6 Anatomical findings of OHSS

Severe hyperstimulation happens with large amounts of fluid retention and low urine output occurs. Several factors independently increase the risk of developing severe OHSS.

These include an age under 30, polycystic ovaries, or high basal antral follicle count on ultrasound, rapidly rising or high serum estradiol, previous history of OHSS, large number of small follicles (8–12 mm) detected by ultrasound during ovarian stimulation, use of hCG as opposed to progesterone for luteal phase support after IVF, large number of oocytes retrieved (over 20), and early pregnancy [34].

Ovarian stimulation falls within the category of standardized practices, during which the onset of OHSS is hard to foresee, except for those cases in which women had undergone previous stimulation cycles, or suffered from polycystic ovarian syndrome. Malpractice charges may be leveled, in all likelihood, in cases of underestimation of OHSS and failure to initiate treatment in a timely fashion; fatalities have been recorded in such circumstance, however rarely, mostly associated with thromboembolic events [35–39].

Any disregard of recommended limits in the number of oocyte donation cycles (the ASRM recommends a maximum limit of six cycles of oocyte donation) would carry the high risk of legal claims of negligence against doctors and/or facilities [39–41].

21.3.5 Secondary Infertility Following Ovarian Stimulation

In a 2009 retrospective study, 16.8% of respondents reported some menstrual problems and 9.6% noted infertility problems. Because the mean time since first oocyte donation was 9.4 years, some of these changes may be unrelated to the oocyte donation [30].

The results of this study reinforce the need for increased attention to the health and safety of oocyte donors.

IVF clinics should provide anonymous oocyte donors clear guidelines about requesting outcome information or giving the clinic medical updates to benefit their biological children. Additional long-term studies are needed to ascertain oocyte donors' risks of infertility or cancer. The recommendations of the Ethics Committee of the ASRM are a significant step in the right direction; they need to be translated into clear guidelines that specify new policies in US fertility clinics.

It is worth pointing out that in 2009, the Ethics Committee of the ASRM published a report outlining the interests, obligations, and rights of gamete donors [32]. Such recommendations clearly assert that programs should respect the rights of donors to be informed about legal, medical, and emotional issues involved in gamete donation, that medical updates be provided by donors, and that information sharing about outcomes be facilitated.

It may serve oocyte donors better to have more stringent recommendations, both on a national level and from supranational health care institutions. There is clearly a need for national oocyte donor registries that include records of subsequent and prior fertility problems, and the number of cycles of oocyte retrieval undergone by the donor. This would permit prospective follow-up studies of fertility in oocyte donors after oocyte retrieval.

As for long-term risks for oocyte donors, only isolated case reports have suggested a possible cancer connection. A large cohort with long-term follow-up, such as an oocyte donor registry, as mentioned before, is necessary to obtain and compare meaningful data [42].

On the other hand, back in 2001, Caligara et al. already recommended the establishment of a world registry for oocyte donors to detect both adverse effects of oocyte donation and to provide a thorough assessment of long-term risks, such as an increased incidence of premature ovarian failure (POF), ovarian cancer, or breast cancer. To date, no such data have been published [43].

However, IVF and egg donation are relatively new procedures: these areas of medicine are still under-researched.

Charles L. Shapiro, director of translational breast cancer research for Mount Sinai Health System, said: "The bulk of the literature on this topic says there is no relationship between IVF, hormone priming or egg harvesting and increasing risk of breast cancer. It's usually not one factor that causes breast cancer, but a whole host of different circumstances, most of which we don't know about." Other researchers, however, seem to differ. Anthony Caruso, director of A Bella Baby OBGYN in Chicago and consultant to the Center for Bioethics and Culture network has pointed out that "High-estrogen states generated artificially for women are potentially putting them at a greater risk for estrogen-related cancers" [44]. Fauser and Velasco in a recent editorial published on Reproductive BioMedicine Online reminded that "… the absence of appropriate data, it is not possible to state with absolute certainty that volunteering as an oocyte donor will not increase breast cancer or other health risks. Indeed, the absence of proof is not the same as the proof of absence…" [45].

Such a dearth of available data is likely due to a certain degree of caution in the assessment of possible causal relationships between repeated oocyte donation cycles and the onset of neoplastic syndromes, yet at the same time, it makes it even more pressing to comply with the ASRM-recommended maximum limits in donation cycles, which is a key factor in preventing litigation based on the exceeding of such limits.

21.3.6 Psychological Risks and Psychological Damages in Donors

When a woman chooses to donate her eggs for use in the in vitro fertilization (IVF) process or scientific research, it is a very personal decision that might entail a variety of psychological implications. Lawson et al. have observed that here is a whole psychology about why a woman decides to do this and what she thinks and feels about being an oocyte donor [46]. And so, in addition to the potential physical risks, however rare they may be, the donation process potentially carries with it a number of psychological risks as well, which can be classified into three broad categories: the psychological aspects of the donor screening process, the psychological aspects of the procedure itself, and a post-donation psychological adjustment to the donation. Relatively few studies have explored the psychology of oocyte donation, and they have generally been small ones, with relatively few subjects. It is nonetheless possible to describe some basic findings about the psychological effects on women who donate their eggs.

Psychological risks to donors can occur in the screening, donation, and post-donation time frames, including psychological distress from being excluded from donating, psychological side effects from medications and retrieval, worry and regret, observed in a minority of donors.

As far as the issues associated with the egg retrieval surgery are concerned, one study of donors conducted by investigators at Dartmouth Medical School found that 83% reported high anxiety on the day of retrieval. Besides this anxiety, donors also listed the daily injections, the frequent travel to the clinic, and pain as the most difficult aspects of the donation process itself [47].

The good news about these potential psychological risks is that they do not appear to carry over past the donation. Once the surgery is done and the medication is out of a woman's system, the psychological symptoms typically appear to vanish.

It seems likely that the potential psychological risks both here and in the screening process will be the same for research donors as they are for women donating their eggs for reproductive purposes [48].

Long-term follow-up studies of donor health, including psychological health, are certainly needed. For the time being, however, there do not seem to be considerable risks of psychological damages directly linked to repeated oocyte donation cycles, hence, litigation arising on this basis is not highly relevant. It is plausible, on the other hand, that psychological distress may be cited in case of adverse outcomes, with psychological suffering stemming from physical damage.

The six-cycle limit recommended by the ASRM ought to be effective enough to minimize the risk of significant and long-lasting psychological fallout.

21.3.7 Pregnancy Expectation Unmet: Is It a Claim Source?

It is estimated that almost 15% of people with a diagnosis of infertility receive treatment at in vitro fertilization units (IVF). Even though there has been a progress in pregnancy rates over the last two decades, live birth rates have not yet reached the desired levels [49]. Among the various factors involved in the formation of pregnancy, there are the age of the woman, the selected treatment protocol, and the reasons of infertility. Even propofol-based anesthetic techniques have been called into question. In fact they have been found to result in significant concentrations of propofol in follicular fluid. Propofol has been shown to have potentially harmful effects on oocyte fertilization (in a mouse model), with some studies suggesting that the dose of propofol administered during anesthesia should be limited, and also that the retrieved oocytes should be cleansed of propofol [50].

Anecdotal reports suggest that certain airborne chemical contaminants and particles, especially volatile organic compounds (VOC), may be toxic to and impair the growth and development of embryos if present in sufficient concentrations in the ambient atmosphere of an IVF incubator [49, 51].

Today, a couple of endocrine biochemical markers and ultrasonographic signs are commonly used, which go a long way in predicting IVF outcomes and determining the gonadotropin doses to be used in ovarian stimulation (OS) [51, 52]. The methods most widely used, and the most reliable, are the ultrasonographic assessment of the primordial antral follicle pool in the early follicular phase and ovarian volume [53]. However, ovarian reserve tests are still inadequate in predicting live birth rates.

For those reasons an unsuccessful procedure, without damage sustained by the patient, would not be enough in and of itself to file a lawsuit and gain compensation in a court of law.

On the other hand, any failure from specialists to inform patients of the dangers entailed in IVF (from the mild manifestations to the severe ones), or their disregarding risk factors, which may result in unfavorable outcomes and damage to patients, would be bound to result in compensation awarded to damaged women under most tort law statutes, as it happened in the cases described above.

21.4 Claims in OPU Published

For illustrating purposes, court cases are reported below that are related to OPU procedures and came to verdict over the past years. A case of negligence and mismanagement led to a patient's death, and a $25 million indemnity payment [54]: a woman with infertility and antiphospholipid antibody syndrome (APA) was advised to have heparin and aspirin therapy in addition to in vitro fertilization. On the day of oocyte retrieval, 18 eggs were harvested. An ultrasound was performed immediately afterward, which showed a large amount of free fluid in the patient's pelvis.

About 3 h later, the patient underwent treatment for APA at another site, during which she became hypotensive. The nurse terminated the therapy and contacted the woman's physician, who arrived about 90 min later.

When he examined the patient, she was lethargic and hallucinating. At that time, her husband, an Ob/Gyn, was contacted. The decedent's husband arrived a short time later and transported the decedent to Holy Redeemer Hospital, which was located approximately 20 min away, later discovering a massive hemoperitoneum (Fig. 21.7).

The decedent's husband and a general surgeon performed surgery to remove blood and clotting from the decedent's abdomen. The decedent was listed in stable condition following the surgery. He transported her to the hospital where he worked and performed emergency surgery. The bleeding was controlled, and the patient was transferred to an ICU postoperatively.

Fig. 21.7 Injury of omental vessel during oocytes retrieval (**a**) and subsequent hemoperitoneum (**b**), in patient in treatment for antiphospholipid antibody syndrome.

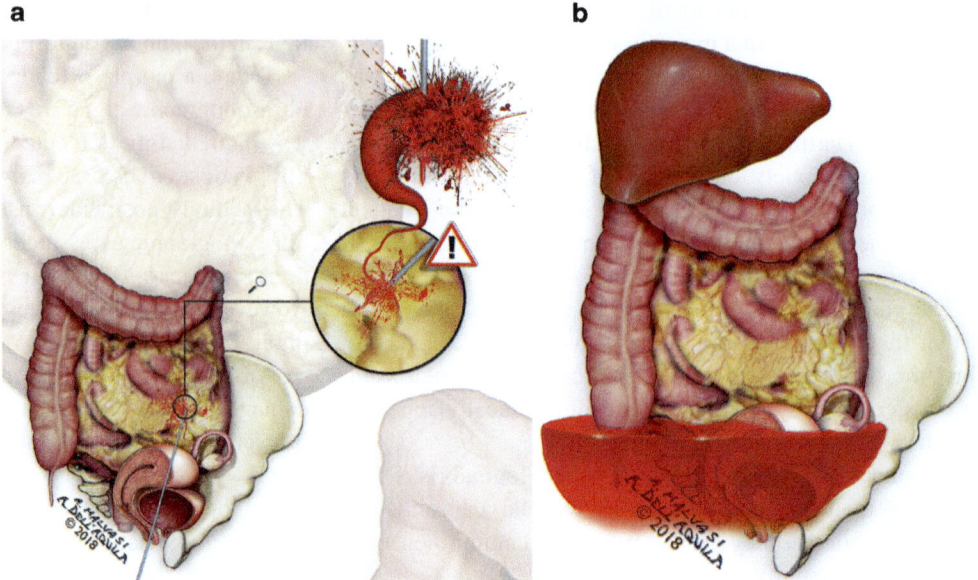

However, 2 days later she suffered a cardiac arrest; 9 days later, she died. The deceased patient's husband decided to sue on grounds of negligence.

In suing, the husband claimed the ultrasound had demonstrated a large amount of blood in his wife's abdomen. Further, he argued that his wife bled for 5 h while under the physician's care. The physician countered that he had not been made aware of the ultrasound findings [55].

The fertility specialists contended that the decedent's husband (third-party defendant) was negligent in transporting the decedent to Holy Redeemer Hospital, rather than allowing the defendants' office staff to call for the patient being taken to an emergency room immediately [56]. The defendants claimed that faster emergency room treatment would have enabled stabilization and faster surgery, if needed. The defendant fertility specialists also asserted that the third-party defendant failed to place the decedent in the intensive care unit following the surgery and failed to properly monitor her, including the taking of chest X-rays and blood gases to check for RDS.

Furthermore, they maintained that since the decedent and her husband were both physicians, they were aware of the risks involved in administering aspirin during egg retrieval, including the possibility of internal bleeding.

The defendant hospital and nurse settled the plaintiff's claim for $5 million prior to trial and the case proceeded against the two defendant fertility specialists and the decedent's husband as a third-party defendant. The jury found each defendant fertility specialist 50% negligent. It found the decedent's husband not negligent. The jury awarded the plaintiff $25 million in damages.

According to attorney Ellen Barton, JD, CPCU, a risk management consultant in Phoenix, MD: "Thus case also points out the need for communication between the referring and primary physicians as the physician patient went back

and forth between them for various treatments and procedures".

While this case is in large part about the practice of medicine, 'there is also a large component of administrative' breakdown. Not only did the defendant physicians not seem to share critical information regarding the patient's condition and subsequent tests, but the referring physician's failure to personally review the ultrasound, relying instead on a technician's oral opinion that 'everything appeared normal' falls below the standard of care. "Thus, the protocols regarding response time by physicians to nursing staff in an outpatient setting should be reviewed so that a patient's condition is not compromised by a lack of or tardy response, as it seems to have been the case here" [57].

A 2014 case of ovarian hyperstimulation syndrome (OHSS) in India, where a 23-year-old died after undergoing an egg-retrieval procedure, sparked protests, and calls for new legislation to protect egg donors in the country.

An initial postmortem report of the 23-year-old Yuma Sherpa, who died after an egg donation procedure at an IVF clinic in Lajpat Nagar on January 29, 2014, has said she sustained internal bleeding in her pelvic region and her ovaries were "hypertrophied." The report has been submitted to the police by AIIMS, and the viscera has been sent for more tests to establish the cause of death.

According to sources, the postmortem has found hematoma or clotting of blood in the peritoneum (stomach cavity), around the uterus and ovaries, indicating internal bleeding. The report has also found her ovaries were "severely hypertrophied" or enlarged. "The ovaries were enlarged due to hormones injected to trigger the ovaries to produce more than the usual number of eggs, since she had undergone a procedure to donate her eggs. We are trying to understand the quantity of hormones that were injected, through viscera tests and chemical and physical examination of the ovary cells to analyse the number of follicles that were formed in the ovary," a source said.

Sources said Sherpa was given general anesthesia in the procedure, and the ovary was probed by a catheter to retrieve the eggs under suction puncture, which has caused internal bleeding. Sources said even the possibility of a reaction from anesthesia had not yet been ruled out. "The procedure was performed under general anaesthesia, many patients have adverse reactions to anaesthesia. Tests on visceral samples will help us establish that," a source said.

Sources confirmed no blood vessels around the ovaries were found to be torn or ruptured in the procedure. Sherpa, the mother of a 3-year-old, had gone to New Life India Fertility Clinic for her first egg donation. She collapsed after the retrieval procedure. When she did not respond to resuscitation efforts, she was taken from the clinic to a hospital in Green Park where she was declared dead on arrival.

When contacted for comments, the medical director of the New Life India Fertility Clinic denied any irregularities. "We are awaiting the post-mortem report. The patient's full consent was taken, she was screened as per procedure and we also conducted all necessary pre-anaesthetic tests. All records have been handed over to police. She lost consciousness suddenly in the recovery room," she said. She added that when the treating team realized that Sherpa was not responding, an ambulance was arranged to have her transported to a Green Park hospital, where the anesthetist from New Life clinic was a consultant. "They also failed to resuscitate her. It appears she had a sudden cardiac arrest. We are also awaiting the post-mortem report to find out what went wrong," the medical director added.

Sherpa's husband had made a PCR call from the Green Park hospital after she was declared dead, on the basis of which a complaint was filed by the police.

A medical board was constituted at All India Institute of Medical Sciences (AIIMS) under the chairmanship of a professor of forensic medicine to conduct the postmortem. "The preliminary report has stated certain physical findings in the body. We are waiting for the viscera report to establish the final cause of death. We will initiate investigations after we get the viscera report," a police officer said.

In oocyte donation procedures, hormones known as gonadotropins are administered to the donor during her menstrual cycle to boost ovaries to produce a number of eggs, against the normal production of one follicle that matures into an egg every month. Doctors say in rare cases this can lead to a condition of ovarian hyperstimulation syndrome (OHSS), which leads to a cascade of reactions when the ovary is stimulated very strongly to produce an excess of eggs.

"While mild to moderate OHSS can happen in 8–10 percent cases, severe OHSS cases are very rare, and between 1–3 percent. I think at AIIMS our incidence will be less than

1 percent," an IVF specialist from AIIMS said. The dosage of the hormones is determined by doctors on the basis of the patient's BMI, ovarian reserve, and hormone levels. Doctors said OHSS can also be prevented by screening tests for donors, like identifying levels of some hormones like AMH and checking the ovarian reserve of the patient. "If the patient has high Anti-Müllerian Hormone (AMH) levels, or very high ovarian reserves, or number of eggs, she should ideally not be used as a donor, because such women have a tendency to go into OHSS with stimulation," the AIIMS doctor explained.

Sudha Sundararaman, national vice president of AIDWA (All India Democratic Women's Association), said the case highlights vulnerability of poverty-stricken women persuaded to donate without counseling, monitoring, or assessment of their suitability. "The ministry of health and family welfare must immediately draft a law to regulate this profit-making industry," she said [58].

21.5 Prospects of Stricter Rules

In many developing countries, the lack of regulation and extreme poverty has resulted in a substantial increase in the number of fertility clinics and brokers that cater to foreigners searching for IVF treatments. What could be defined as a "global market for human eggs" has grown exponentially as in vitro fertilization and stem cell technologies have become more widely available, creating a "global shortage of human oocytes."

The expansion of the global marketplace has created increased opportunities to exploit women, while exerting pressure on the market for eggs within the United States and other developed countries.

A comprehensive legislative package is needed in each state that addresses eggs used for research and those used for IVF purposes, closing the major gaps and filling the voids that unethical actors exploit to their financial benefit.

A better alternative would be for each state to allow reasonable compensation for donors of eggs for either purpose, while mandating informed consent and full disclosure of known risks from the surgical procedure and the drug protocols used. States could specify acceptable ranges of compensation and enforce compliance through a statutory mechanism [59].

Additionally, if national registries were created for IVF donors, like those already being used to monitor embryos used for stem cell research, this would facilitate surveillance efforts by requiring providers and clinics to track the disposition of each oocyte utilized and keep donors' medical records, thus aiding researchers who have been trying to identify possible long-term side effects [60, 61].

Currently, no records are kept in the United States of how many times donors donate their eggs.

There is little information or research on the role played by fertility clinics, which appears to be growing; egg-donation agencies, and private brokers profoundly shape the market for human eggs within the United States.

Often, clinics do not keep donors' medical records, making it hard for donors to seek recourse if they experience complications and making it impossible for researchers to effectively monitor donors for long-term side effects such as infertility and higher risk of cancer.

Finally, states should enact legislation prohibiting predatory advertising and mandating compliance with ASRM-recommended guidelines [62]. Enacting such legislation would give donors a remedy that the courts could enforce, while also protecting young donors who may not realize the risk of cancer and other long-term effects are much higher with repetitive donations. In absence of a national consensus on how to address this issue, unethical entities and providers, looking to make a profit, will continue to take advantage of existing gaps in legislation to exploit women. The "bad actors" that are present in any such ill-defined or poorly regulated setting have been taking advantage of the lack of regulation, as well as making a lucrative business of performing risky procedures on women who are unaware of the long-term dangers to their health and fertility. States must take action to address eggs used for research and IVF purposes [63].

Only a wide-ranging legislative solution has any hope of tackling abuses while providing damaged patients with a tenable legal recourse.

References

1. ESHRE Guideline Group on good practice in IVF labs. Revised guidelines for good practice in IVF laboratories (2015) Guideline of the European Society of Human Reproduction and Embryology. December 2015.
2. Cassazione civile, Sezione III, 30 giugno2015, n. 13328. http://dirittocivilecontemporaneo.com/wp-content/uploads/2015/10/n.-13328-del-30-giugno-2015.pdf.
3. Grubb A, Laing J, McHale J. Principles of medical law. New York: Oxford University Press; 2010.
4. Montanari Vergallo G, Busardò FP, Zaami S, Marinelli E. The static evolution of the new Italian code of medical ethics. Eur Rev Med Pharmacol Sci. 2016;20(3):575–80.
5. Law n. 24/2017 "Disposizioni in materia disicurezza delle cure e della persona assistita nonché in materia di responsabilità professionale degli esercenti le professioni sanitarie".
6. Tucker C. Ethical and legal issues arising from the informed consent process in fertility treatments. ABA Health Law Section. Vol. 9, No. 7; March 2013.
7. Cassazione civile, Sezione III, 20 maggio 2016, n. 10414. http://www.altalex.com/documents/news/2016/06/07/intervento-necessario-consenso-informato.
8. Dicker D, Ashkenazi J, Feldberg D, Levy T, Dekel A, Ben Rafael Z. Severe abdominal complications after transvaginal ultrasonographically guided retrieval of oocytes for in vitro fertilization and embryo transfer. Fertil Steril. 1993;59(6):1313–5.
9. Vahratian A. Prevalence of overweight and obesity among women of childbearing age: results from the 2002 National Survey of Family Growth. Matern Child Health J. 2009;13:268–73.
10. Gesink Law DC, Maclehose RF, Longnecker MP. Obesity and time to pregnancy. Hum Reprod. 2007;22:414–20.
11. Mitchell M, Bakos HW, Lane M. Paternal diet-induced obesity impairs embryo development and implantation in the mouse. Fertil Steril. 2011;95(4):1349–53.
12. Tamer Erel C, Senturk LM. The impact of body mass index on assisted reproduction. Curr Opin Obstet Gynecol. 2009;21(3):228–35.
13. Marquard KL, Stephens SM, Jungheim ES, Ratts VS, Odem RR, Lanzendorf S, Moley KH. Polycystic ovary syndrome and maternal obesity affect oocyte size in in vitro vaginal oocyte retrieval. Gynecol Obstet Investig. 2009;67(1):32–5.
14. Robkeor RL. Evidence that obesity alters the quality of oocytes and embryos. Pathophysiology. 2008;15(2):115–21.
15. Jungheim ES, Moley KH. Current knowledge of obesity's effects in the pre- and periconceptional periods and avenues for future research. Am J Obstet Gynecol. 2010;203(6):525–30.
16. Brewer CJ, Balen AH. The adverse effects of obesity on conception and implantation. Reproduction. 2010;140(3):347–64.
17. Purcell SH, Moley KH. The impact of obesity on egg quality. J Assist Reprod Genet. 2011;28(6):517–24.
18. Özaltın S, Kumbasar S, Sa-van K. Evaluation of complications developing during and after transvaginal ultrasound—guided oocyte retrieval. Ginekol Pol. 2018;89(1):1–6.
19. Ayestaran C, Matorras R, Gomez S, Arce D, Rodriguez-Escudero F. Severe bradycardia and bradypnea following vaginal oocyte retrieval: a possible toxic effect of paracervical mepivacaine. Eur J Obstet Gynecol Reprod Biol. 2000;91(1):71–3.
20. Andersen AN, Gianaroli L, Felberbaum R, de Mouzon J, Nygren KG; European IVF-monitoring programme (EIM), European Society of Human Reproduction and Embryology (ESHRE). European IVFmonitoring programme (EIM). Assisted reproductive technology in Europe, 2001. Results generated from European registers by ESHRE. Hum Reprod. 2005;20(5):1158–76.
21. Oyawoye OA, Chander B, Hunter J, Gadir AA. Prevention of ovarian hyperstimulation syndrome by early aspiration of small follicles in hyper-responsive patients with polycystic ovaries during assisted reproductive treatment cycles. Medscape Gen Med. 2005;7(3):60.
22. Ayestaran C, Matorras R, Gomez S, Arce D, Rodriguez-Escudero F. Severe bradycardia and bradypnea following vaginal oocyte retrieval: a possible toxic effect of paracervical mepivacaine. Eur J Obstet Gynecol Reprod Biol. 2000;91(1):71–3.
23. Zaami S, Montanari Vergallo G, Napoletano S, Signore F, Marinelli E. The issue of delivery room infections in the Italian law. A brief comparative study with English and French jurisprudence. J Matern Fetal Neonatal Med. 2017;31(2):1–8.
24. Ragni G, Scarduelli C, Calanna G, Santi G, Benaglia L, Somigliana E. Blood loss during transvaginal oocyte retrieval. Gynecol Obstet Investig. 2009;67(1):32–5.
25. Aragona C, Mohamed MA, Espinola MS, Linari A, Pecorini F, Micara G, Sbracia M. Clinical complications after transvaginal oocyte retrieval in 7,098 IVF cycles. Fertil Steril. 2011;95(1):293–4.
26. Liberty G, Hyman JH, Eldar-Geva T, Latinsky B, Gal M, Margalioth EJ. Ovarian hemorrhage after transvaginal ultrasonographically guided oocyte aspiration: a potentially catastrophic and not so rare complication among lean patients with polycystic ovary syndrome. Fertil Steril. 2008;93(3):874–9.
27. Zaami S, Malvasi A, Marinelli E. Fundal pressure: risk factors in uterine rupture. The issue of liability: complication or malpractice? J Perinat Med. 2018;46(5):567–8.
28. Malvasi A, Montanari Vergallo G, Tinelli A, Marinelli E. Can the intrapartum ultrasonography reduce the legal liability in

dystocic labor and delivery? J Matern Fetal Neonatal Med. 2018;31(8):1108–9.

29. Jayaprakasan K, Herbert M, Moody E, Stewart JA, Murdoch AP. Estimating the risks of ovarian hyperstimulation syndrome (OHSS): implications for egg donation for research. Hum Fertil. 2007;10:183–7.

30. Kramer W, Schneider J, Schultz N. US oocyte donors: a retrospective study of medical and psychosocial issues. Hum Reprod. 2009;24(12):3144–9.

31. American Society for Reproductive Medicine Practice Committee. Repetitive oocyte donation. Fertil Steril. 2008;90(5 Suppl):S194–5.

32. Practice Committee of the American Society for Reproductive Medicine and Practice Committee of the Society for Assisted Reproductive Technology. Repetitive oocyte donation: a committee opinion. Fertil Steril. 2014;102(4):964–6.

33. Bodri D, Guillén JJ, Polo A, Trullenque M, Esteve C, Coll O. Complications related to ovarian stimulation and oocyte retrieval in 4052 oocyte donor cycles. Reprod Biomed Online. 2008;17(2):237–43.

34. Shmorgun D, Claman P, Gysler M, Hemmings R, Cheung AP, Goodrow GJ, Hughes EG, Min JK, Roberts J, Senikas V, Chee-Man Wong B, Young D. The diagnosis and management of ovarian hyperstimulation syndrome. J Obstet Gynaecol Can. 2011;33(11):1156–62.

35. Mozes M, Bogokowsky H, Antebi E, Lunenfeld B, Rabau E, Serr DM, David A, Salomy M. Thromboembolic phenomena after ovarian stimulation with human gonadotrophins. Lancet. 1965;2(7424):1213–5.

36. Cluroe AD, Synek BJ. A fatal case of ovarian hyperstimulation syndrome with cerebral infarction. Pathology. 1995;27(4):344–6.

37. Tang OS, Ng EH, Wai Cheng P, Chung HP. Cortical vein thrombosis misinterpreted as intracranial haemorrhage in severe ovarian hyperstimulation syndrome: case report. Hum Reprod. 2000;15(9):1913–6.

38. Semba S, Moriya T, Youssef EM, Sasano H. An autopsy case of ovarian hyperstimulation syndrome with massive pulmonary edema and pleural effusion. Pathol Int. 2000;50(7):549–52.

39. Kim H-S, Kim M, Seo I-S, Kwon TJ, Ha H, Lee B-w. An autopsy case of severe ovarian hyperstimulation syndrome with multifocal arterial and venous thromboembolism. Korean J Legal Med. 2011;35(1):57–61.

40. Zaami S. Assisted heterologous fertilization and the right of donor conceived children to know their biological origins. Clin Ter. 2018;169(1):39–43.

41. Montanari Vergallo GM, Zaami S, Bruti V, Signore F, Marinelli E. How the legislation in medical assisted procreation has evolved in Italy. Med Law. 2017;36(2):5–28.

42. Montanari VG, Marinelli E, di Luca NM, Zaami S. Gamete donation: are children entitled to know their genetic origins? A comparison of opposing views. The Italian State of Affairs. Eur J Health Law. 2018;25(3):322–37.

43. Ridley J. Being an egg donor gave me terminal cancer. The New York Post. 3 Dec 2015.

44. Fauser BC, Garcia VJ. Breast cancer risk after oocyte donation: should we really be concerned? Reprod Biomed Online. 2017;34(5):439–40.

45. Lawson AK, Klock SC, Pavone ME, Hirshfeld-Cytron J, Smith KN, Kazer RR. A prospective study of depression and anxiety in female fertility preservation and infertility patients. Fertil Steril. 2014;102(5):1377–84.

46. Reindollar RH, Regan MM, Neumann PJ, Levine BS, Thornton KL, Alper MM, Goldman MB. A randomized clinical trial to evaluate optimal treatment for unexplained infertility: the fast track and standard treatment (FASTT) trial. Fertil Steril. 2010;94(3):888–99.

47. Zweifel JE, Rathert MA, Klock SC, Walaski HP, Pritts EA, Olive DL, Lindheim SR. Comparative assessment of pre- and post-donation attitudes towards potential oocyte and embryo disposition and management among ovum donors in an oocyte donation programme. Hum Reprod. 2006;21(5):1325–7.

48. Gonca S, Gün I, Ovayolu A, Şilfeler D, Sofuoğlu K, Özdamar Ö, Yilmaz A, Tunali G. Effect of lower than expected number of oocyte on the IVF results after oocyte-pickup. Int J Clin Exp Med. 2014;7(7):1853–9.

49. Christiaens F, Janssenswillen C, Verborgh C, Moerman I, Devroey P, Van Steirteghem A, Camu F. Propofol concentrations in follicular fluid during general anaesthesia for transvaginal oocyte retrieval. Hum Reprod. 1999;14(2):345–8.

50. Cohen J, Gilligan A, Esposito W, Schimmel T, Dale B. Ambient air and its potential effects on conception in vitro. Hum Reprod. 1997;12(8):1742–9.

51. Cohen J, Gilligan A, Willadsen S. Culture and quality control of embryos. Hum Reprod. 1998;13(Suppl 3):137–44.

52. Cohen J, Jones HW. In vitro fertilization: the first three decades. In: Gardner DK, editor. In vitro fertilization: a practical approach. 1st ed. New York: Informa Healthcare USA Inc.; 2009. p. 1–13.

53. van Loendersloot LL, van Wely M, Limpens J, Bossuyt PM, Repping S, van der Veen F. Predictive factors in in vitro fertilization (IVF): a systematic review and meta-analysis. Hum Reprod Update. 2010;16(6):577–89.

54. Shaban MM, Abdel Moety GA. Role of ultrasonographic markers of ovarian reserve in prediction of IVF and ICSI outcome. Gynecol Endocrinol. 2014;30(4):290–3.

55. Zaami S, Marinelli E, Montanari Vergallo G. Assessing malpractice lawsuits for death or injuries due to amniotic fluid embolism. Clin Ter. 2017;168(3):220–4.

56. Frati P, Foldes-Papp Z, Zaami S, Busardò FP. Amniotic fluid embolism: what level of scientific evidence can be drawn? a systematic review. Curr Pharm Biotechnol. 2013;14(14):1157–62.

57. Laska LL. Medical malpractice verdicts, settlements & experts. April 2002. Philadelphia (Pa) Court Of Common Pleas. OBG Manag. 2002;14(4):86–8.

58. Gorrie JJ. Legal Review and Commentary: OB/GYN patient dies after egg harvest: $30 million verdict and settlements. July 1st 2001. Reference: Tony Matteo, MD, as Adm. of the Estate of Suzanne Wester Matteo, MD v. Jerome Check, MD, and Admed Nazari, MD v. Tony Matteo, MD, Holy Redeemer Hospital and Nurse Newhall, Philadelphia Court of Common Pleas. Case settled. Thomas Kline, Esq., of Philadelphia, for the plaintiff.

59. Egg donor's death: internal bleeding, ovaries severely enlarged, says report. The Indian Report. July 4th 2014.

60. Zaami S, Busardò FP. Elective egg freezing: can you really turn back the clock? Eur Rev Med Pharmacol Sci. 2015;19(19):3537–8.

61. Vergallo GM. Negligence and embryo protection: a new frontier for medical law? Med Law. 2014;33(1):2–13.

62. Levine AD. Self-regulation, compensation, and the ethical recruitment of oocyte donors. Hastings Cent Rep. 2010;40(2):25–36.

63. Cone KL. Family law—egg donation and stem cell research—eggs for sale: the scrambled state of legislation in the human egg market. U Ark Little Rock L Rev. 2012;35:189.

Medically Assisted Procreation: European Legislation and Ensuing Ethical Issues

Gianluca Montanari Vergallo, Simona Zaami, and Radmila Sparic

Contents

The history of artificial fertilization shows that such techniques was originally meant as therapy for infertility in heterosexual couples because the element of biological lineage is no longer the foundational value on which to base procreation. Medically assisted procreation is by now a deeply rooted phenomenon in modern society, and appears to be constantly growing [1].

Artificial procreation, unrelated to sexuality, has profoundly transformed childbearing as a concept in and of itself, and lays the groundwork for the revamping of the very notion of parenthood. Artificial fertilization falls places itself in the setting of the so-called "reproductive revolution" and is characterized by three fundamental traits: the disconnection of procreation from the sexual act, the ability to take steps in order to alter the genetic profile of the newborn and lastly, the ensuing assertion of new figures in the reproductive process (male and female gamete donors, surrogate mothers) [2] (Fig. 22.1).

The newborn is no longer conceived in his or her mother's womb, and the "parents" involved may turn out to be more than two, and not necessarily a mother and a father playing their respective traditional roles. The mother is no longer a

The original version of this chapter was revised. The author, Tom Schneider was removed from the original version. The correction to this chapter can be found at https://doi.org/10.1007/978-3-030-28741-2_23

G. Montanari Vergallo (✉) · S. Zaami
Department of Anatomical, Histological, Forensic and Orthopaedic Sciences, Sapienza University of Rome, Rome, Italy
e-mail: simona.zaami@uniroma1.it

R. Sparic
Clinic for Gynecology and Obstetrics, Clinical Center of Serbia, Belgrade, Serbia
e-mail: radmila@rcub.bg.ac.rs

Fig. 22.1 The artificial fertilization made a "reproductive revolution" with ethical and controversial aspect between restricted (up) and enlarged (down) ethical criteria relationship to culture of different countries

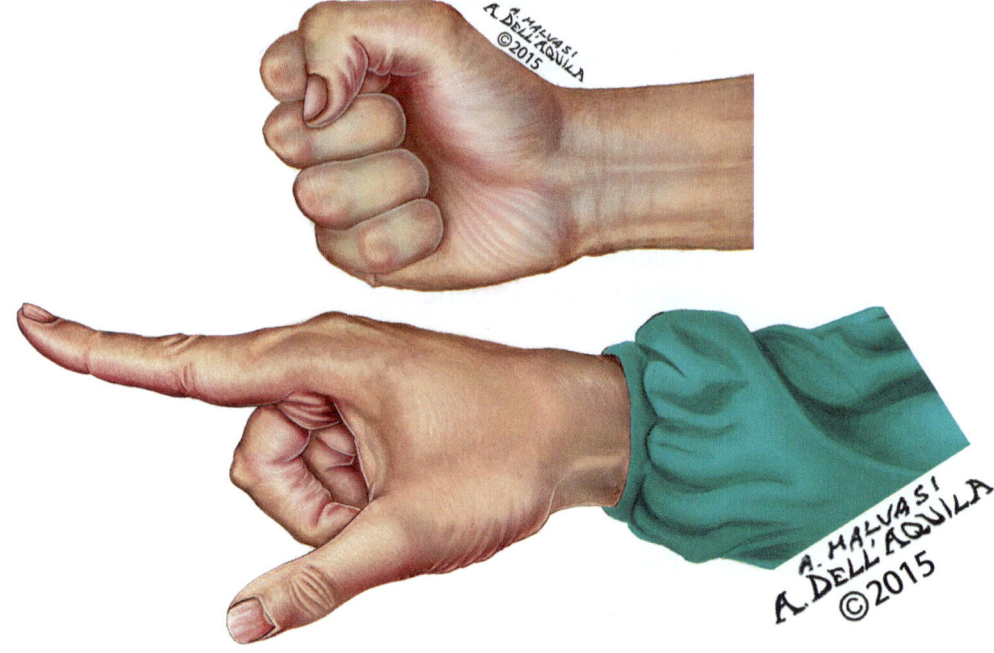

Fig. 22.2 Intrauterine donor sperm insemination

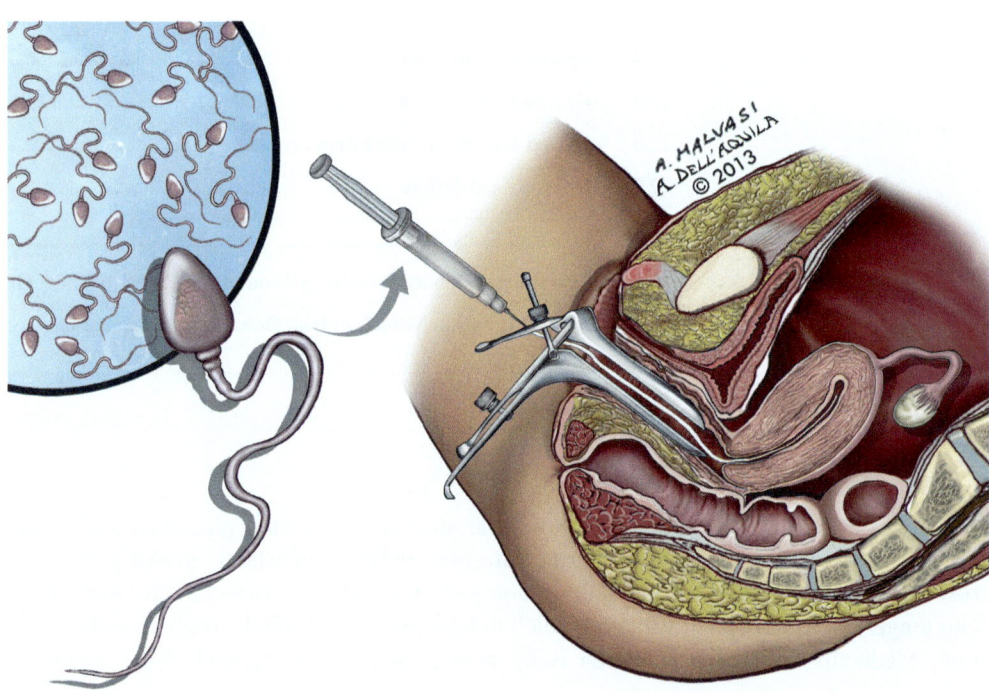

unique entity for each newborn child, rather a genetic mother (who provided the oocyte that was fertilized), a biological one (who carries out gestation and bears the child), and a social one (the person who set in motion the procreative process, without being involved in it from either a genetic or biological standpoint, and will be vested with social parenthood responsibility). The fatherly figure itself is dichotomized into two distinct profiles: a social father and a biological one (i.e., the sperm donor) [3] (Fig. 22.2).

Surrogate motherhood falls within the wider context of medically assisted procreation, although it does not constitute a specific technique in and of itself: the use of multiple procreative procedures represents the "means" by which the various forms of surrogacy are implemented [4].

Surrogacy has grown to become a somewhat widespread practice, and is currently the only choice for women who suffer from sterility, or are otherwise ill, or no longer fertile on account of age, and male homosexual couples who are determined to have children of their own, with a genetic bond to at least either member of the couple. Various kinds of surrogacy are currently in use. By traditional surrogacy, the practice is defined in which the fertilized oocyte belongs to the surrogate mother who bears the child, whereas the sperm is provided by the male in the couple who requested the procedure. In other instances, the surrogate mother is implanted an oocyte that was fertilized by donor sperm (traditional surrogacy and donor sperm); or both gametes may belong to the couple and, after in vitro fertilization, the oocyte is implanted into the surrogate mother's uterus (so-called gestational surrogacy); otherwise, in vitro fertilization may take place between the mother-to-be's oocyte and donor sperm, prior to implantation, (defined as gestational surrogacy and donor sperm); in a different scenario, neither the prospective legal parents nor the surrogate mother may have any genetic tie with the newborn, and an in vitro fertilization procedure is carried out relying on oocyte and sperm both coming from donors (characterized as gestational surrogacy and donor embryo) [5].

No matter how controversial and opposed to it may be, due to its questioning the society's founding principles more than any other procreative process, surrogacy is rather widespread worldwide, and the nations that have legalized it, among which Georgia, Greece, the United Kingdom, Russia, and Ukraine, have drawn women who could not otherwise have a pregnancy, due to sterility or age-related issues [6, 7]. There are then two different ways of approaching reproductive technologies: on the one hand, as a greater power of choice for couples in terms of timing and methods of procreation, on the other hand, as a therapy for sterility.

22.1 European Legislative Framework

In such a complex landscape, with the affirmation of new reproductive rights arising from the development of new assisted reproduction technologies, it is incumbent upon national lawmakers to set up a regulatory framework to outline their scope and define their exact functions. In accordance with the decisions made nationally, parliaments will enact laws and carry out policies that may reflect a permissive, restrictive, or intermediate approach, designed to reconcile all needs and aspirations (Fig. 22.3).

In Europe, medically assisted procreation is regulated ranging from permissive standards (mirrored by regulations in Spain and Britain) and relatively stricter ones (such as those in place in Germany and France). Some countries have no targeted legislation in place, and medically assisted procreation is regulated through general health laws; others still have no legislation at all, but rather rely on "guidelines" that fail to encompass such a crucial aspect of health care from the social, ethical, and legal perspectives [8].

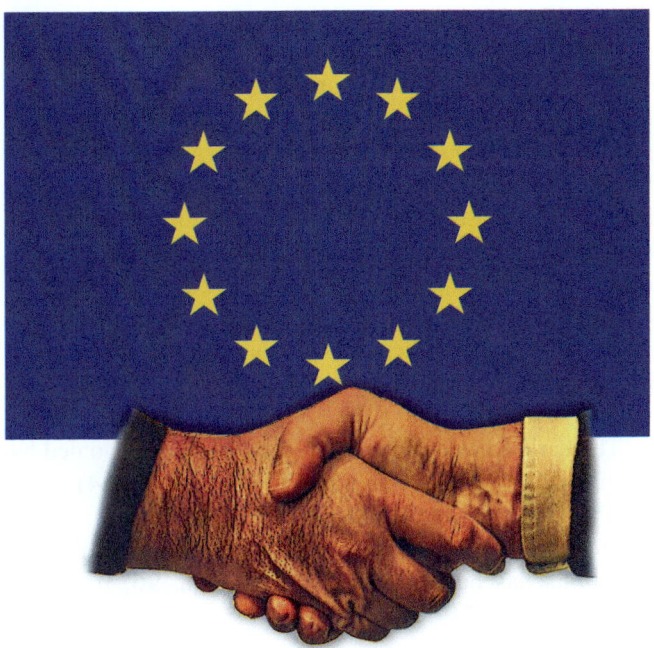

Fig. 22.3 The absence of an European unitary law determines the presence of multiple country legislations

It is worth outlining the fundamental standards governing such a crucial area of medicine in some European Union member states.

22.2 Italian Legislation

In Italy law n. 40, passed on 19th February 2004, containing "norms regulating medically-assisted procreation" allows heterosexual couples, either married or unmarried, with sterility or infertility issues, to avail themselves of medically assisted procreation procedures. Resorting to such techniques is only legal once it has been proved that the issues leading to the couple's inability to have a pregnancy cannot be solved otherwise. Sterility and/or infertility must be medically documented. In its previous form, the law banned heterologous fertilization (in article 4) and embryo research (article 13). Provisions only allowed clinical research and trials for the purpose of preserving the health and development of the embryos used. It banned the following practices:

1. Eugenic selection of embryos and gametes
2. Cloning via nuclear transfer
3. Fertilization of a human gamete with one from different species, i.e., the attempted creation of human–animal hybrids and chimeras

Twelve years after the law's enactment, several court rulings on the merits, at both a national and European level, have voided some of its restrictive provisions: the ban on cryopreservation of embryos, along with the limit of three embryos for each implantation, has been amended by ruling n. 151, from 8th May 2009; according to the court, gynecologists should execute the fertilization of a greater number of embryo than strictly necessary for implantation, based on the most updated and accredited technical and scientific standards. In such a way, a greater amount of zygotes can be used, thus giving hope to those couples who have lower-quality embryos. The embryos produced but not implanted out of medical choice must be stored via cryopreservation [9, 10].

- The ban on heterologous fertilization has been voided by ruling n. 162, from 10th June 2015 [11] (Fig. 22.4).
- The prohibition to access assisted procreation techniques for fertile couples carrying severe genetic conditions has been repealed by ruling n. 96, from 5th June 2016 [12].

The above cited rulings confirm that embryo protection is essential, and it should not be achieved through bans and restrictions, but rather with the harmonization of women's health as they undergo the treatments.

22.3 French Legislation

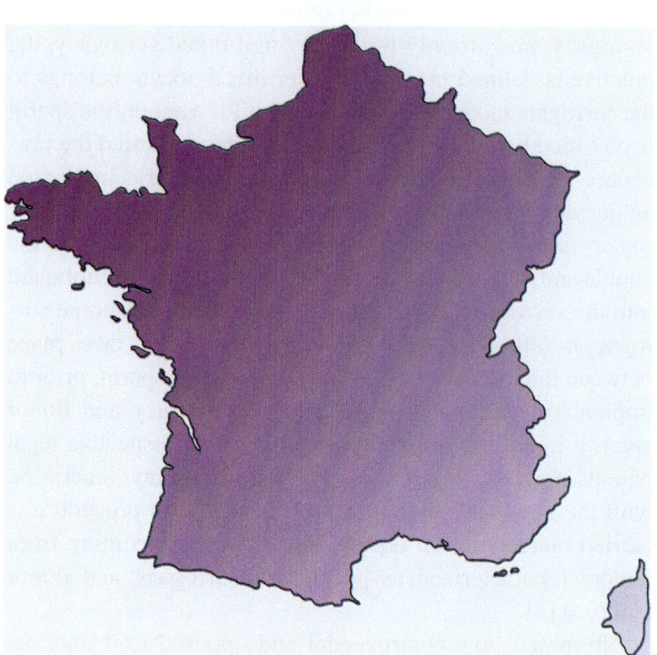

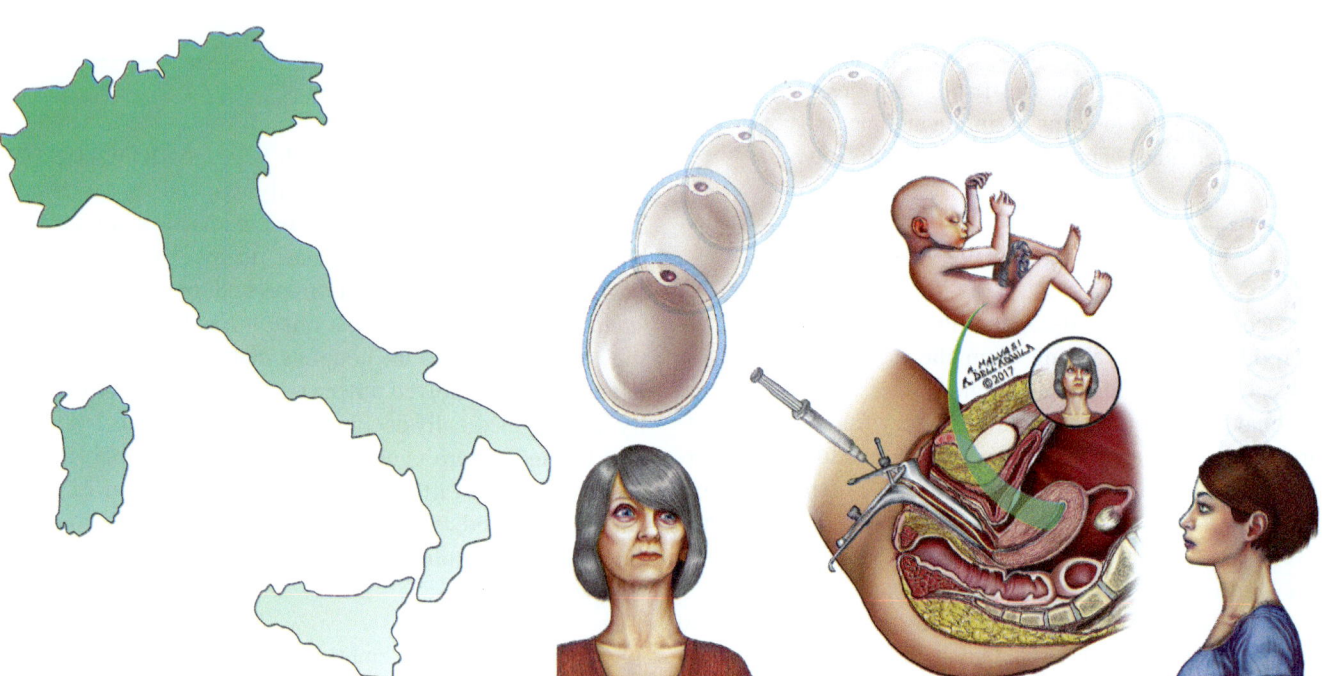

Fig. 22.4 The ban on heterologous fertilization has been voided by ruling n. 162, from 10th June 2015

France has opted for a therapeutic approach to assisted procreation, as a means to solve sterility and infertility cases or avert the risk of passing on hereditary diseases. Access to medically assisted procreation is legal for heterosexual married couples, or those who entered into a civil union, thus barring singles and same-sex couples. Donation is regulated by the public health care code, which mandates that consent be granted by both donors and receivers. Article L. 1244-2, subsection 1 of the same code makes consent from sperm and oocyte donors mandatory, as is that from the couple's other member. Consent, privately drafted and signed (registered by a notary or a civil court, the so-called Tribunal de grande instance) may be withdrawn at any time prior to treatment. France has thus adopted an intermediate approach, half way between a liberal and conservative one, in that it allows access to medically assisted procreation, while banning preimplantation diagnosis, in order to treat pathological infertility or avert the transmission to children of hereditary severe conditions carried by parents. Particularly, article 311-19 c.c., in keeping with the principle of donor anonymity as an element of donation gratuity, asserts that "no parental ties shall be established between donors and children born from medically assisted procreation" and that consent granted by sterile or infertile couples entails the ban on any action aimed at questioning parenthood, whether legal or biological. Embryo and gamete donation is legal [13–15].

22.4   Spanish Legislation

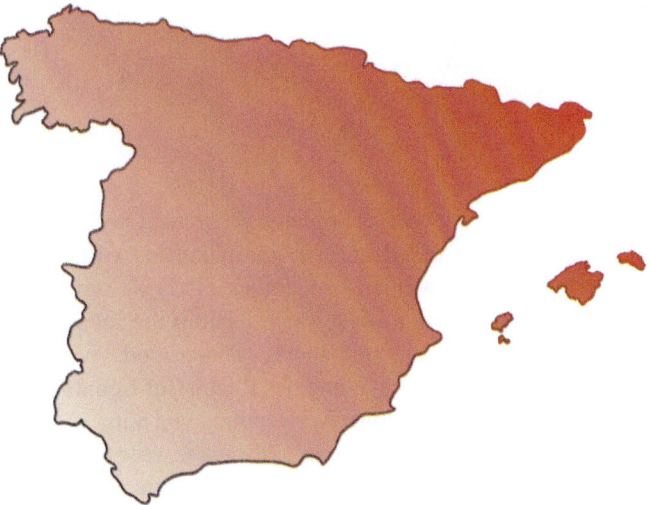

In Spain, a rather permissive set of regulations is in place (Fig. 22.5). Sterility or infertility do not constitute requirements for accessing heterologous fertilization, which is deemed to be simply an alternative procreation technique, in additional to the natural methods. Law n. 35 of 1988 had already legalized all assisted procreation techniques, including heterologous fertilization. All women, whether married,

in civil unions or singles were allowed to resort to the procedures. Such a legislative framework has been kept standing by the new law n. 14/2006 and its subsequent versions. The law makes it possible for public health care to intervene in cases of sterility or other "specific clinical conditions." That is the reason why several regions have included single women, or lesbian couples, even not sterile ones, who cannot have a pregnancy on account of "specific conditions," as stated by the law. In 2013, the Health Care Ministry has enforced further criteria to be met: women should not be over 40 (or over 38, in case of artificial fertilization) and men should not be over 50 [16, 17].

The law allows free, consensual, and anonymous donation. In fact, one of the law's guiding principles is the ban on any form of trade and commercialization of human body parts and cells, along with donor anonymity and guaranteed privacy in terms of personal data and door identity [18].

22.5   German Legislation

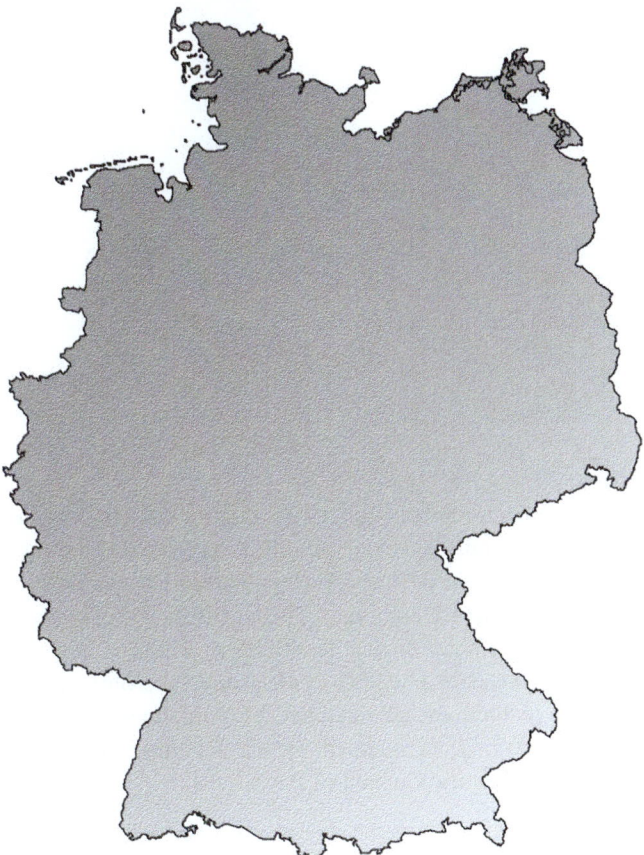

Germany's established policies on the issue appear to be remarkably restrictive (Fig. 22.6). Although there is specific piece of legislation regulating medically assisted procreation in German codes, there has been a law designed for the preservation of embryos (Embryonenschutzgesetz—ESchG for

Fig. 22.5 In Spain, a rather permissive set of regulations is in place

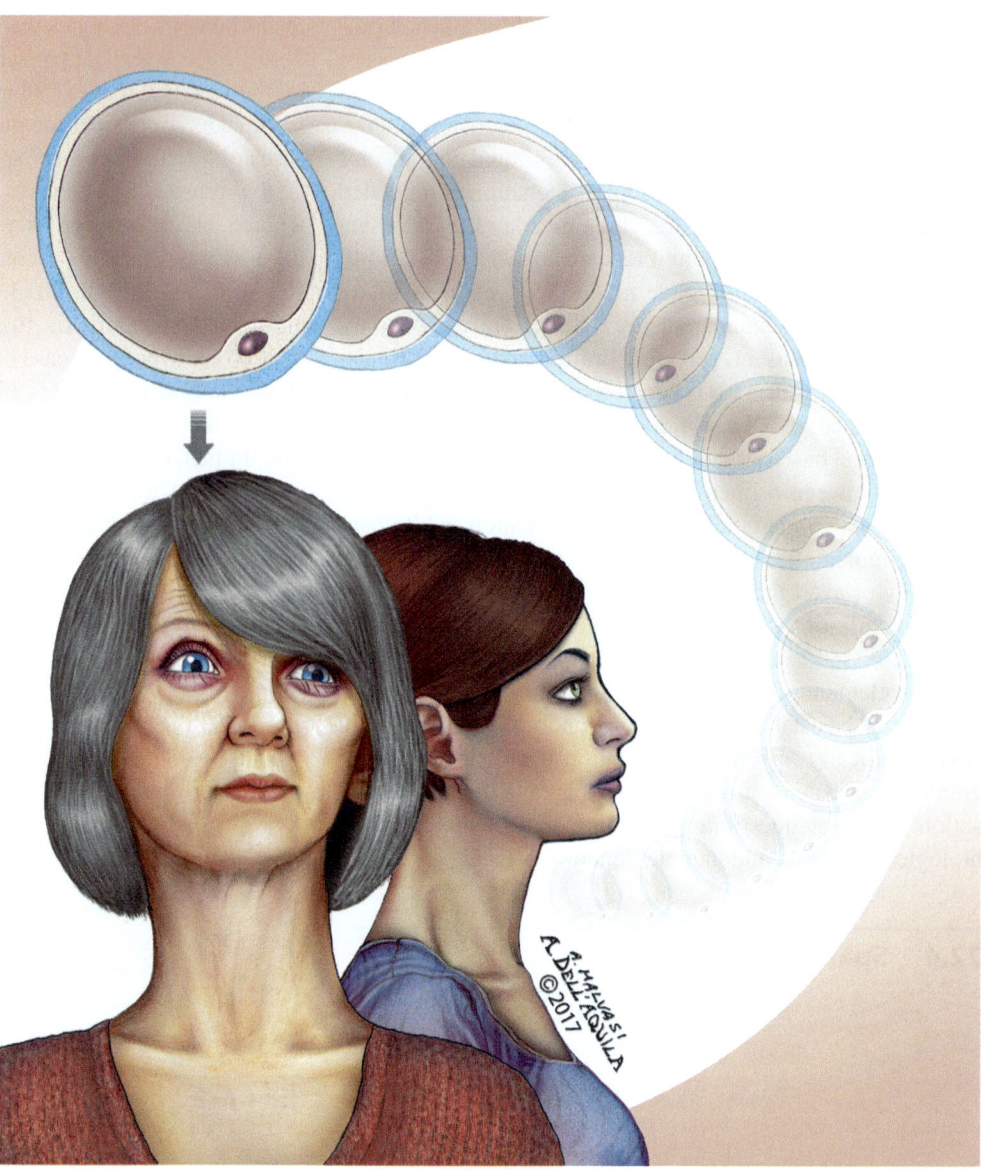

short) since December 13th 1990. Such a law, in keeping with the constitutional principle of life protection, is aimed at averting embryo destruction (it is therefore illegal to produce supernumerary embryos). The legislation does not specifically target heterologous fertilization, which is however banned by the same law [19]. In Germany, heterologous fertilization techniques are regulated by guidelines issued on 17th February 2006, outlined by the scientific committee within the Scientific Council of Physicians.

The EschG bans and criminally prosecutes both oocyte donation (i.e., the fertilization of an ovum that will not be implanted into the woman to whom it belongs) and surrogacy, since the newborn's best interest entails the consistency of genetic, biological, and social motherhood. With the release of "Gesetz zur Regelung des Rechts auf Kenntnis der Abstammung bei heterologer Verwendung von Samen" (Law enforcing the right to know one's origins in cases of sperm donor-conceived children), the German parliament has regu-

Fig. 22.6 Germany's established policies on the issue appear to be remarkably restrictive

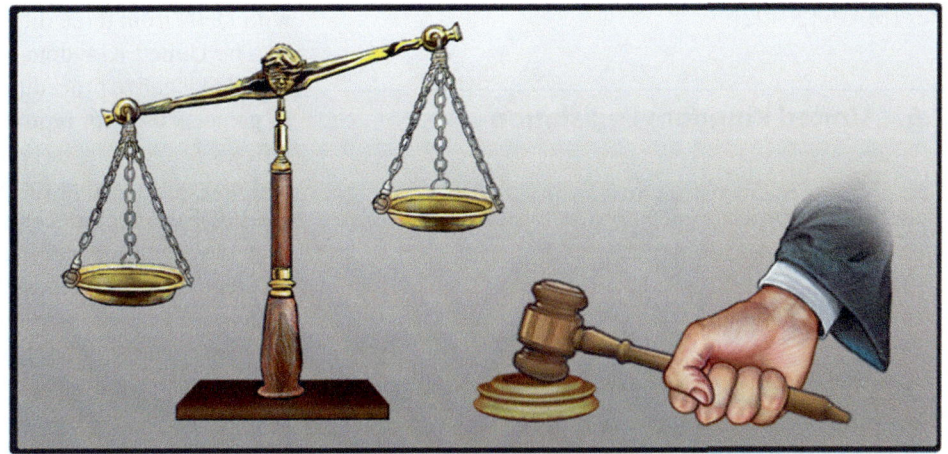

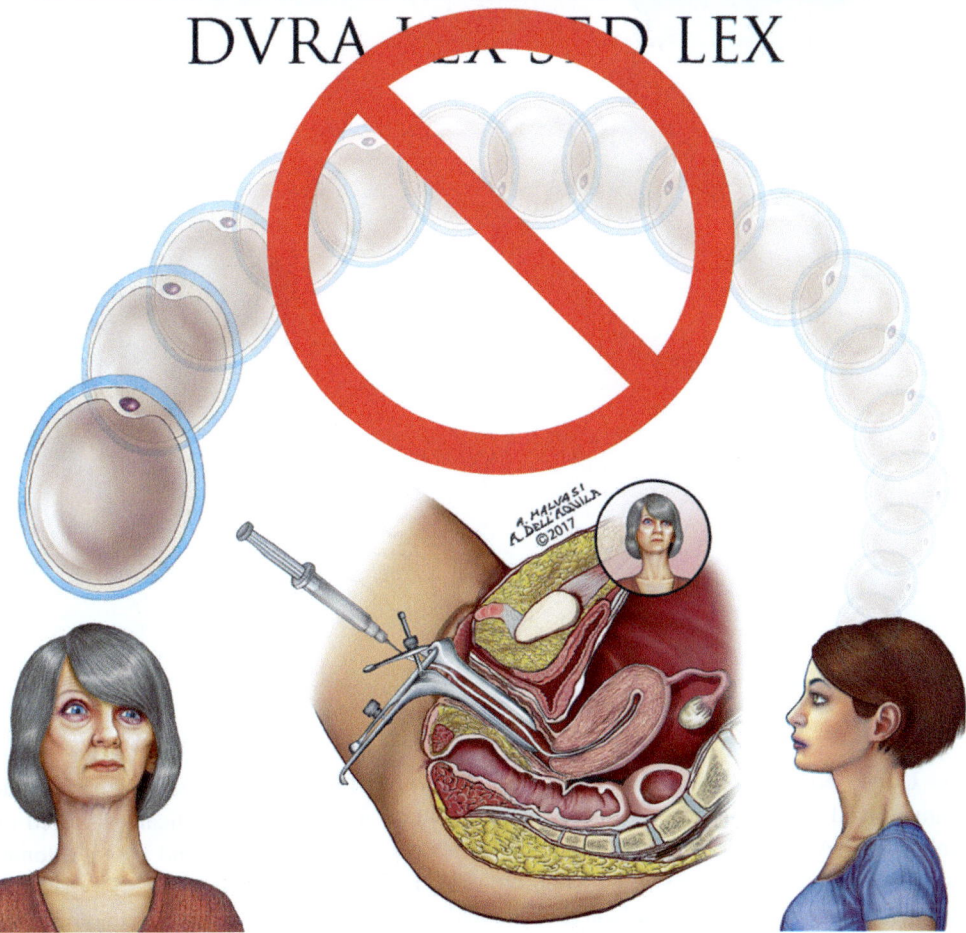

lated the practice of sperm donation for reproductive purposes (MAP) [20–22].

22.6 United Kingdom Legislation

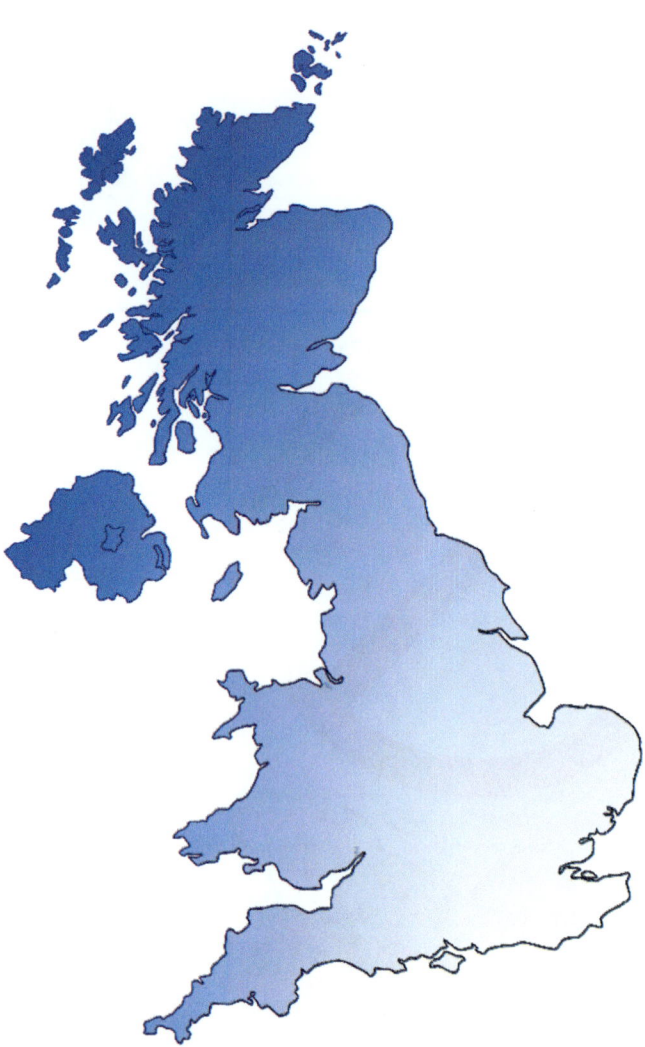

The United Kingdom has adopted a model that could be characterized as permissive. The Human Fertilisation and Embryology Act of 1990 (HFEA) is the first legislative exercise governing MAP in the United Kingdom [23]. In 2008, the legislation has been amended via the identically denominated HFEA. Married couples and couples in civil unions may resort to MAP procedures, in addition to singles and homosexual women. In order to gain access to such techniques, donor consent is required in writing, as well as consent from the receivers and their partners, and donation of male gametes, oocytes, and embryos is likewise legal. The British parliament has passed a law legalizing mitochondrial donation, on the heels of a heated public controversy. Both the Catholic and Anglican Churches have taken a stand against mitochondrial donation, stressing the profound ethi-

cal, social and legal implications of creating human embryos with DNA from three different individuals.

The United Kingdom is therefore the first country in the world to legalize procedures aimed at modifying the genome of gametes used for reproduction. The procedure in question utilizes DNA from three individuals, or "genetic" parents, and makes it feasible for women carrying severe mitochondrial diseases to have children without passing on to them such devastating conditions. In vitro fertilization consists of the replacement of flawed mitochondria from the mother with those from another female donor. The danger lurks that such procedures, rather than repair the mitochondrial abnormalities in the oocyte, might make them worse. Scientists do not see that as a particularly significant risk, in light of recent trials on animals and embryos, which appear to buttress the safety of both operations.

22.7 Belgian Legislation

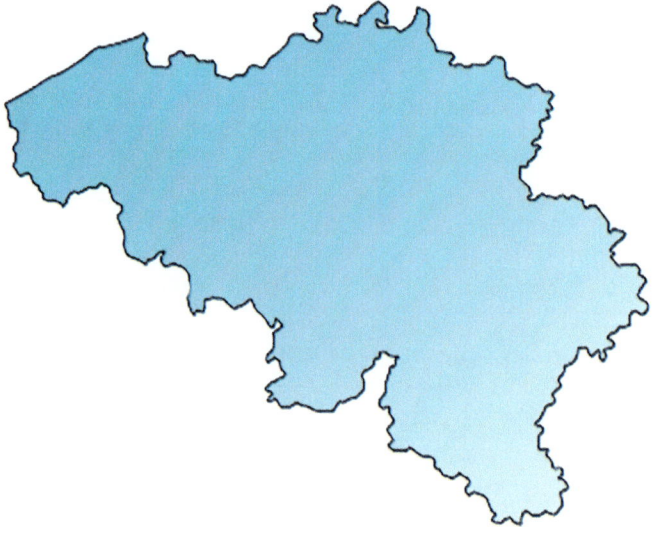

Assisted reproductive procedures in Belgium have been regulated through two main pieces of legislation: the law governing medically assisted procreation and the destination of embryos and gamete donation from 1st July 2007 and the one of in vitro embryo research from 2nd May 2003. Assisted reproductive technologies are usable by homosexual couples and singles as well. An age limit of 45 years has been set for procedures featuring ovarian stimulation, and 47 years in cases of ovum donation. Supernumerary embryos may be stored via cryopreservation for up to 5 years, after which they are destroyed. Parents who have opted for such techniques must sign an agreement with the institution for the use of embryos that have not been implanted in cases of separation, divorce, death of either parent, and whatnot (under article 13). As far as preimplantation genetic diagnosis, there are no legal requirements in place, although it is indirectly regulated by a 2003 law on embryo research, which only allows the practice in cases of high risk of genetic transmission. Sex selection for embryos is only legal for the purpose of preventing gender-related illnesses.

22.7.1 Ethical Issues

Birth in the twenty-first century is defined by a combination of biological and social factors. Such a breakthrough has given rise to an array of ethical, medical, psychological, and legal implications and has caused the juxtaposition of various rights and interests which may be mutually at odds with one another and are all involved in the procreation process: those belonging to parents, children, gamete donors, and family members. Practices such as heterologous fertilization, embryo donation, and surrogacy call for a comprehensive reflection on several matters that are worth being further discussed and elaborated on, the procedures through which informed consent is gained, for instance, or the right of donor-conceived children to know their origins.

22.7.2 Informed Consent

Informed consent is one of the pivotal principles constituting patient rights, and encompasses health care at any level: medical, hospital, and emergency care. Valid consent calls for thorough and suitable information, which has to be provided through the establishment of a doctor–patient relationship in which both parties are integral parts. Their interactions should not be limited to the individual medical procedure, but should rather include the therapeutic pathway in its entirety, and ought to deal with diagnosis, prognosis, benefits, and possible risks inherent to diagnostic screening and treatments prescribed, in addition to possible alternatives and consequences of a refusal or discontinuation of a given therapy or testing (art. 1, Subsection 3). Doctors should take it upon themselves to guide patients through the treatments, making sure that all relevant information is correctly understood, so that a sensible decision can be made.

Self-determination, therefore, entails a thorough, clear, and exhaustive information process in order to lay the groundwork for a truly awareness-based informed consent.

Thus, self-determination entails, and is bound to, the provision of thorough and exhaustive information so that consent can be granted on the basis of self-awareness.

It is therefore essential for prospective parents who undergo such procedures to be thoroughly informed of all aspects related to them. In order to meet this need, the Italian Ministry of Justice, in cooperation with the Ministry of Health, has issued decree n. 265, on 28th December 2016, a set of regulations targeted to the manifestation of a patient's wish to access MA techniques, in pursuance of article 6, subsection 3, within law m. 40 from 19th February 2004 [24]. Doctors should expound upon all techniques that are potentially usable, including MAP and heterologous fertilization, the possibility that either one partner may donate gametes, the operational stages of each technique, particularly in terms of their degree of invasiveness in male and female patients [25, 26]. The level of commitment on the part of prospective parents should also be discussed in depth, with regards to the timing and duration needed to bring the treatment to completion, possible pharmacological therapies necessary, clinical and instrumental screening to be discharged, subsequent checks and hospitalization, including outpatient. Expounding upon possible unwanted side effects with regards to a given treatment is key, in addition to the likelihood of success for various techniques, such as a live birth; further remarks should be made about the risks to mother and newborn, either verified or assumed, and verifiable in scientific literature, and the risks associated with MAP heterologous procedures [27]. Furthermore, it is important to make patients aware of the possibility to store male and female gametes via cryopreservation, for the purpose of future fertilization treatments, and even donation for heterologous fertilization. Psychological repercussions for applicants, couples, and children should not be overlooked. Moreover, it should be brought up that applicants may withdraw their consent until embryo implantation takes place, and the doctor in charge of the ward may refuse to proceed only on medical grounds, to be documented in writing. It is advisable that doctors discuss the ethical issues stemming from the use of MAP techniques. Thus, doctors are required to discharge their duties with regards to preservation of patients' health, which duties may not be shirked on conscientious objection grounds [28]. Italian jurisprudence has shown a certain degree of harshness toward doctors in terms of their obligation to provide information that overstep the bounds of medical professional duties. Thus, the duty of doctors is not merely to point out a fetal anomaly detected by

Table 22.1 Topics to be expounded upon in a solid informed consent process

Elements
Description of procedure or treatment
Explanation of risks and benefits
Description of possible alternative treatments
Description of foreseeable outcome in case of refraining from any therapy
Description of short-term consequences of treatment, including length and recovery challenges
Description of foreseeable long-term consequences of treatment, including possible permanent alterations

means of testing, but rather it includes further screening as to the consequences of such anomaly, the verification ratio, the possible impact on the quality of the parents' and children's lives [29] (Table 22.1).

22.8 The Ethical Debate Revolving Around the Right to Know One's Biological Origins

Within the scenarios outlined above, the opportunity to regulate access to identity data on the methods of procreation has been debated with increased regularity. There are several options available, as far as procreation is concerned: secrecy, partial anonymity, and full disclosure of information identifying gamete donors. Being a donor-conceived child entails the imposition of a family status unlike the one to which he or she would be entitled. A challenging ethical debate is the one centered on the right of donor-conceived children to have access to information to their genetic origins. Considering how widespread such techniques have become, it is reasonable to assume that the number of people who may be keen to exercise such a right will gradually increase [30, 31].

Firstly, it is worth clarifying that those conceived via MAP procedures are entitled to know exactly about the peculiarities of their births. Information therefore constitutes a starting point. It is obviously up to the parents to inform their children, if they wish to do so. Same-sex parents are bound to explain to their children that they were donor conceived [32]. That is not necessarily the case for heterosexual families, since the involvement of third parties, the donors, does not show up in any documentation. In such instances, donor-conceived children are unaware that they were conceived via the external intervention of a stranger, since they were raised by their social parents.

If the social-legal parents decide that it's best to keep it secret, they should inform relatives and friends of their choice, so as to prevent their children from finding out accidentally, which would make them feel betrayed and may even lose trust in their parents [33]. Most couples who choose to keep their child's biological origins secret are driven by their unwillingness to generate confusion in their child genetic and social parenthood. Explaining such events to a child is undoubtedly complicated, because it entails information as to the parents' sexuality, the difference between natural parenthood and one based on affection and voluntarism, and the medical procedures performed. In addition to that motivation, parents may also be concerned with preserving their child from any kind of social and family discrimination which may stem from their not being considered their parents' biological children, and which may in turn cause psychological and social distress and trauma. In our

view, however, although the choice to conceal the truth appears to be in keeping with the emotional intimacy of the family, it also seems hypocritical and hard to sustain at the communicative level. Several studies have been conducted on the psychological implications arising from the decision to inform one's son or daughter of those circumstances, and they ultimately concluded that there is no right or wrong decision in absolute terms. Even though the law establishes who the father is from a legal standpoint, the symbolic presence of a donor, or biological parent, cannot be underestimated [34]. The fundamental question, and one that is everything but easily answered, is: should gamete donors be allowed to keep anonymity or should their identities be disclosed? An undisputed obligation exists to allow these individuals access to gamete donors' medical records and genetic background, given that such news may be of the utmost importance in the case of hereditary diseases.

Various studies have come to diametrically different conclusions. Some researchers contend that donor-conceived children should be entitled to gain access to all information available on donors, including identity and address, in light of the psychological and social consequences that a child would suffer should he or she were to find out about siblings who live in different families and in different places. Denying such information may bring about complex identity-related issues, psychological imbalances described as "genealogical bewilderment."

Arguments in favor of anonymity, conversely, focus on the need to protect a donor's private and family life, in particular when he already has children and solid family ties. Undoubtedly, the revelation of a child born from a donation possibly happened long before and under different family conditions may well give rise to traumatic repercussions on the "newly-found" donor and his family [35]. Anonymity, moreover, certainly incentivizes gamete donation. If anonymity were no longer guaranteed, many potential donors would probably backtrack on their purpose lest they be tracked down by their "children" long after. Such a theory is borne out by data from countries where anonymity has been repealed: the number of donors has decreased in those countries, whereas it has increased in countries that still enforce it. Nonetheless, research has shown that gamete donation can be fostered and enhanced through adequate recruitment strategies and campaigns that appeal to potential donors' altruistic motivations [36, 37].

It is even more contentious whether someone's wish to know his or her biological origins may warrant allowing those born from medically assisted procreation techniques to know the donor's identity, or even their relatives, or whether such data should be kept partially secret, while divulging different, less sensitive ones (a donor's profession, hobbies, etc.). Such a quandary has been dealt with through varying pieces of legislation in different countries. According to a survey conducted by the International Federation of Fertility Societies in 2013, gamete donor anonymity has been gradually dismissed by more and more countries, leaning toward a system of greater transparency.

It is certainly a hot-button issue, and encompasses different ethical, moral, social, and legal ramifications, depending on whose rights should be deserving of more protection: allowing donor-conceived children to know their origins, according to the principle of "favor veritatis" (truthfulness in family relations, parenthood in particular), or prioritizing the right of gamete donors to stay anonymous.

22.9 Ethical Issues in Mitochondrial Donation

The possibility to fix genetic mitochondrial abnormalities raises relevant ethical and moral quandaries [38, 39]. The most serious concern is about the potential harmfulness of such procedures to the newborn, thus dooming him or her to life-long sufferings. Mitochondrial replacement is supposed to stave off the onset of extremely serious diseases, caused by mitochondrial anomalies, yet the transfer of genetic material from an oocyte to another [40] may eventually prove noxious, unpredictably doing more harm than good (Fig. 22.7).

In fact, the newborn child could present different types of organellar genome (one from the mother, another one from the donor), also known as mitochondrial heteroplasmy, which might trigger serious illnesses in the child [41] and future offspring. Further research is then much needed in order to verify that the coexistence of multiple mitochondrial DNA variants in a single source, albeit in minimal amount, does not cause biological damage, in the medium and long terms especially. A further issue should not be hastily dismissed: such procedures, involving the transfer of genetic material have the potential of causing problems that may not be immediately detectable, manifesting themselves as the individual grows older, with unforeseeable consequences. Furthermore, the risks of damages to the newborn inherent to such mitochondrial replacement therapies may be blunted by conducting genetic testing on the embryo, before and after implantation in uterus. After the transfer, in absence of genetic abnormalities, the woman could bring her pregnancy to term. If, on the other hand, anomalies in the genetic codes are found, the patient might choose to terminate her pregnancy.

There are fears that, irrespective of their actual effectiveness and safety, such processes involving mitochondrial DNA could lead to the increase of parental figures, thus creating an element of novelty and difficulty for the children. It arguably does not appear to be ethical for a couple to seek to fulfill their urges with respect to parenthood through procedures that could weaken the sense of identity of child thus born, possibly leading to the creation of various existential frames of reference. Doubts are also raised by the possibility

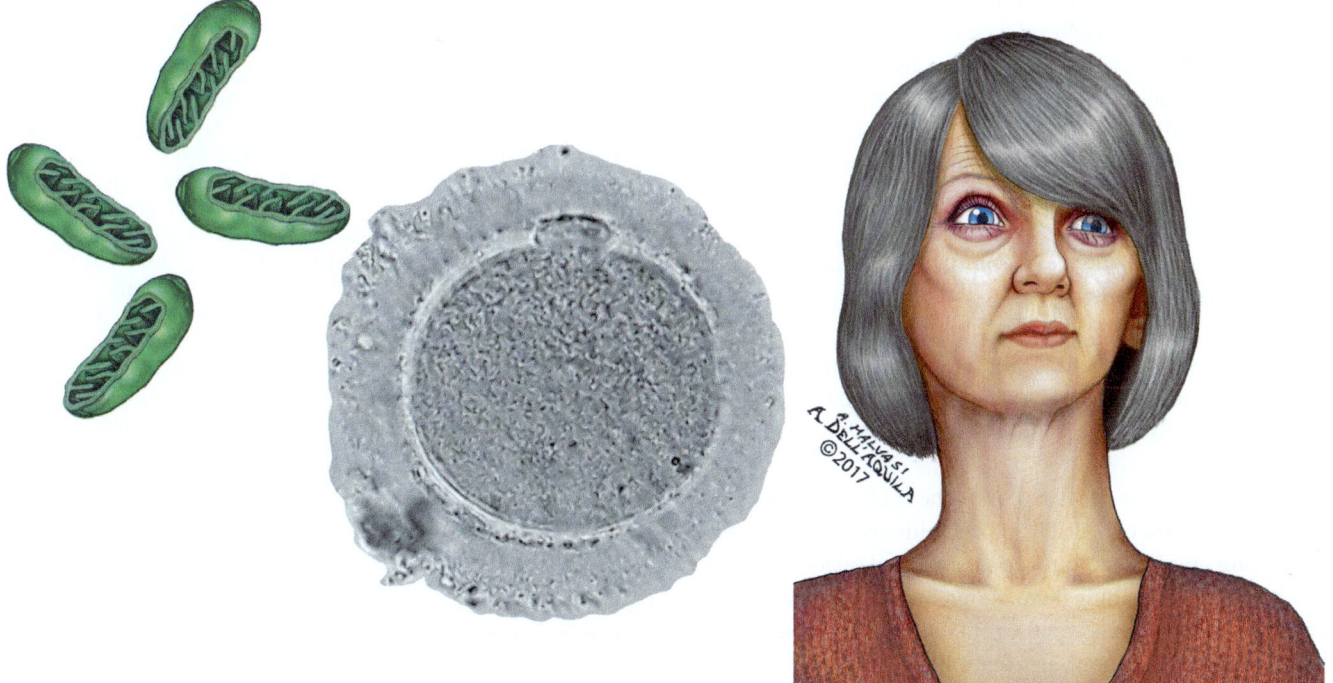

Fig. 22.7 Mitochondrial replacement is supposed to stave off the onset of extremely serious diseases

to prevent some diseases through the alteration of the fetus's genetic code. A risk exists, in fact, that procedures aimed at correcting the mitochondrial DNA could end up manipulating, along with the genome, the very identity of the baby yet to be born. A further issue arises from the inheriting, on the part of the newborn child, of genome from three different parties [42]. In that case, the main concern is that mtDNA replacement procedures lead to an abnormal increase of parental figures, casting the child in a distressing situation, from a psychological standpoint. There will be, in fact, three adults with genetic ties to the baby [43, 44].

Similar techniques could end up leading to new attempts at human cloning, or the creation of man–animal hybrids, which are currently banned practices on account of their being spiteful for human dignity from the genetic identity perspective, its uniqueness, and biological diversity. They are banned, moreover, because they would entail the overstepping of boundaries that define human specificity; although some theoreticians might find that scenario desirable, in order to produce "subhuman" beings, or humanoids (e.g., the so-called "humanzee"), employable in repetitive or unpleasant jobs, as guinea pigs for research purposes or organ harvesting for transplants [45].

Surrogacy itself arguably constitutes an insult to the dignity of women and children alike. It cheapens the dignity of women, because it discounts her role to a mere reproductive organ, akin to a human incubator, even more so if paid; it belittles the newborn child too, in that it reduces him or her to an object of negotiation and even legal claims (as it has already occurred); the baby's actual status, in fact, depends on the compliance on the part of the undersigned with a contract clauses (there have been cases of newborn children that were turned down, since they did not live up to the buyers' expectations) and may even develop identity issues, feeling like the child of too many parents, exposing him or her to the risk of psychophysical development damages due to a warped.

22.10 Conclusions

Innovations in the realm of genetics open up new horizons, in which childbirth seems to be untied to mating, making procreation no longer a natural and spontaneous occurrence.

A solution to the problem cannot be found in an approach based on a lax or, conversely, a prohibitionist strategy (either embracing any kinds of procedures without adequate checks and balances or banning them altogether, encouraging underground illegal practices and profitable criminal trafficking) but should rather oversee, in a careful and thoughtful fashion, the unstoppable and desirable scientific advancements, while

waiting for clearly defined legislation devised to take into account and sensibly regulate the countless issues in the field.

First and foremost, we believe the enactment of legislation to be necessary, both at a European and international level, specifically designed to effectively govern the implementation of such innovative practices, prioritizing the rights of those yet to be born, who are third parties in the overblown notion of "procreation," by a thorough analysis of any possible psycho-social repercussions of assisted reproduction technologies on children.

References

1. Ognibene F. Boom di "figli dell'eterologa" e record di bimbi concepiti in provetta. https://www.avvenire.it/famiglia-e-vita/pagine/figli-dell-eterologa-e-record-di-bambini-in-provetta.
2. Daar Judith F. Accessing reproductive technologies: invisible barriers, indelible harms. Berkeley J Gend Law Justice. 2008;23:18–82.
3. Jouve de la Barreda N. Biomedical perspective of the surrogate motherhood. Cuad Bioet. 2017;28(93):153–62.
4. Aparisi Miralles Á. Surrogate motherhood and woman dignity. Cuad Bioet. 2017;28(93):163–75.
5. Frati P, Busardò FP, Vergallo GM, Pacchiarotti A, Fineschi V. Surrogate motherhood: where Italy is now and where Europe is going. Can the genetic mother be considered the legal mother? J Forensic Legal Med. 2015;30:4–8.
6. Angeli E. The challenge on abortion and assisted reproductive technologies in Europe. Comp Eur Polit. 2009;7(1):56.
7. Nielsen I. Legal consensus and divergence in Europe in the area of assisted conception—room for harmonisation? In: Evans D, Pickering N, (a cura di). Creating the child. The Ethics, Law and Practice of Assisted Procreation, The Hague; 1996. p. 305.
8. White & Case LLP. European laws governing in vitro fertilization. New York; 2009. http://www.federa.org.pl/dokumenty_pdf/invitro/jbf_European_laws_governing_in_vitro_fertilization%5B2%5D.pdf.
9. Zaami S, Busardò FP. Elective egg freezing: can you really turn back the clock? Eur Rev Med Pharmacol Sci. 2015;19(19):3537–8.
10. Montanari Vergallo G. Negligence and embryo protection: a new frontier for medical law? Med Law. 2014;33:2–13.
11. Montanari Vergallo G, Zaami S, Bruti V, Signore F, Marinelli E. How the legislation on medically assisted procreation has evolved in Italy. Med Law. 2017;36(2):5–28.
12. Malvasi A, Signore F, Napoletano S, et al. 2014-2017. How medically assisted reproduction changed in Italy. A short comparative synthesis with European countries. Clin Ter. 2017;168(4):e248–52.
13. Loi sur la bioéthique n. 2011—814 del 7 luglio 2011, Assemblee Nationale, Rapport n. 3111 fait au nom de la Commission spéciale chargée d'examiner le projet de loi relatif à la bioéthique (n. 2911) par J. Leonetti, 26 gennaio 2011, Vol. 1, p. 17. www.assemblee-nationale.fr/13/rapports/r3111-tI.asp.
14. Conseil D'Etat, La révision des lois de bioéthique. Etude adoptée par l'assemblée générale plénière le 9 avril 2009, La documentation française, Parigi, 2009, 53. www.ladocumentationfrancaise.fr/var/storage/rapportspublics/094000288/0000.pdf.
15. Loi relative à la procreation médicalementassistée et à la destination des embryons surnuméraires et de gametes. http://www.ieb-eib.org/nl/pdf/l-20070706-pma.pdf.
16. Jiménez Munoz FJ. La reproduccion asistida y su régimen jurìdico. Madrid; 2012.

17. Luna Serrano A. Comparacion en materia de filiation por reproduccion asistida entre los derechos espanol e italiano, in Icade, Revista cuatrimestral de las Facultades de derecho y Ciencias Economicas y Empresariales. 2012;87:170.
18. Instituto Bernabeu. Legislation in Spain and Europe. http://www.institutobernabeu.com/en/4-14/international-patient/legislation-in-spain-and-europe/. Accessed 20 July 2015.
19. Augst C. Regulating dangerous futures: the German Embryo Protection Act of 1990—legislation in risk society. Soc Leg Stud. 2000;9(2):205–26.
20. Deutsch E. Assisted procreation in German law. In: Evans D, Pickering N, editors. Creating the child: the ethics, law, and practice of assisted procreation. Neil Pickering: Martinus Nijhoff Publishers; 1996. p. 333.
21. Brown E. The dilemmas of German bioethics. J Technol Soc. 2004;5:37–53.
22. Arnold R. Questioni giuridiche in merito alla fecondazione artificiale nel diritto tedesco. In: Casonato C, Frosini TE (a cura di). La fecondazione assistita nel diritto comparato. Torino; 2006. p. 5.
23. Parliament of the UK. Human Fertilisation and Embryology Act 1990. http://www.legislation.gov.uk/ukpga/1990/37/contents.
24. Decree 28th December 2016, n. 265.
25. Lo B, Chou V, Cedars MI, Gates E. Informed consent in human oocyte, embryo, and embryonic stem cell research. Fertil Steril. 2004;82(3):559–63.
26. Hill D, Jaeger A. Informed consent in embryo research. Reprod Biomed Online. 2005;10(Suppl 2):40.
27. Nelson E, Mykitiuk R, Nisker J. Informed consent to donate embryos for research purposes. J Obstet Gynaecol Can. 2008;30(9):824–36.
28. Montanari Vergallo G, Zaami S, Di Luca NM, et al. The conscientious objection: debate on emergency contraception. Clin Ter. 2017;168(2):113–9.
29. Allan S. Commercial surrogate and child: ethical issues, regulatory approaches, and suggestions for change. Working paper May 30, 2014. http://ssrn.com/abstract=2431142.
30. Ergas Y. Babies without borders: human rights, human dignity, and the regulation of international commercial surrogacy. Emory Int Law Rev. 2013;27:124–5.
31. Ravitsky V. The right to know one's genetic origins and cross-border medically assisted reproduction. Isr J Health Policy Res. 2017;6:3.
32. Zaami S. Assisted heterologous fertilization and the right of donor conceived children to know their biological origins. Clin Ter. 2018;169(1):39–43.
33. Leighton K. The right to know genetic origins: a harmful value. Hast Cent Rep. 2014;44(4):5–6.
34. Montanari Vergallo G, Marinelli E, di Luca NM, Zaami S. Gamete donation: are children entitled to know their genetic origins? A comparison of opposing views. The Italian state of affairs. Eur J Health Law. 2018;25:1–16.
35. De Melo-Martín I. The ethics of anonymous gamete donation: is there a right to know one's genetic origins? Hast Cent Rep. 2014;44(2):28–35.
36. Ravitsky V. Autonomous choice and the right to know one's genetic origins. Hast Cent Rep. 2014;44(2):36–7.
37. Gong D, Liu YL, Zheng Z, Tian YF, Li Z. An overview on ethical issues about sperm donation. Asian J Androl. 2009;11:645–52.
38. Tachibana M. Mitochondrial gene replacement in primate offspring and embryonic stem cells. Nature. 2009;461(7262):367–72.
39. Bredenoord AL, Braude P. Ethics of mitochondrial gene replacement: from bench to bedside. Br Med J. 2010;341:c6021.
40. Nuffield Council on Bioethics. Novel techniques for the prevention of mitochondrial DNA disorders: an ethical review. 2012.
41. Graumann S, Haker H. Some conceptual and ethical comments on egg cell nuclear transfer. Politics Life Sci. 1998;17(1):16–8.
42. Parliamentary Office of Science and Technology (House of Parliament), Preventing Mitochondrial Disease. p. 3–23. https://www.parliament.uk/documents/post/postpn431_Preventing_Mitochondrial_Disease.pdf.
43. Anton A. Ethical issues of new techniques to avoid mitochondrial disease, Ethics and Law Advisory Committee (HFEA), 8 giugno 2011, paper number ELAC (06/11)1. p. 1–13.
44. Taylor F., Three-parent embryos for mitochondrial disorders. Christian Medical Fellowship Files, 51, Summer 2013. http://www.cmf.org.uk/publications/content.asp?context=article&id=26082.
45. Baylis F. The ethics of creating children with three genetic parents. Reprod Biomed Online. 2013;26:531–4.

Correction to: Medically Assisted Procreation: European Legislation and Ensuing Ethical Issues

Gianluca Montanari Vergallo, Simona Zaami,
and Radmila Sparic

Correction to:
Chapter 22 in: A. Malvasi, D. Baldini (eds.), *Pick Up and Oocyte Management*,
https://doi.org/10.1007/978-3-030-28741-2_22

The original version of this chapter was revised. The author, Tom Schneider was removed from the original version.

The updated online version of this chapter can be found at
https://doi.org/10.1007/978-3-030-28741-2_22

The manufacturer's authorised representative in the EU is Springer
Nature Customer Service Centre GmbH, Europaplatz 3, 69115 Heidelberg,
Germany. If you have any concerns regarding our products, please
contact ProductSafety@springernature.com

Printed and bound by CPI Group (UK) Ltd, Croydon, CR0 4YY

24/04/2026

02096377-0001